PRACTICAL OBSTETRIC ANESTHESIA

PRACTICAL OBSTETRIC ANESTHESIA

David M. Dewan, M.D.
Professor of Anesthesia
Obstetric and Gynecologic Anesthesia
Bowman Gray School of Medicine
Wake Forest University
Winston-Salem, North Carolina

David D. Hood, M.D.
Associate Professor of Anesthesia
Obstetric and Gynecologic Anesthesia
Bowman Gray School of Medicine
Wake Forest University
Winston-Salem, North Carolina

W.B. Saunders Company
A Division of Harcourt Brace & Company
Philadelphia London Toronto
Montreal Sydney Tokyo

W.B. SAUNDERS COMPANY
A Division of Harcourt Brace & Company

The Curtis Center
Independence Square West
Philadelphia, Pennsylvania 19106

Library of Congress Cataloging-in-Publication Data

Practical obstetric anesthesia / [edited by] David M. Dewan, David D. Hood. —1st ed.

p. cm.

ISBN 0–7216–3658–6

1. Anesthesia in obstetrics. I. Dewan, David M. II. Hood, David D.
DNLM: 1. Anesthesia, Obstetrical. WO 450 P895 1997]

RG 732.P73 1997 617.9′682—dc20

DNLM/DLC 96–6053

PRACTICAL OBSTETRIC ANESTHESIA ISBN 0–7216–3658–6

Printed in the United States of America.

Last digit is the print number: 9 8 7 6 5 4 3 2 1

Contributors

Brenda L. Berkebile, M.D.
Instructor of Anesthesiology, Finch University of Health Sciences, The Chicago Medical School; Associate Attending, Department of Anesthesiology; Director of Obstetric Anesthesia, Mount Sinai Hospital Medical Center, Chicago, Illinois
Anesthesia for Vaginal Delivery Following Cesarean Birth

Robert C. Chantigian, M.D.
Assistant Professor of Anesthesiology, Mayo Medical School; Director of Obstetric Anesthesiology, Mayo Clinic, Rochester, Minnesota
Resuscitation/Critical Care

Theodore G. Cheek, Ph.D.
Associate Professor of Anesthesia and Obstetrics and Gynecology; Director of Obstetric Anesthesia, Hospital of the University of Pennsylvania, Philadelphia, Pennsylvania
Analgesia for Labor

Robert D'Angelo, M.D.
Assistant Professor, Division of Obstetrical Anesthesia, Wake Forest University, Bowman Gray School of Medicine, Winston-Salem, North Carolina
Anesthesia for Forceps Deliveries

David M. Dewan, M.D.
Professor of Anesthesia, Head, Section on Obstetric and Gynecologic Anesthesia, Wake Forest University, Bowman Gray School of Medicine, Winston-Salem, North Carolina
Philosophy; Shoulder Dystocia; Anesthesia for the Morbidly Obese Pregnant Patient; Medical-Legal Aspects of Obstetric Anesthesia

M. Joanne Douglas, M.D., F.R.C.P.(C.)
Head, Department of Anaesthesia, and Head, Division of Obstetric Anaesthesia, British Columbia Women's Hospital and The University of British Columbia, Vancouver, British Columbia, Canada
Complex Medical Problems

Richard P. Driver, Jr., M.D.
Assistant Professor and Co-Director of Obstetric Anesthesia, West Virginia University; Assistant Professor and Co-Director of Obstetric Anesthesia, Ruby Memorial Hospital, Morgantown, West Virginia
Practical Obstetric Physiology

James C. Eisenach, M.D.
Professor and Chair for Anesthesia Research, Wake Forest University, Bowman Gray School of Medicine, Winston-Salem, North Carolina
Postoperative Analgesia in Obstetrics

I. David Elstein, B.S., M.D.
Chief Anesthesiologist, Creedmore Psychiatric Medical Center, Queens, New York
Anesthesia for Non–Birth-Related Surgery During Pregnancy

Brett B. Gutsche, M.D.
Professor of Anesthesia and Obstetrics and Gynecology, Hospital of the University of Pennsylvania, Philadelphia, Pennsylvania
Analgesia for Labor

Deborah L. Holden, M.D.
Assistant Professor, Wake Forest University, Bowman Gray School of Medicine, Winston-Salem, North Carolina
Anesthesia for Cesarean Section

David D. Hood, M.D.
Associate Professor of Anesthesia, Wake Forest University, Bowman Gray School of Medicine, Winston-Salem, North Carolina
Outcome; Preeclampsia

Marc A. Huntoon, M.D.
Assistant Professor of Anesthesiology, Medical College of Ohio, Toledo, Ohio
Embolic Disease in Pregnancy

Ashok Jayaram, M.B., B.S., F.F.A.R.C.S.I.
Assistant Professor, Oregon Health Sciences University; Attending Anesthesiologist, Oregon Health Sciences University Hospital, Portland, Oregon
Practical Obstetric Pharmacology

BettyLou Koffel, M.D.
Associate Professor of Anesthesiology, Boston University School of Medicine; Attending Anesthesiologist, Boston City Hospital, Boston, Massachusetts
Complicated Obstetrics—Management Considerations: Fetal Stress, Premature Fetus, Breech/Twins

Joseph J. Kryc, M.D.
Associate Professor of Clinical Anesthesiology, Associate Professor of Obstetrics and Gynecology, Vice Chairman, Department of Anesthesiology, Maricopa Medical Center (A major teaching affiliate of the University of Arizona, Tucson), Pheonix, Arizona
Evaluation of the Pregnant Patient: Preoperative Concerns

Andrew M. Malinow, M.D.
Associate Professor of Anesthesiology, Obstetrics and Gynecology, University of Maryland School of Medicine; Director of Obstetric Anesthesia, Associate Vice Chair, Development, Department of Anesthesiology, University of Maryland Medical Center, Baltimore, Maryland
Complicated Obstetrics—Management Considerations: Fetal Stress, Premature Fetus, Breech/Twins

Gertie F. Marx, M.D.
Professor of Anesthesiology, Albert Einstein College of Medicine; Attending Anesthesiologist, Hospitals Affiliated with Albert Einstein College of Medicine, Bronx, New York
Anesthesia for Non–Birth-Related Surgery During Pregnancy

Medge D. Owen, M.D.
Assistant Professor of Anesthesia, Wake Forest University, Bowman Gray School of Medicine, Winston-Salem, North Carolina
Anesthesia for the Bleeding Obstetric Patient

Mary Louise Steward, B.Sc., M.Sc., M.D., F.R.C.P.(C.)
Assistant Professor, University of Southern California, Los Angeles, California
Cardiovascular Disease

Connie E. Taylor, M.D.
Assistant Professor, Department of Anesthesiology, Tulane Hospital and Clinic, New Orleans, Louisiana
Anesthesia in the Febrile Parturient

Desmond Writer, M.B., F.R.C.A., F.R.C.P.(C.)
Professor, Departments of Anesthesia and Obstetrics and Gynaecology, Dalhousie University; Staff Anaesthetist, IWK—Grace Health Centre, Halifax, Nova Scotia, Canada
Diabetes in Pregnancy

Preface

The impetus for *Practical Obstetric Anesthesia* was both serendipitous and fortuitous. In 1978, after a number of years of debate, our community consolidated all obstetric services in one hospital. Prior to 1978, the services were divided, by and large, between two sites. The medical school provided services for approximately 1000 deliveries, and the community hospital provided services for approximately 3000 deliveries annually. The needs of neither institution were being met. One thousand deliveries were insufficient for quality resident training and inadequate for obstetric research. At the community hospital, full-time obstetric anesthesia coverage was not available and only emergency obstetric anesthesia services were provided. The merging of these obstetric services provided the larger patient base necessary to justify 24-hour-a-day dedicated anesthesia services.

During the initial year following consolidation, there were approximately 4000 deliveries and a 25% labor epidural analgesia rate, as well as approximately 1000 gynecologic procedures performed in the obstetric suite. Unanticipated growth occurred, and in 1993, an enlarged perinatal suite opened. By 1995, approximately 5700 women delivered in the enlarged obstetric suite and the epidural analgesia rate increased to between 75 and 80%. The cesarean section rate approximated 21%, with regional anesthesia used in 95% of operations. Nearly 3000 gynecologic operations are now performed annually in this combined obstetric-gynecologic suite.

As an academic anesthesia department, the missions of the obstetric anesthesiologists necessarily remained consistent throughout the years of growth: provision of quality patient care, resident training, and clinical and basic research. During the earlier years, with infrequent patient care demands, meeting the mission requirements with fewer available personnel than presently available was relatively easy. However, as the size of service and patient care demands grew, providing timely and efficient care became key to allowing ample time for accomplishing the secondary missions of resident teaching and research.

Thus, the serendipitous thought process directed at efficiency and practicality allowed us to maintain our academic missions and is now fortuitous as we enter today's managed care environment and intensify our efforts to become increasingly cost efficient. Therefore, when selecting authors to contribute to this text, we attempted to identify individuals with a perspective consistent with the provision of efficient and practical care. We also hopefully identified individuals with an understanding of the obstetrician's perspective and needs. The ability for both obstetric and anesthesia services to recognize the validity of the other's perspective has been key to encouraging the growth in our service and promoting the *team* concept that has fortunately evolved at our institution. We hope the readers will develop a feel that providing timely, efficient, appropriate care makes everyone a winner, including the patient.

David M. Dewan
David D. Hood

Contents

ONE

Philosophy

David M. Dewan, M.D.

Obstetric anesthesia has historically been an area of disinterest and sometimes overtly disliked by anesthesia providers. This outlook, compounded by the frequent remote location of obstetric suites documented in the previous obstetric staffing survey,[1] has sometimes led to inadequate coverage potentially contributing to poor maternal and fetal outcomes. In contrast to the historical neglect of labor and delivery, recent trends suggest greater patient and hospital administration demands for more complete anesthesia coverage for obstetric patients. As hospitals attempt to become "full service" and gain a market edge, the provision of 24-hour "epidural services" becomes a marketing tool. Unfortunately, many obstetric units, because of their small size, may not provide a volume of service justifying full-time anesthesia coverage and are considered "cost ineffective" by anesthesia providers. Unless the service is subsidized by the hospital, it is clearly much more cost effective for the anesthesia provider to deliver surgical anesthesia in the operating room rather than provide "labor" intensive care in the small obstetric suite. Ironically, high-volume services also create problems by presenting workloads that can exceed the capacity of the anesthesia care team to provide timely, safe care. These dichotomies may explain, in part, an older report that documented increased maternal mortality in very small and very large obstetric units when compared with units of medium size.[2] The pressures may worsen. The soon-to-be-published obstetric anesthesia staffing survey reveals that 25% of obstetric anesthesia providers have been denied payment for labor epidural analgesia.[3] If, in this emerging economic environment, this payment practice continues, pressures militgating against full-time obstetric coverage may intensify.

Viewed in this context, quality medical care can be defined by four parameters: mortality, morbidity, utility, and prognosis.[4] Otherwise stated, the ideal obstetric anesthesia service should first limit maternal-fetal morbidity and mortality, a philosophy consistent with other anesthesia services. In today's environment, there should also be utility, which weighs the relative importance of side effects and benefits—for example, while spinal narcotics may offer a less "labor-intensive" anesthetic for some parturients, this benefit may be outweighed by the disadvantage of not having a potentially extant surgical epidural anesthetic in high-risk parturients. Finally, prognosis attempts to address the allocation of financial and human resources. What is the "wisest" expenditure of human and financial resources? Cost-efficient services are likely to be deemed wise expenditures. At the editors' institution, an obstetric service of nearly 6000 deliveries, a recurring question is: Should the unit have the capacity to perform one, two, or three simultaneous cesarean sections, 24 hours a day? Otherwise stated, do we staff for peaks, valleys, or average numbers of occurrences?

The editors hope that *Practical Obstetric Anesthesia* offers a framework of obstetric anesthesia care that allows obstetric anesthesia care providers to deliver "quality" care effectively in this environment. The text starts with the premise that the obstetric patient deserves quality care consistent with the goals that poor maternal and fetal outcomes must be minimized. The fundamental principles necessary to minimize maternal mortality are known. The lessons learned are outlined in Dr. David Hood's chapter on morbidity and mortality. Applying these principles in today's practice environment is the challenge.

The early portions of the text attempt to define and delineate the unique risks of the obstetric patient and describe in practical terms why the pregnant patient is physiologically and pharmacologically unique. The editors particularly hope the presentation identifies areas where these differences are clinically significant and of more than academic interest. For example, although the obstetric patient may require less local anesthetic to establish surgical anesthesia than the nonobstetric patient, in the framework of slow and fractionated administration of local anesthetic administration, this difference becomes less clinically relevant. Dr. Joseph Kryc delineates the important aspects of obstetric patient evaluation that are essential for allowing the anesthesia team to assess significant newborn and maternal risks that may alter the anesthetic plan. Understanding these risks, however, will have little impact unless the subsequently delivered care occurs in a safe environment. Simply stated, the quality of anesthesia services in the obstetric suite should not differ from the quality of services delivered in the surgical operating suite. Equipment, standards, and the personnel providing coverage should be comparable. In this regard, Dr. Kryc also addresses the primary concerns for anesthesiologists evaluating the environment in which they work.

The editors hope such chapters as "Analgesia for the Laboring Patient," which addresses how to deliver care, effectively treat both "utility" and "prognosis." In today's environment, knowing how to do an epidural is not sufficient. For both the patient and the anesthesia provider, utility is important. For example, what should the anesthesia provider do with an imperfect block? Repetitive redosing can be a "time-inefficient" use of personnel and unacceptable from the patient's perspective. Early problem resolution is best for all. Some options for resolution may be better than others. Although the addition of narcotic to the anesthetic may be "utilitarian" and an appropriate choice in terms of allocation of human resources, morbidity may be worse if the block is insufficient for a subsequently required cesarean section. "How to do it" safely, efficiently, and importantly, proactively are essential components of this text.

The latter chapters address the complicated obstetric patient and provide practical guidelines for supplying the same safe, efficient, quality care for high-risk patients that is recommended for low-risk patients. Sometimes the options are different. For example, spinal anesthesia may be the best anesthetic for a normal parturient undergoing cesarean section but is of little value if the surgery outlasts the anesthetic, as may occur in morbidly obese patients. Finally, Dr. Robert Chantigian and Dr. James Eisenach discuss care of the newborn and postoperative pain management. They answer questions about the role of the anesthesia provider in newborn resuscitation and the choices for postoperative pain management in this patient population.

In summary, the editors hope the authors in this text provide a practical framework for delivering safe, time-effective, cost-effective anesthetic care. As a new era in medicine is entered, obstetric anesthesia will remain a vital concern for hospitals and patients. Flexibility, appropriate anesthetic selection, and effective utilization of personnel will be the cornerstones of success.

REFERENCES

1. Gibbs CP, Krischer J, Peckham B, et al: Obstetric anesthesia: A national survey. Anesthesiology 65:298–306, 1986.
2. Kaunitz A, Grimes D, Hughes J, et al: Maternal deaths in the United States by size of hospital. Obstet Gynecol 64:311–314, 1984.
3. Hawkins J: Personal communication, 1996.
4. Kaplan RM: Application of a general health policy model in the American health care crisis. J R Soc Med 86:277–281, 1993.

TWO

Outcome

David D. Hood, M.D.

Obstetric anesthesia outcome is a broad topic deserving extensive discussion. In many respects, each chapter in this text provides the specific, practical outcome information that most anesthesiologists need on a given topic. This chapter, in contrast, takes a global, somewhat philosophical approach to the topic of outcome. In addition, some practical approaches to both differential diagnosis and treatment are presented for topics that are not discussed in other chapters.

MATERNAL MORTALITY

Since the mid-1970s, maternal mortality rates have dramatically fallen. Improved understanding of pathophysiology and improved medical care account for this reduction in maternal risk. Similarly, the maternal risk of death due to anesthesia complications has also fallen dramatically, however, at a rate that exceeds the improvements noted in the overall maternal death rate. Although anesthesia complications resulting in maternal death are less frequent, the lessons learned from the past must be emphasized to further reduce maternal risks for anesthesia-related death. This section discusses these lessons and recommends a practical approach for minimizing the risk of maternal death related to anesthesia.

Maternal mortality is traditionally divided into three classifications. *Direct* deaths are those related directly to obstetric causes, that is, complications resulting from pregnancy (e.g., uterine hemorrhage and anesthesia for labor or cesarean section). *Indirect* causes of death are deaths due to preexisting disease or disease developing during pregnancy and unrelated to obstetric causes. Preexisting diseases causing maternal death, although further aggravated by pregnancy, are nevertheless classified as *indirect*. *Fortuitous* deaths are those that are unrelated to pregnancy or preexisting disease (e.g., from accidents).

Although maternal death is usually attributed to one primary cause, there may be indirect, contributory causes. For example, hemorrhage may be the primary cause of death, but severe preeclampsia, placental abruption, and less-than-adequate resuscitation by the anesthesia provider may be indirect contributory causes.

By international agreement, deaths that occur within 42 days of delivery are classified as *maternal*. Because approximately 15% of maternal deaths occur more than 42 days postpartum, many authors extend the classification period to 6 months or 1 year. Comparison of mortality statistics is therefore often difficult, since tabulating periods vary.

Although collection of maternal mortality statistics began in 1915 in the United States, reports are published intermittently and frequently contain insufficient detail to judge the appropriateness of the assigned causes of death. In contrast, consistent, detailed, triennial maternal mortality reports have been published in

TABLE 2–1
Direct Maternal Deaths by Cause, Rates per Million Estimated Pregnancies, England and Wales, 1970–1990

Period	Pulmonary Embolism	Hypertensive Disease	Anesthesia	Amniotic Fluid Embolism	Hemorrhage	Sepsis	Ruptured Uterus	Other Direct Causes	All Deaths*
1970–1972	17.6	14.9	12.8	4.8	10.4	10.4	3.8	6.9	81.9
1973–1975	12.8	13.2	10.5	5.4	8.1	7.4	4.3	8.5	70.1
1976–1978	18.5	12.5	11.6	4.7	10.3	6.5	6.0	8.2	78.4
1979–1981†	9.0	14.2	8.7	7.1	5.5	3.1	1.6	7.5	56.6
1982–1984	10.0	10.0	7.2	5.6	3.6	1.0	1.2	8.4	46.6
1985–1987	9.1	9.4	1.9	3.4	3.8	2.3	1.9	7.5	39.4
1988–1990‡	8.0	8.6	1.0	3.5	7.3	2.1	0.7	8.3	39.4

*Excludes abortion and ectopic pregnancy.
†Includes two other direct deaths omitted in the 1976–1978 report.
‡Patient care was judged substandard in almost 50% of maternal deaths.
Data from Hibbard BM, Anderson MM, O'Drife JO, et al: Report on Confidential Enquiries into Maternal Deaths in the United Kingdom, 1988–1990, 36th ed. London, Department of Health and Social Security, Reports on Health and Social Subjects, 1994.

the United Kingdom since 1952. These relatively large, recurring reports contribute significantly to the understanding of the causes of maternal death.

Table 2–1 lists the causes of maternal death in the United Kingdom during the period 1970 to 1990. Several findings and trends are apparent. First, care was judged substandard in almost 50% of all maternal deaths in the most recent report. This finding confirms that, despite the dramatic reductions in maternal death rates, further improvement is possible. Second, the incidence of fatal hypertensive disease complications and pulmonary embolism has stabilized but still accounts for a large percentage of maternal deaths. Third, hemorrhagic death rates nearly doubled in the last triennial report. Noteworthy for the anesthesiologist is the fact that the four leading causes of maternal death—hypertensive disease, pulmonary embolism, hemorrhage, and amniotic fluid embolism—are complications that may require the care of an anesthesiologist. These obstetric complications should serve as a "red flag" for the anesthesia provider and demand the utmost vigilance. Finally, despite dramatic reduction in anesthesia-related deaths, many of the direct and indirect anesthesia-related maternal deaths are still associated in part or in whole to substandard care, indicating that a further decline in anesthesia-related maternal death rates can be achieved by improved anesthesia care.

Preventing Anesthesia-Related Maternal Death

The changes in anesthesia care adopted since the mid-1970s are due largely to the detailed analysis of anesthesia-related maternal deaths reported in the United Kingdom triennial maternal mortality reports (Confidential Enquiries into Maternal Deaths [CEMD]). U.S. reports of anesthesia-related maternal death have, for the most part, confirmed the conclusions noted in the English reports. Reviewing the critical conclusions of these reports illustrates the anesthesia care that is necessary to minimize risk of maternal death.

Prior to the 1980s, the most common cause of anesthesia-related maternal death was gastric aspiration, often associated with mask inhalational anesthesia. During the late 1970s, the implications of gastric acid volume and pH were investigated, and the effectiveness of various antacid prophylaxis regimens examined and applied to the obstetric population. Routine rapid-sequence tracheal intubation with concurrent cricoid pressure was additionally advocated to reduce the risk of fatal gastric aspirations.

Particulate antacids, an early attempt at antacid prophylaxis, did not appear to reduce morbidity.[1–3] The 1982–1984 CEMD[1] reported that six of seven women suffering fatal gastric aspiration received *particulate antacid therapy*. Consensus developed that nonparticulate antacids, such as 0.3-M sodium citrate, administered immediately prior to initiating cesarean section anesthesia, would reduce the morbidity of gastric aspiration and, unlike particulate antacids, do not appear to cause direct pulmonary injury.

By necessity, other measures in addition to antacid prophylaxis have also been advocated to reduce the risks of gastric aspiration. Although sodium citrate is highly reliable at raising the gastric pH, it is effective for less than 60 minutes.[4] In many hospitals where surgical operating times are prolonged, sodium citrate's short duration of action places the parturient at risk for aspiration at the end of the operation or in the recovery room. For these reasons, some authorities recommend utilizing H_2 blockers, such as ranitidine, with a long duration of action, for patients who are at high risk for cesarean section. In addition, some authorities recommend placing an oral gastric tube intraoperatively during use of general anesthetics, emptying the stomach. In this instance, the rationale is that H_2 blockers do not reduce the gastric volume that is initially present while sodium citrate's effectiveness will wane prematurely. However, these ancillary measures are not routinely practiced, and their contribution to reducing maternal deaths secondary to gastric aspiration is unknown. While inexpensive prophylaxis with sodium citrate is mandated, additional interventions should be considered for those patients who are at unusual risk for emergency cesarean section.

In summary, increased awareness of the risks for fatal maternal gastric aspiration resulted in an intensive worldwide educational campaign that emphasized this danger and the need for antacid prophylaxis combined with protection of the airway via tracheal intubation with a cuffed endotracheal tube. Slowly, practice patterns changed and gastric aspiration fell from its place as the number one cause of anesthesia-related maternal death.

The 1982–1984 triennial CEMD[1] illustrated an incomplete application of the other lesson for preventing maternal deaths from gastric aspiration: rapid-sequence tracheal intubation with continuous cricoid pressure. Difficulty managing the airway and tracheal intubation became the number one cause of death (Table 2–2). Instead of receiving mask inhalational general anesthesia for cesarean section, tracheal intubation was routinely attempted, but often without appropriate training to perform the

TABLE 2–2
Causes of Maternal Deaths Directly Attributed to Anesthesia, England and Wales, 1982–1984

Cause	Number	Percentage
Difficult intubation	11	58
Gastric aspiration	2*	
Esophageal intubation	4	
Failed intubation and inadequate ventilation	3	
Obstructed endotracheal tube	2	
Gastric aspiration	5*	27
Mask general anesthesia	1	
Probable gastric aspiration with respiratory distress at the end of operation	2	
Excessive postoperative sedation	1	
Induction of general anesthesia with cricoid pressure	1	
Anesthesia machine failure	1	5
Ventilator disconnect and patient unattended	1	5
Total spinal following epidural analgesia redose, patient unattended	1	5
Total maternal deaths	**19**	**100**

*Six of seven patients received particulate antacids (as opposed to nonparticulate antacids).

Data from Turnbull AC, Tindall VR, Beard RW, et al: Report on Confidential Enquiries into Maternal Deaths in England and Wales, 1982–1984, 35th ed. London, Department of Health and Social Security, Reports on Health and Social Subjects, 1989.

TABLE 2–3
Management of the Parturient's Airway—Lessons Learned

1. Consider all parturients at risk for gastric aspiration.
2. Evaluate all patients' airways for possible difficulty in intubating the trachea, *before induction of general anesthesia.*
3. Administer clear antacid such as sodium citrate 0.3 M, 30 ml immediately before induction of anesthesia. Consider prophylactic H_2 blockers such as ranitidine.
4. Apply correct cricoid pressure before loss of consciousness and release only after verification of correct placement of the endotracheal tube.
5. Apply a "failed intubation drill" on encountering difficult intubation.
   a. Drill must be learned before encountering difficult intubation.
   b. Drill must include mask ventilation with oxygen and continued cricoid pressure rather than continued attempts to place an endotracheal tube despite maternal hypoxemia.
6. Plan for the management of a difficult intubation when it is anticipated. This should include the prospective involvement of additional experienced anesthesia providers and alternative intubation methods such as bronchoscopy.
7. Use end-tidal CO_2 monitoring to verify correct placement of the endotracheal tube.
8. Use continuous pulse oximetry to help in diagnosing endobronchial intubation.
9. Most importantly, avoid general anesthesia and difficult intubation by using well-performed regional anesthesia.

technique safely. Table 2–3 lists some of the lessons learned in the 1980s concerning management of the parturient's airway.

The author's group believes that lesson 9, listed in Table 2–3, which recommends using regional anesthesia instead of general anesthesia, is the factor that has contributed most to improved maternal outcome and reduced maternal anesthesia deaths. Increased use of regional anesthesia has been emphasized in the United Kingdom, and spinal anesthesia usage today is much more common worldwide compared with its use in the 1970s. Although the percentage of cesarean sections performed under regional anesthesia is not reported in the England and Wales reports, a survey of anesthetic methods in the U.S. workforce was recently presented and supports the contention that use of general anesthesia for cesarean section is markedly reduced compared with the early 1980s. Hawkins and colleagues[5] reported that the use of general anesthesia for cesarean section in the United States fell by nearly 60% between 1981 and 1992. This survey found that general anesthesia was used, on average, 17% of the time in 1992 compared with 41% of the time in 1981. This reduction in the use of general anesthesia occurred in both small and large hospital practices. Similar reductions in the use of general anesthesia probably occurred in the United Kingdom during the same time period.

Other measures advocated to decrease maternal mortality associated with general anesthesia have no doubt contributed to the dramatic reductions in anesthesia risk. These measures include end-tidal CO_2 monitoring to exclude placement of the endotracheal tube in the esophagus and continuous-pulse oximetry to help recognize earlier maternal hypoxemia, as might occur with endobronchial intubation.

Regional anesthesia safety has also improved since the mid-1970s. Many reports suggest that bupivacaine is more cardiotoxic than other local anesthetics, and since its introduction in the United States in 1973, at least 44 maternal cardiac arrests attributed to bupivacaine toxicity following intravenous (IV) injections have been reported.[6, 7] Subsequent to these reports of maternal cardiac arrest, several modifications in anesthetic technique were adopted and have apparently reduced the incidence of bupivacaine myocardial toxicity. The increased awareness of the potential for maternal cardiac arrest following accidental IV injection of local anesthetics has led to better methods to identify intravenous injection. In addition, and probably more importantly, the injection of epidural local anesthetics is today usually divided into portions, or fractionated. Fractionation of doses prevents the accidental intravenous injection of large, potentially lethal boluses of local anesthetics.

Other safety measures designed to prevent regional anesthesia morbidity/mortality have also been adopted. A better awareness of aorta caval syndrome and the importance of routine uterine displacement during epidural and spinal anesthesia reduced the incidence of severe hypotension. The incidence of accidental "total spinal" during epidural anesthesia has been substantially lessened by "testing" with a small dose of "epidural" local anesthetic. This dose is sufficient to produce a recognizable spinal block if the local anesthetic is injected intrathecally, but insufficient to produce total spinal anesthesia.

As mentioned previously, avoidable factors and substandard care are still substantial contributors to direct and indirect anesthesia-related maternal deaths. The most glaring category identified is substandard care provided in the recovery room or postanesthesia care unit (PACU). To minimize maternal anesthesia mortality vigilance must continue in the recovery room. U.S. standards now dictate that the level of postoperative care rendered after cesarean delivery must be comparable to the care following nonobstetric operations and includes routine pulse oximetry, supplementary oxygen until pulse oximetry demonstrates safe oxygen discontinuation despite pain therapy. In the author's group's practice, incremental IV morphine is administered until the patient is comfortable and oxyhemoglobin saturation must remain above 90% for 30 minutes following the last dose of morphine.

The author believes the previously discussed changes in anesthesia practice effectively reduce maternal mortality and must become routine. These changes, combined with improvements in postoperative care, must be instituted to further reduce maternal risk for anesthesia-related death. Nevertheless, the author's group firmly believes that increased utilization of regional anesthesia remains the most significant contributor to the improved maternal mortality statistics. Regional anesthesia should be strongly encouraged, even for those patients who seem to be at low risk for having difficult airways. Remember, emergency cesarean sections consistently associate with increased risk of maternal death.

PERINATAL MORTALITY

Perinatal mortality rates have fallen dramatically since the mid-1970s. Certainly, changes in perinatal and neonatal care account for almost all of the improvements in perinatal death rates. Contributions from improvements in anesthesia practice are unknown and probably insignificant.

OBSTETRIC ANESTHESIA MORBIDITY

Morbidity can be divided into perinatal and maternal. Assessment of perinatal morbidity is extremely difficult. Alterations in fetal heart rate (FHR), neonatal acidosis, depressed Apgar scores, and the most nebulous of all, changes in neurobehavioral scores, are frequent outcomes used to evaluate new obstetric anesthesia drugs or techniques. The following discussion focuses on the practical assessment of the significance of these morbidities and outcomes.

Perinatal Morbidity

Common perinatal assessment tools—such as Apgar scores, FHR tracing analysis, scalp and umbilical cord pH values, and neurobehavioral scores—unless extremely abnormal, poorly predict outcome. Unfortunately, these assessment tools that can measure minor differences that are of little clinical significance are nonetheless used to recommend changes in anesthetic practice. The practitioner should be wary of this trap. Avoiding theoretical concerns should not dictate performing a riskier anesthetic.

The most common measurement of potential neonatal morbidity is the Apgar score. Unfortunately, the predictive accuracy of the Apgar score for longterm outcome is suspect. For example, low Apgar scores can indicate an asphyxiated infant or may simply reflect coincident problems such as prematurity, drug effects, congenital anomalies, sepsis, or poor resuscitation efforts. Clearly, many factors other than anesthetic interventions influence Apgar scores. Viewed from this perspective, it should not be surprising that very low Apgar scores (<3) correlate with higher neonatal death rates, particularly among premature infants.[8] In contrast, the import of low Apgar scores in surviving infants is often grossly overestimated. Physicians, when asked to estimate the likelihood of normal outcome in surviving infants with 5- and 10-minute Apgar scores less than 3, overestimated handicap 10-fold.[9] In fact, a low 1-minute Apgar score has almost no predictive efficacy, unless accompanied by a low 5-minute score. Obviously, other ancillary assessments are needed in addition to a low Apgar score to improve predictive ability. Whereas low Apgar scores accompanied by hypoxia and acidosis demand close attention and follow-up, a low 1-minute Apgar score without acidosis or hypoxemia may simply reflect sedation from the effects of nitrous oxide and require less scrutiny. In summary, Apgar scores can be used to assess the adequacy of neonatal resuscitation or indicate the need for further in-depth evaluation. Be wary of statistically significant reductions in Apgar scores that do not reflect worse clinical outcomes!

Continuous electronic FHR monitoring is a common and somewhat controversial measurement of intrapartum fetal well-being. A normal FHR tracing predicts a nondepressed infant with 99% accuracy (5-minute Apgar score > 6). The opposite is not true. FHR patterns thought to characterize loss of fetal well-being associate with normal infants in 50% of cases.[10] This should not be surprising, since obstetricians often cannot agree when an FHR tracing indicates stress requiring immediate delivery. In one study, one third of experienced obstetricians could not agree when to continue monitoring or proceed to immediate delivery.[11] Not surprisingly, in one study, follow-up of children for 6 to 9 years after delivery could not correlate neurologic/cognitive development with abnormal FHR tracings.[12]

Practically speaking, since ominous changes in FHR tracings cannot be correlated with long-term morbidity, *minor, transient* changes in FHR tracings occurring after initiating epidural analgesia should be viewed from this perspective. This does not mean that the anesthesia practitioner should ignore the FHR tracing but, rather, should place appropriate importance on observed patterns. Measuring the effects of drugs on the FHR is important. For instance, transient changes in FHR variability can follow induction of epidural analgesia but do not associate with fetal acidosis/hypoxia. However, knowing that these FHR alterations may occur following epidural analgesia without altering fetal well-being is vital and aids the obstetrician's interpretation of the significance of the FHR changes. Abandoning epidural analgesia out of fear that these changes in FHR tracings might occur would not be appropriate.

Fetal scalp pH or umbilical cord blood pH is used to identify and document fetal stress. However, only severely depressed pH values correlate with morbidity. Abnormal pH values require ancillary assessments, such as arterial umbilical cord oxygenation, to better interpret the significance of pH values. From a practical perspective, minor alterations in pH attributed to anesthesia techniques are probably of little clinical significance, particularly when neonatal hypoxemia is absent.

In this author's opinion, no neonatal assessment test is more overrated and overvalued than the neurobehavior score. On one occasion, an acceptable analgesic was essentially abandoned for years based on one abnormal neurobehavioral score report. In 1974, Scanlon and associates reported that babies were "floppy but alert" after their mothers received epidural lidocaine for treatment of labor pain.[13] This report led to the virtual abandonment of lidocaine utilization for epidural anesthesia in obstetrics. It was not until the 1980s that other investigators, repeating the initial study, failed to confirm Scanlon's original findings.[14] Epidural lidocaine is now judged safe for use in obstetrics.

The problem with the neurobehavioral examination is that this scoring system assesses subtle newborn behavioral reflexes. Although these tests purportedly reflect drug effects on the newborn, *no* long-term studies associate these subtle findings with morbidity. Since severely depressed Apgar scores correlate poorly with morbidity, why should subtly "depressed" neurobehavioral scores correlate with morbidity? "Measured decrements" in neurobehavioral tests—which do not influence neonatal survival or ability to breast feed—disappearing within 24 hours have little clinical importance. Only large differences in neurobehavioral-type scores persisting for 24 hours, should be considered as *potentially* clinically significant. Unfortunately, the U.S. Food and Drug Administration now requires neurobehavioral assessments as part of an obstetric drug evaluation, even though what constitutes clinically significant decrements in neurobehavioral scores is unknown.

Nevertheless, maintain perspective! These perinatal assessment tools have improved care by stimulating anesthetic technique modifications that potentially improve clinical outcome. For example, untreated or inadequately treated maternal hypotension often associates with depressed, acidotic neonates. Application of uterine displacement, early treatment of hypotension with ephedrine and prophylactic "IV prehydration" have reduced most episodes of hypotension to transient, easily treated episodes with good neonatal outcome. Unfortunately, we have overcompensated. The principles of maternal hypotension prevention have been extrapolated to extremes. Dramatically changing current anesthetic practice to lessen the incidence of *transient* hypotension following regional anesthesia induction without documenting any improvement in *clinical* neonatal morbidity is not warranted. For example, some practitioners extended the known beneficial effects of prehydration to the point that they refuse to induce regional anesthesia if there is a perceived lack of time to infuse the "required preload" for fear of transient hypotension. Prehydration prior to epidural or spinal anesthesia does lessen the incidence of hypotension; however, rigid, arbitrary volume requirements are not always rational and may deny the mother a safer regional anesthetic on the basis of theoretical contraindications.

Another example of the extension of questionably significant clinical findings into everyday anesthesia technique is the practice of administering 50% or greater inspired maternal oxygen concentrations during general anesthesia for cesarean section. This practice pattern was adopted on the basis of studies that reported "improved" 1-minute Apgar scores and shorter neonatal "time-to-sustained respirations" compared with lower inspired oxygen concentrations. However, whether 70% inspired nitrous oxide produces more neonatal morbidity than 50% nitrous oxide is questionable. The increased neonatal depression attributable to 70% nitrous oxide, if real, will be transient and more correctly reflects neonatal sedation, and rapidly disappears in the first few minutes in life. One could invoke the theoretical benefit of greater fetal/neonatal oxygen content in the blood and potentially greater neonatal reserve to withstand stress. However, this is a theoretical benefit without any clinical evidence that increased newborn oxygen reserve improves neonatal outcome. As a result, a practice pattern has been established without good science.

In summary, the emerging medical practice environment in the United States is emphasizing outcome-based studies. It is no longer affordable to abandon clinical practices for new, usually more expensive, practices and drugs on the basis of assessments with little or no predictive efficacy. Future studies will need to verify outcome and morbidity improvements before new anesthetic techniques and drugs are widely accepted and adopted.

Maternal Morbidity

Increased incidences of forceps and cesarean deliveries have been attributed to epidural labor analgesia. See Chapters 6 and 7 for discussions of this morbidity. In addition, three other categories of maternal morbidity are commonly attributed to regional anesthesia in the parturient: complaints of headache, backache, and rarely, neurologic deficit. The author's group's practical approach to these complications is discussed.

Headache

Table 2–4 lists the differential diagnosis of postpartum headache. The anesthesiologist is frequently asked to evaluate headache in the postpartum period and must be able to recognize not only headaches related to anesthesia but also other serious complications manifesting with headaches. This section presents a practical approach to evaluating postpartum headache.

Start by remembering that 39% of women suffer headache, unrelated to anesthesia, in the first week postpartum.[15] For the anesthesiologist, the first goal is to separate anesthesia-related headaches from headaches due to other causes.

Postdural Puncture Headache

Patients with known dural punctures, particularly large-gauge needle punctures, should be evaluated with a high index of suspicion which begins with the anesthesia record. At the Bowman Gray School of Medicine, the author's group documents the number of epidural needle advancements during block placement as well as the height and degree of sensory/motor blockade resulting from the epidural local anesthetic. Accidental, *unrecognized* dural puncture does occur. Indirect evidence such as multiple epidural needle placement attempts or exaggerated spread of epidural blocks, in combination with a clearly postural headache, support the diagnosis of postdural puncture headache (PDPHA). The defining symptom of PDPHA is exacerbation of symptoms when the patient moves from supine to sitting or standing. Unless postural, consider other etiologies. Although the headache should immediately improve when the patient assumes the supine position, it may not totally disappear. PDPHAs usually occur in the first or second postpartum day, but

TABLE 2–4
Differential Diagnosis of Postpartum Headache

Diagnosis	Symptoms
Positional Headaches	
1. Postdural puncture headache (PDPHA)	Improved or absent when supine. Patient may have nausea, vomiting, or visual or hearing changes. History of dural puncture helps make the diagnosis.
2. Pneumocephalus	Usually within hours of dural puncture. History of using loss of resistance with air.
3. Cortical vein thrombosis	Severe throbbing headache with nausea/vomiting and sweating. May have seizures, focal neurologic signs, or signs of increased intracranial pressure (ICP).
Nonpositional Headaches	
1. Nonspecific headache	Diagnosis of exclusion, may have component of neck/head muscle spasm.
2. Caffeine withdrawal	History of routine caffeine intake with none recently.
3. Sinus headache	Pain over sinuses. Patient may be allergic or bacterial. Upright position improves symptoms.
4. Preeclampsia	Hypertension may not necessarily be severe.
5. Flu or viral syndrome	May be accompanied by fever, myalgia.
6. Hypertensive encephalopathy	Significant hypertension. Diagnosis of preeclampsia not necessary.
7. Migraine headache	Similar to other episodes of migraine headache, but not necessarily as severe.
8. Lactation headache	Occurs during breast feeding.
9. Meningitis	Fever, nuchal rigidity, lethargy, seizures, rash, and other classic signs.
10. Subdural hematoma	May be preceded by PDPHA symptoms. Signs of increased ICP are present.
11. Intracerebal hemorrhage	Sudden severe headache, signs of increased ICP.
12. Brain tumor	Variable but usually signs of increased ICP.
13. Pseudotumor cerebri	Headache and visual changes.

may rarely appear after 7 days; most last less than one week.[16]

Decreased cerebrospinal fluid (CSF) volume and intracranial pressure contribute significantly to the postural symptoms and are thought secondary to continued CSF leakage through the dural puncture. Support for this etiology exists because epidural blood patch (EBP) immediately increases CSF pressure and headache symptoms frequently lessen or resolve shortly after EBP. Although other methods of increasing CSF pressure such as epidural saline infusions and abdominal binders have been used as therapy, evidence does not support their efficacy. Cerebral vasodilatation, probably in response to low CSF pressure, may also contribute to the headache and responds to cerebral vasoconstricting drugs such as caffeine and methyl xanthine. Both of these drugs have been reported to *transiently* reduce headache symptoms. Although these drugs will occasionally be efficacious when attempting to lessen a mild headache, EBP is the most reliable "cure" of PDPHA.

Other symptoms that may accompany PDPHA include nausea and vomiting and hearing or visual changes. In the author's group's practice, women manifesting hearing or visual changes are *strongly* encouraged to receive an EBP. The author's group believes that these latter symptoms may be indicative of significant cranial nerve stretching that, if left untreated, may cause hearing or visual changes to persist after headache resolution.

Epidural Blood Patch

Most authors report approximately 90% cure rates of PDPHA following EBP. EBP is so reliable, before performing a second EBP, reassess the headache attempting to ensure that it is a

PDPHA and not another type of postpartum headache. Both the timing and the blood volume most appropriate for successful EBP are controversial and may depend as much on philosophy as on science.

Szeinfeld and coworkers,[17] using technetium-labeled red blood cells, injected blood into the epidural space, using as an end-point, back, buttock, or leg pain. The mean injected blood volume was approximately 15 ml, which spread over nine spinal segments. Approximately two thirds of the blood volume spread cephalad. Therefore, when confronted with multiple puncture sites, the EBP should be administered at or below the lowest puncture. Other reports have used arbitrary blood volumes, ranging from 3 ml to 20 ml of blood;[18, 19] however, most authors use 10 to 15 ml. Back pain is the most common complication of EBP. Abouleish and colleagues,[20] in a long-term follow-up of EBP, found that 35% of women reported back pain during the first 48 hours after EBP and 16% reported persistent back pain with a mean duration of 27 days. Other more serious complaints such as severe nerve root irritation or radiculopathy rarely occur.

The timing of EBP administration is controversial. Some studies report 54 to 71% failure rates when therapeutic EBP is administered within 24 hours of headache onset, compared with 4% failure rates when delayed for 24 hours.[21, 22] Other authors believe that prophylactic EBP through a functioning epidural catheter is justifiable, since up to 70 to 80% of accidental dural punctures occurring with epidural needles result in PDPHA. Nonetheless, failure rates following prophylactic EBP approximate 20%.[23–25]

Technique of Epidural Blood Patch. If prophylactic EBP is planned, it should be administered through an existing epidural catheter only after all signs of local anesthetic blockade have resolved. A "total spinal block" has been reported when prophylactic EBP was administered before the residual local anesthetic block resolved.[26] The hypothesized mechanism of this total spinal block was that the EBP increased spinal CSF pressure, moving residual local anesthetic cephalad. Furthermore, sensory function is necessary to allow the patient to report pain during EBP so that the injection can be stopped in a timely manner (usually 10 to 20 ml of blood).

Although some institutions administer prophylactic EBP, anesthesiologists at the author's institution do not. First, the author's group is concerned about the possibility of administering blood through a contaminated epidural catheter. Epidural catheter contamination is particularly likely after prolonged labors and multiple catheter reinjections. Although the risk is low, the published experience of prophylactic EBP through epidural catheters is insufficient to characterize the risks for blood contamination when compared with the thousands of therapeutic EBPs performed as a second procedure. Second, prophylactic EBP subjects 100% of women to the risks of post-EBP back/neck pain, when only 50% would require EBP if evaluated 24 to 48 hours after dural puncture.[27] Finally, although EBP performed in women with persistent symptoms lasting for more than 24 hours is 90 to 95% successful on first treatment, prophylactic EBP has a 20% failure rate necessitating a second EBP.

The author performs EBP using the following technique. The author assures that the patient is afebrile. Using sterile technique, the needle is placed into the epidural space at or below the lowest visible skin puncture. Twenty milliliters of blood is drawn sterilely from the arm and slowly injected through the epidural needle until the patient reports feeling mild back, neck, or leg discomfort. If pain occurs before the injection is complete, the author stops the injection, waits 1 minute, then continues the injection until the patient reports return of the back fullness/discomfort sensation. Most patients tolerate only 12- to 15-ml; however, some will receive 20 ml without reporting any discomfort. Performing the EBP in this fashion allows the blood injection volume to be customized to the patient's apparent epidural space compliance and avoids the pitfalls of arbitrarily injecting volumes that may be too little in some patients and too much in others, leading to increased failure rates or increased risks for significant back/neck pain following the procedure. Following blood injection the patient remains supine for 30 to 60 minutes, then gradually sits upright. Whereas many patients report immediate significant improvement or resolution of headache symptoms, others require at least 24 hours before headache symptoms resolve. Back and neck muscle spasm may require 1 to 2 days to resolve. If the PDPHA symptoms remain constant or worsen after 24 to 48 hours, the author will consider a second EBP after searching for other headache causes.

Some investigations report that a previous dural puncture increases the risk for epidural failure in subsequent pregnancies.[28] This reported epidural failure risk increased independent of the patient receiving an EBP. The author's group's experience at Bowman Gray School of Medicine is dissimilar.[29] The author's group evaluated 47 women in labor receiving epidural analgesia with a history of previous wet tap. Epidural success rates were similar to those in 500 control patients. In addition, previous EBP for PDPHA did not change epidural success rates.

Other causes of *positional headaches* are *pneumoencephalus* and, rarely, *cortical vein thrombosis.* Pneumoencephalus occurs when air used to indicate epidural loss of resistance is accidentally injected into the subarachnoid space. Onset of headache is almost immediate and is very short-lived (several hours) unless large amounts of air were injected. The author's group discourages injecting large volumes of "epidural" air to avoid the possibility of producing a significant pneumoencephalus if accidentally injected intrathecally.

Cortical Vein Thrombosis

Cortical vein thrombosis may occur in the hypercoagulable postpartum period and lead to focal neurologic deficits, seizures, cerebral infarction, and coma. Women with cortical vein thrombosis may have symptoms that can be confused with PDPHA and have received EBP.[30, 31] Gewirtz and associates[31] suggest that the symptoms consistent with cortical vein thrombosis are severe postural throbbing headache, nausea/vomiting, and sweating. Women with these symptoms should have a neurology consultation to exclude the diagnosis before receiving EBP. Prevention of seizure with antiepileptic drugs is the primary therapy.

Nonpositional Headaches

Although nonpositional headaches are very common in the postpartum period and usually unrelated to anesthesia, the anesthesiologist can often help with the diagnosis. Table 2–4 lists types of nonpositional headaches and common associated symptoms.

Backache

Backache commonly follows delivery. Grove[32] found that 40% of parturients delivering without regional anesthesia complained of in-hospital back pain that resolved within 6 days. Nonetheless, parturients and anesthesiologists often attribute postdelivery back pain to regional anesthesia. Indeed, some older retrospective studies support this belief and identify statistical associations of epidural analgesia/anesthesia with risks of backache.[33, 34] However, in addition to the inherent problems of retrospective surveys, these surveys were performed when relatively high concentrations of epidural local anesthetics (e.g., bupivacaine 0.375–0.5%) were routinely used. These concentrations of local anesthetics commonly produce significant motor blockade which could allow excessive stretching of muscles and ligaments or permit accidental malposition of the parturient. However, more recently, Breen and coworkers[35] prospectively studied 1042 women and found that the incidence of backache 1 to 2 months following delivery was approximately 44% regardless of whether epidural anesthesia was used. In contrast to older studies, women in this study received epidural analgesia during labor using dilute concentrations of bupivacaine (0.04–0.125%). The most common factors associated with new-onset backache persisting 1 to 2 months postpartum were greater weight and short stature. Women developing back pain during pregnancy were also more likely to report persistent back pain 1 to 2 months after delivery. Most importantly, no association was found between postpartum back pain and epidural anesthesia, number of attempts at epidural placement, duration of second stage, birth weight, or mode of delivery. Although epidural anesthesia is unlikely to cause backache in the immediate postpartum period, persistent, severe back pain must be evaluated to separate potentially serious complications of regional anesthesia from benign backache.

Localized bruising and minimal-to-moderate pain over the epidural insertion site are common. Difficult epidural placement, involving multiple needle punctures predispose to this type of temporary backache. Nonsteroidal analgesics, heat, and mobilization facilitate pain resolution.

Moderate-to-severe pain, particularly pain of

increasing severity that is localized to the lumbar region of the back, may represent the initial presenting symptoms of space-occupying lesions such as an epidural hematoma or abscess. Both of these extremely rare complications usually present with complaints of localized back pain that increases in severity with progressive degrees of sensory and motor deficits developing below the lesion. Epidural or spinal abscess usually presents with fever, malaise, and backache, progressing to bowel/bladder dysfunction and, in the late period, lower extremity pain, weakness, and paralysis 1 to 2 weeks following the anesthetic.[36, 37] Most epidural hematomas are spontaneous, but those associated with regional anesthesia can present hours or days after the anesthetic. Although usually associated with altered coagulation, the degree of coagulopathy necessary to increase the risk of this complication in association with regional anesthesia is unknown. Nevertheless, anticoagulation therapy and diseases associated with altered coagulation should be "Red Flags" for the anesthesia provider.[38–41]

Remember, successful treatment of spinal or epidural abscess or hematoma requires early diagnosis and decompressive laminectomy within 6 to 12 hours of the onset of symptoms. Severe back pain unresponsive to analgesics and heat mandates serial physical examinations until symptoms lessen or the physical examination indicates developing neurologic symptoms. In this situation, early neurology or neurosurgery consultation is prudent, and magnetic resonance imaging (MRI) is now the definitive radiologic study to confirm the diagnosis.

Neurologic Deficits

Transient neurologic deficits presenting in the postpartum period are not unusual. The usual causes are: (1) obstetric neurologic injuries, (2) injuries associated with patient positioning, and (3) anesthesia-related injuries.

Obstetric and Patient Position Neurologic Injuries

Lumbosacral nerves may be damaged directly and compressed between the descending fetal head and the sacrum. This neurologic injury is thought to be more likely with abnormal fetal presentations, significant fetal macrosomia, or maternal-fetal disproportion. Figure 2–1 illustrates peripheral nerves that may be injured in the pelvis by the fetal head.

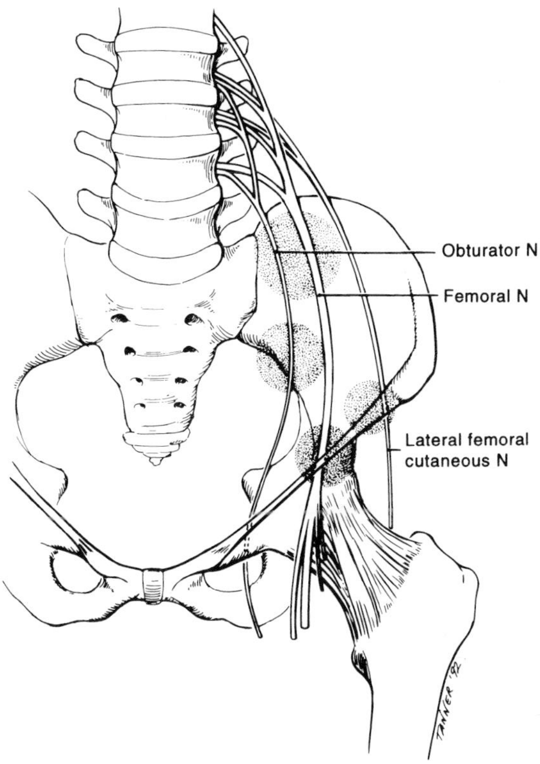

Figure 2–1. Schematic of the paths of nerves in the pelvis that may be injured by pressure during labor and delivery. (From Redick LF: Maternal perinatal nerve palsies. Clin Obstet Gynecol 12:1–5, 1992.)

Postpartum footdrop is a relatively common obstetric neurologic injury. The injury is usually unilateral, and occurs on the side opposite the fetal occiput.[42] Stirrups injury to the common peroneal nerve at the neck of the fibula may also result in postpartum footdrop. Improper leg positioning and prolonged stirrup use predispose to injury. Physical examination reveals decreased pinprick perception along the lateral surface of the lower leg and the dorsal surface of the foot. Weakness of ankle dorsiflexion and eversion is also apparent. This neurologic deficit usually resolves within several weeks.

The fetal head may also injure other pelvic nerves, most commonly femoral or obturator nerves. Abnormal fetal presentations (transverse lie or occiput posterior) fetal macrosomia, and prolonged labor increase the likelihood of postpartum neuropathy. Injury is secondary to fetal head compression of the lumbar plexus in the pelvis, and causes unilateral or bilateral nerve injury (see Fig. 2–1). Twenty-five percent of femoral or obturator nerve injuries are bilateral and may be mistaken for an intraspinal injury or lesion.[42] Clues to the diagnosis are the development of sudden pain or muscle spasm during labor. Femoral neuropathy also associates with decreased sensation in the nerves' distribution, diminished or absent patellar reflex, and while the patient may walk satisfactorily on a level surface, climbing stairs may prove difficult. Obturator neuropathy has associated hip adduction and rotation weakness and may have decreased sensation along the upper inner thigh.[42]

Intraoperative nerve injury may also occur and be attributed to anesthesia. At the author's institution, several instances of ilioinguinal nerve or lateral femoral cutaneous nerve deficits have followed cesarean section when the obstetrician used a low Phannenstiel incision. Deficits have occurred following both general and regional anesthesia and were attributed to operative injury.

Prolonged, exaggerated hip flexion and external rotation during the second stage cause postpartum femoral neuropathy.[43, 44] Epidural analgesia during the second stage of labor may allow this extreme positioning, since the parturient is unlikely to complain of discomfort. Encouraging the parturient to relax her hip flexion between contractions may decrease the risk of nerve injury.

Permanent postpartum paresis in one or both lower limbs has occurred after delivery in women who have not received an anesthetic. A Nigerian report of 34 patients with postpartum palsy revealed that 85% of cases were transient with partial or complete recovery, whereas 15% of patients had permanent neurologic injury.[45] None of the women suffering permanent neurologic palsies received regional anesthesia.[46]

In addition to the previously discussed etiologies for postpartum nerve injury, permanent spinal cord or cauda equina injury may manifest postpartum. One explanation for this rare neurologic catastrophe is that in 15% of the population the ascending iliac artery provides a significant contribution to the blood flow of the tip of the conus medullaris and the cauda equina.[47] Difficult or traumatic delivery may impair this blood flow and place this population at risk for permanent spinal cord or cauda equina injury.

Anesthesia-Related Neurologic Injuries

Ong and colleagues[48] reviewed the outcome of 23,927 deliveries and noted a postpartum paresthesia and motor dysfunction rate of 18.9/10,000 deliveries. All neurologic injuries were transient, lasting less than 72 hours. Whereas the overall incidence of neurologic deficit following epidural anesthesia was similar to that following general anesthesia, women who delivered without anesthesia demonstrated less risk for postpartum neurologic deficits (Table 2–5). Consistent with other reports, women who experienced difficult/prolonged deliveries, especially those delivered with forceps, were more likely to have postpartum neurologic deficit and also more likely to receive epidural or general anesthesia. Overall, there is little evidence that the increased incidence of transient neurologic

TABLE 2–5
Transient Postpartum Sensory and Motor Deficits Following 23,875 Deliveries, 1975–1983

Anesthetic/Analgesic Technique	Number of Deliveries	Number of Neurologic Deficits	Incidence per 10,000 Deliveries
None	8198	2	2.4
Inhalational analgesia only	4766	3	6.3
Epidural anesthesia	9403	34	36.2*
General anesthesia	864	3	34.7*
Other	596	3	50.3
Total	23,872	45	18.9

*$p < .001$, when compared with no analgesia/anesthesia.

Data from Ong BY, Cohen MM, Esmail A, et al: Paresthesias and motor dysfunction after labor and delivery. Anesth Analg 66:18–22, 1987.

deficit in women receiving epidural anesthesia is *directly caused by* epidural anesthesia.

Spinal cord infarction has been attributed to the addition of epinephrine to spinal and epidural local anesthetics. Although epidural epinephrine is a venoconstricting agent in the epidural space, slowing systemic local anesthetic absorption, there is good evidence that spinal epinephrine does not cause spinal cord vasoconstriction and reduce spinal cord blood flow.[49–51] Postpartum spinal cord ischemia or infarction is more likely due to severe hypotension, anterior spinal artery syndrome, or other spinal arteriovenous malformations.

Direct spinal cord or nerve root injury can occur secondary to needle or catheter laceration. The author's group has noted in the laboratory that it is surprisingly easy to accidentally thread an 18-gauge spinal catheter into the spinal cord of an anesthetized sheep. Similar complications have occurred in anesthetized humans, resulting in significant morbidity. In awake patients, sudden, severe lancinating pain occurring during needle or catheter advancement should serve as a warning to immediately stop the placement attempt. Depending on the severity of pain and its persistence, either the regional anesthetic should be abandoned or another interspace (usually lower) should be elected for needle placement.

Other regional anesthetic misadventures can occur. Injection of contaminated solutions or unintended harmful substances into the epidural or spinal space has caused both temporary and permanent sequela. Vigilance is required to ensure strict aseptic technique and injection of the intended drug. Finally, neurologic deficits can result from complications such as infection, hematoma, and untreated PDPHA, as discussed earlier in this chapter.

SUMMARY

As mentioned in the introduction, the topic of outcome is broad and complicated. This chapter discussed both the lessons learned to minimize anesthesia-related maternal mortality and some aspects of *clinically significant* perinatal and maternal morbidity. The lesson that most reduces risks for anesthesia-related maternal mortality is to perform regional anesthesia for cesarean section when possible. In the future, outcome studies must focus on anesthetic practices and techniques that improve *clinically significant* morbidity outcomes.

TEN PRACTICAL POINTS

1. Regional anesthesia associates with fewer maternal deaths than general anesthesia.
2. Establish postcesarean section postanesthesia care standards resembling nonobstetric postanesthesia standards.
3. Apgar scores poorly predict long-term outcome.
4. Consider the diagnosis of cortical vein thrombosis when the patient complains of severe throbbing postural headache accompanied by nausea, vomiting, and sweating.
5. Epidural anesthesia does not increase the frequency of postpartum backache.
6. Severe back pain or neurologic symptoms in the early postpartum period require further evaluation.
7. Most postpartum neurologic deficits are related to delivery, *not* regional anesthesia.
8. The incidence of neurologic deficit following regional anesthesia is similar to that following general anesthesia.
9. Prolonged hip flexion during the second stage of delivery may result in femoral nerve deficits.
10. History of dural puncture with an epidural needle or treatment with an epidural blood patch does not influence success in subsequent epidural anesthetics.

REFERENCES

1. Turnbull AC, Tindall VR, Beard RW, et al: Report on Confidential Enquiries into Maternal Deaths in England and Wales 1982–1984, 35th ed. London, Department of Health and Social Security, Reports on Health and Social Subjects, 1989.
2. Bond VK, Stoelting RK, Gupta CD: Pulmonary aspiration syndrome after inhalation of gastric fluid containing antacids. Anesthesiology 51:452–453, 1979.
3. Cohen SE: Aspiration syndromes in pregnancy. Anesthesiology 51:375–377, 1979.
4. O'Sullivan G, Harrison BJ, Bullingham RE: The use of radiotelemetry techniques for the in vivo assessment of antacids. Anaesthesia 39:987–995, 1984.
5. Hawkins JL, Gibbs CP, Orleans M, Schmid K: Obstetric anesthesia workforce survey—1992 ver-

sus 1981 [Abstract]. Anesthesiology 81:A1128, 1994.
6. Albright GA: Cardiac arrest following regional anesthesia with etidocaine or bupivacaine [Editorial]. Anesthesiology 51:285–287, 1979.
7. Albright GA: Local anesthetics. *In* Albright GA, Ferguson JEI, Joyce THI, et al (eds): Anesthesia in Obstetrics. Boston, Butterworths, 1986, p 115.
8. Nelson KB, Ellenberg JH: Antecedents of cerebral palsy. Multivariate analysis of risk. N Engl J Med 315:81–86, 1986.
9. Paneth N, Fox HE: The relationship of Apgar score to neurologic handicap: A survey of clinicians. Obstet Gynecol 61:547–550, 1983.
10. Paul RH, Suidan AK, Yeh S, et al: Clinical fetal monitoring. VII. The evaluation and significance of intrapartum baseline FHR variability. Am J Obstet Gynecol 123:206–210, 1975.
11. Cohen AB, Klapholz H, Thompson MS: Electronic fetal monitoring and clinical practice. A survey of obstetric opinion. Med Decis Making 2:79–95, 1982.
12. Painter MJ, Scott M, Hirsch RP, et al: Fetal heart rate patterns during labor: Neurologic and cognitive development at six to nine years of age. Am J Obstet Gynecol 159:854–858, 1988.
13. Scanlon JW, Brown WU Jr, Weiss JB, Alper MH: Neurobehavioral responses of newborn infants after maternal epidural anesthesia. Anesthesiology 40:121–128, 1974.
14. Abboud TK, Sarkis F, Blikian A, et al: Lack of adverse neonatal neurobehavioral effects of lidocaine. Anesth Analg 62:473–475, 1983.
15. Stein G, Morton J, Marsh A, et al: Headaches after childbirth. Acta Neurol Scand 69:74–79, 1984.
16. Vandam LD, Dripps RD: Long-term follow-up of patients who received 10,098 spinal anesthetics. JAMA 161:586–591, 1956.
17. Szeinfeld M, Ihmeidan IH, Moser MM, et al: Epidural blood patch: Evaluation of the volume and spread of blood injected into the epidural space. Anesthesiology 64:820–822, 1986.
18. Gormley J: Treatment of postspinal headache. Anesthesiology 21:565–566, 1960.
19. Crawford JS: Experiences with epidural blood patch. Anaesthesia 35:513–515, 1980.
20. Abouleish E, de la Vega S, Blendinger I, Tio TO: Long-term follow-up of epidural blood patch. Anesth Analg 54:459–463, 1975.
21. Colonna-Romano P, Shapiro BE: Unintentional dural puncture and prophylactic epidural blood patch in obstetrics. Anesth Analg 69:522–523, 1989.
22. Ackerman WE, Juneja MM, Kaczorowski DM: The attenuation of postdural puncture headache with a prophylactic blood patch in labor patients [Abstract]. Anesth Analg 68:S1, 1989.
23. Ackerman WE, Juneja MM, Kaczorowski DM: Prophylactic epidural blood patch for the prevention of postdural puncture headache in the parturient. Anesth Rev 17:45–49, 1990.
24. Cheek TG, Banner R, Sauter J, Gutsche BB: Prophylactic extradural blood patch is effective. Br J Anaesth 61:340–342, 1988.
25. Quaynor H, Corbey M: Extradural blood patch—Why delay? Br J Anaesth 57:538–540, 1985.
26. Leivers D: Total spinal anesthesia following early prophylactic epidural blood patch. Anesthesiology 73:1287–1289, 1990.
27. Norris MC, Leighton BL, DeSimone CA: Needle bevel direction and headache after inadvertent dural puncture. Anesthesiology 70:729–731, 1989.
28. Ong BY, Graham CR, Ringaert KRA, et al: Impaired epidural analgesia after dural puncture with and without subsequent blood patch. Anesth Analg 70:76–79, 1990.
29. Blanche R, Eisenach JC, Tuttle R, Dewan DM: Previous wet tap does not reduce success rate of labor epidural analgesia. Anesth Analg 79:291–294, 1994.
30. Siegle JH, Dewan DM, James FM III: Cerebral infarction following spinal anesthesia for cesarean section. Anesth Analg 61:390–392, 1982.
31. Gewirtz EC, Costin M, Marx GF: Cortical vein thrombosis may mimic postdural puncture headache. Reg Anesth 12:188–190, 1987.
32. Grove LH: Backache, headache and bladder dysfunction after delivery. Br J Anaesth 45:1147–1149, 1973.
33. Russell R, Groves P, Taub N, et al: Assessing long-term backache after childbirth. Br Med J 306:1299–1303, 1993.
34. MacArthur C, Lewis M, Knox EG: Investigation of long-term problems after obstetric epidural anaesthesia [See comments]. Br Med J 304:1279–1282, 1992.
35. Breen TW, Ransil BJ, Groves PA, Oriol NE: Factors associated with back pain after childbirth. Anesthesiology 81:29–34, 1994.
36. Danner RL, Hartman BJ: Update on spinal epidural abscess: 35 cases and review of the literature. Rev Infect Dis 9:265–274, 1987.
37. Bromage PR: Masked mischief [Editorial; comment]. Reg Anesth 18:143–144, 1993.
38. Owens EL, Kasten GW, Hessel EA II: Spinal subarachnoid hematoma after lumbar puncture and heparinization: A case report, review of the literature, and discussion of anesthetic implications. Anesth Analg 65:1201–1207, 1986.
39. Gingrich TF: Spinal epidural hematoma following continuous epidural anesthesia. Anesthesiology 29:162–163, 1968.
40. Onishchuk JL, Carlsson C: Epidural hematoma

associated with epidural anesthesia: Complications of anticoagulant therapy. Anesthesiology 77:1221–1223, 1992.
41. Butler AB, Green CD: Haematoma following epidural anaesthesia. Can Anaesth Soc J 17:635–639, 1970.
42. Donaldson JO: Neurology of Pregnancy. Philadelphia, WB Saunders, 1989.
43. Redick LF: Maternal perinatal nerve palsies. Postgrad Obstet Gynecol 12:1–6, 1992.
44. Vargo MM, Robinson LR, Nicholas JJ, Rulin MC: Postpartum femoral neuropathy: Relic of an earlier era? Arch Phys Med Rehabil 71:591–596, 1990.
45. Bademosi O, Osuntokun BO, Van de Werd HJ, et al: Obstetric neuropraxia in the Nigerian African. Int J Gynaecol Obstet 17:611–614, 1980.
46. Bromage PR: Neurologic complications of labor, delivery, and regional anesthesia, *In* Chestnut DH (ed): Obstetric Anesthesia: Principles and Practice. St. Louis, CV Mosby, 1994, pp 621–639.
47. Lazorthes G, Poulhes J, Bastide G, et al: La vascularisation de la moelle épin ière. Rev Neurol (Paris) 106:535–557, 1962.
48. Ong BY, Cohen MM, Esmail A, et al: Paresthesias and motor dysfunction after labor and delivery. Anesth Analg 66:18–22, 1987.
49. Porter SS, Albin MS, Watson WA, et al: Spinal cord and cerebral blood flow responses to subarachnoid injection of local anesthetics with and without epinephrine. Acta Anaesthesiol Scand 29:330–338, 1985.
50. Kozody R, Palahniuk RJ, Wade JG, et al: The effect of subarachnoid epinephrine and phenylephrine on spinal cord blood flow. Can Anaesth Soc J 31:503–508, 1984.
51. Dohi S, Takeshima R, Naito H: Spinal cord blood flow during spinal anesthesia in dogs: The effects of tetracaine, epinephrine, acute blood loss, and hypercapnia. Anesth Analg 66:599–606, 1987.

THREE

Evaluation of the Pregnant Patient: Preoperative Concerns

Joseph J. Kryc, M.D.

An integral part of obstetric care during the intrapartum period is the relief of pain associated with labor. Individuals responsible for the administration of anesthesia in the obstetric patient must be familiar with the monitoring techniques of the maternal-fetal unit, as well as with the physiologic changes of pregnancy and the anesthetic implications of these changes. In addition, optimal care requires a basic understanding of the medical, surgical, and obstetric problems that complicate pregnancy. Thus, evaluation of the pregnant patient prior to the induction of anesthesia for labor and delivery is essential. Equally important is continued assessment of the patient throughout labor, as a significant percentage of maternal-fetal problems develop at this time.

Fetal monitoring has evolved from relatively simple procedures to sophisticated techniques involving ultrasonic imaging, Doppler ultrasound, direct sampling of fetal tissue and fluids, and complex biophysical profiles. Similar advances have occurred with maternal monitoring capabilities. This chapter provides a description of the techniques used to assess the status of the mother and fetus prior to delivery. An understanding of these techniques enables the obstetric anesthesiologist to more accurately anticipate the obstetrician's and parturient's needs and develop a comprehensive anesthetic plan for the intrapartum period.

ANTEPARTUM EVALUATION

Prenatal Care

Routine prenatal care is the oldest and most common monitoring technique used to evaluate the obstetric patient. Early prenatal care is an important factor in determining a favorable outcome for both the mother and the baby. During the first prenatal visit, the obstetrician's major goals are to evaluate the status of the mother and fetus, determine fetal gestational age, and initiate an obstetric care plan.[1] A comprehensive history and physical examination are, therefore, a vital part of the first visit (Fig. 3–1). A review of the patient's past medical, surgical, and obstetric history assists in identifying potential risk factors that may influence the course of pregnancy. A thorough gynecologic and menstrual history detailing the length and duration of each menstrual cycle, its regularity, and the date of the last menstrual period dates the pregnancy. Accurately assessing the gestational age at the first visit is important, because treatment of complications developing later in pregnancy is frequently based on the estimated gestational age of the fetus. The physical examination should include a comprehensive evaluation of all organ systems, with particular emphasis on the reproductive system. A Pap smear and cervical cultures, as well as a description of the bony architecture of the pelvis and an estimation of

ACOG ANTEPARTUM RECORD

DATE ____________

NAME ____________ (LAST) (FIRST) (MIDDLE)

ID # ____________ HOSPITAL OF DELIVERY ____________

NEWBORN'S PHYSICIAN ____________ REFERRED BY ____________

FINAL EDD ____________

BIRTH DATE MO DAY YR	AGE	RACE	MARITAL STATUS S M W D SEP	ADDRESS:
OCCUPATION ☐ HOMEMAKER ☐ OUTSIDE WORK ☐ STUDENT ______ Type of Work			EDUCATION (LAST GRADE COMPLETED)	ZIP: PHONE: (H) (O) INSURANCE CARRIER/MEDICAID #
EMERGENCY CONTACT:			RELATIONSHIP:	PHONE:

TOTAL PREG	FULL TERM	PREMATURE	ABORTIONS INDUCED	ABORTIONS SPONTANEOUS	ECTOPICS	MULTIPLE BIRTHS	LIVING

MENSTRUAL HISTORY

LMP ☐ DEFINITE ☐ APPROXIMATE (MONTH KNOWN) ☐ UNKNOWN ☐ NORMAL AMOUNT/DURATION

MENSES MONTHLY ☐ YES ☐ NO PRIOR MENSES ______ DATE

FREQUENCY: Q ______ DAYS ON BCP'S AT CONCEPT. ☐ YES ☐ NO

MENARCHE ______(AGE ONSET) hCG + ____/____/____

PAST PREGNANCIES (LAST SIX)

DATE MO / YR	GA WEEKS	LENGTH OF LABOR	BIRTH WEIGHT	TYPE DELIVERY	ANES.	PLACE OF DELIVERY	PERINATAL MORTALITY YES / NO	TREATMENT PRETERM LABOR YES / NO	COMMENTS / COMPLICATIONS

PAST MEDICAL HISTORY

	O Neg + Pos.	DETAIL POSITIVE REMARKS INCLUDE DATE & TREATMENT
1. DIABETES		
2. HYPERTENSION		
3. HEART DISEASE		
4. RHEUMATIC FEVER		
5. MITRAL VALVE PROLAPSE		
6. KIDNEY DISEASE / UTI		
7. NEUROLOGIC/EPILEPSY		
8. PSYCHIATRIC		
9. HEPATITIS / LIVER DISEASE		
10. VARICOSITIES / PHLEBITIS		
11. THYROID DYSFUNCTION		
12. MAJOR ACCIDENTS		
13. HISTORY OF BLOOD TRANSFUS.		

	AMT/DAY PREPREG	AMT/DAY PREG	#YRS USE
14. TOBACCO			
15. ALCOHOL			

	O Neg + Pos.	DETAIL POSITIVE REMARKS INCLUDE DATE & TREATMENT
16. Rh SENSITIZED		
17. TUBERCULOSIS		
18. ASTHMA		
19. ALLERGIES (DRUGS)		
20. GYN SURGERY		
21. OPERATIONS / HOSPITALIZATIONS (YEAR & REASON)		
22. ANESTHETIC COMPLICATIONS		
23. HISTORY OF ABNORMAL PAP		
24. UTERINE ANOMALY		
25. INFERTILITY		
26. IN UTERO DES EXPOSURE		
27. STREET DRUGS		
28. OTHER		

COMMENTS: ____________

Figure 3–1. Antepartum record—History and physical examination. (Reprinted with permission from the American College of Obstetricians and Gynecologists. Washington, DC © 1989.)

the size and consistency of the uterus, are important aspects of the pelvic examination (Fig. 3–2). Abnormalities detected during this examination may influence the timing or the mode of delivery. Baseline laboratory studies consisting of a complete blood count, Venereal Disease Research Laboratory (VDRL), rubella titer, antibody titers, hepatitis screen, and blood type and Rh are routinely obtained during this visit and periodically repeated throughout pregnancy (Fig. 3–3). Additional laboratory studies are selectively ordered when indicated, de-

GENETICS SCREENING
INCLUDES PATIENT, BABY'S FATHER, OR ANYONE IN EITHER FAMILY WITH:

	YES	NO		YES	NO
1. PATIENT'S AGE ≥ 35 YEARS			10. HUNTINGTON CHOREA		
2. THALASSEMIA (ITALIAN, GREEK, MEDITERRANEAN, OR ORIENTAL BACKGROUND): MCV < 80			11. MENTAL RETARDATION		
			IF YES, WAS PERSON TESTED FOR FRAGILE X?		
3. NEURAL TUBE DEFECT (MENINGOMYELOCELE, OPEN SPINE, OR ANENCEPHALY)			12. OTHER INHERITED GENETIC OR CHROMOSOMAL DISORDER		
4. DOWN SYNDROME			13. PATIENT OR BABY'S FATHER HAD A CHILD WITH BIRTH DEFECTS NOT LISTED ABOVE		
5. TAY-SACHS (EG, JEWISH BACKGROUND)					
6. SICKLE CELL DISEASE OR TRAIT			14. ≥3 FIRST-TRIMESTER SPONTANEOUS ABORTIONS, OR A STILLBIRTH		
7. HEMOPHILIA			15. MEDICATIONS OR STREET DRUGS SINCE LAST MENSTRUAL PERIOD		
8. MUSCULAR DYSTROPHY			IF YES, AGENT(S):		
9. CYSTIC FIBROSIS			16. OTHER SIGNIFICANT FAMILY HISTORY (SEE COMMENTS)		

COMMENTS: ____________________

INFECTION HISTORY	YES	NO		YES	NO
			4. PATIENT OR PARTNER HAVE HISTORY OF GENITAL HERPES		
1. HIGH RISK AIDS			5. RASH OR VIRAL ILLNESS SINCE LAST MENSTRUAL PERIOD		
2. HIGH RISK HEPATITIS B			6. HISTORY OF STD, GC, CHLAMYDIA, HPV, SYPHILIS		
3. LIVE WITH SOMEONE WITH TB OR EXPOSED TO TB			7. OTHER (SEE COMMENTS)		

COMMENTS: ____________________

INTERVIEWER'S SIGNATURE ____________________

INITIAL PHYSICAL EXAMINATION

DATE ____/____/____ PREPREGNANCY WEIGHT ________ HEIGHT ________ BP________

1. HEENT	☐ NORMAL	☐ ABNORMAL	12. VULVA	☐ NORMAL	☐ CONDYLOMA	☐ LESIONS
2. FUNDI	☐ NORMAL	☐ ABNORMAL	13. VAGINA	☐ NORMAL	☐ INFLAMMATION	☐ DISCHARGE
3. TEETH	☐ NORMAL	☐ ABNORMAL	14. CERVIX	☐ NORMAL	☐ INFLAMMATION	☐ LESIONS
4. THYROID	☐ NORMAL	☐ ABNORMAL	15. UTERUS	☐ NORMAL	☐ ABNORMAL	☐ FIBROIDS
5. BREASTS	☐ NORMAL	☐ ABNORMAL	16. ADNEXA	☐ NORMAL	☐ MASS	
6. LUNGS	☐ NORMAL	☐ ABNORMAL	17. RECTUM	☐ NORMAL	☐ ABNORMAL	
7. HEART	☐ NORMAL	☐ ABNORMAL	18. DIAGONAL CONJUGATE	☐ REACHED	☐ NO	________ CM
8. ABDOMEN	☐ NORMAL	☐ ABNORMAL	19. SPINES	☐ AVERAGE	☐ PROMINENT	☐ BLUNT
9. EXTREMITIES	☐ NORMAL	☐ ABNORMAL	20. SACRUM	☐ CONCAVE	☐ STRAIGHT	☐ ANTERIOR
10. SKIN	☐ NORMAL	☐ ABNORMAL	21. ARCH	☐ NORMAL	☐ WIDE	☐ NARROW
11. LYMPH NODES	☐ NORMAL	☐ ABNORMAL	22. GYNECOID PELVIC TYPE	☐ YES	☐ NO	

COMMENTS (Number and explain abnormals): ____________________

EXAM BY ____________________

Figure 3–2. Antepartum record—History and physical examination. (Reprinted with permission from the American College of Obstetricians and Gynecologists. Washington, DC © 1989.)

LABORATORY AND EDUCATION

INITIAL LABS	DATE	RESULT	REVIEWED
BLOOD TYPE	/ /	A B AB O	
Rh TYPE	/ /		
ANTIBODY SCREEN	/ /		
HCT/HGB	/ /	______ % ______ g/dl	
PAP SMEAR	/ /	NORMAL / ABNORMAL / _____	
RUBELLA	/ /		
VDRL	/ /		
GC	/ /		
URINE CULTURE/SCREEN	/ /		
HBsAg	/ /		
8–18-WEEK LABS (WHEN INDICATED)	DATE	RESULT	
ULTRASOUND	/ /		
MSAFP	/ /	____________MOM	
AMNIO/CVS	/ /		
KARYOTYPE	/ /	46, XX OR 46, XY / OTHER____	
ALPHA-FETOPROTEIN	/ /	NORMAL____ ABNORMAL____	
24–28-WEEK LABS (WHEN INDICATED)	DATE	RESULT	
HCT/HGB	/ /	______ % ______ g/dl	
DIABETES SCREEN	/ /	1 HR____________	
GTT (IF SCREEN ABNORMAL)	/ /	____FBS ____1 HR ____2 HR ____3 HR	
Rh ANTIBODY SCREEN	/ /		
RhIg GIVEN (28 WKS)	/ /	SIGNATURE ____________	
32–36-WEEK LABS (WHEN INDICATED)	DATE	RESULT	
ULTRASOUND	/ /		
VDRL	/ /		
GC	/ /		
HCT/HGB	/ /	______ % ______ g/dl	
OPTIONAL LAB (HIGH-RISK GROUPS)	DATE	RESULT	
HIV	/ /		
HGB ELECTROPHORESIS	/ /	AA AS SS AC SC AF ↑A_2	
CHLAMYDIA	/ /		
OTHER	/ /		

COMMENTS/ADDITIONAL LAB

PLANS/EDUCATION (COUNSELED ☐)

- ☐ ANESTHESIA PLANS ____________
- ☐ TOXOPLASMOSIS PRECAUTIONS (CATS/RAW MEAT) ____________
- ☐ CHILDBIRTH CLASSES ____________
- ☐ PHYSICAL ACTIVITY ____________
- ☐ PREMATURE LABOR SIGNS ____________
- ☐ NUTRITION COUNSELING ____________
- ☐ BREAST OR BOTTLE FEEDING ____________
- ☐ NEWBORN CAR SEAT ____________
- ☐ POSTPARTUM BIRTH CONTROL ____________
- ☐ ENVIRONMENTAL/WORK HAZARDS ____________
- ☐ TUBAL STERILIZATION ____________
- ☐ VBAC COUNSELING ____________
- ☐ CIRCUMCISION ____________
- ☐ TRAVEL ____________

REQUESTS ____________

TUBAL STERILIZATION	DATE	INITIALS
CONSENT SIGNED	____/____/____	________

AA128 1 /1

Figure 3–3. Antepartum record—Baseline laboratory tests and suggested follow-up. (Reprinted with permission from the American College of Obstetricians and Gynecologists. Washington, DC © 1989.)

pending on information obtained during the history and physical evaluation, genetic screens, amniocentesis, and human immunodeficiency virus testing.

During the second trimester, hemoglobin/hematocrit and antibody titers are usually repeated. In addition, patients undergo *screening* for the presence of diabetes mellitus. During the third trimester, the hemoglobin/hematocrit is again repeated.

Routine prenatal care traditionally consists of timed visits approximately 4 weeks apart throughout the first 7 months of pregnancy. Visits increase to every other week until the last month, when patients are seen on a weekly basis. During these visits, information concerning the general health of the mother and the status of the pregnancy is obtained. When the patient approaches term, pelvic examinations are often performed on a weekly basis to confirm the presenting part, identify the station of the presenting part, and determine the consistency, effacement, and dilatation of the cervix (Fig. 3–4).

The prenatal record is an important source of information for the anesthesia care team. It describes concisely the patient's past history and physical status and documents the course of the current pregnancy. A review of the prenatal record quickly alerts the practitioner to concurrent medical or obstetric complications that may influence anesthetic management during the peripartum period. Problems frequently encountered during the antepartum period include bleeding and anemia, cardiovascular disease, endocrine disorders, and premature rupture of the membranes. (For a complete description of these conditions, please refer to individual chapters.)

A precise definition of anemia during pregnancy is uncertain since a variety of factors (e.g., altitude, sex, race) influence red cell volume. At term, a hemoglobin concentration of 10.0 gm/dl is usually recognized as the normal lower limit. Acute hemorrhage and iron deficiency are two of the most common causes of anemia during pregnancy. Less frequent causes include hemoglobinopathies, megaloblastic anemia (most frequently folate deficiency), and acquired hemolytic anemias (pregnancy-induced hemolytic anemia; paroxysmal nocturnal anemia; hemolysis, elevated liver enzymes, and low platelet count [HELLP syndrome]). Importantly, the anesthesia provider must distinguish between patients with chronic anemia and those with an acute hemorrhage and possible coagulopathy. The obstetric record aids the anesthesia provider in making this important distinction.

Coagulation defects in the pregnant patient are not uncommon. Coagulopathies may be primarily hematologic (idiopathic thrombocytopenic purpura and von Willebrand's disease) or secondary to a complication of pregnancy (pregnancy-induced hypertension [PIH] and abruptio placentae). After evaluating the record and prior to the institution of a regional anesthetic, the patient's ability to clot should be evaluated with a thorough history and appropriate laboratory studies when indicated. A platelet count or bleeding time is frequently used to screen patients prior to induction of anesthesia. If either of these tests is abnormal or the history is suggestive of extensive bleeding, a complete evaluation of coagulation is warranted (e.g., prothrombin time, partial thromboplastin time, fibrinogen, and fibrin degradation products).

Approximately 7% of all pregnancies are associated with hypertension. The incidence varies but it appears more prevalent in lower socioeconomic populations. An elevated blood pressure in a pregnant patient prior to the 20th week of gestation is usually due to chronic hypertension and may be a manifestation of a variety of disorders. In contrast, PIH and preeclampsia are rarely diagnosed before the 20th week of gestation. PIH is frequently encountered in primiparous women at the extremes of reproductive age (e.g., teenagers and women over 35 years old) and in older multiparous patients with preexisting medical problems such as diabetes mellitus, hypertensive disease, collagen vascular disorders, and multifetal gestation. PIH is characterized by an elevated blood pressure, proteinuria, and excessive weight gain. Regardless of the etiology, hypertensive women have a higher incidence of perinatal morbidity and mortality owing to uteroplacental insufficiency and prematurity that increases with the severity and duration of hypertension. The obstetric record is an invaluable source of information for distinguishing among various hypertensive causes that may have significantly different implications for the anesthesia care team.

A variety of endocrine disorders may complicate pregnancy. Diabetes mellitus is the most

ACOG ANTEPARTUM RECORD

NAME ____
LAST FIRST MIDDLE

DRUG ALLERGY:
ANESTHESIA CONSULT PLANNED ☐ YES ☐ NO

PROBLEMS/PLANS	MEDICATION LIST:	Start date	Stop date
1.	1.		
2.	2.		
3.	3.		
4.	4.		

EDD CONFIRMATION		18–20-WEEK EDD UPDATE:	
INITIAL EDD:		QUICKENING	____/____/____ + 22 WKS = ____/____/____
LMP	____/____/____ = EDD ____/____/____	FUNDAL HT. AT UMBIL.	____/____/____ + 20 WKS = ____/____/____
INITIAL EXAM	____/____/____ = ____ WKS = EDD ____/____/____	FHT W/FETOSCOPE	____/____/____ + 20 WKS = ____/____/____
ULTRASOUND	____/____/____ = ____ WKS = EDD ____/____/____	ULTRASOUND	____/____/____ = ____ WKS = ____/____/____
INITIAL EDD	____/____/____ INITIALED BY __________	FINAL EDD	____/____/____ INITIALED BY __________

32–34-WEEK EDD–UTERINE SIZE CONCORDANCE (±4 OR MORE CM SUGGESTS THE NEED FOR ULTRASOUND EVALUATION)

VISIT DATE (YEAR ______)																
WEEKS GEST. (BEST EST.)																
FUNDAL HEIGHT (CM)																
FHR PRESENT: F=FETOSCOPE D=DOPTONE																
FETAL MOVEMENT: +=PRESENT O=ABSENT																
PREMATURITY: SIGNS/SYMPTOMS:* +=PRESENT O=ABSENT																
CERVIX EXAM (DIL./EFF./STA.)																
BLOOD PRESSURE:	INITIAL															
	REPEAT															
EDEMA +=PRESENT O=ABSENT																
WEIGHT (PREPREG: ________)																
CUMULATIVE WEIGHT GAIN																
URINE (GLUCOSE/ ALBUMIN/KETONES)																
NEXT APPOINTMENT																
PROVIDER (INITIALS)																
TEST REMINDERS		8–18 WEEKS CVS/AMNIO/MSAFP					24–28 WEEKS GLUCOSE SCREEN/Rhlg									

COMMENTS: ____

*For example: vaginal bleeding, discharge, cramps, contractions, pelvic pressure.

Figure 3–4. Antepartum record—Initial and subsequent prenatal visits. (Reprinted with permission from the American College of Obstetricians and Gynecologists. Washington, DC © 1989.)

common and may be extremely difficult to control owing to insulin resistance caused by placental hormones. Maternal effects of diabetes include a fourfold increase in PIH, more cesarean sections owing to fetal macrosomia, postpartum hemorrhage, and polyhydramnios. Fetal and neonatal effects of diabetes include higher perinatal death rates, increased numbers of major congenital anomalies, and increased morbidity owing to metabolic derangements such as hypoglycemia and hypocalcemia. Poorly controlled diabetic mothers prone to frequent ketoacidosis or with associated PIH experience a perinatal mortality rate of approximately 20%. Maternal mortality in this group of patients increases 10-fold when compared with nondiabetic pregnant patients.

The anesthetic management of a pregnant diabetic patient is very challenging. Macrosomic infants are common in patients with gestational diabetes and in patients with insulin-dependent diabetes of short duration. Shoulder dystocias occur commonly in this patient population, and macrosomic infants with estimated weights greater than 4000 gm are usually delivered by cesarean section. Placental vascular insufficiency is often encountered in patients with insulin-dependent diabetes of long duration. These patients commonly experience intrauterine growth retardation, chronic hypoxia, fetal distress, and premature delivery. Blood glucose concentrations require close control during labor to prevent neonatal hypoglycemia following delivery. Anesthetic considerations for these patients should include the use of dextrose-free solutions for acute hydration prior to induction of anesthesia; avoidance of hypotension, as neonatal depression is more severe in these patients if hypotension occurs; adequate anesthesia and pelvic relaxation at the time of vaginal delivery; preparations for the immediate induction of general anesthesia should a severe dystocia occur; and the immediate availability of neonatal resuscitation equipment and personnel skilled in the management of these infants. In summary, the early detection of diabetes is important to the mother and fetus. This information is equally important for the obstetric, neonatal, and anesthetic care teams, as it enables them to devise an appropriate plan for delivery.

Cardiovascular disease complicates less than 1% of pregnancies. Irrespective of cause, a favorable outcome is based on several factors, including an adequate cardiac reserve, the stress placed on the heart during pregnancy (e.g., PIH), and the quality and consistency of medical care. During pregnancy, attention should be directed toward the prevention and early recognition and treatment of congestive heart failure, as these patients often experience chronic hypoxemia and polycythemia that are associated with intrauterine growth retardation and fetal wastage.

Cardiac decompensation occurs most commonly in the immediate postpartum period, and a history of congestive heart failure documented prior to term indicates a fragile state and a greater likelihood of decompensation in the peripartum period. Although vaginal delivery is often preferred, there is an increased incidence of cesarean section in these patients and anesthetic plans must remain flexible. In addition, the ability to perform invasive monitoring, cardiovascular support, operative intervention, and neonatal resuscitation must be immediately available.

A variety of sexually transmitted diseases may have an impact on both the mother and the fetus during pregnancy. Diagnosis is accomplished with the use of blood tests (VDRL, acquired immunodeficiency syndrome [AIDS]), cervical cultures (gonorrhea, chlamydia, and herpes simplex type II), and cytologic examination (Pap smear). When active disease is present, delivery by cesarean section is common. Although there is substantial evidence linking vaginal and cervical infections with occult chorioamnionitis and premature rupture of the membranes, the use of regional anesthesia for labor and delivery is not contraindicated unless fulminant maternal infection is present.

Risk Scoring

Considerable attention has been directed toward identifying the patient at risk during pregnancy. Risk-scoring techniques developed in the early 1960s attempted to identify perinatal events associated with poor neonatal outcomes.[2, 3] However, the usefulness of these systems is difficult to determine, as a significant portion of patients experience adverse outcomes during pregnancy despite low-risk scores.[4] In a study by Rayburn and associates, only one third of 168 infants admitted to the newborn intensive care unit were anticipated based on risk factors assigned during the antepartum period.[5] Despite deficiencies, risk assessment continues as an integral part of prenatal care.[6] When used as a broad screening device, risk assessment identifies patients requiring additional surveillance (Table 3–1).

FETAL SCREENING TECHNIQUES

Historically, the fetus was regarded as an extension of the maternal organism, and it was believed that optimal maternal care guaranteed good fetal outcome. Advances in technology and a better understanding of the maternal-fetal unit altered this perception. The fetus is a second patient capable of experiencing serious risks independent of the mother. A variety of diagnostic techniques have been developed to assess the status of the fetus in utero. Understanding the obstetric significance of these tests and their implications is vitally important in determining the anesthetic management of these patients.

Placental Hormone Analysis

The use of placental hormones, such as human placental lactogen and estrogen (e.g., estriol), illustrates early attempts to evaluate fetal well-being.[7] In high-risk patients, placental hormone levels were measured in maternal serum or urine samples at periodic intervals during the last trimester of pregnancy. A deterioration of placental function and fetal status was thought to exist when these values decreased. Subsequent studies revealed that these tests were probably of little value in identifying the fetus at risk. In fact, they may have led to erroneous premature intervention on the part of the obstetrician. As a result, alternative technologies were developed.[8]

Amniocentesis

Amniocentesis is performed by placing a needle percutaneously through the maternal abdominal wall into the amniotic sac (Fig. 3–5). Developing the ability to perform this procedure without excessive risk to the mother or fetus had a significant effect on obstetric care. Amniocentesis was initially used to diagnose and manage hemolytic disease of the newborn. Currently, it is *also* used for genetic screening in early pregnancy and for assessment of fetal pulmonary maturity prior to delivery.

Surfactant-active phospholipids (lecithin, sphingomyelin, and phosphatidylglycerol [PG])

TABLE 3–1
High-Risk Factors

Medical Problems	Obstetric Problems
Cardiovascular and renal	Poor obstetric history
Heart disease—AHA classes I–IV	Maternal age
Chronic hypertension	<16 years old
Pregnancy-induced hypertension	>35 years old
Anemia	Previous congenital anomalies
Metabolic	Multiple gestation
Diabetes mellitus	Intrauterine growth retardation
Thyroid disease	Third trimester bleeding
Miscellaneous	Oligohydramnios or polyhydramnios
Pulmonary disease	Prematurity
Hepatic disease	Abnormal fetal presentation
Sexually transmitted diseases	Premature rupture of membranes
Convulsive disorders	Chorioamnionitis
Smoking >1 pack/day	Fetal distress
Substance abuse	Postterm >42 weeks
	Previous stillbirths
	Infant >10 pounds

Abbreviation: AHA = American Heart Association.

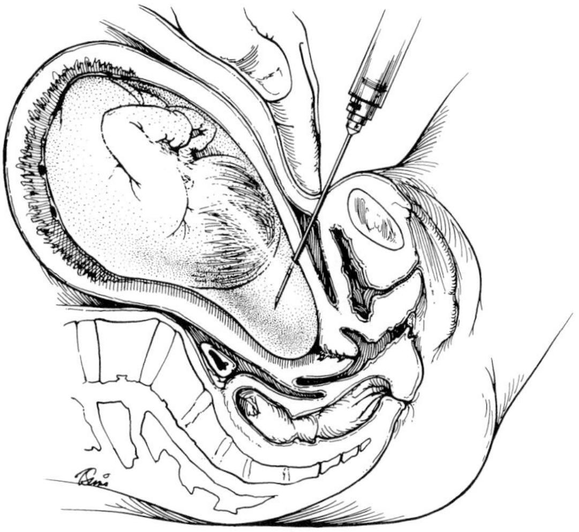

Figure 3–5. Suprapubic amniocentesis. (From Cunningham FG: Placental hormones. *In* Cunningham FG, MacDonald PC, Gant NF [eds]: Williams Obstetrics, 18th ed. East Norwalk, CT, Appleton & Lange, 1989.)

present in amniotic fluid prevent alveolar collapse and the development of hyaline membrane disease in the neonate.[9, 10]

Prior to 34 weeks' gestation, the concentrations of lecithin and sphingomyelin in the amniotic fluid are similar. After 34 weeks, the concentration of lecithin relative to sphingomyelin increases. The lecithin/sphingomyelin (L/S) ratio is commonly used to determine fetal lung maturity and the potential risk of neonatal respiratory distress syndrome (RDS). An L/S ratio greater than 2 is associated with a very low incidence of RDS. In contrast, 40% of neonates develop RDS if the L/S ratio is between 1.5 and 2, and more than 75% are affected if the ratio is less than 1.5.[11]

In a fetus that is metabolically compromised (e.g., if the mother has diabetes), an L/S ratio greater than 2 is not as predictive of fetal lung maturity as in the normal fetus. The presence of PG, which enhances the activities of surfactant, provides additional assurance that the possibility of respiratory distress in these patients is limited.[12] In many facilities, the laboratory report includes the L/S ratio and the presence or absence of PG.

The major risks associated with amniocentesis are trauma, infection, abortion, and preterm labor. If the procedure is performed in early pregnancy (e.g., for genetic screening), there appears to be little fetal risk. Fetal trauma is more common when the volume of amniotic fluid is small compared with the size of the fetus. This situation is generally encountered late in pregnancy when amniocentesis is used to assess fetal maturity.

The anesthesia provider should understand that at the time of delivery, intubation and neonatal resuscitation are often required when the L/S ratio is low and PG is absent. Thus equipment and personnel skilled in neonatal resuscitation should be immediately available to manage the neonate at birth, an effort requiring coordination among all members of the perinatal team.

Chorionic Villus Sampling

Chorionic villus sampling has become a widely used alternative to amniocentesis for genetic screening. With this technique, fetal cells can be obtained earlier in gestation for genetic evaluation. Hereditary disorders are diagnosed sooner, and if the pregnancy is to be electively terminated, the procedure may be performed earlier and with greater maternal safety.

Villus sampling is often performed using a transvaginal approach. When the cervix is visualized, a small suction catheter is placed into the cervical canal and advanced to the placenta and a sample is obtained (Fig. 3–6). Complications associated with villus sampling occur infrequently. When compared with amniocentesis, the incidence of spontaneous abortions is not increased; however, there is a greater frequency of chorioamnionitis with septicemia and shock.[13]

Amniocentesis and chorionic villus sampling are office procedures and do not require anesthesia assistance. However, anesthesia may be required if the patient becomes septic or threatens abortion and evacuation of the uterus is necessary.

Percutaneous Umbilical Blood Sampling

Percutaneous umbilical blood sampling (PUBS) was initially used for the diagnosis and treatment of hemolytic disease of the newborn.[14] Indications for this procedure now include the diagnosis of congenital disease, fetal

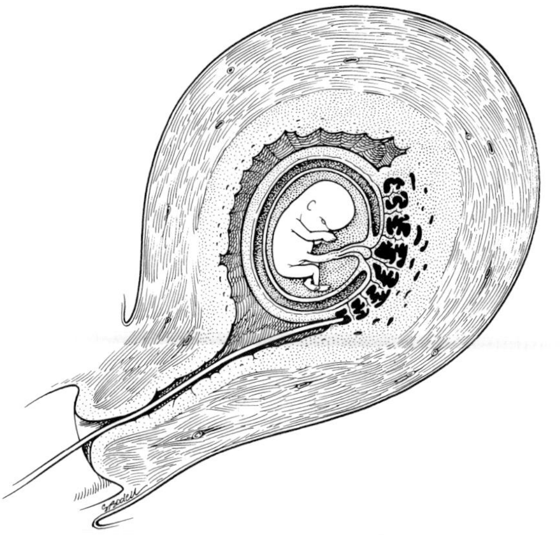

Figure 3–6. Transcervical chorionic villus sampling. (From Cunningham FG: Techniques to evaluate fetal health. *In* Cunningham FG, MacDonald PC, Gant NF [eds]: Williams Obstetrics, 18th ed. East Norwalk, CT, Appleton & Lange, 1989.)

infections, and hypoxia and treatment of fetal blood abnormalities.

PUBS is performed in a manner similar to that for amniocentesis. A needle is placed percutaneously through the maternal abdominal wall into the amniotic sac. Real-time ultrasound is then used to guide the tip of the needle into the umbilical vein (Fig. 3–7). After a sample of fetal blood is obtained, the needle is withdrawn. The fetal heart rate (FHR) is monitored for a short period of time following the procedure, as bleeding from the umbilical cord is common but usually limited.

PUBS is an office procedure when used for genetic screening in early pregnancy. When used for intrauterine blood transfusions late in pregnancy, it is performed in the obstetric suite with anesthesia assistance, as emergent intervention on behalf of the fetus may be required. Infants delivered under these conditions are frequently stressed and premature and may require extensive resuscitative efforts.

ULTRASONOGRAPHY AND DOPPLER ULTRASOUND

The use of sound waves to examine the intrauterine environment greatly expanded the practice of obstetrics. Ultrasonographic techniques can supply vital information concerning fetal status and assist in the management of the high-risk patient.

Real-time ultrasonography is a technique that incorporates motion into the imaging process. This is accomplished with the use of a linear array of piezo crystals that generates and receives sound waves in a phased manner. A visual display generated by the phased echoes creates an image with motion.

Fetal surveillance using real-time ultrasonography identified a variety of intrauterine fetal events (e.g., breathing, heartbeat, limb, and trunk movements) that led to the development of the biophysical profile.

The Doppler effect, another form of ultrasound, is an investigational tool used to evaluate fetal well-being. An example of this type of technology is the pocket Doppler stethoscope. It is based on the principle that the frequency of sound changes as it moves toward or away from an object.[15]

Doppler ultrasound is used in a variety of experimental situations to calculate the absolute amount of blood flowing through a vessel. However, in the clinical setting, the absolute blood flow is difficult to determine, since the angle at which the sound wave enters the vessel is frequently unknown. Utilizing a ratio of the height of the systolic and diastolic peaks circumvents this problem.[16] The systolic/diastolic ratio is calculated by dividing the maximal systolic Doppler shift by the end-diastolic shift. The normal range for this ratio is less than 3. Other commonly used indices are the Pourcelot or resistance index, and the pulsatility index, both of which supply information similar to the systolic/diastolic ratio but require more sophisticated digitalized waveform analysis.

Doppler ultrasound provides an indirect measurement of vascular resistance in the fetal villous circulation. Increased vascular resistance decreases end-diastolic flow in the umbilical cord, which raises the systolic/diastolic ratio. The measurement of umbilical artery waveforms has been used successfully to identify fetal intrauterine growth retardation associated with placental insufficiency. However, the usefulness of this technique in the antenatal assessment of the postmature fetus is limited, as an increase in placental vascular resistance does not appear

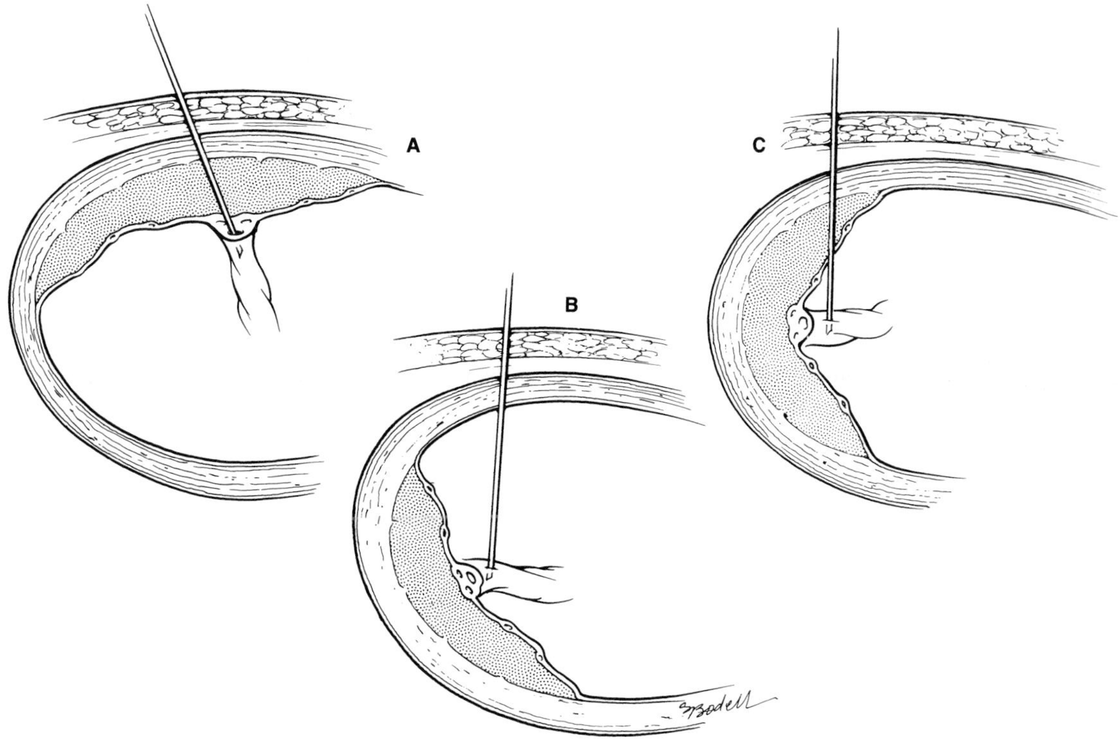

Figure 3–7. Percutaneous umbilical cord sampling. *A,* If the placenta is located on the anterior uterine wall, the needle may traverse the placenta. *B,* If the placenta is located on the posterior uterine wall, the needle usually passes through the amniotic fluid before entering the umbilical cord. *C,* If the placenta is located on the lateral uterine wall, the needle may pass through both the amniotic fluid and the placenta before entering the umbilical cord. (From Queenan JT, King JC: Intrauterine transfusion for severe RH-EBF: Past and future. Contemp OB/GYN 30:51, 1987.)

to play a major role in the pathophysiologic process.[17, 18] Abnormal umbilical artery waveforms can often be identified before changes in the biophysical profile and are associated with significant fetal risk.[19]

An increase in placental vascular resistance has been documented in patients with the supine hypotensive syndrome and in some patients receiving epinephrine in local anesthetics used for regional anesthesia.[20, 21] If epidural anesthesia is well managed and hypotension avoided, placental vascular resistance and the umbilical artery waveforms are not significantly affected.[22]

THE CONTRACTION STRESS TEST AND THE NONSTRESS TEST

Uteroplacental blood flow at term is approximately 700 ml/min, representing 10% of the maternal cardiac output. A majority of blood (70 to 90%) entering the uterine artery passes through the intervillous space. Importantly, uteroplacental perfusion is not autoregulated. Therefore, perfusion is directly proportional to pressure.

There are a variety of maternal disorders (e.g., PIH, chronic hypertension, and diabetes) associated with increased vascular resistance and decreased placental perfusion that result in intrauterine growth retardation and fetal hypoxia/asphyxia.

Historically, the FHR has been used exclusively to identify the "at-risk" fetus. As early as 1800, a decrease in the FHR following a contraction was considered an ominous sign for the fetus.[23] Abdominal auscultation remained the primary method for evaluating the FHR until the 1960s when the concept of continuous electronic FHR monitoring was introduced.

Labor represents a stress to the fetus as uterine contractions temporarily decrease uteroplacental perfusion and fetal oxygen delivery. During uterine contractions, intramural pressure increases and occludes venous channels in the placental bed. This increases venous back pressure and decreases uterine blood flow. If intramural pressure exceeds the pressure in the spiral arteries, uterine perfusion ceases. The brief suspension of oxygen delivery does not affect a fetus with adequate reserves. However, in the compromised fetus, the possibility of hypoxia during contractions increases. Continuous FHR monitoring with simultaneous recording of intrauterine pressure provides a mechanism for identifying FHR patterns and allows correlation of these patterns with contractions.

In 1972, Ray and colleagues, using experience obtained from intrapartum fetal monitoring, introduced the oxytocin challenge test (contraction stress test [CST]) for antepartum fetal surveillance.[24] The CST evaluates the ability of the fetus to tolerate the "stress" of uterine contractions. The test is performed by attaching an external ultrasound transducer and tocographic unit to the maternal abdomen and recording the FHR and uterine activity for 15 to 20 minutes (Table 3–2). The CST requires considerable time to perform and is not applicable to all patients. Contraindications include threatened preterm labor, third trimester bleeding, polyhydramnios, multifetal gestation, premature rupture of the membranes, and previous classic cesarean section.

The CST utilizes contractions that occur spontaneously or are induced with an oxytocin infusion. In the mid-1980s, several reports described nipple stimulation as an alternative method for inducing uterine contractions.[25, 26] In theory, nipple stimulation triggers the oxytocin release from the posterior pituitary. Despite the absence of a certain physiologic explanation, there is a high degree of success when nipple stimulation is used to induce uterine contractions. When compared with an oxytocin infusion, nipple stimulation produces satisfactory uterine contractions in a shorter period of time, can be accomplished without an intravenous infusion, and is more acceptable to the patient.[27–29] However, it is also associated with uterine hyperstimulation in some patients.[30]

A negative CST does not guarantee continued fetal health. However, evidence demonstrates that placental reserves are adequate to maintain fetal viability for approximately 1 week following a negative test. If fetal death occurs within 1 week of a negative CST, it is a false-negative test, which accounts for approximately 8% of all negative CSTs.[31]

A positive CST suggests fetal stress and occurs when late decelerations (discussed later) follow the induced contractions. If a CST is positive and the fetus is not in jeopardy, the test is falsely positive. Approximately 50% of all positive CSTs are false-positive tests. The CST is, therefore, useful for predicting fetal well-being but not for predicting fetal compromise. In an effort to

TABLE 3–2
Interpretation of the Contraction Stress Test

Result	Findings	Actions
Negative	At least three contractions within a 10-minute span, with each contraction lasting at least 40 sec, and having no late decelerations of the fetal heart rate	Repeat in 1 week or sooner as indicated Additional biophysical profile as indicated
Positive	Consistent and persistent late decelerations of the fetal heart rate	Additional biophysical profile Consider delivery
Suspicious	Inconsistent late decelerations that do not persist with subsequent contractions	Additional biophysical profile Repeat in 24 hr
Hyperstimulation	If uterine contractions are more frequent than every 2 min or last longer than 90 sec or persistent uterine hypertonus is suspected	Repeat in 24 hr
Unsatisfactory	The frequency of contractions is less than three in a 10-min period	Repeat in 24 hr

prevent premature intervention based on a positive CST, other tests, such as the biophysical profile, are used to further assess fetal status.

The nonstress test (NST) is based on the observation that fetal movement is associated with a transient acceleration of the FHR. In the healthy fetus, movement and heart rate accelerations occur at frequent intervals. In the compromised fetus, movement occurs infrequently and may not be associated with changes in the FHR.

The NST is performed by placing an ultrasonic transducer on the maternal abdomen and recording the FHR. Each time the mother perceives a fetal movement, she presses a button that places a mark on the recording. The period of time immediately following fetal movement is then evaluated for FHR accelerations. An NST is considered reactive when two or more fetal movements are accompanied by an FHR acceleration of at least 15 beats per minute. In addition, the accelerations must last at least 15 seconds and occur within a 20-minute span. An NST is interpreted as nonreactive when there are no FHR accelerations during a 40-minute period. The NST is easy to perform; is less time-consuming, less costly, and easier to interpret than the CST; and has no contraindications.

Techniques such as acoustic stimulation and feeding the mother prior to testing are used to enhance fetal activity and shorten the time required to perform the NST.[32, 33] However, there appears to be no benefit derived from this practice and more rigorous testing is recommended before its routine clinical use.[34, 35]

The NST or CST is used to identify potential fetal problems in those pregnancies determined to be at risk. Since the NST is easy to perform, it is often used as the initial screening test. If the NST is reactive, pregnancy is allowed to continue with subsequent testing performed at weekly intervals. More frequent testing is recommended in patients with complex problems associated with pregnancy (e.g., diabetes, hypertension). A nonreactive NST requires further evaluation with either a CST or a biophysical profile.

A fetus with a nonreactive NST, a positive CST, or an abnormal biophysical profile frequently experiences difficulty during labor and delivery. Abnormal FHR patterns may be intensified by maternal position and hypotension, both of which may be influenced by anesthesia. For example, abnormal tests increase the likelihood of cesarean section for fetal distress. Therefore, adequate preparations for emergency operative delivery and neonatal resuscitation are important considerations for the anesthesia team.

THE BIOPHYSICAL PROFILE

The improved outcome of high-risk pregnancies is a result of prevention and early recognition of intrauterine fetal asphyxia.

Current attention focuses on using a variety of fetal biophysical activities that are regulated by the fetal central nervous system and attempt to identify the fetus at risk (Table 3–3). Therefore, the presence of a given activity is indirect evidence of an intact and functioning central nervous system. Nerve impulses that initiate different fetal activities are located in the brain at distinct anatomic sites that appear to exhibit varying degrees of sensitivity to hypoxemia. In the human fetus, progressive hypoxia produces a gradual loss of biophysical activity. Biophysical activities that appear first during fetal neurodevelopment are least sensitive to hypoxemia, whereas those appearing later demonstrate a greater sensitivity (Table 3–4).

Fetal movement is probably the oldest and most widely used biophysical activity employed

TABLE 3–3
Biophysical Parameters Evaluated by Ultrasound

Generalized activities
Gross body movements
Breathing movements
Fetal tone
Specific activities
Sucking
Swallowing
Micturition
Reflex activities
Fetal eye movements and sleep states
Fetal heart rate
Umbilical vessel flow
Intrauterine environment
Amniotic fluid volume
Placental architecture and grade
Cord condition

TABLE 3–4
Fetal Central Nervous System Centers

Parameter	Center	Neurodevelopment	Effects of Hypoxia
			↑
Fetal tone	Cortex	(Early)	(Late)
Fetal movement	Cortex-nuclear		
		Embryogenesis	Hypoxia
Fetal breathing movements	Surface of fourth ventricle		
Fetal heart rate variability	Posterior hypothalamic medulla	(Late)	(Early)
		↓	

From Vintzileos AM, Campbell WA, Ingardia CJ, Nochimson DJ: The fetal biophysical profile and its predictive value. Reprinted with permission from The American College of Obstetricians and Gynecologists (Obstetrics and Gynecology, 1983, Vol 62, pp 271–278).

to assess the fetus. It is simple and inexpensive to assess and does not require a great amount of technical skill or equipment. Fetal movement increases throughout early pregnancy and plateaus at approximately 32 weeks' gestation, then remains constant until term. Although adverse fetal outcomes are associated with diminished fetal movement, the incidence of fetal problems during labor is low unless diminished movement is accompanied by other risk factors.[36, 37] Patient complaints of decreased fetal activity should be further evaluated with an NST or a CST. If these tests are abnormal, a biophysical profile should be performed.[38, 39]

Fetal breathing in utero is a component of normal fetal development. The duration and frequency of fetal breathing increases during the last 10 weeks of pregnancy and appears to be influenced to some degree by circadian rhythms.[40] The presence of fetal breathing is a reasonable indicator of fetal well-being. However, if breathing is absent, only 50% of infants are depressed or asphyxiated at birth.[41] Fetal tachypnea and prolonged absence of breathing have also been described; however, the exact meaning of these events is unknown.[42, 43]

Normal fetal tone is associated with active flexion and deflexion of the limbs and opening and closing of the hand. Fetal hypotonia is characterized by a loss of fist formation, unclasped hands, and deflexion of the limbs. Poor fetal tone is associated with a high incidence of fetal distress in labor and low 5-minute Apgar scores.[37]

Although ultrasonic placental grading is not a biophysical activity, it is used in some scoring systems. Since the placenta is of fetal origin, its composition may reflect the condition of the fetus. Grannum and coworkers evaluated the relationship between fetal pulmonary maturity and ultrasonic changes of the placenta as it matures. They discovered that an adequate L/S ratio is consistently present when a mature placenta is identified ultrasonically. However, placental maturity may not indicate a term pregnancy. When maternal complications exist during pregnancy, placental maturity accelerates and occurs earlier in gestation (Table 3–5).[44]

Oligohydramnios is associated with a variety of adverse fetal outcomes such as intrauterine growth retardation, dysmaturity syndrome, postmaturity, and major congenital fetal anomalies involving the genitourinary tract.[45, 46] In addition, meconium staining, low 1-minute and 5-minute Apgar scores, and the incidence of cesarean section for fetal distress increase in this patient population.

The amount of amniotic fluid that correlates with oligohydramnios and poor fetal outcome has not been clearly established. A single pocket of amniotic fluid less than 1 cm in diameter was initially used to diagnose oligohydramnios. However, more precise information can be obtained with the use of the amniotic fluid index (AFI). This technique divides the maternal abdomen into four quadrants and measures the largest pocket of fluid in each quadrant. The AFI is the sum of these measurements. An AFI less than or equal to 5 cm suggests oligohydramnios.[47, 48] The AFI increases progressively

TABLE 3–5
Placental Grade

Grade 0	Smooth, unbroken chorionic plate Homogeneous placenta No echogenic activity Commonly seen early gestation
Grade 1	Chorionic plate well defined Nondescript echo activity in body of placenta Represents earliest maturation changes of placenta
Grade 2	Marked indentations of chorionic plate Lack of homogeneity of placenta Increased echo activity in body of placenta represents a greater maturation of placenta
Grade 3	Chorionic plate interrupted with indentations and irregular densities with acoustic shadowing Body of placenta divided into compartments represents a mature placenta Maturity may be accelerated by maternal pathology

until midpregnancy, remains stable until the 38th week, then gradually decreases.[49, 50] At term, a normal AFI is approximately 12 cm.

When a single biophysical activity is normal, it is generally a good predictor of fetal well-being. However, if an activity is absent or abnormal, it may represent either a normal rest state or central nervous system depression. Variations of biophysical activities range in duration from 20 to 80 minutes.[41] The high false-positive rate encountered when using a single variable to evaluate the fetus suggests that normal periodicity is the most common cause of absent activity. Accuracy improves when several biophysical activities are used simultaneously.

In 1981, Manning reported using several biophysical activities as a profile to evaluate fetal status (Table 3–6). Active intervention or the conservative management of the pregnancy was determined by a score obtained during the test (Table 3–7).[51, 52] Subsequent studies verified the predictive value of the biophysical profile as well as its universal applicability and ease of performance.

TABLE 3–6
Biophysical Profile Scoring

Parameter	Findings	Normal	Abnormal
Antepartum fetal heart rate testing nonstress test	Reactive nonstress test	2	0
Fetal breathing	One or more episodes within 30 min, lasting 30 sec or more	2	0
Fetal movements	Three or more discrete body or limb movements within 30 min	2	0
Fetal tone	One or more episodes of limb extension with return to flexion within 30 min	2	0
Amniotic fluid volume	Adequate volume defined as one or more 1 cm or larger pocket of fluid in two perpendicular planes	2	0

From Manning FA: Fetal biophysical profile scoring: A prospective study in 1,184 high-risk patients. Am J Obstet Gynecol 140:290, 1981.

TABLE 3–7
Biophysical Profile Score and Recommended Management

Score	Interpretation	Recommended Management
10	Nonasphyxiated fetus	Repeat test weekly
8/10 Normal fluid	Nonasphyxiated fetus	As above
6	Suspect chronic fetal asphyxia	Consider delivery as soon as possible 1. If: Amniotic fluid abnormal—Deliver 2. If: Amniotic fluid normal, greater than 36 weeks, favorable cervix—Deliver 3. If: Less than 36 weeks' EGA or L/S ratio <2 or cervix not favorable—Repeat test in 24 hr 4. If: Repeat test <6—Deliver If: Repeat test >6—Observe and repeat test as above
4	Probable fetal asphyxia	Repeat test same day If: Repeat score <6—Deliver If: Repeat score >6—As above
0–2	Fetal asphyxia	Immediate delivery

Abbreviations: EGA = estimated gestational age; L/S = lecithin/sphingomyelin.
From Manning FA: Fetal assessment based on fetal biophysical profile scoring experience in 19,221 referred high-risk pregnancies. II. An analysis of false-negative fetal deaths. Am J Obstet Gynecol 157:880–883, 1987.

INTRAPARTUM SURVEILLANCE OF THE FETUS

Fetal Scalp Blood Sampling

Fetal blood may be sampled intrapartum by making a small incision in the fetal scalp or presenting part and collecting blood in a capillary tube. Since this requires direct access to the presenting part, this procedure is limited to use in women with ruptured membranes. During labor, placental perfusion decreases during each uterine contraction, subjecting the fetus to recurrent episodes of impaired placental gas exchange and relative hypoxia. As labor progresses, there is a gradual increase in fetal P_{CO_2} and a decrease in fetal pH and P_{O_2} (Table 3–8). Although continuous measurement of fetal P_{O_2} and P_{CO_2} is attractive and potentially useful, the interpretation of these data and their relationship to fetal outcome has not been determined.

The pH of fetal blood offers an additional surveillance technique in a compromised fetus with an abnormal FHR tracing. Decreased fetal pH occurs as a *late* sign of hypoxia and may not accurately reflect acute hypoxic episodes. In addition, fetal pH may be influenced by maternal acidosis, sampling during uterine contractions, and sampling late in labor. Rooth and associates recommend that fetal pH be compared with maternal pH and a diagnosis of fetal acidosis entertained if a difference of greater than or equal to 0.02 pH units exists.[23] A fetal pH of 7.20 to 7.25 is associated with good fetal outcomes, whereas a fetal pH of less than 7.20 indicates fetal acidosis necessitating immediate delivery (Table 3–9).[53]

Umbilical cord blood pH and gas measurements are routine at the author's facility and many other hospitals throughout the United States. They serve an educational purpose and help distinguish birth asphyxia (hypoxia, hypercapnia, and low pH) from other factors causing low Apgar scores (e.g., drugs) (Table 3–10).

Fetal Heart Rate

Early in gestation, the FHR averages 150 beats per minute (bpm). It decreases during the third

TABLE 3–8
Fetal Scalp Blood Values in Labor

Scalp Blood Value	Early Labor	Late Labor
pH	7.33 ± 0.03	7.29 ± 0.04
P_{O_2} (torr)	21.8 ± 2.6	16.5 ± 1.4
P_{CO_2} (torr)	44.0 ± 4.05	46.3 ± 4.2

TABLE 3–9
Fetal Scalp Blood Values and Acidosis

Scalp Blood Value	Normal	Metabolic Acidosis	Respiratory Acidosis
pH	≥7.25	<7.25	<7.25
Po_2 (torr)	≥20	Variable	<20
Pco_2 (torr)	≤50	>50	>50
HCO_3^- (mMol/L)	≥20	<20	<20
BE (mMol/L)	<−6	>−6	<−6

Abbreviation BE = base excess.

trimester and at term ranges from 120 to 160 bpm. Although the fetal myocardium is innervated by both the sympathetic and the parasympathetic nervous systems, the latter is more influential in utero. Parasympathetic tone increases throughout gestation and is responsible for the beat-to-beat variability of the FHR. During episodes of acute hypoxia, parasympathetic tone predominates and produces fetal bradycardia.[54]

Traditionally, the FHR was monitored with a stethoscope every 15 minutes during labor. In the early 1960s, Hon and colleagues introduced continuous electronic FHR monitoring during labor using either an external (noninvasive) or an internal (invasive) technique.[63]

External FHR monitoring uses a Doppler ultrasound transducer placed on the maternal abdomen. Sound waves generated by the transducer are directed toward the fetal heart. Movement of the ventricular wall reflects the signal back to the transducer where it is interpreted as a cardiac event. Although it is easy to use, Doppler ultrasound lacks the sensitivity to detect beat-to-beat variability. Uterine contractions are identified externally with a tocodynamometer, a small pressure sensor, placed on the maternal abdomen. Physical changes of the contracting uterus are converted into an electrical signal, which is processed and displayed on the recorder. External uterine monitoring displays the frequency and duration of contractions, but not the intensity. Internal FHR monitoring uses a small electrode attached to the presenting part and is the most sensitive technique available for evaluating beat-to-beat variability. Internal uterine contractions are detected with the use of an open-ended, fluid-filled plastic catheter placed within the uterine cavity. Pressure generated by a contraction is transmitted through the column of fluid to a pressure sensor where it is converted to an electrical signal and displayed on a recorder. This technique accurately determines the frequency, duration, *and* intensity of uterine contractions.

TABLE 3–10
Fetal Scalp pH and Management of Labor

Fetal Scalp pH	Recommendations
pH > 7.25	Observe labor
pH between 7.20 and 7.25	Observe labor Repeat scalp pH in 30 min
pH < 7.20	Repeat scalp pH Prepare for immediate delivery

Fetal Heart Rate Patterns

FHR patterns can be classified into two major groups: the baseline FHR (i.e., the heart rate between uterine contractions) and the periodic FHR (i.e., the change in the heart rate associated with contractions).

The normal baseline FHR ranges from 120 to 160 bpm. Fetal heart rates exceeding 160 bpm define fetal tachycardia. Mild tachycardia exists when the FHR is between 160 and 180 bpm and severe tachycardia exists when the rate is greater than 180 bpm. Persistent baseline fetal tachycardia may reflect maternal or fetal complications such as maternal fever, chorioamnionitis, fetal tachyarrhythmias, extreme prematurity, and thyrotoxicosis.

Fetal bradycardia occurs when a baseline FHR is less than 120 bpm. Bradycardia is mild when the FHR is between 100 and 120 bpm. Baseline FHRs between 60 and 100 bpm are regarded as moderate to severe and reflect severe fetal compromise. Fetal bradycardia may also be associated with congenital heart blocks, viral infections of the fetus, and maternal hypotension.

FHR variability consists of two components—short-term and long-term beat-to-beat variability. Short-term variability measures the time interval between the same points of successive cardiac electrical events (Fig. 3–8*A* and *B*).

Since the cardiac cycle is not fixed, beat-to-beat variation occurs normally and probably represents a continuous interaction of the fetal cerebral cortex and other areas of the brain with the cardiac regulatory center in the medulla. Absent beat-to-beat variability may indicate fetal sleep, the effect of maternal medications, or severe fetal compromise (Fig. 3–8*C* and *D*).

Long-term variability is an irregular sinusoidal oscillation of 6 to 10 bpm with a normal frequency of 3 to 6 cycles per minute (Fig. 3–8*A* and *C*). Although fetal death has been associated with sinusoidal oscillations exceeding 25 bpm, this pattern has also been described following drug administration during labor (alphaprodine and butorphanol) with no apparent adverse fetal effects.

Periodic changes in the FHR occur in association with uterine contractions and are either uniform or nonuniform in appearance (Fig. 3–9).

Early decelerations represent a uniform pattern whose onset, nadir, and recovery coincide with the onset, peak, and end of a uterine contraction (see Fig. 3–9). The cause most likely relates to reflex vagal activity caused by either mild hypoxia or transient increases in intracranial pressure associated with head compression. Abnormal fetal outcomes are uncommon when early decelerations are mild. However, severe decelerations or the presence of meconium requires further evaluation (e.g., fetal scalp pH).

Late decelerations also represent a uniform pattern; however, the onset, nadir, and recovery occur after the onset, peak, and end of a uterine contraction (see Fig. 3–9). They are classified as reflex and nonreflex decelerations. Reflex late decelerations typically occur in response to maternal hypotension. This is associated with reduced uterine blood flow and fetal oxygen deprivation. Fetal hypoxia increases fetal vagal tone and the characteristic late deceleration pattern appears. During reflex late decelerations, the FHR demonstrates good beat-to-beat variability and the pattern returns to normal when maternal hypotension is corrected.

Nonreflex late decelerations are due to fetal myocardial hypoxia. During contractions, the

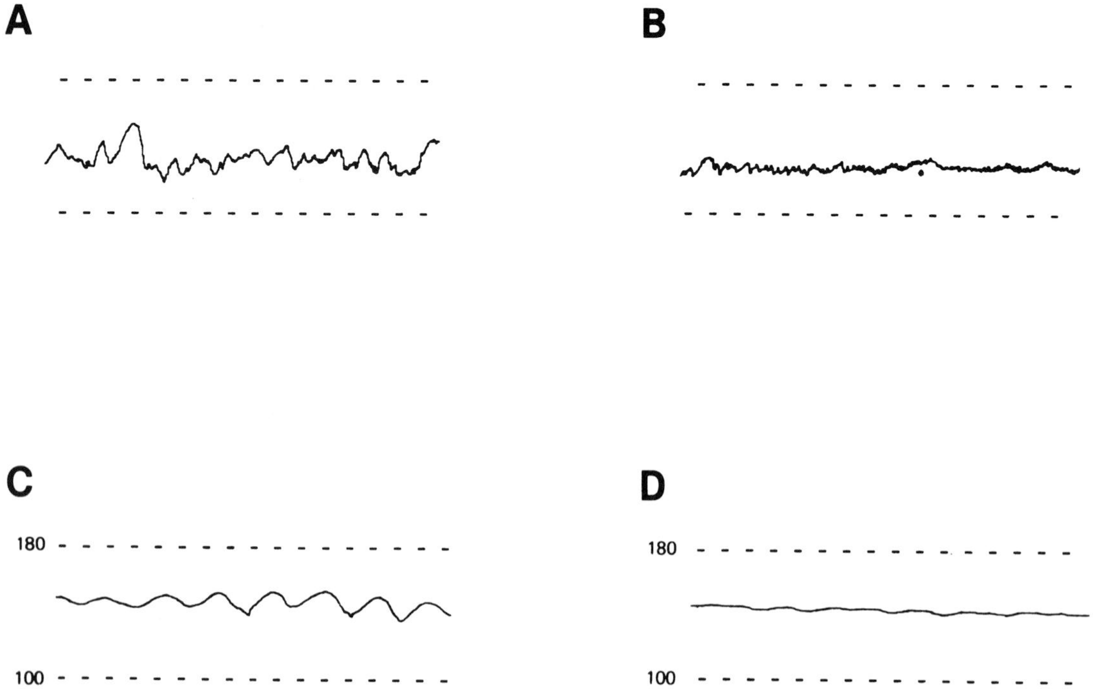

Figure 3–8. Fetal heart rate variability. *A*, Normal short-term variability (STV) and concurrent long-term variability (LTV). *B*, STV without LTV. *C*, LTV without STV. *D*, Absent STV and LTV may indicate severe fetal compromise. (From Zanini B, Paul RH, Huey JR: Intrapartum fetal heart rate: Correlation with scalp pH in the preterm fetus. Am J Obstet Gynecol 136:43–47, 1980.)

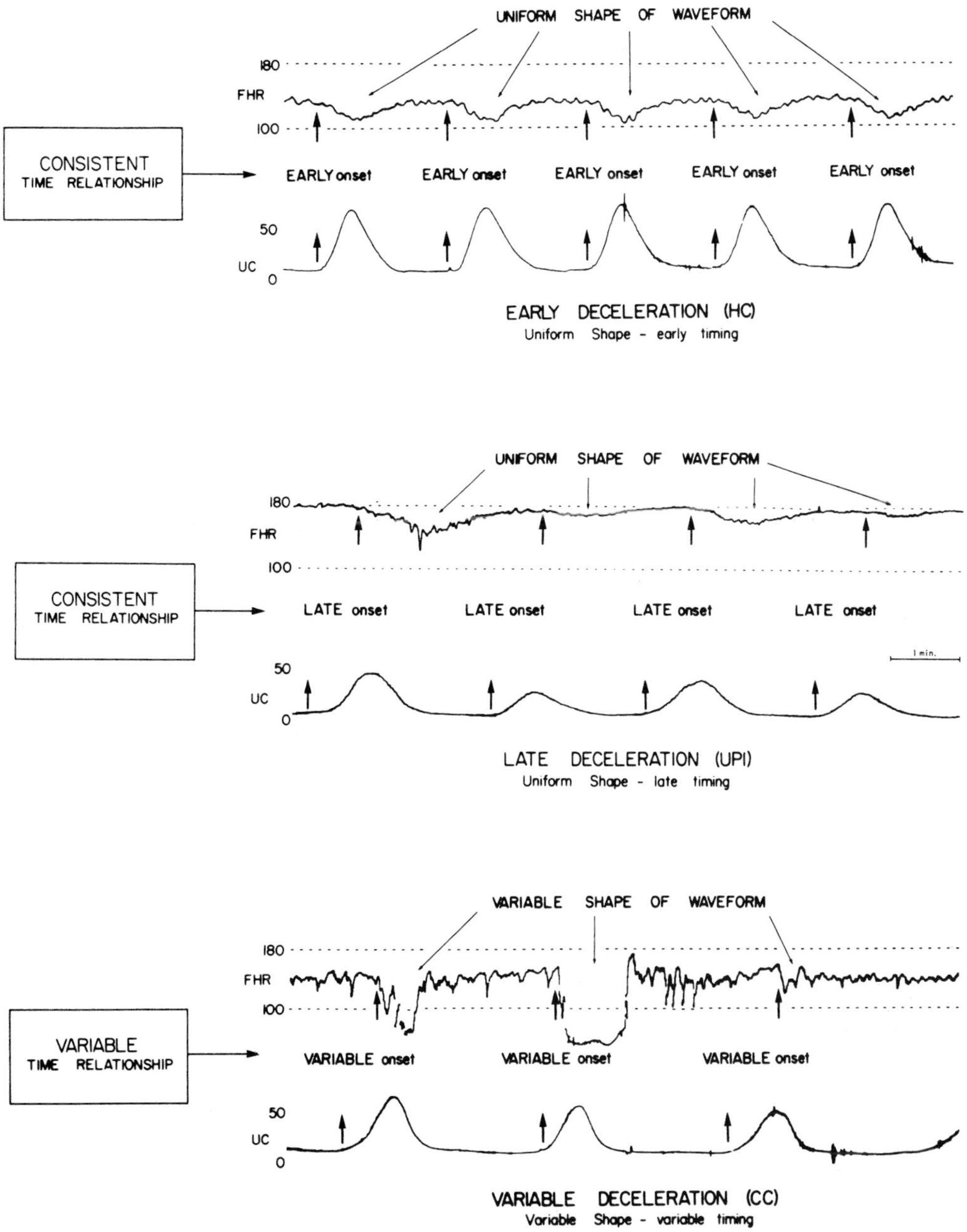

Figure 3–9. Patterns of fetal heart rate decelerations. (*Abbreviations:* HC = head compression; UPI = uteroplacental insufficiency; CC = cord compression.) (From Hon EH: An Atlas of Fetal Heart Rate Patterns. New Haven, CT, Harty, 1968.)

fetal oxygen supply is insufficient to support cardiac function, producing progressive myocardial decompensation. Vagal tone increases, and depending on the severity of hypoxia, beat-to-beat variability decreases or disappears. Nonreflex late decelerations are associated with uteroplacental insufficiency, intrauterine growth retardation, and prolonged asphyxia during pregnancy.

Variable or nonuniform decelerations are characterized by a lack of uniformity in the duration and shape of the deceleration accompanying uterine contractions (see Fig. 3–9). Most commonly, the FHR decreases abruptly and precipitously with the onset of a contraction and rapidly returns to baseline following the contraction. Severe variable decelerations may progress to late decelerations or, in contrast to the previous description, may demonstrate a mixed pattern of variable onset and delayed return to baseline when related to contractions. Variable decelerations occur in response to umbilical cord compression and are the most frequent type of deceleration pattern encountered during labor.

The major treatment goals for persistent abnormal FHR patterns are to alleviate fetal stress and improve fetal oxygenation. This is best achieved by turning the mother on her side and administering oxygen. Fluids and vasopressors are beneficial if maternal hypotension is present. Tocolytic agents may be considered in women with tonic uterine contractions. Treatment is directed at improving uteroplacental perfusion and fetal oxygenation.

INTRAPARTUM MATERNAL MONITORING

Prior to the mid-19th century, physicians typically relied on their senses as a means of evaluating physiologic processes. During the past century, a variety of mechanical devices and techniques were developed that enhanced the ability of the clinician in detecting physiologic alterations. If viewed as mechanisms for collecting data or as extensions of the senses, monitors may identify trends that lead to adverse outcomes and assist in early problem recognition. They do not eliminate critical events. To be of any value, a monitor or a monitoring technique requires evaluation and interpretation of data, as well as supervision of changes associated with intervention.[55]

Instruments and techniques that are easy to use and alert the clinician to impending problems often become "the standard of care" despite a lack of data demonstrating improved outcome or a favorable cost/benefit analysis. However, several studies have now been published that provide data supporting these beliefs.[56, 57]

The question of appropriate monitoring during anesthesia has been controversial since the first recorded anesthetic death in 1848.[58] In the United States, approximately 2000 anesthetic deaths occur annually.[56] In the obstetric population, anesthesia-related maternal mortality represents 5 to 10% of all maternal deaths, with failed intubation and aspiration of gastric contents accounting for 50% of these deaths.

In 1984, Cooper and coworkers investigated the frequency and types of human errors, and equipment failures associated with adverse outcomes during anesthesia.[57] Critical incidents that could easily lead to hypoxia and severe patient outcomes occurred so frequently that the authors recommended applying minimal monitoring standards to be used during the administration of anesthesia. Subsequently, the American Society of Anesthesiologists developed a national monitoring operating room standard (Table 3–11). Epidural anesthesia for labor was excluded, as the risks in this setting were judged to be extremely low.[59] In 1988, the American Society of Anesthesiologists published guidelines for the use of regional anesthesia in obstetrics and addressed the issue of monitoring in this patient population (Table 3–12).

A common pathway of many anesthetic mishaps appears to be desaturation of arterial blood. The development of pulse oximetry in 1974 greatly advanced the measurement of oxygen saturation and the detection of hypoxia. The amount of light absorbed by oxygenated and reduced hemoglobin, at specific wavelengths, forms the basis for estimating oxygen saturation of hemoglobin. A pulse oximeter is a device that transmits and receives light at specified wavelengths through vessel-rich areas such as the ear lobe or finger. The amount of light absorbed at each wavelength is calculated electronically and is displayed as the percent saturation of hemoglobin. Pulse oximetry decreases the incidence and duration of oxygen desaturation, which occurs in a variety of clinical settings. In the obstetric suite, a pulse oximeter is often used to assess maternal oxygen saturation during operative procedures, evaluate fetal oxygenation during labor, and assess the effectiveness of neonatal resuscitation.[60–62] However, it is not widely used in patients in labor.

Consumer demand for more aesthetic surroundings and fewer restrictions during labor and delivery has resulted in more family members participating in the birthing process. This has led to a proliferation of birthing rooms and labor, delivery, and recovery rooms (LDRs) where a parturient remains active and mobile until late in labor. What constitutes appropriate

TABLE 3–11
Standards for Basic Intraoperative Monitoring

Standard I

Qualified anesthesia personnel shall be present in the room throughout the conduct of all general anesthetics, regional anesthetics, and monitored anesthesia care.

Standard II

During all anesthetics, the patient's oxygenation, ventilation, circulation, and temperature shall be continually evaluated.

Oxygenation

Objective

To ensure adequate oxygen concentration in the inspired gas and the blood during all anesthetics.

Methods

1. Inspired gas: During every administration of general anesthesia using an anesthesia machine, the concentration of oxygen in the patient breathing system shall be measured by an oxygen analyzer with a low oxygen concentration limit alarm in use.
2. Blood oxygenation: During all anesthetics, a quantitative method of assessing oxygenation such as a pulse oximetry shall be employed. Adequate illumination and exposure of the patient are necessary to assess color.

Ventilation

Objective

To ensure adequate ventilation of the patient during all anesthetics.

Methods

1. Every patient receiving general anesthesia shall have the adequacy of ventilation continually evaluated. While qualitative clinical signs such as chest excursion, observation of the reservoir breathing bag, and auscultation of breath sound may be adequate, quantitative monitoring of the CO_2 content and/or volume of expired gas is encouraged.
2. When an endotracheal tube is inserted, its correct positioning in the trachea must be verified by clinical assessment and by identification of carbon dioxide in the expired gas. End-tidal CO_2 analysis, in use from the time of endotracheal tube placement, is encouraged.
3. When ventilation is controlled by a mechanical ventilator, there shall be in continuous use a device that is capable of detecting disconnection of components of the breathing system. The device must give an audible signal when its alarm threshold is exceeded.
4. During regional anesthesia and monitored anesthesia care, the adequacy of ventilation shall be evaluated, at least by continual observation of qualitative clinical signs.

Circulation

Objective

To ensure the adequacy of the patient's circulatory function during all anesthetics.

Methods

1. Every patient receiving anesthesia shall have the electrocardiogram continuously displayed from the beginning of anesthesia until preparing to leave the anesthetizing location.
2. Every patient receiving anesthesia shall have arterial blood pressure and heart rate determined and evaluated at least every five minutes.
3. Every patient receiving anesthesia shall have, in addition to the above, circulatory function continually evaluated by at least one of the following: palpation of a pulse, auscultation of heart sounds, monitoring of a tracing of intra-arterial pressure, ultrasound peripheral pulse monitoring, or pulse plethysmography or oximetry.

Body Temperature

Objective

To aid in the maintenance of appropriate body temperature during all anesthetics.

Methods

There shall be readily available a means to continuously measure the patient's temperature. When changes in body temperature are intended, anticipated, or suspected, the temperature shall be measured.

Excerpts from ASA Standards for Basic Intra-Operative Monitoring. Approved by the ASA House of Delegates 10/21/86, Amended 10/23/90, Effective 1/1/91. Reprinted with permission of the American Society of Anesthesiologists, Park Ridge, Illinois 60068–3189.

TABLE 3–12
Guidelines for Regional Anesthesia in Obstetrics

Guideline I

Regional anesthesia should be initiated and maintained only in locations in which appropriate resuscitation equipment and drugs are immediately available to manage procedurally related problems.

Guideline II

Regional anesthesia should be initiated by a physician with appropriate privileges and maintained by or under the medical direction of such an individual.

Guideline III

Regional anesthesia should not be administered until:

1. The patient has been examined by a qualified individual; and
2. The maternal and fetal status and progress of labor have been evaluated by a physician with privileges in obstetrics who is readily available to supervise the labor and manage any obstetric complications that may arise.

Guideline IV

An intravenous infusion should be established before the initiation of regional anesthesia and maintained throughout the duration of the regional anesthetic.

Guideline V

Regional anesthesia for labor and/or vaginal delivery requires that the parturient's vital signs and the fetal heart rate be monitored and documented by a qualified individual. Additional monitoring appropriate to the clinical condition of the parturient and the fetus should be employed when indicated. When extensive regional blockade is administered for complicated vaginal delivery, the standards for basic intraoperative monitoring should be applied.

Guideline VI

Regional anesthesia for cesarean delivery requires that the standards for basic intraoperative monitoring be applied and that a physician with privileges in obstetrics be immediately available.

Guideline VII

Qualified personnel, other than the anesthesiologist attending the mother, should be immediately available to assume responsibility for resuscitation of the newborn.

Guideline VIII

A physician with appropriate privileges should remain readily available during the regional anesthetic to manage anesthetic complications until the patient's postanesthesia condition is satisfactory and stable.

Guideline IX

All patients recovering from regional anesthesia should receive appropriate postanesthesia care following cesarean delivery and/or extensive regional blockade; the standards for postanesthesia care should be applied.

Guideline X

There should be a policy to ensure the availability in the facility of a physician to manage complications and to provide cardiopulmonary resuscitation for patients receiving postanesthesia care.

Excerpts from ASA Guidelines for Regional Anesthesia in Obstetrics. Approved by the ASA House of Delegates 10/12/88, Amended 10/30/91. Reprinted with permission of the American Society of Anesthesiologists, Park Ridge, Illinois 60068–3189.

maternal-fetal monitoring in this setting has not been defined. In the author's hospital, vital signs (blood pressure and pulse) and fetal heart tones are recorded every 30 minutes throughout labor. When epidural anesthesia is used for pain relief, continuous FHR monitoring (internal/external) is initiated prior to induction. Vital signs (blood pressure and pulse) are recorded frequently for 20 minutes following injection, then every 15 minutes throughout labor. Pulse oximetry and cardiac monitoring are *not* used routinely. Additional monitoring (e.g., electrocardiography and pulse oximetry) is used only if maternal-fetal circumstances warrant it.

Patients delivering in the traditional delivery-operating rooms of the obstetric suite are monitored in a manner consistent with policies and procedures in the main operating room. This includes the use of a cardiac monitor, pulse oximeter, a noninvasive blood pressure cuff, end-tidal carbon dioxide monitor, temperature monitor, and a stethoscope.

Anesthesia and the Obstetric Suite

Traditionally, the obstetric suite is designed with well-defined areas for labor, delivery, and recovery. In this setting anesthesia monitors and equipment are confined to the delivery rooms, which, in many institutions, are used for both vaginal and cesarean deliveries. Many hospitals throughout the United States are replacing conventional obstetric suites with LDRs or with labor, delivery, recovery, and postpartum rooms (LDRPs). This design enables the parturient to labor, deliver, and recover in one area. In some cases, the room also serves as the postpartum room.

In a conventional obstetric suite, the management of anesthesia during labor is easy to accomplish, as patients are contained in a small area. However, in a facility with LDRs, the obstetric anesthesia team may need to provide coverage for a very large area. This influences not only the obstetric management of the parturient but the anesthetic management as well. These rooms should be used only for spontaneous vaginal or elective low-outlet forceps deliveries. If difficulties are anticipated during delivery, the patient should be transferred to a traditional delivery room or operating room where better anesthesia facilities exist.

In the author's hospital, each LDR has a separate oxygen and vacuum supply for the mother and neonate. Equipment necessary for neonatal resuscitation is stored in an area separate from the LDR and moved into the room and warmed prior to delivery. Each unit has an adequate supply of suction bulbs, oral airways, masks, laryngoscopes, batteries, light bulbs, oral endotracheal tubes, suction catheters, and medication (e.g., atropine, naloxone, sodium bicarbonate, and epinephrine).

A neonatal team is responsible for all neonatal resuscitation. In addition, nurses assigned to labor and delivery are certified in neonatal advanced life support and advanced cardiac life support and are responsible for resuscitation until the neonatal team arrives. The obstetric anesthesiologist may provide assistance if necessary; however, his or her primary responsibility is to provide care to the mother.

Equipment for emergency maternal resuscitation should be available in each LDR. At the author's facility, this includes an oxygen delivery system and an adequate supply of oral airways, nasopharyngeal airways, masks, and suction catheters. In addition, each regional anesthetic cart contains laryngoscopes, batteries, light bulbs, oral endotracheal tubes, and medications (e.g., ephedrine, succinylcholine, and sodium thiopental). Emergency transtracheal insufflation equipment is immediately available in the anesthesia work room and in each of the delivery rooms.

Epidural anesthesia is the most common procedure performed in the LDRs. Infrequently, intrathecal opioids are used in conjunction with epidural anesthesia in selected patients. The use of spinal anesthesia for delivery is limited to the delivery-operating rooms where greater support is available should complications occur.

Recovery of a postpartum patient in an LDR(P) or obstetric postanesthesia care unit (PACU) requires that policies and procedures are consistent with standards established by the PACU of the main operating room and implemented by personnel trained and skilled in the management of these patients (Table 3–13).

At the author's facility each of the operating rooms in the obstetric suite is equipped with a late-model anesthesia machine and ventilator, a cardiac monitor capable of extensive invasive monitoring, a pulse oximeter, a capnograph, an electronic temperature monitor, and an oxygen analyzer. All of the equipment is on a preventive maintenance schedule and is interchangeable with equipment in the operating room. In addition, each room has a designated neonatal resuscitation area and is supplied with an anesthesia cart that contains airway equipment, laryngoscopes, medications, syringes, needles, fluids, and other devices. Fiberoptic equipment is available in the main operating room.

Philosophies and Concerns in the Obstetric Suite

The guidelines published by the American College of Obstetricians and Gynecologists (ACOG) and the American Society of Anesthesiologists state that prior to the administration of

TABLE 3-13
Standards for Postanesthesia Care

Standard I

All patients who have received general anesthesia, regional anesthesia, or monitored anesthesia care shall receive appropriate postanesthesia management.

Standard II

A patient transported to the PACU shall be accompanied by a member of the anesthesia care team who is knowledgeable about the patient's condition. The patient shall be continually evaluated and treated during transport with monitoring and support appropriate to the patient's condition.

Standard III

Upon arrival in the PACU, the patient shall be reevaluated and a verbal report provided to the responsible PACU nurse by the member of the anesthesia care team who accompanies the patient.

Standard IV

The patient's condition shall be evaluated continually in the PACU.

Standard V

A physician is responsible for the discharge of the patient from the PACU.

Abbreviation: PACU = postanesthesia care unit.

Excerpts from ASA Standards for Postanesthesia Care. Approved by the ASA House of Delegates 10/12/88, Amended 10/23/90, Effective 10/30/91. Reprinted with permission of the American Society of Anesthesiologists, Park Ridge, Illinois 60068-3189.

regional anesthesia the "maternal and fetal status and progress of labor have been evaluated by a physician with privileges in obstetrics who is readily available to supervise the labor and manage any obstetric complications that may arise." The term "readily available" was chosen to allow for some institutional variation.

In many tertiary perinatal centers, obstetric residents and interns staff labor and delivery. However, in smaller facilities, this capability does not exist. Although attention is focused on the presence of an obstetrician during the administration of anesthesia, the author's opinion is that the more important issue is the in-house presence of an obstetrician when a patient in labor is admitted to the obstetric suite. As previously indicated, a significant portion of patients experience adverse outcomes during the intrapartum period. Quick response to an unanticipated event is important to the mother and fetus. Therefore, when a problem is identified, every effort should be made to minimize the time to delivery. Despite the advantages offered by in-house obstetric coverage, this may be impractical in many small institutions. These institutions should select staffing patterns consistent with ACOG Guidelines and good patient care.

In some institutions, the reinjection of an epidural anesthetic for labor and delivery is performed by the labor nurse. In many states, this practice is limited by nursing practice standards and regulated by law. At the author's facility, an anesthesia provider is in the immediate vicinity of labor and delivery at all times. If a parturient is not placed on a continuous infusion, the epidural is redosed by anesthesia personnel. The author's opinion is that the management of all anesthetics should be the responsibility of individuals trained and skilled in anesthesia.

PREANESTHETIC ASSESSMENT

A careful review of the prenatal record is an important aspect of obstetric anesthesia care. Information regarding the current pregnancy helps the anesthesia provider focus on problem areas during the preanesthetic interview. When a woman in labor is admitted to the obstetric suite, a member of the anesthesia care team should perform a preanesthetic assessment prior to the administration of anesthesia. The interview consists of three parts: A brief history and physical examination; a discussion of techniques available to relieve pain and the risks and complications of these techniques; and an opportunity to ask questions. The history and physical examination provide information useful to the anesthesia provider regarding the choice of anesthetic techniques (e.g., intrathecal opioids and spinal or epidural anesthesia), preparations for delivery (e.g., prematurity, twins, infant of a diabetic mother, postmature, and fetal distress), and potential problems that may arise if emergent operative delivery with general anesthesia is required (e.g., difficult airway, short neck, and loose teeth). A discussion of analgesia techniques includes a description of systemic medications, how they are administered during labor (e.g., small intermittent doses, limited use prior to delivery), and their effects on the mother and fetus (e.g., minimal pain relief at the peak of contractions, sedation of mother and fetus); a description of regional anesthetic techniques (e.g., epidural or spinal), and associated risks and complications (poor block, dural puncture, intravenous injection, paralysis, and need for general anesthesia); and a description of general anesthesia and associated risks and complications (e.g., sore throat following intubation, aspiration, and death). The anesthesia provider explains that general anesthesia may be required in the event of a maternal or fetal emergency despite the presence of a functioning epidural, as sufficient time may not be available to achieve surgical anesthesia with that technique.

Informed consent with written documentation is required at the author's facility. Therefore, a signed permit is obtained from the patient, her parents, or her legal guardian, prior to the administration of anesthesia. Written permits are not required at all institutions; however, it is important to document that a discussion of anesthetic techniques and a description of the risks and complications occurred. In many states, the potential for liability to members of the obstetric anesthesia care team continues through the 21st birthday of the child. Accurate and complete documentation of events occurring during the intrapartum period is, therefore, important. Not infrequently, a mother receives systemic medication prior to a preanesthetic assessment and then requests regional anesthesia. If the patient is alert and oriented between contractions, a preanesthetic interview will be performed, informed consent obtained, and anesthesia administered. However, if the patient is sedated or falls asleep between contractions the anesthesia provider will wait for the effects of the medication to subside before interviewing the patient and administering anesthesia, unless circumstances warrant immediate intervention.

Additional problems may arise if a pregnant patient is considered a minor and not recognized as an emancipated individual by the state. The laws governing the rights of a minor are not consistent throughout the United States. Therefore, physicians practicing obstetric anesthesia should be familiar with the laws pertaining to minors in their state. Informed consent must be obtained from the patient's parents or legal guardian if the minor is not recognized as emancipated. In addition, the proposed anesthetic technique and associated risks and complications should be discussed with the patient and written documentation placed in the chart.

A written record is maintained for every patient receiving anesthesia during labor and delivery (Fig. 3–10). Information regarding the position of the patient when anesthesia was administered, fetal heart tones, technique, location, difficulty and complications encountered, test dose, induction dose, and final level of anesthesia is recorded. Vital signs (blood pressure, pulse, and respirations) are recorded every 2 minutes for five times, then every 5 minutes for two times during induction and reinjections. Blood pressure and pulse are subsequently recorded every 15 minutes.

CONCLUSION

The management of anesthesia in the obstetric patient is greatly influenced by the physiologic and pathologic processes associated with pregnancy. A basic understanding of these processes and their interactions is important to the obstetric anesthesiologist. A thorough review of the prenatal record and comprehensive preanesthetic assessment provides significant information regarding the status of the parturient. Problems identified by these sources will help the obstetric anesthesiologist anticipate maternal-fetal complications and identify the need for additional maternal-fetal monitoring during labor and delivery.

The ability to identify the fetus at risk has been enhanced by a better understanding of the intrauterine environment and the use of sophisticated monitoring techniques. Information regarding the fetal status assists in the selection, administration, and maintenance of anesthesia and organization of neonatal support following delivery. A coordinated effort involving the obstetrician, anesthesiologist, and neonatologist will ensure the best possible outcome for each patient.

TEN PRACTICAL POINTS

1. The prenatal record serves as a vital resource for identification of the high-risk parturient and fetus.

MARICOPA MEDICAL CENTER
2601 E. ROOSEVELT, PHOENIX, ARIZONA 85008

OBSTETRICAL ANESTHESIA RECORD

Name

PID

dob

IMPRINT OR PRINT

Pre-op Diagnosis:

Procedure:

Time												TOTAL
O_2												
AGENTS												
POSITION												

Date ______

	start	end	duration
Anesthesia			
Surgery			

OR # ______ Machine # ______

Anesthesiologist
Attending ______

Symbols:
V/Λ BP
• P
X Induction
⊙ Incision
⊗ Leave OR

240, 220, 200, 180, 160, 140, 120, 100, 80, 60, 40, 20, 0

Block
Type ______
Needle ______
Lot # ______
Interspace ______
Attempts ______
Blood ___ CSF ___
Parathesia's ______

Resident/CRNA ______
Obstetrician ______
Resident ______
Preanesthetic evaluation reviewed:
Resident/CRNA Initial ______ Attending Initial ______
Age ______ Ht ______ Wt ______
BP ______ P ______
PMH ______
Meds ______
Allergy ______
ASA ______ Hgb ______ Hct ______ K+ ______
System ______
Mask ______ Airway O / N
Tube size ______ O / N Cuff y / n
Direct / Blind / Fiberoptic Blade ______
Difficulty ______
Eye Protection ______
MONITORS (circle all used) ECG NIBP
TEMP (esoph / rectal / ______
stethoscope (precordial / esoph.) SaO_2, FiO_2, $ETCO_2$, agent monitor, SvO_2, EEG, nerve stimulator, Doppler
Other ______

Event												
MONITORS: ECG												
TEMP												
FiO_2												
SaO_2												
$ETCO_2$												
FHR												
RESP TV / R / PIP Ⓢ/Ⓐ/Ⓒ												
FLUIDS												
Estimated Blood Loss												
Urine Output												

TOTALS

NEONATAL DATA		
TIME		
SEX		
APGAR 1"		
APGAR 5"		
MECONIUM	☐	☐
LARYNGOSCOPY	☐	☐
TRACH SUCTION	☐	☐
RESUSCITATION	☐	☐
NICU NURSE	☐	☐
NEONATOLOGIST	☐	☐

Comments:

EPID CATH:
Left in ______
Removed intact at ______

PACU:
BP ______ P ______
R ______ SaO_2 ______
Page ______ of ______

CHART COPY

081 5129 4-91

Figure 3–10. Obstetrical anesthesia record.

2. "High-risk" pregnancies increase the likelihood of anesthetic intervention.

3. One third of "low-risk" pregnancies become high-risk intrapartum, emphasizing the need for continued evaluation of the parturient throughout labor.

4. The nonstress test and contraction stress test accurately predict fetal well-being but not fetal distress.

5. The biophysical profile consists of several biophysical activities that predict fetal risk.

6. A fetal scalp pH of less than 7.2 indicates fetal compromise and necessitates immediate delivery.

7. Equipment in the obstetric operating room should be consistent with that in the main operating room.

8. Limit procedures performed in LDRs and LDRPs to spontaneous vaginal deliveries and elective low-outlet forceps deliveries.

9. An L/S ratio of greater than 2 in the presence of PG indicates fetal pulmonary maturity.

10. Review the prenatal record and perform a preanesthetic assessment prior to the administration of anesthesia.

REFERENCES

1. Cunningham FG, MacDonald PC, Gant NF: Part IV. Management of normal pregnancy: Prenatal care. *In* Cunningham FG, MacDonald PC, Gant NF (eds): Williams Obstetrics, 18th ed. East Norwalk, CT, Appleton & Lange, 1989, pp 257–275.
2. Hobel CJ, Merkatz IR: High-risk scoring. *In* Sciarra JJ, Depp R, Eschenbach DA (eds): Gynecology and Obstetrics, Vol 3. Philadelphia, Harper & Row, 1982, pp 1–8.
3. Hobel CJ, Hyvarinen MA, Okada DM, Oh W: Prenatal and intrapartum high-risk screening. I. Prediction of the high-risk neonate. Am J Obstet Gynecol 117:1–9, 1973.
4. Fortney JA, Whitehorne EW: The development of an index of high-risk pregnancy. Am J Obstet Gynecol 143:501–508, 1982.
5. Rayburn WF, Anderson CW, O'Shaughnessy RW, Ruckman WP: Predictability of the distressed term infant. Am J Obstet Gynecol 140:489–491, 1981.
6. Frigoletto FD, Little GA: Guidelines for Perinatal Care, 2nd ed. Elk Grove Village, IL, American Academy of Pediatrics and American College of Obstetricians and Gynecologists, 1988.
7. Cunningham FG, MacDonald PC, Gant NF: Part I. Placental hormones. *In* Cunningham FG, MacDonald PC, Gant NF (eds): Williams Obstetrics, 18th ed. East Norwalk, CT, Appleton & Lange, 1989, pp 67–85.
8. Duenhoelter JH, Whalley PJ, MacDonald PC: An analysis of the utility of plasma immunoreactive estrogen measurements in determining delivery time of gravidas with the fetus considered at high risk. Am J Obstet Gynecol 125:889–898, 1976.
9. Gluck L, Kulovich MV, Borer RC Jr, et al: Diagnosis of the respiratory distress syndrome by amniocentesis. Am J Obstet Gynecol 109:440–445, 1971.
10. Gluck L, Kulovich MV: Lecithin/sphingomyelin ratios in amniotic fluid in normal and abnormal pregnancy. Am J Obstet Gynecol 115:539–546, 1973.
11. Harvy D, Parkinson CE, Campbell S: Risk of respiratory distress syndrome. Lancet 1:42, 1975.
12. Whittle MJ, Wilson AI, Whitfield CR, et al: Amniotic fluid phosphatidylglycerol and the lecithin/sphingomyelin ratio in the assessment of fetal lung maturity. Br J Obstet Gynaecol 89:727–732, 1982.
13. Pritchard JA, MacDonald PC: Part VIII. Congenital malformations and inherited disorders. *In* Cunningham FG, MacDonald PC, Gant NF (eds): Williams Obstetrics, 18th ed. East Norwalk, CT, Appleton & Lange, 1989, pp 561–591.
14. Bang J, Brock JE, Trolle D: Ultrasound guided fetal intravenous transfusion for severe rhesus hemolytic disease. Br Med J 284:373–374, 1982.
15. Trudinger BJ, Giles WB, Cook CM: Flow velocity wave forms and the maternal, uteroplacental and fetal umbilical placental circulations. Am J Obstet Gynecol 152:155–163, 1985.
16. Pritchard JA, MacDonald PC: Part IV. Techniques to evaluate fetal health. *In* Cunningham FG, MacDonald PC, Gant NF (eds): Williams Obstetrics, 18th ed. East Norwalk, CT, Appleton & Lange, 1989, pp 277–305.
17. Berkowitz GS, Mehalek KE, Chitkara U, et al: Doppler umbilical velocimetry and the prediction of adverse outcome in pregnancies at risk for intrauterine growth retardation. Obstet Gynecol 71:742–746, 1988.
18. Guidetti DA, Divon MY, Cavalieri RL, et al: Fetal umbilical artery flow velocimetry in post date pregnancies. Am J Obstet Gynecol 157:1521–1523, 1987.
19. Divon MY, Girz BA, Lieblich R, Langer O: Clinical management of the fetus with markedly diminished umbilical artery and diastolic flow. Am J Obstet Gynecol 161:1523–1527, 1989.
20. Pirhonen JP, Eikola RU: Uterine and umbilical velocity wave forms in the supine hypotension syndrome. Obstet Gynecol 76:176–179, 1990.
21. Hughes AB, Devoe LD, Wakefield MC, Metheny WP: The effects of epidural anesthesia on the

Doppler velocimetry of the umbilical and uterine arteries in normal term labor. Obstet Gynecol 75:809–812, 1990.
22. Marx GF, Edelstein ID, Schuss M, et al: Effects of epidural block with lignocaine and lignocaine adrenaline on umbilical artery velocity wave ratios. Br J Obstet Gynaecol 97:517–520, 1990.
23. Rooth G, McBride R, Ivy BJ: Fetal and maternal pH measurements. Acta Obstet Gynaecol Scand 52:47–50, 1973.
24. Ray M, Freeman R, Pine S, Hesselgesser R: Clinical experience with the oxytocin challenge test. Am J Obstet Gynecol 114:1–9, 1972.
25. Lenke RK, Nemes JM: Use of nipple stimulation to obtain contraction stress test. Obstet Gynecol 63:345–348, 1984.
26. Capelass EL, Mann LI: Use of breast stimulation for antepartum stress testing. Obstet Gynecol 64:641–645, 1984.
27. Lipitz S, Barkai G, Rabinovici J, Mashiach S: Breast stimulation test and oxytocin challenge test in fetal surveillance: A prospective randomized study. Am J Obstet Gynecol 151:1178–1181, 1987.
28. Oki EY, Keegan KA, Freemen RK, Dorchester WL: The breast-stimulated contraction stress test. J Reprod Med 12:919–923, 1987.
29. Rosenzweig BA, Levy JS, Schipiour P, Blumenthal PD: Comparison of the nipple stimulation and exogenous oxytocin contraction stress test: A randomized prospective study. J Reprod Med 34:950–954, 1989.
30. Hill WC, Moenning RK, Katz N, Kitzmiller JZ: Characteristics of uterine activity during the breast stimulation stress test. Obstet Gynecol 64:489–492, 1984.
31. Thaker SB, Berkelman RL: Assessing the diagnostic accuracy and efficacy of selective antepartum fetal surveillance techniques. Obstet Gynecol Surv 41:121–141, 1986.
32. Castillo RA, Devoe LD, Arthur M, et al: The preterm non-stress test: Effects of gestational age and length of study. Am J Obstet Gynecol 160:172–175, 1989.
33. Smith CV, Phelan JP, Platt LD, et al: Fetal acoustic stimulation testing. II. A randomized clinical comparison with a non-stress test. Am J Obstet Gynecol 155:131–134, 1986.
34. Romero R, Mazor M, Hobbins JC: A critical appraisal of fetal acoustic stimulation as an antenatal test for fetal well-being. Obstet Gynecol 71:781–786, 1988.
35. Devoe LD, Gardner P, Arnold P, Searle N: The effects of laboratory acoustic stimulation on baseline fetal heart rate in term pregnancy. Am J Obstet Gynecol 160:1086–1090, 1986.
36. Connors G, Natale R, Nasello-Patterson C: Maternally perceived fetal activity from 24 weeks' gestation to term in normal and at risk pregnancies. Am J Obstet Gynecol 158:294–299, 1988.
37. Manning FA, Platt LD, Sipos L: Antepartum fetal evaluation: Development of a biophysical profile score. Am J Obstet Gynecol 136:787–795, 1980.
38. Egertsen SC, Benedetti TJ: Maternal response to daily fetal movement counting in primary care settings. Am J Perinatol 4:327–330, 1987.
39. Ahn MO, Phelan JP, Smith CV, et al: Antepartum fetal surveillance in the patient with decreased fetal movement. Am J Obstet Gynecol 157:860–864, 1987.
40. Patrick J, Campbell K, Carmichael L, et al: Patterns of human fetal breathing during the last 10 weeks of pregnancy. Obstet Gynecol 56:24–30, 1980.
41. Brar HS, Platt LD, Devore GR: Biophysical profiles. Clin Obstet Gynecol 30:936, 1987.
42. Duff P, Sanders R, Hayashi RH: Intrauterine tachypnea—A sign of fetal distress? Am J Obstet Gynecol 142:1054–1056, 1982.
43. Manning FA, Herman M, Boyce D, Carter LJ: Intrauterine fetal tachypnea. Obstet Gynecol 58:398–400, 1981.
44. Grannum PAT, Berkowitz RL, Hobbins JC: The ultrasonic changes in the maturing placenta and their relation to fetal pulmonic maturity. Am J Obstet Gynecol 133:915–922, 1979.
45. Chamberlain PF, Manning FA, Morrison I, et al: Ultrasound evaluation of amniotic fluid volume. II. The relationship of increased amniotic fluid volume to perinatal outcome. Am J Obstet Gynecol 150:250–254, 1984.
46. Phelan JP, Platt LD, Yeh S, et al: The role of ultrasound assessment of amniotic fluid volume in the management of the postdate pregnancy. Am J Obstet Gynecol 151:304–308, 1985.
47. Rutherford SE, Phelan JP, Smith CV, Jacobs N: The four-quadrant assessment of amniotic fluid volume: An adjunct to antepartum fetal heart rate testing. Obstet Gynecol 70:353–356, 1987.
48. Shamoys SM, Sivkin M, Dery C, et al: Amniotic fluid index: An appropriate predictor of perinatal outcome. Am J Perinatol 7:266–269, 1990.
49. Phelan JP, Ahn MY, Smith CV, et al: Amniotic fluid index measurements during pregnancy. J Reprod Med 32:601–604, 1987.
50. Phelan JP, Smith CV, Broussard P, Small M: Amniotic fluid volume assessment with the four quadrant technique at 36–42 weeks' gestation. J Reprod Med 32:540–542, 1987.
51. Manning FA, Morrison I, Harman CR, Menticoglou SM: The abnormal fetal biophysical profile score. V. Predictive accuracy according to score composition. Am J Obstet Gynecol 162:918–927, 1990.
52. Manning FA, Harman CR, Morrison I, et al: Fetal assessment based on fetal biophysical profile

scoring. IV. An analysis of perinatal morbidity and mortality. Am J Obstet Gynecol 162:703–709, 1990.

53. Zalar W, Quilligan EJ: The influence of scalp sampling on the cesarean section rate for fetal distress. Am J Obstet Gynecol 135:239–246, 1979.

54. Parer JT: Fetal heart rate. *In* Creasy RK, Resnick R (eds): Maternal-Fetal Medicine: Principles and Practice, 2nd ed. Philadelphia, WB Saunders, 1989, pp 314–343.

55. Gravenstein JS: Essential monitoring through different lenses. J Clin Monit 2:22–29, 1986.

56. Epstein RM: Morbidity and mortality from anesthesia [Editorial]. Anesthesiology 49:388–389, 1979.

57. Cooper JB, Newbower RS, Kitz RJ: An analysis of major errors and equipment failures in anesthesia management: Considerations for prevention and detection. Anesthesiology 60:34–42, 1984.

58. Beecher HK: The first anesthesia death with some remarks suggested by it on the fields of the laboratory and the clinic and appraisal of new anesthetic agents. Anesthesiology 2:443, 1941.

59. Eichhorn JH, Cooper JB, Cullen DJ, et al: Standards for monitoring during anesthesia at Harvard Medical School. JAMA 256:1017–1020, 1986.

60. Bowes WA, Corke BC, Hulka J: Pulse oximetry: A review of the theory, accuracy, and clinical applications. Obstet Gynecol 74:541–546, 1989.

61. Sendak MJ, Harris AP, Donham RT: Use of pulse oximetry to assess arterial oxygen saturation during newborn resuscitation. Crit Care Med 14:739–740, 1986.

62. Maxwell L, Harris A, Sendak M, Donham R: Monitoring the resuscitation of preterm infants in the delivery room using pulse oximetry. Clin Pediatr 26:18–20, 1987.

63. Freeman RK, Garite TJ, Nageotte MP (eds): Fetal Heart Rate Monitoring, 2nd ed. Baltimore, Williams & Wilkins, 1991, p. 2.

FOUR

Practical Obstetric Physiology

Richard P. Driver, Jr., M.D.

The physiologic and anatomic changes occurring during pregnancy alter our concepts of what constitutes human "normality." A resetting of homeostatic mechanisms results in a new physiologic equilibrium that addresses the needs of the developing fetus and prepares the maternal physiologic reserves necessary to meet the stresses imposed by labor and delivery. This unique physiology demands an altered approach to the administration of anesthesia and perioperative patient management. When preparing to administer anesthesia, the physiologic and anatomic changes that occur in pregnancy must be considered in order to optimize uterine blood flow and fetal oxygen delivery and provide safe anesthesia.

This chapter (1) provides an overview of the aspects of maternal physiologic adaptations to pregnancy that are pertinent to anesthetic management for either abdominal or vaginal delivery, (2) describes how manipulation of maternal physiology can positively or negatively affect the fetus, and (3) provides an outline of normal maternal physiologic changes to assist in making patient management decisions.

MATERNAL PHYSIOLOGIC CHANGES

Pulmonary System

Upper Respiratory Tract

The pulmonary system of the parturient, from nares to alveolus, undergoes anatomic and functional changes. Venous engorgement and mucosal edema develop and involve the nasopharynx, oropharynx, glottic structures, vocal cords, and trachea.[1] Risks of airway obstruction and difficult intubation are increased secondary to increased soft tissue mass. Upper airway caliber often declines, requiring a smaller-than-average endotracheal tube. Endotracheal tubes of 7.0 mm are routinely used by most practitioners. Furthermore, trauma to the venous-engorged nasopharynx and oropharynx, occurring during nasotracheal or orotracheal intubation, can cause severe bleeding, obstructing visualization and causing hemoaspiration. Nasotracheal intubation is rarely performed during pregnancy because of the increased potential for bleeding.

Chest and Thorax

The breasts of the parturient increase in volume, potentially up to 800 ml per breast owing to hormonally mediated hypertrophy of glandular tissue.[2] Redundant breast tissue tends to shift cephalad when the patient is in the supine position, owing to the downward slope of the upper thorax, potentially obstructing maneuvering room for insertion of a laryngoscope. The increased anteroposterior (AP) diameter of the chest (see the discussion later in this chapter) increases the downward slope of the thorax, exaggerating this problem. Short-handled laryngoscopes allow increased range of movement during laryngoscope insertion.

The diaphragm elevates by as much as 4 cm

during pregnancy and the costophrenic angle increases from 68 to 103 degrees.[3,4] Chest circumference increases from 5 to 7 cm as a consequence of an increased AP diameter.[5] Because of this compensatory increase in AP diameter, diaphragmatic elevation secondary to the enlarging uterus does not decrease vital capacity. Tidal breathing becomes increasingly diaphragmatic as the enlarging uterus distorts and stretches the abdominal musculature. The accessory role of the abdominal musculature in respiration is eliminated, which potentially limits the increase in minute ventilation in response to stress.

These anatomic changes make endotracheal intubation and mask ventilation more difficult, and the increased chest wall weight may impede mask ventilation. Airway management is critical, and the leading causes of anesthesia-related morbidity and mortality in pregnancy result from complications associated with failure to intubate and with inability to maintain a patent airway for ventilation.[6,7] Careful evaluation of airway anatomy is indicated, and a heightened vigilance for potential airway disasters is essential.

TABLE 4–1
Major Pulmonary Alterations in Pregnancy

Parameter	Direction	Magnitude (%)
Tidal volume	Increased	40
Respiratory rate	Increased or unchanged	
Minute volume	Increased	40
FRC	Decreased	20
ERV	Decreased	15
Residual volume	Decreased	20
FEV_1	Unchanged	
MEF	Unchanged	

Abbreviations: FRC = functional residual capacity; ERV = expiratory reserve volume; FEV_1 = forced expiratory volume in 1 sec; MEF = maximal expiratory flow.

Data from American College of Obstetricians and Gynecologists, 1985; Pernoll et al, 1975; Prowse and Gaensler, 1965; Clapp et al, 1988; Baldwin et al, 1977; and Weinberger et al, 1980.

Indices of Pulmonary Function

Reserve volume, expiratory reserve volume, and functional residual capacity (FRC) decrease approximately 20% during pregnancy (Table 4–1). From a practical standpoint, the most significant change in lung volume is the decrease in FRC. Decreased FRC reduces the time between apnea and arterial oxygen desaturation secondary to a reduced oxygen "reservoir" in the lung. Increased oxygen consumption occurring in pregnancy accentuates this rapid decline.[8] Indeed, very rapid arterial oxygen desaturation can occur during the induction of general anesthesia.[9] After 1 minute of apnea, Archer and Marx[9] demonstrated a twofold greater decrease in arterial Pa_{O_2} in parturients compared with gynecologic controls (30% vs. 12% decrease). Byrne and colleagues documented a progressive decrease in times required to denitrogenate as gestation increased from 13 to 42 weeks.[10]

Tidal volume increases significantly during pregnancy and is the major factor responsible for the 40% increase in minute ventilation observed in pregnancy.[11–13] In contrast, the respiratory rate has been shown to be either unchanged or mildly elevated during pregnancy, and contributes little to the increased minute ventilation. Increased minute ventilation has been attributed either to direct stimulation of the respiratory center by elevated progesterone levels or to a heightened respiratory center sensitivity to PCO_2.[14,15] Regardless, the increased work of breathing associated with increased minute ventilation contributes significantly to the increased maternal metabolism occurring during pregnancy.

Since closing volume remains constant in pregnancy, reduced FRC increases the propensity for small airway closure.[16] As with all patients, airway closure may worsen when patients assume the supine position, which causes further decreases in lung volume secondary to elevation of the diaphragm by abdominal contents. If airway closure becomes problematic, maintaining the patient in a sitting or semisitting position and administering supplemental O_2 will lessen the potential for maternal hypoxemia. Baraka and coworkers documented that the head-up position extends the duration of apnea that can take place before desaturation occurs in nonpregnant patients.[17]

The effects of pregnancy on large and small airways appears to be minimal. Although some authors suggest decreased airway resistance during pregnancy, indices of large airway function (forced expiratory volume in 1 sec [FEV_1] and FEV_1/forced vital capacity [FVC] [FEV_1%]) and small airway function (maximal expiratory flow rate [MEFR]) are unchanged by pregnancy.[18–20]

Pulmonary and Acid-Base Physiology

Increased minute ventilation decreases arterial P_{CO_2} and normal maternal values range from 27 to 32 mmHg. This is an important maternal adaptation, since CO_2 diffusion is concentration-dependent. Reduced maternal arterial P_{CO_2} allows more efficient fetal transfer of CO_2 secondary to the larger concentration gradient between fetal and maternal blood (Table 4–2). Increased renal HCO_3 excretion prevents the development of frank alkalemia from the relative respiratory alkalosis. However, acid-base compensation is not complete and maternal pH reflects a slight alkalotic shift, which is clinically insignificant. However, further increases in minute ventilation, precipitated by the stress and pain of labor, may cause further increased respiratory alkalosis and frank alkalemia. In this setting, pain-free intervals between contractions may result in hypoventilation secondary to decreased respiratory drive in response to CO_2.[21, 22] In theory, maternal hypoxemia can occur during these periods. In response to this intermittent hypoxemia, a leftward shift in the oxyhemoglobin dissociation curve occurs, further decreasing O_2 delivery and resulting in fetal hypoxemia and fetal distress.[23] This effect can be ameliorated by adequate epidural analgesia, which interrupts pain transmission and prevents the hyperventilatory response to pain.[22] It is unclear whether this scenario is of consequence in uncompromised pregnancies.

Finally, there is a modest increase in arterial P_{O_2} as a consequence of increased maternal minute ventilation.[9] A small increase in Sp_{O_2} may occur and augment fetal O_2 delivery.

Cardiovascular System

Cardiac Output

The increased maternal cardiac output required to meet expanded maternal and fetal metabolic needs is central to most other cardiovascular adaptations occurring during pregnancy. The increased cardiac output is not uniformly distributed, rather, it is "consumed" by organ systems with accelerated metabolic needs (Table 4–3). Although the absolute quantity of blood flow to an organ system is not reduced during pregnancy, the percentage of total cardiac output to a particular organ may show a relative decrease.

Increased uterine blood flow may consume 15% of total cardiac output. Consequently, rapid exsanguination can occur during uncontrolled uterine hemorrhage. Other organs that have significant increases in blood flow during pregnancy include the kidneys, skin, brain, breasts, and coronary arteries.[24] Breast blood flow increases, allowing tissue hypertrophy and preparation for lactation. Increased coronary artery blood flow meets the metabolic requirements of increased cardiac work. Increased renal blood flow aids the elimination of the additional load of waste products generated by maternal and fetal metabolism, whereas increased cutaneous blood flow facilitates dissipa-

TABLE 4–2
Maternal-Fetal Blood Gas Transport

	pH	P_{CO_2} (mmHg)	P_{O_2} (mmHg)	H_{CO_3}	Sp_{O_2} (%)
Nonpregnant	7.37–7.44	35–45	80–100	22–26	98
Maternal artery	7.40–7.45	27–32	102–108	18–20	98
Umbilical vein	7.30–7.35	38–42	26–32	NM	70
Umbilical artery	7.24–7.29	48–54	12–18	NM	28

Abbreviation: NM = not directly measured in literature.

Data from Rosa M: Pediatrics: Physiology and practice. *In* Proceedings of "Mastery of Anesthesia Basics." New York, Montefiore Medical Center, Albert Einstein College of Medicine, 1992; and Gomella LG: Blood gasses and acid-base disorders. *In* Gomella LG (ed): Clinician's Pocket Reference, 7th ed. East Norwalk, CT, Appleton & Lange, 1993, p. 134.

TABLE 4–3
Average Changes in Blood Flow Distribution During Pregnancy

Uterus	Increased blood flow by approx 500 ml/min May reach 800 ml/min in some individuals
Skin	Increased blood flow by 300–400 ml/min
Renal	Increased blood flow by approximately 400 ml/min
Breast	Increased blood flow by approximately 200 ml/min
Cardiac	Not quantified

Total would require an approximate 1.5–1.8 L/min increase in cardiac output

Data from American College of Obstetricians and Gynecologists: CREOG Basic Science Monograph. Maternal Physiology. Washington, DC, ACOG, 1985.

tion of the excess heat generated from increased body metabolism. Increased cutaneous blood flow is, at least in part, responsible for the increase in the incidence of spider angiomata and palmar erythema observed during pregnancy.[25] Venodilatation may assist in securing venous access.

The reported increase in cardiac output varies slightly among studies but averages 1.8 L/min, or an approximate 30% increase over nonpregnant values (Table 4–4).[26, 27] Both increased stroke volume and increased heart rate contribute to the increase. However, the contribution to elevated cardiac output from stroke volume and heart rate varies with gestation, with a progressive rise in heart rate and a relatively decreasing contribution from stroke volume as pregnancy progresses toward term.[28] Increased stroke volume is achieved in part by increased left ventricular volumes.[29] There does not appear to be any change in ejection fraction, as both left ventricular end-diastolic volume and left ventricular end-systolic volume increase similarly.[30] Ejection fraction is therefore a valuable and reliable indicator of left ventricular function during pregnancy. Evidence conflicts as to whether there is a compensatory hypertrophy of the left ventricular wall in response to the increased cardiac chamber volumes.[29–31]

TABLE 4–4
Maternal Cardiovascular Parameters*

Parameter	Vector	Nonpregnant	Pregnant	% Change	Nadir/Max
HR (beats/min)	Increased	68	85	20	
SBP (mmHg)	No change	106–117	103–113		
DBP (mmHg)	Decreased	65–75	55–65	14	16–24 wk
MAP (mmHg)	No change	80–120			
CVP-RAP (mmHg)	No change	10	10		
CVP-fem (mmHg)	Increased	10	25	250	Term
SVR (dynes·cm·sec^{-5})	Decreased	1275	900	30	
PVR (dynes·cm·sec^{-5})	Decreased	119	78	34	
PAP (mmHg)	No change	15–30/4–12			
PCWP (mmHg)	No change	5–12			
CO (L/min)	Increased	5.1	6.9	27	Term
SV (ml)	Increased	75	81	8	
LVEDV (ml)	Increased				
EjF (%)	No change				
LVSWI (gm·m/m^2)	No change	45–60			
Heart size	Increased			12	

Abbreviations: HR = heart rate; SBP = systolic blood pressure; DBP = diastolic blood pressure; MAP = mean arterial pressure; CVP-RAP = central venous pressure-right atrial pressure; CVP-fem = CVP-femoral vein; SVR = systemic vascular resistance; PVR = pulmonary vascular resistance; PAP = pulmonary artery pressure; PCWP = pulmonary capillary wedge pressure; CO = cardiac output; SV = stroke volume; LVEDV = left ventricular end-diastolic volume; EjF = ejection fraction; LVSWI = left ventricular stroke work index.

Data from American College of Obstetricians and Gynecologists, 1985; Katz et al, 1978; Robson et al, 1987; Equimokhai et al, 1982; Mabie et al, 1994; Clark et al, 1989; McLennan, 1943; MacGillvray et al, 1969; and Lake, 1992.

Cardiac output rises rapidly during the first trimester and then continues to rise at a slower rate. Although there are conflicting data, cardiac output likely continues to rise until term[30] rather than peaking at 20 to 24 weeks' gestation as previously suggested.[32] Importantly, further increases in cardiac output occur during labor, as much as an additional 45% over nonpregnant values.[33] In addition, each contraction can result in a 300- to 500-ml "autotransfusion" of volume from the uterine vascular bed into the central circulation, causing further increased preload and a 10 to 15% increase in cardiac output.[33] The greatest increase in cardiac output occurs immediately following delivery secondary to the relief of caval obstruction and increased preload. This increased preload may produce an additional 10 to 20% increase in cardiac output[34] and perhaps as much as 80%.[35] This progressive increase in cardiac output during gestation and the acute increases in cardiac output that occur during labor, delivery, and the immediate postpartum period may unmask underlying cardiac pathology, which was subclinical earlier in the pregnancy, and produce acute cardiopulmonary decompensation. Rather than feeling relieved with impending delivery, the clinician should maintain heightened vigilance through delivery and the first 2 hours postpartum. Remember, the cardiovascular response to labor can be blunted by the administration of epidural analgesia. However, extreme caution must be exercised in patients with cardiac lesions in whom afterload reduction may be contraindicated.

Cardiac Function and Cardiac Indices

Cardiac function during pregnancy is determined primarily by preload, afterload, and contractility. The contractile state of the myocardium is not affected significantly by pregnancy, with authors noting either no change or a modest increase in contractility.[26, 29, 36] However, preload can be severely and rapidly decreased by compression of the vena cava by the gravid uterus, producing decreased venous return, acute maternal hypotension, decreased uterine perfusion, and if uncorrected, fetal distress.[37–39] (See "Uterine Perfusion and Aortocaval Syndrome," later in this chapter.) In the absence of aortocaval compression, right atrial pressure (RAP) resembles nonpregnant values.[40] However, venous pressures in the lower extremities increase, reflecting continuous partial vena caval occlusion (Fig. 4–1).[41] This obstruction of venous flow from the lower extremities probably contributes significantly to the increased risk of thromboembolic pulmonary embolus during pregnancy. Normal RAPs, despite the partial obstruction of venous return from the lower extremities, may be a reflection of increased plasma volume in pregnancy.

Both systemic vascular resistance (SVR) and pulmonary vascular resistance (PVR) decrease during pregnancy, suggesting decreased afterload to the right and left sides of the heart. Decreased vascular resistance mediated at the tissue level enhances forward blood flow and tissue perfusion. Several proposed mechanisms include prostaglandins,[42] decreased circulating levels of atrial natriuretic peptide,[43] decreased vascular sensitivity to angiotensin II, and increased uteroplacental conductance.[44] The decrease in SVR has been implicated as the initial cardiovascular adaptation in pregnancy that precipitates increases in heart rate and intravascular volume expansion.[45] Pregnant patients demonstrate a greater decrease in blood pressure in response to sympathectomy, which may be related to the decrease in vascular resistance or to further reductions in cardiac preload.

Systemic blood pressures vary with gestation. Although systolic blood pressure remains relatively constant throughout pregnancy, diastolic blood pressure falls during the first and second trimesters, reaching a nadir between 16 to 24 weeks. Diastolic pressure averages 55 to 65 mmHg during this period. After 24 to 26 weeks, diastolic pressure progressively increases and may reach nonpregnant values by term.[3, 46] Low diastolic pressure can mask the onset of hypertension associated with preeclampsia. For example, a diastolic pressure of 70 mmHg measured at 24 weeks' gestation could be an early sign of impending preeclampsia.

Although PVR decreases, pulmonary capillary wedge pressure (PCWP) and pulmonary artery systolic and diastolic pressures remain at nonpregnant values.[36] Since flow is dependent on the ratio of pressure to resistance, unchanged pulmonary blood pressure represents increased blood flow and volume through the pulmonary

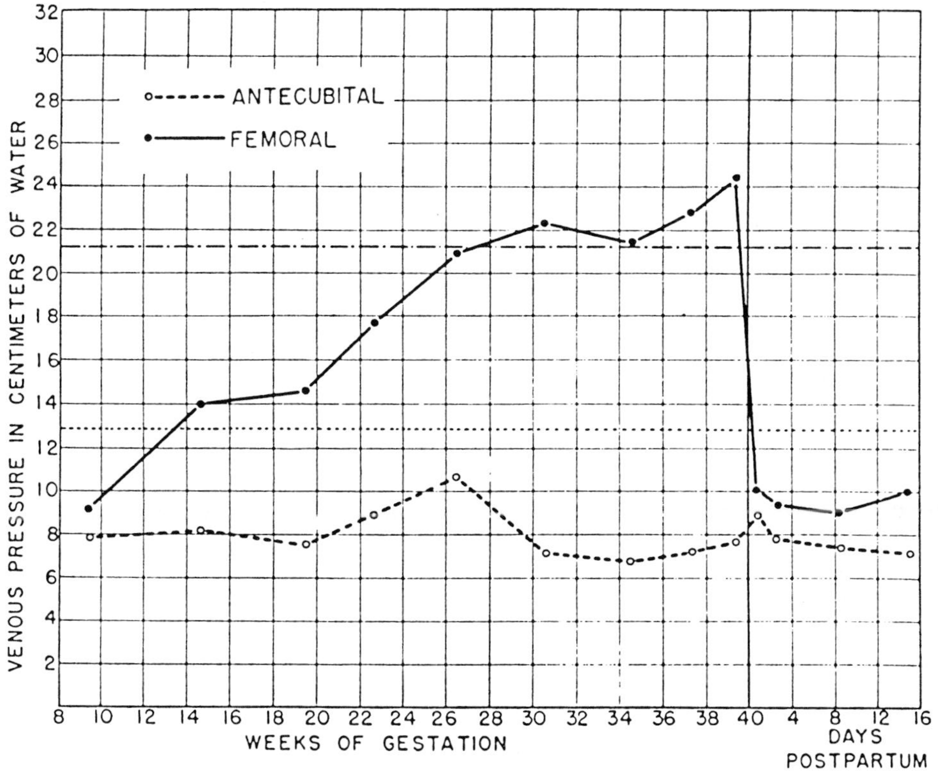

Figure 4–1. Serial changes in antecubital and femoral venous blood pressure throughout normal pregnancy and early puerperium. These measurements were made on women in the supine position. (From McLennan CE: Antecubital and femoral venous pressure in normal and toxemia pregnancy. Am J Obstet Gynecol 45:568, 1943.)

vasculature consistent with the increased cardiac output. Despite maintaining nonpregnant values of PCWP, the parturient is more susceptible to serous transudation and development of pulmonary edema owing to a decrease in colloid oncotic pressure (see "Plasma Volume and Hematology," later in this chapter).[36, 47]

In summary, cardiac output, left ventricular end-diastolic volume, heart rate, and stroke volume increase in pregnancy, and ejection fraction, pulmonary artery pressure, PCWP, and RAP appear unaltered. Maternal cardiovascular parameters are summarized in Table 4–4.

Uterine Perfusion and Aortocaval Syndrome

The uterine vasculature is nearly maximally vasodilated throughout pregnancy. As a consequence, any decrease in maternal mean arterial pressure (MAP) decreases uterine perfusion. Sensitivity to α_1-adrenergic stimulation is maintained, and α_1-adrenergic stimulation produces constriction of the uterine vasculature and decreased uterine perfusion. This occurs despite increased maternal MAPs accompanying α_1-adrenergic stimulation. For this reason, indirect-acting positive inotropes and chronotropes such as ephedrine are preferred over α_1 agonists such as phenylephrine for blood pressure support during pregnancy. However, in the face of prolonged, unresponsive, or life-threatening hypotension during pregnancy, α_1 agonists should not be withheld over concerns for uterine perfusion. Indeed, Moran and associates documented the safety of phenylephrine, when used in small incremental bolus injections, in healthy, nonlaboring parturients.[48]

Uterine contractions reduce blood flow through the uterine vascular bed, regardless of maternal blood pressure, by vessel compression. Intermittent interruption of blood flow and oxygen delivery is the basis of some fetal heart rate decelerations associated with contractions. Fetal hypoxemia can result from profound or prolonged maternal hypotension, prolonged or frequent uterine contractions, uterine tetany, or α_1-adrenergic stimulation, especially in the face of preexisting placental insufficiency.

Aortocaval Syndrome

Cardiac preload can be severely and rapidly reduced in the pregnant patient by compression of the vena cava by the gravid uterus. Acute reductions in cardiac preload will result in the rapid onset of maternal hypotension. As discussed previously, because the uteroplacental vasculature cannot compensate by further vasodilatation, hypotension decreases uteroplacental perfusion.[49–51] Importantly, abdominal aortic compression can also occur and resemble coarctation of the aorta. Thus, decreased uterine artery pressures can occur despite the presence of normal maternal brachial blood pressure in the arm. Therefore, uterine displacement is vital and not dependent on apparently normal maternal blood pressure.

Although the aortocaval syndrome is classically described as occurring after the 20th week of gestation, partial vena caval compression likely occurs prior to this time. Placing the patient in 15 degrees of left lateral tilt (left uterine displacement [LUD]) treats or prevents the syndrome. Increased abdominal mass (e.g., obesity, multiple gestations) accentuates caval occlusion and may require additional uterine deflection. Lateral decubitus positioning or, ultimately, knee-chest position results in the greatest unloading of the vena cava and can be employed when fetal distress continues despite LUD. Although LUD has been shown to be superior to right uterine displacement (RUD),[52] occasionally, some patients respond better to RUD than to LUD. Aortocaval compression may also be worsened by bearing down efforts during the second stage of labor.[53]

Although most supine nonanesthetized patients do not demonstrate clinical hypotension prior to the 20th week, reductions in preload may accompany initiation of general or regional anesthesia. Regional anesthesia can reduce preload by producing a sympathectomy, and during general anesthesia, the increase in intrathoracic pressure that accompanies positive-pressure ventilation reduces preload. Uterine displacement should be considered during anesthesia after the 12th week of pregnancy.

Changes in Clinical Examination and Laboratory Data

The increased intracardiac volume and blood flow that occur during pregnancy cause changes that would be considered abnormal in nonpregnant patients. Echocardiography examination reveals enlargement of all four cardiac chambers and in valvular annular diameters.[54] Between 12 and 20 weeks' gestation, greater than 90% of all patients develop physiologic systolic murmurs.[55] Multivalvular regurgitation has been identified including the tricuspid (>90% incidence), pulmonic (>90% incidence), and mitral (>20% incidence) valves on echocardiography.[54] However, diastolic murmurs are heard infrequently, suggesting that pulmonic regurgitation is mild and not detectable by auscultation. Diastolic murmurs, considered to be potentially pathologic by most practitioners, occur in less than 20% of pregnant patients.[55] Wide splitting of S_1 is also found on auscultation in the majority of patients as well as a loud S_3 and occasionally S_4.[55, 56] Other than the potential pathology associated with diastolic murmurs, few cardiac auscultatory changes developing during pregnancy are noteworthy.

Several benign electrocardiogram changes occur during pregnancy. There may be up to a 15- to 20-degree left axis deviation resulting from cephalad displacement of the heart by the elevation of the diaphragm. Increased irregularity in cardiac rhythm is seen, including ventricular extrasystoles and supraventricular tachycardia. Alterations of cardiac rhythms may be the result of atrial enlargement and stretching of cardiac conduction pathways. Loss of Q waves in Lead aVF (augmented unipolar lead, left leg) and inversion or flattening of T waves in Lead III have also been reported.[3]

Chest roentgenography often shows an increase in cardiac silhouette size suggestive of left ventricular hypertrophy. Increased pulmonary vascular markings may also be evident. These changes should not be of concern in the absence of clinical symptoms.

Homeostasis

Plasma Volume and Hematology

One of the most important maternal adaptations during pregnancy is the expansion of plasma volume and the increase in red blood cell mass. Expanded blood volume allows increased flow to hypermetabolic organ systems without reducing blood flow to other organs. Although hemoglobin concentration decreases, cardiac output is increased, producing a net increase in substrate delivery to the tissues. Indeed, the reduced hematocrit may enhance tissue oxygen delivery by reducing blood viscosity and increasing microcirculatory flow.

Intravascular volume increases progressively starting around the 10th week of gestation and becomes maximal between the 30 and the 34th weeks of gestation.[57] There is no evidence of further increases after this time.[57] The mean increase in plasma volume is approximately 50% but there is a wide range of reported increases, varying between 20 and 100%.[57]

Red blood cell mass begins to increase at approximately the 10th week of gestation. Without iron supplementation, the increase averages 15 to 20%; iron supplements result in an approximate 30% increase in red cell mass.[27] The red blood cell mass continues to rise throughout pregnancy and peaks at term.

Decreased hemoglobin concentration may make the diagnosis of iron-deficiency anemia problematic. Mean corpuscular volume is the best indicator of true anemia during pregnancy. However, the average life of a red blood cell is 120 days, and changes in corpuscular volume take time to accumulate, potentially delaying diagnosis. A mean corpuscular volume of 82 mm^3 or greater is not associated with true iron-deficiency anemia.[3] Most obstetricians recommend iron supplementation during pregnancy because the greater hemoglobin concentrations that result provide the parturient greater reserves in case of complications during labor and delivery.

The proportionately greater increase in intravascular volume when compared with that of red blood cell mass results in a decline in serum hemoglobin concentrations and explains the apparent anemia observed during pregnancy. As discussed, red blood cell mass increases throughout pregnancy, whereas expansion of plasma volume peaks at 30 to 34 weeks. Thus, hemoglobin concentration is lowest at 30 to 34 weeks, corresponding to the plateau in volume expansion. Despite the decrease in serum hemoglobin concentration, oxygen delivery is maintained or increased owing to the increase in cardiac output and tissue perfusion. Most importantly, the reported average blood losses of 500 ml for vaginal delivery and 1000 ml for cesarean delivery are easily tolerated by most healthy patients.[58–60]

Alterations in platelet and leukocyte concentrations also occur during pregnancy. Platelet count is uniformly reported to be decreased during pregnancy.[58, 61, 62] Decreases in platelet count appear to occur progressively during gestation, with a nadir of approximately 260,000/μl at term.[61, 62] Increased mean platelet volume is consistent with a younger platelet population and suggests a decrease in platelet lifespan in pregnancy.[63] The decrease in platelet count does not affect bleeding time and hemostasis.[62]

Pregnancy is associated with a mild leukocytosis, with a mean leukocyte count of 9500/mm^3 during the first trimester and 10,500/mm^3 after the 12th week of gestation and may rise as high 16,000/mm^3.[58] Further increases occur with the onset of labor. An increased white blood cell count complicates the diagnosis of infection and the response to antibiotic therapy.

Serum Electrolytes, Proteins, and Viscosity

Expansion of plasma volume occurs in early pregnancy, and numerous changes in serum composition occur concomitantly. There is a 14% decrease in serum colloid oncotic pressure, representing an increase in the quantity of free water relative to proteins and electrolytes.[64] Decreased oncotic pressure is partially responsible for the edema noted during pregnancy as well as the increased propensity of parturients to develop pulmonary edema. Serum sodium concentration decreases, and it has been postulated that there is a "resetting" of central osmoreceptors necessary to maintain the expanded plasma volume. Changes in serum electrolyte composition are summarized in Table 4–5. Ionized serum calcium concentrations do not decrease in pregnancy despite a decrease in total calcium concentration, likely owing to the concomitant decrease in serum albumin concentration.[65]

There is also a relative decrease in the serum concentration of most proteins. However, the absolute mass of these proteins may increase or remain constant because of the expanded plasma volume. Of particular interest to the anesthesiologist are decreases in the concentra-

TABLE 4–5
Alterations in Major Serum Electrolytes

Electrolyte	Nonpregnant	Vector	Pregnant
Na^+	140 mEq/L	Decrease	137 mEq/L
K^+	3.9 mEq/L	Decrease	3.6 mEq/L
Cl^-		No change	
HCO_3^{-2}	24 mEq/L	Decrease	20 mEq/L
Ca^{2+}	10.2 mg/dL	Decrease	9.2 mg/dl
Mg^{2+}	2.1 mg/dl	Decrease	1.6 mg/dl
Zn^{2+}	883 mg/L	Decrease	635 mg/L
Cu^{2+}	1.14 mg/L	Increase	2.03 mg/L
PO_4^{-2}		No change	

Data from American College of Obstetricians and Gynecologists: CREOG Basic Science Monograph. Maternal Physiology. Washington, DC, ACOG, 1985; and Pitkin RM, Gebhart MP: Serum calcium concentrations in human pregnancy. Am J Obstet Gynecol 127:775, 1977.

tions of serum albumin and plasma cholinesterase.[66–69] A decrease in serum albumin results in less of a "reservoir" for the binding of protein-bound drugs. In theory, this may result in increased serum concentrations of highly protein-bound anesthetic agents such as sodium thiopental and cause an increased clinical effect. Practically, this is of little consequence. Reductions in plasma cholinesterase activity in pregnancy are discussed further under "Neuromuscular Function," later in this chapter.

The decreased concentrations of serum proteins in conjunction with decreased erythrocyte concentrations contribute to a decrease in blood viscosity that may enhance tissue oxygen delivery by increasing flow through the microcirculation.

Hemostasis and Fibrinolysis

Pregnancy is often referred to as a "hypercoagulable" state. Whether initiation of clot formation is more likely to occur during pregnancy is controversial. What is certain is that many clotting factors, especially fibrinogen, increase during pregnancy. Elevated clotting factors provide abundant substrate when the clotting system is activated, ensuring a reserve of materials involved in clot formation. This is an important maternal adaptation and helps to achieve maternal hemostasis postdelivery. Other clotting factors that increase during pregnancy include VII, VIII, IX, and X.[70–72] A slight increase in levels of Factor II occurs, whereas Factors XI and XIII decrease.

Pulmonary embolism is the leading cause of death in obstetric patients. Thrombus formation in the lower extremities may be related to the increased concentrations in clotting factors combined with the elevated femoral venous pressures and venous stasis secondary to vena caval compression. The relative contribution of clotting mechanisms versus venous stasis to the increased frequency of pulmonary embolism is unclear.

Glucose Metabolism and Endocrine Function

Glucose metabolism changes significantly during pregnancy and is an important maternal adaptation that provides optimal growth conditions for the fetus. Glucose transport across the placenta is concentration-dependent and driven by maternal serum glucose concentrations. The maternal system develops a relative state of insulin resistance to provide a greater glucose concentration gradient. Decreased peripheral tissue sensitivity to insulin[14] or circulating placental hormones, or both, probably account for the insulin resistance. As a result, a given carbohydrate load produces higher peak maternal serum glucose concentrations, which remain elevated for a longer period of time compared with those of the nonpregnant state.[73] The combined increases in concentration gradient and in duration of serum glucose elevation drive glucose across the placenta for fetal use (Fig. 4–2). Insulin resistance helps to explain the phenomena of gestational diabetes mellitus and the usual exacerbation of diabetes mellitus during pregnancy. Delivery and extraction of the placenta rapidly reverse the effects and make it difficult to predict postdelivery insulin requirements. Severe maternal hypoglycemia can occur if predelivery insulin dosing regimens are continued postdelivery or perioperatively. Conversely, continued fetal extraction of maternal serum glucose in the presence of maternal fasting will result in glucose concentrations lower than those of fasting nonpregnant patients.[74] Overt hypoglycemia usually does not occur. Administration of intravenous dextrose or insulin in

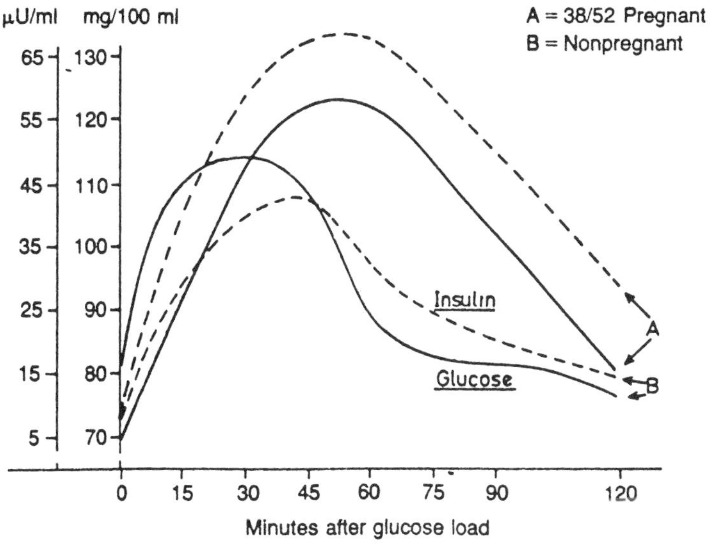

Figure 4–2. Mean plasma glucose and insulin concentrations following a 50-gm oral glucose load in healthy women at 38 weeks of normal pregnancy and the same women 12 weeks' postdelivery (labeled "Nonpregnant"). (From American College of Obstetricians and Gynecologists: CREOG Basic Science Monograph. Maternal Physiology. Washington, DC, ACOG, © 1985.)

the immediate "predelivery" period in diabetic patients should be guided by blood sugar values.

Although glucose readily crosses the placenta, maternal insulin does not. Fetal serum glucose concentrations depend solely on the secretion of fetal insulin in response to a maternal glucose load. Thus, neonatal hypoglycemia may occur postdelivery after stimulation of fetal insulin secretion by elevated maternal blood glucose concentrations followed by abrupt removal of the maternal glucose supply by delivery. Care must be taken with maternal glucose administration immediately preceding delivery to prevent iatrogenic maternal hyperglycemia and reactive neonatal hypoglycemia.

The anterior pituitary gland enlarges during pregnancy, suggesting increased secretion of trophic hormones.[75] There is an increase in free cortisol in pregnancy despite a doubling in the serum concentrations of corticosteroid-binding globulin.[76, 77] Elevated cortisol may be an adaptation to meet the added stresses of pregnancy, labor, and delivery.

Thyroid function is unchanged during pregnancy. Free triiodothyronine (T_3) and thyroxine (T_4) concentrations are similar to those of the nonpregnant state.[78] Thyroid-binding globulin concentrations increase during pregnancy, which alters the result of the free T_4 index. The concentration of free T_4 has therefore become the standard for assessing thyroid function during pregnancy.[79] A progressive rise in parathyroid hormone occurs during pregnancy that may exceed 135% of nonpregnant values.[80]

Neurologic and Anesthetic Changes During Pregnancy

Neuronal Sensitivity

Pregnant patients exhibit increased sensitivity to anesthetic agents compared with their nonpregnant counterparts. This phenomenon occurs with both volatile anesthetic agents and local anesthetics, but not with narcotics, barbiturates, and benzodiazepines. The minimal alveolar concentration (MAC) of volatile anesthetic agents declines approximately 40% and is not agent-specific.[81, 82] Increased neuronal sensitivity during regional blockade has been demonstrated during epidural and spinal anesthesia as well as median nerve blockade.[83–85] Reduced drug requirements for local anesthetics for spinal and epidural anesthesia occur early in pregnancy and do not appear related to physical alteration of the spinal or epidural space.[83]

The mechanism for reduced anesthetic requirements during pregnancy remains unclear and may be multifactorial. Proposed mechanisms include increased serum and central nervous system progesterone concentrations, increased β endorphins, decreased serum bicarbonate levels, and an additive or synergistic effect of several of these factors. Serum and cerebrospinal fluid progesterone levels increase during pregnancy.[86, 87] Progesterone possesses inherent anesthetic properties and intravenous administration can produce sedation, and high progesterone concentrations result in loss of consciousness.[88, 89] Indeed, progesterone decreases volatile anesthetic requirements in animals.[90] Increased serum β endorphins and endorphin-like substances in pregnancy may have an additive effect with anesthetic agents and may be responsible for the "hyperanalgesic" state of pregnancy.[91, 92] Narcotic antagonists oppose the analgesic state observed during pregnancy, implicating opioid receptor involvement in the reduced MAC requirements of pregnancy.[91] Finally, decreased serum bicarbonate increases the fraction of un-ionized local anesthetic and has been proposed as a mechanism for increased neuronal sensitivity to local anesthetics.

These observations notwithstanding, the changes in anesthetic potency in pregnancy have little effect on the conduct of general anesthesia and regional anesthesia during pregnancy. As with any patient, volatile anesthetic concentrations are titrated to the physiologic responses of the patient. However, practitioners should be aware of these changes and vigilance must be maintained. Changes in depth of anesthesia will be more rapid owing to the reduction in FRC discussed earlier, and a greater anesthetic effect will occur at a given alveolar concentration because of the increased sensitivity of pregnant patients to volatile anesthetics.

Similarly, safe epidural anesthesia requires drug titration to achieve the desired dermatomal level of blockade. Although reducing local anesthetic doses for subarachnoid block, particularly with lidocaine and tetracaine, is warranted, this precaution appears questionable for bupivacaine since the author's group routinely uses 12 to 15 mg of bupivacaine for cesarean section. Remember, the cephalad spread of anesthesia during subarachnoid block also depends on the degree of thoracic kyphosis and possible placement of the spinal needle on the caudad versus cephalad slopes of the lumbar lordosis may lead to lesser or greater local anesthetic spread, respectively. Furthermore, increased abdominal pressure and engorgement of epidural veins increase pressure within the epidural space during pregnancy. Because epidural space pressure frequently exceeds atmospheric pressure, the hanging drop technique for identifying the epidural space is a poor choice in obstetric anesthesia.[93] In addition, the engorgement of epidural veins due to venous shunting from the caval system may increase the incidence of intravenous epidural catheter insertion during pregnancy. Finally, the effects of intra-abdominal pressure are evidenced by the greater spread of spinal anesthesia among twin pregnancies compared with singleton pregnancies.[94] In summary, an awareness of the potential for exaggerated response to local anesthetics is the key to safety.

Neuromuscular Function

The action of nondepolarizing neuromuscular blockers is not appreciably affected by pregnancy. As discussed previously, plasma cholinesterase activity declines between 25 and 30% at term, with further reductions occurring in the immediate postpartum period.[67–69] Decreased plasma pseudocholinesterase concentration may result in a slight increase in the duration of action of succinylcholine at term; however, the significance of this effect remains controversial.[69] The duration of action of succinylcholine is clearly increased in the postpartum period, likely due to a reduction in the volume of distribution occurring after delivery.[69] However, any increase in duration of action that may occur at term is minimal, and the concerns of performing a rapid-sequence induction and establishing an airway supersede the consideration of the potential for a slight increase in duration of action.

Gastrointestinal System

The anesthetic implications of changes occurring in the gastrointestinal system during pregnancy remain one of the most controversial subjects in obstetric anesthesia. Conflicting reports concerning gastric volume, pressure, and pH have been published over the years. Various theories relating to displacement and disruption of the lower esophageal sphincter have also been proposed. Much of the older data support increased gastric volume and decreased gastric pH during pregnancy.[95–98] The increased incidence of heartburn observed during pregnancy highly suggests diminution in lower esophageal sphincter efficiency in pregnancy. Decreased barrier pressure appears to occur early in pregnancy independent of gastric pressure.[99] More recent evidence suggests that it is unlikely that gastric pH and volume are increased solely by pregnancy.[100] Traditional teaching states that gastric emptying is delayed in the peripartum period and for at least 2 hours and up to 18 hours postpartum. Increased sympathetic tone and catecholamine release associated with the pain of labor as well as narcotic administration may be responsible for this purported peripartum decrease in gastric emptying. However, one study reports that the percentage of patients presenting for postpartum tubal ligation between 1 and 45 hours postdelivery who had gastric contents exceeding 25 ml and with a pH of less than 2.5 did not differ from control nonpregnant patients.[101] Nevertheless, adequate non-narcotic analgesia may improve gastric emptying during labor. There is some direct evidence for this postulate, since gastric emptying times are faster in patients receiving bupivicaine epidural analgesia than in those patients receiving narcotic-bupivicaine epidural analgesia during labor.[102] This is not surprising, since intravenous narcotics delay gastric emptying,[103, 104] and both intravenous narcotics and anticholinergics decrease lower esophageal sphincter tone.[103, 104] Until this conflicting scientific evidence is resolved, pregnant patients should be treated as being at risk for aspiration and they require the appropriate protective maneuvers discussed subsequently.

Since insurance data clearly indicate an increased risk of pulmonary aspiration of gastric contents during anesthesia in pregnancy, endotracheal intubation, either by rapid-sequence induction or by awake intubation in those patients with potentially difficult airways, remains the standard of care during general anesthesia. During rapid-sequence induction, succinylcholine increases lower esophageal sphincter pressure proportionately to the accompanying rise in intragastric pressure. Succinylcholine remains the muscle relaxant of choice for rapid-sequence inductions during pregnancy. Minimal preoperative preparation should include 30 ml oral 0.3 M sodium citrate. Histamine blockers and metoclopramide may be considered for high-risk patients.

Renal System

Renal plasma flow and glomerular filtration rate (GFR) both increase markedly in response to the expanded intravascular volume and the increased metabolic load associated with pregnancy. Estimates of these increases range from 50 to 75% and have been identified as early as 16 weeks' gestation.[105, 106] Increased renal filtration does not appear to appreciably affect the duration of action of any anesthetic drugs that undergo renal excretion.

Glycosuria occurs frequently in pregnant patients despite normal serum glucose levels.[107] Glycosuria does not reliably indicate maternal pathology. However, the presence of protein in the urine should be viewed with suspicion, especially when more than 200 to 300 mg of protein is collected in 24 hours.[3, 27]

Plasma levels of bicarbonate, creatinine, and blood urea nitrogen (BUN) decrease during pregnancy. Increased excretion of bicarbonate partially compensates for the respiratory alkalosis that occurs early in pregnancy. This compensation is not complete, resulting in a slight alkalemia in pregnancy with an average pH ranging from 7.40 to 7.44.[3] Serum bicarbonate level averages 20 mEq/L with a range from 18 to 22 mEq/L.[3] Serum creatinine and BUN decrease throughout pregnancy in a nonlinear fashion. These decreases begin prior to the increase observed in GFR, making it unclear whether the decreased BUN and creatinine result from increased renal excretion or from alterations in maternal protein metabolism. It is important to note that BUN and creatinine levels that would be considered "normal" in nonpregnancy may be considered elevated in pregnancy and could represent renal compromise.

CLINICAL IMPLICATIONS OF MATERNAL PHYSIOLOGIC CHANGES

General Anesthesia for Cesarean Section

The physiologic implications of the administration of general anesthesia are outlined in Table 4–6. Maternal physiologic alterations may increase the likelihood of difficult intubation. The author's group chooses to avoid these potential problems by the preferential use of regional anesthesia when not contraindicated. When general anesthesia is indicated, a short-handled laryngoscope and a maximum of a 7-mm endotracheal tube should be used to facilitate intubation.[108] A plan or algorithm for failed intubation and the necessary emergency equipment to carry out the plan should be readily at hand, and these are discussed in Chapter 7.

Maximal denitrogenation/preoxygenation prior to induction of anesthesia is critical. The combined effects of decreased FRC and in-

TABLE 4–6
Implications of Maternal Physiologic Alterations on the Administration of General Anesthesia

Physiologic Alteration	Interventions
Increased difficulty of endotracheal intubation	Short-handled laryngoscope
Airway edema	Smaller endotracheal tube
Venous engorgement	Failed intubation protocol and emergency airway equipment in operating room
Soft tissue obstruction (breasts, chest shape)	
Rapid arterial oxygen desaturation	Preoxygenation for 3–5 min
Increased metabolic needs and oxygen consumption	Titrate N_2O to keep Spo_2 >96%
Maternal	More rapid denitrogenation possible owing to decreased FRC
Fetal	
Decreased FRC	
Increased risk of aspiration of pulmonary contents and aspiration pneumonitis	Rapid-sequence induction with cricoid pressure or awake intubation
Increased intragastric pressure	Prophylactic nonparticulate antacid
Decreased intragastric pH	
Possible decreased LES tone	
Altered response to volatile anesthetics	Reduced volatile anesthetic requirements and careful titration required compared with "nonpregnant" patients
Decreased MAC	
More rapid uptake	
Decreased FRC	
More rapid F_A/F_I rate of rise	
Muscular effects of progesterone	Defasciculation with nondepolarizing muscle relaxants not routinely necessary
Decreased postoperative myalgia	

Abbreviations: FRC = functional residual capacity; LES = lower esophageal sphincter; MAC = minimal alveolar concentration.

creased oxygen consumption result in rapid arterial oxygen desaturation during apnea. Total washout of lung N_2 with 100% O_2 for 3 to 5 minutes prior to induction of general anesthesia is indicated.

The MAC of halogenated agents is reduced in pregnancy. Also, F_A/F_I (the ratio of alveolar gas concentration to inspired gas concentration) rate of rise of potent inhalational agents is increased owing to the decrease in FRC. Consequently, the onset of action of the potent inhalational anesthetics is more rapid, with a greater physiologic effect at lower concentrations. Overdosage and hypotension can occur if potent agents are used as part of a "routine" and not titrated to clinical effect.

Regional Anesthesia for Cesarean Section and Labor

The physiologic implications of the administration of regional anesthesia during pregnancy are summarized in Table 4–7.

Shunting of blood return from the lower extremities through collateral venous conduits results in engorgement of the epidural veins. This engorgement, in theory, can result in an increased incidence of intravenous cannulation by the epidural catheter. Inserting catheters between contractions may decrease the likelihood of intravenous catheter placement. However, this rationale has never been tested.

Neuronal sensitivity to local anesthetics is increased during pregnancy. During epidural anesthesia, local anesthetics should be titrated to achieve the desired clinical effect, and a wide variation in dosage requirements should be expected. During spinal anesthesia, a reduction in total dosage should be considered.

Pregnant patients are more prone to develop hypotension in response to sympathectomy when compared with nonpregnant patients. Uterine displacement should be maintained at all times. The incidence and severity of hypotension may be blunted by a 10- to 15-ml/kg intra-

TABLE 4–7
Implications of Maternal Physiologic Alterations on the Administration of Regional Anesthesia

Physiologic Alteration	Interventions
Increased neuronal sensitivity to local anesthetics or decreased volume of epidural space	Epidural titrated fractionally to effect Dosage requirements may be decreased SAB dosage may need to be decreased Increased lumbar lordosis may enhance cephalad spread and head and neck should be elevated after SAB placement
Aortocaval compression resulting in epidural venous engorgement	Increased incidence of epidural catheters placed intravenously, which may be reduced by catheter insertion between contractions
Aortocaval compression resulting in reduced preload and exaggerated hypotensive response to sympathectomy	Preload IV crystalloid prior to regional anesthesia 10–15 ml/kg Maintain uterine displacement at all times

Abbreviation: SAB = subarachnoid block.

venous preload of crystalloid. The benefit of this intervention has been recently brought into question. However, in the absence of maternal contraindications, fluid loading remains a reasonable precaution.

Maternal Physiologic Adaptations and Clinical Management

The implications of maternal physiologic adaptations during pregnancy are summarized in Table 4–8.

The uterine vasculature is normally nearly maximally vasodilated and uteroplacental perfusion directly correlates with MAP. Decreases in MAP should be treated promptly and aggressively to maintain perfusion and prevent fetal hypoxia. Nominally, a 20 to 30% decrease in MAP warrants treatment; however, less substantial decreases in MAP may result in signs of fetal distress in an already compromised fetus. Indirect-acting vasopressors with minimal α_1 activity are the agents of choice. Ephedrine is the most commonly used of these agents.

An acute reduction in preload can occur from vena caval occlusion in the supine position, resulting in maternal hypotension, decreased uterine blood flow, and fetal hypoxia (supine hypotension syndrome). Abdominal aortic compression can occur to a lesser degree and contribute to placental hypoperfusion. Intravascular volume loading and vasopressors may be used to improve uterine perfusion; however, the primary treatment remains unloading of the vena cava by lateral uterine displacement.

The endocrine changes that occur in pregnancy result in a relative resistance to insulin, altered response to a glucose load, and the propensity for the development of gestational diabetes mellitus. These changes may rapidly reverse after delivery, and insulin requirements are unpredictable. Use of routine predelivery insulin dosages may result in hypoglycemia postpartum. Insulin should be withheld preoperatively and serum glucose treated on an as-needed basis intraoperatively. Postoperatively, patients should be placed on sliding-scale insulin coverage.

TEN PRACTICAL POINTS

1. Decreased functional residual capacity and increased oxygen consumption during pregnancy result in rapid arterial oxygen desaturation during apnea.
2. The uterine vascular bed is maximally dilated during pregnancy. Reductions in blood pressure reduce uterine blood flow.
3. Although plasma cholinesterase activity declines 25 to 30% during pregnancy, this should not influence succinylcholine dose selection.
4. The maternal insulin requirements may fall abruptly following delivery. Titrate insulin administration accordingly.
5. Utilize left uterine displacement to maintain cardiac output.

TABLE 4–8
Management of Maternal Physiology and Uterine Blood Flow

Physiologic Alteration	Intervention
Acute reduction in preload from aortocaval compression resulting in maternal hypotension or fetal hypoxia	Uterine displacement LUD after 20 wk EGA Alternate uterine displacement if unresponsive to LUD; maternal knee chest position allows maximal caval and umbilical cord unloading Vasopressors Ephedrine Avoid alpha$_1$-agonists when possible. Alpha$_1$-agonists are indicated with profound maternal hypotension. Intravascular volume expansion to increase cardiac preload
Uteroplacental perfusion directly correlates with maternal MAP	Decreases in MAP should be treated promptly and aggressively to maintain uterine perfusion and prevent fetal hypoxia. Treat as above
More prone to hypoxemia Decrease in FRC in the supine position Closing capacity may impinge on tidal volume Hypoxemia exaggerated by obesity and underlying pulmonary pathology	Maintain low therapeutic threshold for prophylactic oxygen administration during regional anesthetics and prior to delivery Pulmonary unloading by semisitting position
Propensity for development of diabetes mellitus and gestational diabetes mellitus owing to circulating placental hormones	Rapid recovery from "diabetic" effects of placental hormones postdelivery Preoperative insulin administration should be based on blood sugar values Postoperative insulin requirements are rapidly reduced and unpredictable; an insulin sliding scale should be used postoperatively
Expansion of intravascular volume and increase in red blood cell mass **Ample substrate for clot formation owing to "overpriming" of the clotting cascade with clotting factors**	Average blood loss of 500–1000 ml for vaginal and cesarean delivery well tolerated
Increased GFR and renal plasma flow **Decreased BUN and creatinine**	Glycosuria—often normal Proteinuria—potentially pathologic Nonpregnant "normal" values of BUN and creatinine may represent frank elevations during pregnancy

Abbreviations: LUD = left uterine displacement; EGA = estimated gestational age; MAP = mean arterial pressure; FRC = functional residual capacity; GFR = glomerular filtration rate; BUN = blood urea nitrogen.

6. Increased sensitivity of pregnant patients to the potent inhalation agents and the more rapid rise in alveolar gas concentration increase the potential for patient overdose.
7. Avoid nasotracheal intubation during pregnancy.
8. Serum creatinine or blood urea nitrogen levels decrease during pregnancy.
9. Proteinuria, not glycosuria, indicates maternal pathology.
10. Pregnancy increases sensitivity to local anesthetics.

REFERENCES

1. Mackenzie AI: Laryngeal oedema complicating obstetric anaesthesia. Anaesthesia 33:271, 1978.
2. Hytten FE, Leitch I: Preparation for breast feeding. *In* Hytten FE, Leitch I (eds): The Physiology of Human Pregnancy. Oxford, Blackwell, 1971, p 234.
3. American College of Obstetricians and Gynecologists: CREOG Basic Science Monograph. Maternal Physiology. Washington, DC, ACOG, 1985.
4. Thomson KJ, Cohen ME: Studies on the circula-

tion in pregnancy. II. Vital capacity observations in normal pregnant women. Surg Gynecol Obstet 66:591, 1938.
5. Gilroy RJ, Mangura BT, Lavietes MH: Rib cage and abdominal volume displacement during breathing in pregnancy. Am Rev Respir Dis 137:668, 1988.
6. Report on Confidential Enquiries into Maternal Deaths in England and Wales, 1982–1984. No. 34. London, Her Majesty's Stationery Office, 1989.
7. Report on Confidential Enquiries into Maternal Deaths in England and Wales, 1979–1981. No. 29. London, Her Majesty's Stationery Office, 1986.
8. Clapp JF III: Oxygen consumption during treadmill exercise before, during and after pregnancy. Am J Obstet Gynecol 161:1458, 1989.
9. Archer GW Jr, Marx GF: Arterial oxygen tension during apnea in parturient women. Br J Anaesth 46:358, 1974.
10. Byrne F, Oduro-Dominah A, Kipling R: The effect of pregnancy on pulmonary nitrogen wash out. A study of preoxygenation. Anesthesia 42:148, 1987.
11. Pernoll ML, Metcalf J, Kovach PA, et al: Ventilation during rest and exercise in pregnancy and postpartum. Respir Physiol 25:295, 1975.
12. Prowse CM, Gaensler EAZ: Respiratory acid-base changes during pregnancy. Anesthesia 26:382, 1965.
13. Clapp JF, Seaward BL, Sleamaker RH, Hiser J: Maternal physiologic adaptations to early human pregnancy. Am J Obstet Gynecol 159:1456, 1988.
14. Skatrud JB, Dempsey JA, Kaiser DG: Ventilatory response to medroxyprogesterone acetate in normal subjects: Time course and mechanism. J Appl Physiol 44:939, 1978.
15. Lyons HA, Antonio R: The sensitivity of the respiratory center in pregnancy and after the administration of progesterone. Trans Assoc Am Physicians 72:173, 1959.
16. Holdcroft A, Bevan DR, O'Sullivan JC, et al: Airway closure and pregnancy. Anesthesia 32:517, 1977.
17. Baraka AS, Hanna MT, Jabbour SI, et al: Preoxygenization of pregnant and nonpregnant women in the head up versus supine position. Anesth Analg 75:757, 1992.
18. Baldwin GR, Moorthi DS, Welton JA, et al: New lung functions and pregnancy. Am J Obstet Gynecol 127:235, 1977.
19. Weinberger SE, Weiss ST, Cohen WR, et al: Pregnancy and the lung. Am Rev Respir Dis 121:559, 1980.
20. Milne JA, Mills RJ, Howie AD, Pack AI: Large airways function during normal pregnancy. Br J Obstet Gynaecol 84:448, 1977.
21. Hagerdall M, Morgan CW, Sumner AE, Gutsche BB: Minute ventilation and oxygen consumption during labor with epidural analgesia. Anesthesiology 59:425, 1983.
22. Sangoul F, Fox GS, Houle GL: Effect of regional analgesia on maternal oxygen consumption during the first stage of labor. Am J Obstet Gynecol 121:1080, 1975.
23. Huch A, Huch R, Schneider H, Rooth G: Continuous transcutaneous monitoring of fetal oxygen tension during labour. Br J Obstet Gynaecol (Suppl) 84:1, 1977.
24. McAnolty JH, Netcalfe J, Ueland K: Heart disease in pregnancy. *In* Hurst JN (ed): The Heart, 6th ed. New York, McGraw-Hill, 1985, p 1383.
25. Bean WB, Cogswell R, Dexter M, Embick JF: Vascular changes of the skin in pregnancy. Vascular spiders and palmar erythema. Surg Gynecol Obstet 88:739, 1949.
26. Katz R, Karliner JS, Resnik R: Effect of a natural volume overload state (pregnancy) on left ventricular performance in normal human subjects. Circulation 58:434, 1978.
27. Hytten FE, Lind T: Indices of cardiovascular function. *In* Hytten FE, Lind T (eds): Diagnostic Indices in Pregnancy. Basel, Documenta Geigy, 1973.
28. Ueland K, Novy MJ, Peterson EN, et al: Maternal cardiovascular dynamics. IV. The influence of gestational age on the maternal cardiovascular response to posture and exercise. Am J Obstet Gynecol 104:856, 1969.
29. Robson SC, Hunter S, Moore M, Dunlop W: Haemodynamic changes during the puerperium: A Doppler and M-mode echocardiographic study. Br J Obstet Gynaecol 94:1028, 1987.
30. Equimokhai M, Davison JM, Philips PR, Dunlop W: Non-postural serial changes in renal function during the third trimester of normal human pregnancy. Br J Obstet Gynaecol 88:465, 1982.
31. Mabie WC, DiSessa TG, Crocker LG, et al: A longitudinal study of cardiac output in normal human pregnancy. Am J Obstet Gynecol 170:849, 1994.
32. Elkayam U, Gleicher N: Cardiovascular physiology of pregnancy. *In* Elkayam U, Gleicher N (eds): Cardiovascular Problems in Pregnancy. Diagnosis and Management of Maternal and Fetal Disease. New York, Alan R. Liss, 1982, p 5.
33. Ueland K, Hansen JM: Maternal cardiovascular dynamics. III. Labor and delivery under local and caudal analgesia. Am J Obstet Gynecol 103:8, 1963.
34. Metcalfe J: The maternal heart in the postpartum period. Am J Cardiol 12:439, 1963.
35. Hansen JM, Ueland K: The influence of caudal

analgesia on cardiovascular dynamics during labor and delivery. Acta Anaesthesiol Scand 23:449, 1966.
36. Clark SL, Cotton DB, Lee W, et al: Central hemodynamic assessment of normal term pregnancy. Am J Obstet Gynecol 161:1439, 1989.
37. Howard BK, Goodson JH, Mengert WF: Supine hypotension syndrome in late pregnancy. Obstet Gynecol 1:371, 1953.
38. Kerr MG: The mechanical effects of the gravid uterus in late pregnancy. J Obstet Gynaecol Br Comm 72:513, 1965.
39. Kerr MG, Scott DB, Samuel E: Studies of the inferior vena cava in late pregnancy. Br Med J 1:532, 1964.
40. O'Driscoll K, McCarthy JR: Abruptio placentae and central venous pressures. J Obstet Gynaecol Br Comm 73:923, 1966.
41. McLennan CE: Antecubital and femoral venous pressure in normal and toxemia pregnancy. Am J Obstet Gynecol 45:568, 1943.
42. Goodman RP, Killon AP, Barsh AR, Branch RA: Prostacyclin production during pregnancy: Comparison during normal pregnancy and pregnancy complicated by hypertension. Am J Obstet Gynecol 132:817, 1982.
43. Thomsen JK, Fogh-Andersen N, Jaszczak P, Giese J: Atrial natriuretic peptide (ANP) decrease during normal pregnancy as related to hemodynamic changes and volume regulation. Acta Obstet Gynecol Scand 72:2, 1993.
44. Curran-Everett D, Morris KG Jr, Moore LG: Regional circulatory contributions to increased systemic vascular conductance of pregnancy. Am J Physiol 261:H1842, 1991.
45. Duvekott J, Emile C, Pieters F, et al: Early pregnancy changes in hemodynamics and volume homeostasis are consecutive adjustments triggered by a primary fall in systemic vascular tone. Am J Obstet Gynecol 169:1382, 1993.
46. MacGillvray I, Rose GA, Rowe B: Blood pressure survey in pregnancy. Clin Sci 37:395, 1969.
47. MacLennan FM, MacDonald AF, Campbell DM: Lung water during the puerperium. Anaesthesia 42:141, 1987.
48. Moran DH, Berillo M, LaPorta RF, et al: Phenylephrine and the prevention of hypotension following spinal analgesia for cesarean delivery. J Clin Anesth 3:301, 1991.
49. Bieniarz I, Crottogini JJ, Curachet E: Aortocaval compression by the uterus in late human pregnancy. Am J Obstet Gynecol 100:203, 1968.
50. Marx GF: Aortocaval compression: Incidence and prevention. Bull N Y Acad Med 50:443, 1974.
51. Abitbol MM: Aortic compression and uterine blood flow during pregnancy. Obstet Gynecol 55:5, 1977.
52. Buley RJR, Downing JW, Brock-Utne JG, Cuerden C: Right versus left lateral tilt for caesarean section. Br J Anaesth 49:1009, 1977.
53. Bassell GM, Humayun SG, Marx GF: Maternal bearing down efforts—Another fetal risk? Obstet Gynecol 56:39, 1980.
54. Campos O, Andrade JL, Bocanegra J, et al: Physiologic multivalvular regurgitation during pregnancy: A longitudinal Doppler echocardiographic study. Int J Cardiol 40:3, 1993.
55. Cutforth R, MacDonald MB: Heart sounds and murmurs in pregnancy. Am Heart J 71:741, 1966.
56. O'Rourke RA, Ewy GA, Marcus FI: Cardiac auscultation in pregnancy. Med Ann DC 39:92, 1970.
57. Pritchard JA: Changes in blood volume during pregnancy and delivery. Anesthesiology 26:393, 1965.
58. Pritchard JA, Baldwin RM, Dickey JC, et al: Blood volume changes in pregnancy and the peurperium. II. Red blood cell loss and changes in apparent blood volume during and following vaginal delivery, cesarean section and cesarean section plus cesarean hysterectomy. Am J Obstet Gynecol 84:1271, 1962.
59. DeLeeuw NKM, Lowenstein L, Tucker EC, et al: Correlation of red cell loss at delivery with changes in red cell mass. Am J Obstet Gynecol 100:192, 1968.
60. Euland K: Maternal cardiovascular dynamics. VII. Intrapartum blood volume changes. Am J Obstet Gynecol 126:671, 1976.
61. Sejeny SA, Eastman RD, Baker SR: Platelet counts during normal pregnancy. J Clin Pathol 28:812, 1975.
62. Pitkin RM, Witte DL: Platelet and leukocyte counts during normal pregnancy. JAMA 242:2696, 1979.
63. Fay RA, Hughes AO, Farron NT: Platelets in pregnancy: Hyperdestruction in pregnancy. Obstet Gynecol 61:239, 1983.
64. Oian P, Maltau JM, Noddeland H, Fadness HO: Oedema: Preventing mechanisms in subcutaneous tissue of normal pregnant women. Br J Obstet Gynaecol 92:1113, 1985.
65. Pitkin RM, Gebhart MP: Serum calcium concentrations in human pregnancy. Am J Obstet Gynecol 127:775, 1977.
66. McNair RD, Jaynes RV: Alterations in liver function during normal pregnancy. Am J Obstet Gynecol 80:500, 1960.
67. Shnider SM: Serum cholinesterase activity during pregnancy, labor and puerperium. Anesthesiology 26:335, 1965.
68. Blitt CD, Petty WC, Alberternst EE, Wright BJ: Correlation of plasma cholinesterase activity

and duration of action of succinylcholine during pregnancy. Anesth Analg 56:78, 1977.
69. Leighton BL, Cheek TG, Gross JB, et al: Succinylcholine pharmacodynamics in peripartum patients. Anesthesiology 64:202, 1986.
70. Talbert LM, Langdell RD: Normal values of certain factors in the blood clotting mechanism in pregnancy. Am J Obstet Gynecol 90:44, 1964.
71. Kasper CK, Hoag MS, Aggelar PM, Stone S: Blood clotting factors in pregnancy: Factor VIII concentrations in normal and AHF-deficient women. Obstet Gynecol 24:242, 1964.
72. Coopland A, Alkjaersig N, Fletcher AP: Reduction in plasma factor XIII (fibrin stabilization factor) concentration during pregnancy. J Lab Clin Med 73:144, 1969.
73. O'Sullivan JB, Mahan CM: Criteria for the oral glucose tolerance test in pregnancy. Diabetes 13:278, 1964.
74. Felig P, Lynch V: Starvation in human pregnancy: Hypoglycemia, hypoinsulinemia, and hyperketonemia. Science 170:990, 1970.
75. Gonzalez JG, Elizondo G, Saldivar D, et al: Pituitary gland growth during normal pregnancy: An in vivo study using magnetic resonance imaging. Am J Med 85:217, 1988.
76. Rosenthal HE, Slaunwhite WR Jr, Sandberg AA: Transcortin: A corticosteroid-binding protein of plasma. X. Cortisol and progesterone interplay and unbound levels of these steroids in pregnancy. J Clin Endocrinol Metab 29:352, 1969.
77. Doc RP, Fernandez R, Seal US: Measurement of corticosteroid-binding globulin in man. J Clin Endocrinol Metab 24:1029, 1964.
78. Harada A, Hershman JM, Reed AW, et al: Comparison of thyroid hormone concentrations in the sera of pregnant women. J Clin Endocrinol Metab 48:793, 1979.
79. Chopra IJ, Van Herle AJ, Chua Teco GN, et al: Serum-free thyroxine in thyroidal and nonthyroidal illnesses: A comparison of measurements by radioimmunoassay, equilibrium dialysis, and free thyrocine index. J Clin Endocrinol Metab 51:135, 1980.
80. Pitkin RM, Reynolds WA, Williams GA, Hargis GK: Calcium metabolism in normal pregnancy: A longitudinal study. Am J Obstet Gynecol 133:781, 1979.
81. Palahniuk RJ, Shnider SM, Eger EI II: Pregnancy decreases the requirements for inhaled anesthetic agents. Anesthesiology 41:82, 1974.
82. Gin T, Chan MTV: Decreased alveolar concentration of isoflurane in pregnant humans. Anesthesiology 81:829, 1994.
83. Fagraeus L, Urban B, Bromage P: Spread of epidural analgesia in early pregnancy. Anesthesiology 58:184, 1983.
84. Bromage P: Physiology and pharmacology of epidural analgesia. Anesthesiology 28:592, 1967.
85. Butterworth JF, Walker FO, Lyzak SZ: Pregnancy increases median nerve susceptibility to lidocaine. Anesthesiology 72:692, 1990.
86. Yannone ME, McCurcy JR, Goldfein A: Plasma progesterone levels in normal pregnancy, labor and the puerperium. II. Clinical data. Am J Obstet Gynecol 101:1058, 1968.
87. Datta S, Hurley RJ, Naulty SJ, et al: Plasma and cerebrospinal fluid progesterone levels in pregnant and nonpregnant women. Anesth Analg 65:950, 1986.
88. Selye H: Studies concerning the anesthetic action of steroid hormones. J Pharmacol Exp Ther 73:127, 1941.
89. Merryman W: Progesterone "anesthesia" in human subjects. J Clin Endocrinol Metab 14:1567, 1954.
90. Datta S, Migliozzi RP, Flanagan HL, Krieger NR: Chronically administered progesterone decreases halothane requirements in rabbits. Anesth Analg 68:46, 1989.
91. Gintzler AR: Endorphin-mediated increases in pain threshold during pregnancy. Science 210:193, 1980.
92. Csontos K, Rust M, Halt V, et al: Elevated beta-endorphin levels in pregnant women and their neonates. Life Sci 25:835, 1979.
93. Galbert MW, Marx GF: Extradural pressures in the parturient patient. Anesthesiology 40:499, 1974.
94. Jawan B, Lee JH, Chong ZK, Chang CS: Spread of spinal anesthesia for cesarean section in singleton and twin pregnancies. Br J Anaesth 7:639, 1993.
95. Christofides ND, Ghatei MA, Bloom SR, et al: Decreased plasma motilin concentrations in pregnancy. Br Med J 285:1453, 1982.
96. Davison JS, Davison MC, Hay DM: Gastric emptying time in late pregnancy and labour. J Obstet Gynaecol Br Comm 77:37, 1970.
97. Murray FA, Eishine JP, Fielding J: Gastric secretion in pregnancy. J Obstet Gynaecol Br Emp 64:373, 1957.
98. Hunt JN, Murray FA: Gastric function in pregnancy. J Obstet Gynaecol Br Emp 65:78, 1957.
99. Jones MJ, Mitchell RWD, Hindocha N, James RH: The lower esophageal sphincter in the first trimester of pregnancy: Comparison of supine with lithotomy positions. Br J Anaesth 61:475, 1988.
100. Whitehead EM, Smith M, Dean Y, O'Sullivan G: An evaluation of gastric emptying times in pregnancy and the puerperium. Anaesthesia 48:53, 1993.
101. James CF, Gibbs CP, Banner T: Postpartum peri-

operative risk of aspiration phenomena. Anesthesiology 61:756, 1984.

102. Ewah B, Yau K, King M, et al: Effect of epidural opioids on gastric emptying in labour. Int J Obstet Anaesth 2:125, 1993.
103. Hall AW, Moosa AR, Clark J, et al: The effect of premedication drugs on the lower esophageal high pressure zone and reflux status in rhesus monkeys and man. Gut 16:347, 1975.
104. Brock-Utne JG, Rubin J, Welman S, et al: The effect of glycopyrrolate [Robinol] on the lower esophageal sphincter. Can Anaesth Soc J 25:144, 1978.
105. Dunlop W: Serial changes in renal haemodynamics during normal human pregnancy. Br J Obstet Gynaecol 88:1, 1981.
106. Dignam WJ, Titus P, Assali NS: Renal function in human pregnancy. I. Changes in glomerular filtration rate and renal plasma flow. Proc Soc Exp Biol Med 97:512, 1958.
107. Davison JM, Hytten FE: The effect of pregnancy on the renal handling of glucose. J Obstet Gynaecol Br Comm 82:374, 1975.
108. Datta S, Briwa J: Modified laryngoscope for endotracheal intubation of obese patients. Anesth Analg 60:120, 1981.
109. Rosa M: Pediatrics: Physiology and practice. *In* Proceedings of "Mastery of Anesthesia Basics." New York, Montefiore Medical Center, Albert Einstein College of Medicine, 1992.
110. Gomella LG: Blood gases and acid-base disorders. *In* Gomella LG (ed): Clinician's Pocket Reference, 7th ed. East Norwalk, CT, Appleton & Lange, 1993, p 134.
111. Lake CL: Cardiovascular anatomy and function. *In* Barash PG, Cullen BF, Stoelting RK (eds): Clinical Anesthesia, 2nd ed. Philadelphia, JB Lippincott, 1992, pp 996, 1005.

FIVE

Practical Obstetric Pharmacology

Ashok Jayaram, M.B., B.S., F.F.A.R.C.S.I.

Pregnancy alters maternal drug response, and maternally administered drugs can cross the placenta and potentially affect the fetus. Following delivery, the neonate, if breast-fed, may be affected by drugs administered to the mother intrapartum and postpartum. This chapter discusses the maternal and fetal effects of drugs commonly utilized by anesthesiologists and obstetricians and offers some practical principles for drug selection and administration.

THE PLACENTA

The placenta forms from maternal and fetal tissues and is the barrier against free drug exchange between mother and fetus. As the invasive trophoblast attaches the blastocyst to the uterus, clefts develop within the mass of trophoblastic cells, forming lacunae that later coalesce to form the intervillous spaces in the developed placenta. Maternal blood from the spiral arteries spurts into these intervillous spaces, providing an exchange interface for maternal and fetal blood (Fig. 5–1). The villi, formed by trophoblastic cells, are perfused by the fetus with fetal blood contained within fetal capillary endothelium. Therefore, maternal blood is separated from fetal blood by only the trophoblast and the fetal capillary endothelium (Fig. 5–2). Thus, it is readily apparent that very little placental barrier exists. Placental circulation may be established as early as the 17th day following fertilization, allowing drug exchange.

FACTORS AFFECTING DRUG TRANSFER (Table 5–1)

Maternal Factors

Drug passage across membrane barriers requires a concentration gradient, with larger gradients, in general, producing greater drug transfer. *Drug dose* is obviously a key factor, and the greater the maternal drug dose, the greater the potential fetal drug accumulation. For example, large dosages of thiopental (TPL) produce greater fetal TPL levels than small dosages. However, maternal *protein-drug binding* may influence drug transfer by reducing the amount of available drug present at the placental exchange site, since only free, unbound drug is available for transfer because of the large molecular size of protein-drug combinations. For example, when a drug is highly bound to albumin, only the free portion of the drug is available for placental transfer. However, with time, equilibration between bound and free drug occurs and maternal and fetal equilibration occurs. Although pregnancy reduces the concentration of both albumin (which binds acidic drugs) and α_1 glycoprotein (which binds basic drugs), these reductions may not directly translate to increased drug transfer. Total body protein may increase compared with that in nonpregnant patients because of the increased blood volume during pregnancy. Furthermore, other physiologic changes of pregnancy including increases in total body water, renal clearance, and altered receptor sensitivity may influence drug passage.

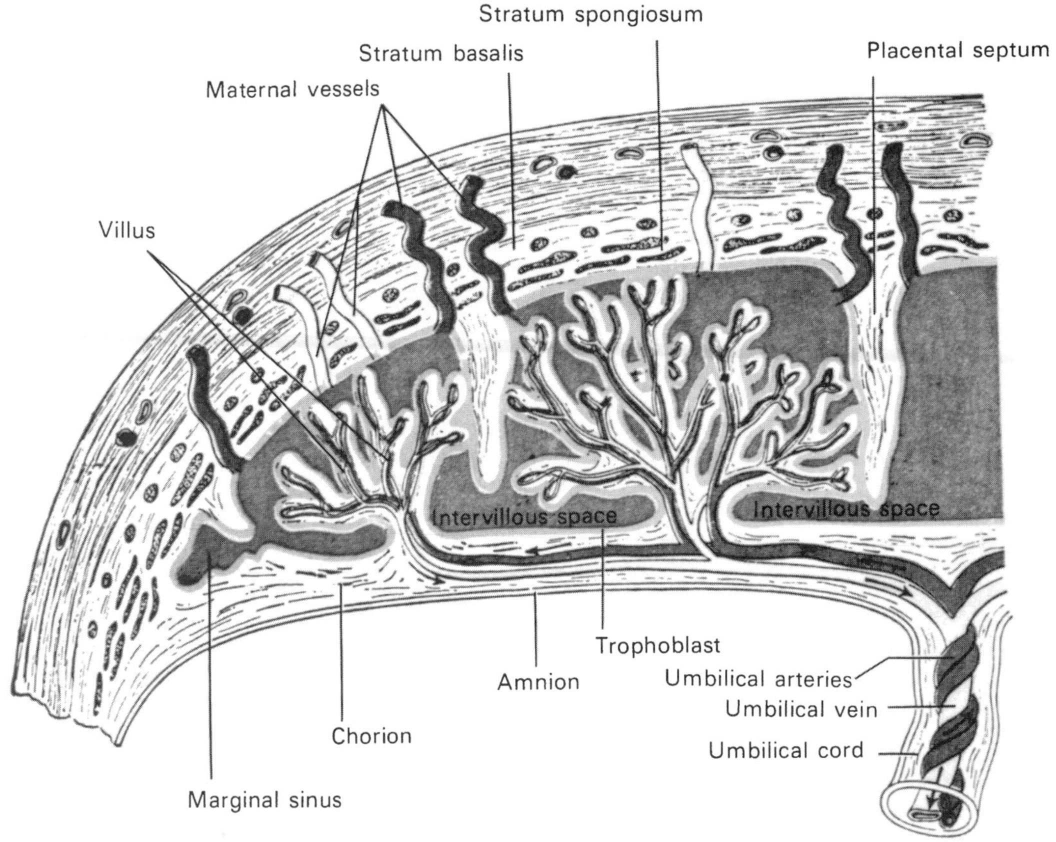

Figure 5–1. Placental circulation. Maternal blood spurts into the intervillous spaces from the spiral arteries. The villi contain fetal vessels. This arrangement is designed to maximize the area available for exchange. (From Clemente CD [ed]: Gray's Anatomy of the Human Body, 30th American ed. Philadelphia, Lea & Febiger, 1985.)

In theory, these changes suggest that dosing regimens should be based on plasma free blood levels; however, these factors are probably of relatively little clinical significance except when extreme variations occur.

Highly charged drugs do not cross the placenta easily. For example, nondepolarizing muscle relaxants may not cross because of their ionization and their large molecular weight. Although maternal blood pH influences the degree of ionization, these changes are of little significance in most patients.

Rapid biotransformation and excretion speed the decline of drug levels at the exchange site and limit placental transfer. For example, succinylcholine is rapidly metabolized by pseudocholinesterase, which limits drug transfer across the placenta. In contrast, maternal pseudocholinesterase deficiency increases the amount of drug presented for placental transfer, with a resultant increased transfer. Drug biotransformation can, however, lead to *active* metabolites, as occurs with the metabolization of meperidine to normeperidine. Thus, biotransformation is not always beneficial.

The *route* of drug administration influences maternal blood levels and, secondarily, placental passage by indirectly altering the concentration gradient. For example, direct intravenous (IV) injection of a local anesthetic produces higher local anesthetic blood levels than when equivalent amounts of local anesthetic are injected within the epidural space. Less transfer occurs following epidural administration. However, these relationships are not always consistent. Peak serum fentanyl levels are similar whether fentanyl is administered epidurally or intravenously. Similarly, local anesthetic blood levels are similar, for identical milligram dosages, whether the local anesthetic is adminis-

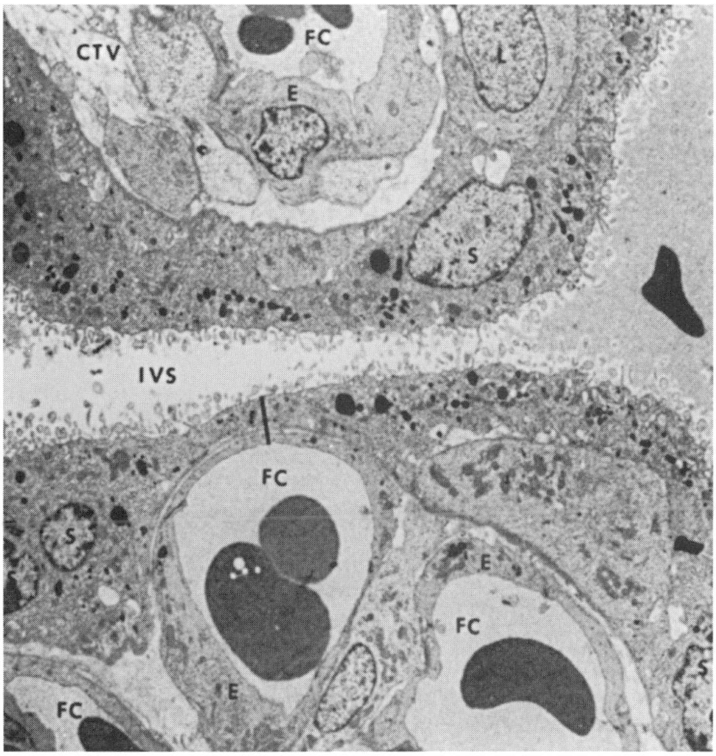

Figure 5–2. Transmission electron micrograph. The *bar* indicates the shortest distance between maternal and fetal blood—two layers of the trophoblast and the fetal capillary endothelium (E). *(Abbreviations:* CTV = connective tissue of villus; FC = fetal capillary; L = Langhans cell nucleus; S = syncytial nuclei; IVS = intervillous space.) (Courtesy of R. M. Wynn, M.D.)

tered subarachnoid or epidurally. Furthermore, *concomitant* drug administration can alter this relationship. For example, peak blood levels of absorbed drug from vascular areas may be reduced by the addition of a vasoconstrictor such as epinephrine.

TABLE 5–1
Factors Affecting the Amount of Drug That Will Reach Fetal Organs

Maternal Factors
Dose
Route of administration
Degree of protein binding
Degree of ionization at plasma pH
Biotransformation and excretion
Uterine contractions
Placental Factors
Concentration gradient
Molecular weight
Lipid solubility
Ionization
Fetal Factors
Fetal perfusion uptake
pH of fetal blood
Fetal biotransformation and excretion

Finally, blood must be delivered to the placental site in order for exchange to occur. Reduced uterine blood flow (UBF) should theoretically reduce drugs' transfer. Blood flow to the placenta declines during uterine contractions, and in theory, intravascular drug injection immediately preceding a uterine contraction should limit the amount reaching the exchange site and transfer. In this instance, the effect is short-lived, since *contractions wane* and continued circulation reexposes the placenta to drug. The clinical significance of reduced uterine blood flow's alteration in drug transfer in daily obstetric anesthesia practice is suspect.

Placental Factors

Drug exchange depends on multiple maternal and fetal factors and the placenta. As discussed previously, concentration gradient, determined by maternal drug dosage, significantly influences placental crossage. For most anesthesia drugs, passive diffusion follows the established concentration gradient. Importantly, exchange across the placenta is bidirectional.

When maternal blood levels fall below fetal levels, diffusion from fetus to mother may occur. In some circumstances, this reverse transfer may improve outcome. For example, if excessive local anesthetic transfer occurred, the decline of maternal blood levels over time would assist the fetus in clearing local anesthetic from its system.

Compounds with molecular weights exceeding 1000 do not cross the placenta easily. However, most anesthetic or obstetric drugs have molecular weights less than 1000 and can be expected to cross the placenta. Finally, higher lipid solubility enhances diffusion, whereas high degrees of ionization impede transfer.

Fetal Factors

Fetal plasma drug concentrations ultimately determine the degree of fetal drug effect. Fetal factors that limit fetal plasma concentration limit drug effects. To a great degree, fetal factors resemble maternal factors.

In the absence of cord compression, which limits transfer to the fetus, *drug uptake* by fetal tissues influences fetal plasma concentration. For example, liver uptake of TPL may limit exposure of the fetal brain to anesthetizing concentrations of TPL by reducing plasma drug concentration. However, the relevance of fetal tissue uptake in determining adverse effects for most drugs is poorly understood at this time.

Decreased fetal blood pH increases the ionization of weak bases such as local anesthetics and, as in the maternal circulation, restricts diffusion across the placenta. In this instance, the ionized compound is trapped in the fetal circulation. This phenomenon is known as *ion trapping*. In theory, local anesthetics such as lidocaine may be trapped in the acidotic fetus. The clinical significance of this phenomenon is also unclear.

Biotransformation and excretion of drugs occur as early as the fifth or sixth week of pregnancy, and the human conceptus exhibits drug-metabolizing enzyme activities that increase as pregnancy advances.[1] Genetic, developmental, and environmental factors can influence fetal enzyme activities and may account for why different fetuses are affected differently by the same chemicals.[2]

Fetal Drug Effects

In the last century, it was widely believed that the conceptus within the womb was in a highly protected environment. It is now known that the conceptus may be affected directly or indirectly. The thalidomide tragedy in the 1960s clearly revealed significant fetal vulnerability for drug-induced teratogenesis. Thalidomide, a sedative administered to mothers in the first trimester of pregnancy, was associated with a high incidence of congenital malformations in the newborn that ultimately led to a better understanding of teratogenesis.

Organogenesis occurs between 15 and 65 days following fertilization, and the fetus is most vulnerable during this period to the direct effect of drug-induced congenital malformations. The central nervous, immune, endocrine, and reproductive systems mature later in pregnancy than other organ systems. Importantly, teratogenesis may occur at doses that are not harmful to the mother. It now appears that the genetic makeup of the conceptus also determines individual susceptibility.[2] Severe malformations may produce fetal death, whereas lesser malformations are evidenced at birth. No anesthetic drug, used in clinical concentrations, is a *proven* teratogen.

In theory, maternally administered drugs might cause premature labor and delivery, leading directly to increased perinatal morbidity and mortality. Despite these concerns, no currently used anesthetic drug, administered in usual clinical doses, has been *proved* to induce premature delivery.

Maternally administered drugs may also indirectly affect the fetus. For example, drugs that decrease uterine blood flow can jeopardize fetal well-being by limiting fetal oxygen supply. Uterine blood flow can be reduced either directly by a constrictive effect on uterine vessels or indirectly by increasing uterine tone (and decreasing perfusion) or decreasing maternal blood pressure and secondarily reducing placental perfusion. Local and general anesthetics, vasopressors, and oxytocics are of particular importance in this regard. The effect of these drugs is discussed later.

Recommendations

Finally, the dilemma remains about how to monitor fetal drug effects and make recommendations. Gross insults produce abortions, stillbirths, or major malformations. In this context, it is important to remember that thalidomide was a profound teratogen and the association was obvious. However, subtler associations like the potential relationship between diazepam and cleft lip/palate may elude firm conclusions.[3] Assessment of the neonate at birth using Apgar scores and neurobehavioral tests attempts to associate more subtle drug effects. Today, although subtle differences may be demonstrated between outcomes by the neurobehavioral testing scores, the significance of these findings is unclear. For the most part, physicians are left to practice utilizing drugs with a long history of safe use.

LOCAL ANESTHETIC DRUGS

Mechanism of Action

Local anesthetics reversibly block conduction in nerves. They diminish the absolute action potential and reduce the rate of rise of this potential. Further, the firing threshold is elevated and the refractory period prolonged. These changes result in smaller and smaller local currents that cannot reach the higher and higher firing threshold and nerve blockade develops.

Sodium influx triggers the action potential. Local anesthetics work by inhibiting this influx through sodium channels. The site of action seems to be within the sodium channel. Access to this site of bonding appears to be from within the nerve for the charged form and through the membrane for the hydrophobic base form. This mode of nerve blockade is important for clinically relevant local anesthetics. However, local anesthetics such as benzocaine, which are essentially nonionized, probably work by membrane expansion and thus shut off the sodium channels. Finally, the biotoxins probably attach to a receptor at the external opening of the sodium channel. This blockade of sodium channels explains axonal and hence peripheral nerve blockade.

However, spinal or epidural anesthesia with local anesthetics may involve inhibition of synaptic transmission as well. Also, apart from sodium channels, other membrane proteins and second messenger systems may also be affected by local anesthetics. So, it may well be that sodium channel inhibition may not be the only mechanism by which local anesthetics produce spinal or epidural anesthesia.[4]

Physiologic and Chemical Characteristics

Local anesthetics, with the exception of prilocaine, are weakly basic tertiary amines. The general structure is: aromatic ring (lipophilic)–intermediate chain–amine (hydrophilic). The linkage between the lipophilic and the hydrophilic portions characterizes local anesthetics as either esters or amines and ultimately determines the way the body disposes of them. Esters are rapidly hydrolyzed by the appropriate esterase (probably plasma cholinesterase), although the liver may participate to some degree in their clearance. Esters have a low toxicity potential because of the rapid breakdown into innocuous metabolites. They do, however, have a greater allergic potential than amides.

Amide local anesthetics are generally more resistant to hydrolysis and require conversion to simpler forms prior to degradation, which takes place in the endoplasmic reticulum of the liver. Hydrolysis of prilocaine, however, results in the formation of *o*-toluidine metabolites, which may cause methemoglobinemia. For this reason, the drug has restricted use in obstetric patients. Lipid solubility and protein binding also influence local anesthetic action (Table 5–2). Greater lipid solubility eases passage across lipoprotein nerve membranes, thus increasing potency. Greater protein binding increases the duration of action of the local anesthetic by

TABLE 5–2
Physicochemical Properties of the Local Anesthetic Agents Commonly Used in Obstetrics

Agent	Lipid Solubility	Protein Binding	pKa
Bupivacaine	340	95%	8.1
Lidocaine	4	65%	7.7
Chloroprocaine	>1	?	9.1
Tetracaine	80	85%	8.6

Adapted from Datta S: Pharmacology of local anesthetic agents. American Society of Anesthesiologists Refresher Courses In Anesthesiology, vol 21. Philadelphia, JB Lippincott, 1993, p 245.

binding the local anesthetic to the receptor protein.

The speed of onset of local anesthetic relates to pKa. (The pKa is the pH at which 50% of the local anesthetic is in an ionized state.) Thus, drugs with a pKa close to body pH will have a greater proportion of un-ionized drug and a more rapid onset of action. Remember, the ionized form of local anesthetic is responsible for blockade. Intracellular pH determines how much local anesthetic resides in the ionized form within the cell. These principles also explain the previously discussed potential for ion trapping of amide local anesthetic in the acidotic fetus.

Systemic Effects and Toxicity

Local anesthetics block conduction in excitable tissues and consequently affect (in addition to peripheral nerves) the function of the central nervous system (CNS), autonomic ganglia, neuromuscular junction, and muscle including the vascular musculature and the myocardium.

Of practical importance are the effects of local anesthetics on the CNS and cardiovascular systems. To a great degree, pregnancy does not alter the manifestations of toxicity, only the sensitivity of the organs to toxicity.

Local anesthetics cross the blood-brain barrier with relative ease, and CNS manifestations are a function of the blood level of local anesthetic. In this context, it is important to realize that the effect of a small intravascular dose injected rapidly will be more profound than that of a much larger dose that is absorbed slowly from the epidural space.

As the blood concentration of local anesthetic increases, symptoms develop—lightheadedness, tinnitus, drowsiness, circumoral tingling and numbness, and blurring of vision—suggesting impending toxicity. On examination, the patient may exhibit the following signs—confusion, nystagmus, slurred speech, muscle tremors, and twitches. All are manifestations of CNS toxicity. If these premonitory signs are ignored or if these signs are the initial result of a large accidental intravascular injection, generalized tonic-clonic convulsions may ensue if the blood level rises. The doses of different agents that produce convulsions in humans are shown in Table 5–3. Remember, bupivacaine affects the heart disproportionately compared with its effects on the CNS. Indeed, with bupivacaine, cardiovascular collapse has immediately followed accidental intravascular injection.[5] Ropivacaine may be a preferable drug in this regard.

TABLE 5–3
Doses of Intravenous Local Anesthetics That Have Been Associated With Convulsions in Humans

Agent	Dose (mg/kg)
Bupivacaine	1.6
Lidocaine	5–7
Chloroprocaine	22.8

Adapted from de Jong RH: Contral nervous system effects. *In* de Jong RH: Local Anesthetics. St. Louis, Mosby–Year Book, 1994, p 273.

Cardiovascular System

Local anesthetics directly affect the contractility, automaticity, conductivity, and rhythmicity of the heart as well as the musculature of the blood vessels. Autonomic blockade consequent to spinal or epidural block also affects cardiovascular system function but is not considered here.

The predominant effect of local anesthetics on the heart is the drugs' influence on the cardiac action potential. The actions of lidocaine and bupivacaine on cardiac electrophysiology have been extensively studied. In brief, there appears to be some difference in their individual effects to account for the fact that lidocaine is antiarrhythmogenic whereas bupivacaine, in toxic doses, causes lethal arrhythmias. Lidocaine has an affinity for sodium channels in the open state, whereas bupivacaine binds more to channels that are inactive. The inactive state follows the open configuration. Since bupivacaine dissociates more slowly than lidocaine, a bupivacaine block persists longer into diastole, affecting impulse conduction and making it easier for reentrant arrhythmias to develop. Taken together and put in simple terms, lidocaine is fast-in and fast-out, whereas bupivacaine is fast-in but slow-out.[6] The electrophysiologic actions of bupivacaine are compounded further by its negative inotropic effect. Finally, bupivacaine cardiotoxicity may have a centrally mediated component.[7]

Pregnancy may enhance bupivacaine toxicity

and narrow the margin between CNS toxicity and cardiovascular collapse.[8] This may be due to progesterone potentiation[9] or altered protein binding in pregnancy leading to greater amounts of the unbound drug.[10]

Methods of prevention and treatment of toxicity are listed in Table 5–4. Bupivacaine toxicity requires further consideration. As far as specific treatment of bupivacaine overdose is concerned, lidocaine has been successfully used for resuscitating a patient who received 750 mg of bupivacaine infiltrated into the scalp.[11] However, an animal study showed that bretylium was more effective than lidocaine.[12] The advent of life-threatening dysrhythmia should be treated with electrical countershock, starting with low doses and increasing appropriately, followed by bretylium 5 to 10 mg/kg every 30 seconds up to a maximal dose of 30 mg/kg. For persistent hypotension and bradycardia, large doses of epinephrine and atropine may be required. In addition, isoproterenol and external pacing should be considered. It is important to realize that successful resuscitation is possible but can take a very long time. Successful resuscitation has included cardiopulmonary bypass with a total bypass time of 1 hour and 30 minutes.[13] In this case, cardiopulmonary bypass itself was not even begun until 1 hour and 40 minutes following onset of ventricular fibrillation, emphasizing that successful resuscitation can be prolonged.

TABLE 5–4
Prevention and Treatment of Local Anesthetic Toxicity

Prevention

Aspirate catheter prior to drug injection
Administer "test dose" of local anesthetic or epinephrine → assess heart rate and elicit possible premonitory CNS signs/symptoms
Administer local anesthetic in 5-ml aliquots, assessing in 1-min–2-min intervals for premonitory CNS signs/symptoms

Treatment

Control convulsions: Thiopental sodium (Pentothal) 50 mg or diazepam 5 mg IV, incrementally; most convulsions are brief and do not require drug treatment
Control airway: Needed for prolonged convulsions; hyperventilate via mask with 100% O_2 until rapid-sequence tracheal intubation (may be facilitated with IV succinylcholine) achieved
Support circulation: Left uterine displacement; consider delivering fetus via cesarean section if restoration of circulation not anticipated <5 min; apply standard CPR/ACLS protocols as appropriate

Abbreviations: CNS = central nervous system; CPR/ACLS = cardiopulmonary resuscitation/advanced cardiac life support.

Specific Local Anesthetic Agents

Lidocaine

Lidocaine's propensity to cause motor blockade and the development of tachyphylaxis mitigate against the routine use of epidural lidocaine for labor analgesia. Early reports of the deleterious effects of lidocaine on neonatal neurobehavioral scores were subsequently disproved. Indeed, because of its lack of cardiac toxicity, lidocaine, usually containing epinephrine or bicarbonate, or both, proves a useful agent for providing cesarean section anesthesia. However, lidocaine without additives produces marginal anesthesia, and frequent signs of impending CNS toxicity accompany large doses.

Reports that suggest that intrathecal 5% hyperbaric spinal lidocaine associates with persistent neurologic deficits have been discussed in a recent editorial.[14] Nevertheless, lidocaine still plays a major role in obstetric anesthesia.

Chloroprocaine

Rapidly metabolized by plasma cholinesterase by both mother and fetus, chloroprocaine has limited placental transfer and is not subject to ion trapping. However, large volumes accidentally injected intrathecally have produced persistent nerve deficits.[60] Subsequent investigation of these cases implicated the preservative (sodium bisulfite), leading to its replacement with sodium ethylenediaminetetraacetic acid (EDTA). Another problem associated with epidural chloroprocaine is backache, which may relate to the newer preservative sodium EDTA. Backache is most common in young, nonpregnant adults and rare during pregnancy. Finally, epidural narcotics work less well if they are given after chloroprocaine. Bupivacaine's effectiveness may be diminished transiently following chloroprocaine administration. Chloroprocaine's rapid onset of block proves very useful for emergent cesarean sections in patients with epidural catheters in situ. The editor's group usually avoids chloroprocaine after accidental dural puncture; whether the practice is warranted is unknown, but it does avoid questions about possible neurotoxicity.

Bupivacaine

Bupivacaine has beome the most common local anesthetic used for epidural labor analgesia. Its sensory blockade usually exceeds motor blockade, and its high degree of protein binding in maternal blood results in less drug transfer to the fetus. Bupivacaine's potential for cardiotoxicity has led to the abandonment of the 0.75% solution for epidural use. The potential for cardiotoxicity has also stimulated the search for less toxic local anesthetics that are long-acting and produce good sensory blocks with little motor blockade.

Ropivacaine

The observation that S(−) bupivacaine was much less cardiotoxic than R(+) bupivacaine indicated the stereospecificity of the cardiac sodium channel binding site. However, for unknown reasons, S(−) bupivacaine was not marketed. Rather, its *N*-propyl homologue (synthesized 40 years earlier) was taken off the shelf and marketed as ropivacaine, the S(−) enantiomer of *N*-propyl pipecolyl xylidine. Ropivacaine has all the desirable properties of bupivacaine including low motor blockade in low concentration, neonatal safety, and no detrimental effect on uteroplacental circulation. Ropivacaine has less cardiotoxicity than bupivacaine.

GENERAL ANESTHETIC AGENTS

Intravenous

Thiopental

First administered in 1934, TPL is the most widely used IV induction agent. Following IV administration, TPL is distributed by the blood to all body tissues and rapidly crosses the placenta. Highly perfused, low-volume tissues such as those in the brain equilibrate rapidly, resulting in rapid loss of consciousness usually in one arm to brain circulation time. Redistribution of TPL from highly perfused tissues to less well perfused tissues such as in muscle terminates the initial effects of the induction dose. Importantly, clearance from the body is slow and does not make a significant contribution to terminating clinical effects. Both mother and fetus rely on redistribution to terminate clinical efforts. Drug dosage, *not* the timing of delivery, determines the degree of newborn depression; that is, very large doses can produce prolonged depression because of saturation of redistribution sites.

The predominant cardiovascular effect of TPL is venodilatation, decreasing preload and potentially resulting in hypotension. In addition, myocardial contractility is depressed, cardiac output decreases, and heart rate increases. Clinically, the depressive effects of TPL are offset by sympathetic stimulation caused by laryngoscopy and intubation. Healthy parturients rarely display hypotension secondary to TPL.

TPL is devoid of effect on the tone of the gravid uterus. The fetal brain is protected from high concentrations of the drug by absorption by the fetal liver and by redistribution in the maternal and fetal tissues. Also, drug present in the umbilical vein is diluted by blood in the inferior vena cava in the fetal circulation. However, a high dose of the drug (8 mg/kg) results in neonatal depression. So, in practice, the dose of TPL in obstetric practice should be between 2.5 and 4.5 mg/kg. Lower doses risk maternal awareness, and higher doses risk newborn depression.

Ketamine

A phencyclidine derivative released for clinical use in 1970, ketamine produces dissociative anesthesia, a cataleptic state with profound analgesia, some maintenance of protective airway reflexes, and no or low recall of surgery during anesthesia. Low-dose, incremental (0.25 mg/kg to a maximum of 1 mg/kg) ketamine produces profound analgesia and doses larger than 1 mg/kg can produce anesthesia.

Ketamine stimulates the cardiovascular system, increasing blood pressure, heart rate, and cardiac output, probably secondary to central stimulation of the sympathetic nervous system. In isolated animal heart preparations, ketamine depresses the myocardium. In theory, severe hypovolemia with accompanying maximal sympathetic stimulation might allow ketamine's depressor effects to appear. Mild hypertension is the norm in healthy, pregnant patients.

Ketamine has minimal effects on central respiratory drive and, more importantly, relaxes bronchial smooth muscle, making it a reasonable choice in asthmatic patients. Neonatal outcome in terms of Apgar scores and umbilical cord gases is comparable with those observed with TPL.

Unfortunately, ketamine associates with a 10 to 30% incidence of emergent reactions—consisting of vivid dreams, out-of-body experiences, and delusions on awakening following anesthesia —and with excitement, confusion, and fear. Emergent reactions are the chief side effect restricting its routine use in clinical practice. Unlike other IV agents, ketamine raises intracranial pressure, which is rarely a consideration in the obstetric population. Mild increases in uterine tone have been noted postpartum, but these do not appear to be clinically relevant.

Etomidate

Etomidate, an imidazole derivative in clinical use since 1972, produces anesthesia through an unknown mechanism that may involve the γ-aminobutyric acid (GABA) system. Etomidate's major advantage is its minimal effect on cardiovascular function in healthy patients and those with compromised myocardial function. Etomidate, however, does not attenuate the cardiovascular response to laryngoscopy and intubation. Because of its favorable pharmacokinetics (short elimination half-life and rapid clearance), arousal time is minimized. A secondary advantage is that etomidate does not associate with histamine release.

Concerns regarding etomidate include its inhibition of adrenal steroid hormone synthesis, believed due to blockade of 11β-hydroxylase and, to a lesser extent 17α-hydroxylase inhibition, leading to decreased glucocorticoid and mineralocorticoid production. In practical terms, the impact of a single induction dose is unknown and thought to be insignificant. However, prolonged infusions of etomidate have been associated with significant morbidity and mortality. Adverse effects during induction include pain on injection, myoclonic movements, and hiccuping. Finally, there is a high incidence of postoperative nausea and vomiting.

Propofol

Propofol, one of a group of alkyl phenols, was recently introduced in clinical practice in the United States but has been available in Europe since the mid-1980s. Propofol is not yet approved for use in obstetric patients in the United States. Its rapid metabolism in the liver to inactive metabolites ensures rapid awakening with little anesthetic hangover. However, this characteristic may have contributed to a high incidence of awareness in a clinical study in which it was used as an induction agent, using a dose of 2.5 mg/kg.[15] Although a continuous infusion following the induction dose could probably avoid awareness, if the induction-to-delivery period were prolonged, neonatal depression might result.

A major advantage of propofol is the low incidence of postoperative nausea and vomiting. Furthermore, by a combination of effects on the upper airway, propofol has been shown to produce favorable conditions for intubating conditions without the use of muscle relaxants. In theory, this property might be useful in conditions when succinylcholine is contraindicated, but in the obstetric patient this technique poses significant hazards.

Hypotension may accompany an induction secondary to both vasodilatation and myocardial depression, but should rarely be a problem in healthy parturients. The second disadvantage to propofol is pain during injection as well as myoclonic movements and, very rarely, thrombophlebitis following injection. At present, the use of propofol for cesarean section must be considered experimental. Many questions concerning dose technique and outcome must be answered before widespread clinical use.

Inhalation Anesthetics

The four most commonly used inhalation agents today are nitrous oxide (N_2O), halothane, isoflurane, and enflurane (Fig. 5–3). Desflurane has not yet been approved for obstetric usage, although its low blood solubility and consequent early awakening make it an attractive agent. Its reported sympathetic system activation could, in theory, reduce uterine blood flow and needs further investigation.

Pregnancy has consistently been shown to reduce the minimal alveolar concentration (MAC)

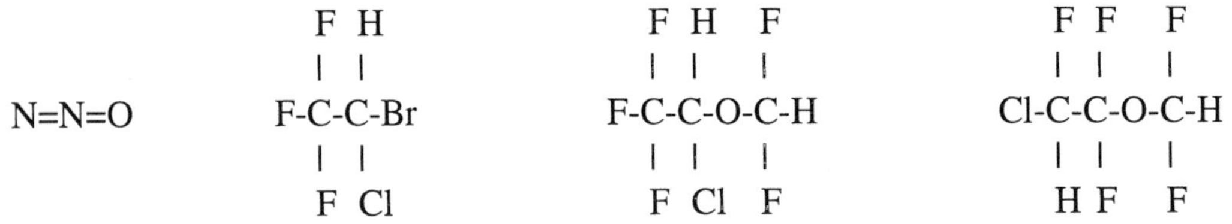

Nitrous Oxide Halothane Isoflurane Enflurane

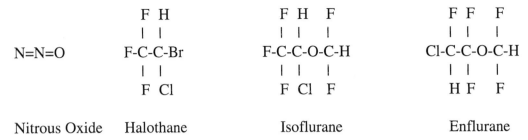

Figure 5–3. The four most commonly used inhalation agents.

for all inhalation agents by approximately 30%. Therefore, remember that lower concentrations than are required in nonpregnant patients are needed to effect the same anesthetic level. Inhalational *analgesia* with either potent agents or N_2O requires careful monitoring of the mother's level of consciousness because of the increased sensitivity. Concentrations of N_2O exceeding 50% may sufficiently depress consciousness to risk airway reflexes, especially when the parturient has received systemic narcotics for labor analgesia. Although all inhalation agents have at some time been used to provide pain relief during labor, their main use today in obstetrics is to supplement anesthesia for operative procedures; they are most commonly administered in concentrations that minimize maternal awareness while producing minimal detrimental indirect or direct effects on neonatal well-being. In this section, evidence from animal, in vitro, and clinical studies is presented to form a practical guide for the clinician.

The placenta, like the blood-brain barrier, permits rapid crossing by the inhaled anesthetic agents and eventual equilibration between mother and fetus. Traditional indications for inhalation anesthetics were the provision of intrapartum analgesia, analgesia for vaginal delivery, and general anesthesia for operative delivery. Utilization for provision of intrapartum analgesia has waned as epidural analgesia use increased and the conversion to labor, delivery, and recovery (LDR) and LDR-postpartum units rendered the intrapartum application impractical. Irrespective of the indication, proper usages requires consideration of the potential adverse effects of the inhalation agents, including direct drug depression, indirect depression secondary to altered maternal hemodynamics, and altered uterine contractility. As with IV agents, the degree and significance of effects relate to the delivered concentration of the agent. In this context, potent inhalation agents are utilized to supplement rather than provide anesthesia for operative procedures, permitting the use of low concentrations that produce minimal neonatal effects, and absent or mild effects on uterine contractility while providing maternal amnesia.

Uterine Contractility

N_2O is devoid of any significant effect on uterine contractility, irrespective of administered concentration. All other inhaled agents in use today inhibit uterine contractility in a dose-related manner. However, when potent anesthetic agents are administered in concentrations of less than 1 MAC, the uterus responds appropriately to oxytocin.[16] Clinically, concentrations of 0.5% halothane, 1% enflurane, and 0.75% isoflurane in combination with 50% N_2O minimize recall, provide adequate fetal oxygenation, and do not produce excessive blood levels at cesarean section.[17, 18] Although controversial, higher concentrations of isoflurane (1 to 1½ MAC) administered in 100% oxygen are reported to have no effect on blood loss following cesarean section.[19] To minimize the issue of uterine contractility depression following delivery, consider deepening anesthesia with IV narcotics and a higher concentration of N_2O and limiting potent agent concentrations to ½ MAC or less following delivery. (See Chapter 7 for a discussion of cesarean section anesthesia.) Profound uterine relaxation, if required, demands concentrations of 2 to 3 MAC.

Fetal Effects and Neonatal Depression

Inhalation agents (small, highly lipid-soluble uncharged molecules) cross the placenta as a direct function of maternal plasma concentration. High maternal concentrations lead to maternal hypotension and high fetal blood levels of the agent and potentially affect fetal well-being. However, if hypotension and reduced maternal cardiac output are avoided, what then? N_2O, a relatively impotent agent, requires high concentrations, up to 70%, to semireliably produce analgesia if unsupplemented. When utilized as an *induction* agent, 21 minutes of exposure to N_2O led to lower 1-minute Apgar scores and slightly lower umbilical artery pH when compared with patients induced with TPL and maintained with 70% N_2O.[20] The latter group had an induction delivery time of 17 minutes and a briefer exposure to N_2O, providing a possible explanation for the findings. Indeed, prolonged exposure (24–43 min) to 70% N_2O results in fetal concentrations approaching maternal levels and associates with lower neonatal Apgar scores.[21] Eighty-seven percent equilibration occurs in 15 to 19 minutes following 50 to 70% N_2O with 5-minute Apgar scores in the 9 to 10 range in all neonates.[22] The lower 1-minute Apgar scores associated with N_2O are more accurately described as sedative rather than depressive effects and are easily reversed with ventilation with 100% O_2. In practical terms, following IV induction of anesthesia, minimize neonatal depression risks by utilizing 50% N_2O until delivery of the baby. Do not use 70% N_2O unless delivery of the infant is probable within 12 to 14 minutes following initiation of N_2O. Inducing anesthesia following the patient's surgical preparation and drape offers advantages that minimize fetal exposure to inhalational agents. Whether administering 50 to 100% maternal oxygen is a better choice when fetal distress exists is controversial.

The potent inhalation agents administered in low concentrations (0.5% halothane, 1% enflurane, or 0.5% isoflurane) and supplemented with 50% N_2O maintain normal maternal and neonatal conditions while reducing risks for maternal awareness. However, higher concentrations (e.g., 0.8% halothane) have been associated with maternal hypotension, which may be detrimental to fetal well-being.[17] Importantly, no practical combination of inhalation agents guarantees maternal amnesia and no newborn depression.

In summary, N_2O concentrations of 50% or less do not detrimentally alter maternal or fetal outcome nor impair uterine contractility. To a great degree, the potent inhalation agents may be used interchangeably at concentrations of less than 1 MAC without adversely altering maternal or neonatal outcome. In theory, the superior pharmacokinetics, low blood solubility, lack of hepatic or renal toxicity, low arrhythmogenic potential, and cardiovascular stability might make isoflurane a better choice in obstetric anesthesia.

Muscle Relaxants

Modern techniques providing general anesthesia for cesarean section are designed for fetal protection at the expense of depth of anesthesia. Muscle relaxants are essential to facilitate rapid-sequence induction and tracheal intubation and provide reliable muscle relaxation during the operative procedures. Easy reversal of effect is desirable when the operative procedure is expected to be brief. Finally, the muscle relaxant should not affect neonatal outcome. To date, no single agent provides all the requisite properties, and a combination of depolarizing and nondepolarizing agents, each with its own advantages and disadvantages, produces the foundation for anesthetic administration.

Depolarizing Muscle Relaxants

Succinylcholine

Succinylcholine, the only depolarizing muscle relaxant in clinical use today, produces neuromuscular blockade by persistent depolarization. Succinylcholine's rapid onset makes it the agent of choice to facilitate endotracheal intubation during rapid-sequence induction. Rapid hydrolysis by pseudocholinesterase, an enzyme found in the liver and in plasma, provides rapid termination of effect. Importantly, pseudocholinesterase is not present at the motor endplate, and succinylcholine's action is terminated by diffusion away from the motor endplate. Although pseudocholinesterase levels decline during pregnancy and reach their nadir shortly postpartum, these effects are of minimal clinical significance and dosage should not be adjusted during pregnancy.

Low lipid solubility and ionization at physiologic pH restrict placental transfer to some degree. If the mother and fetus are both homozygotic for the atypical pseudocholinesterase enzyme, clinically relevant amounts cross the placenta and affect the fetus. In such cases, the newborn will require respiratory support. For most patients, doses of 1 to 2 mg/kg do not affect clinical outcome.

Potentially detrimental side effects may accompany succinylcholine administration, and pregnancy offers no protection from them. Succinylcholine administration may increase intragastric pressure (increasing the risk of aspiration) and cause muscle pain in nonpregnant patients. Although controversial, there may be a concomitant increase in lower esophageal sphincter tone, counteracting the rise of intragastric pressure. Administration of a small dose of nondepolarizing agent prior to administering succinylcholine and the application of cricoid pressure minimize the significance of these effects. Remember, the prior administration of a nondepolarizing agent may necessitate administering a larger dose of succinylcholine with, perhaps, some alteration in the onset and offset of neuromuscular blockade. In addition, the nondepolarizing agent may very rarely cause weakness and increase the risk of aspiration. Finally, bradycardia may occur following repeat drug injections. In the author's group's experience, muscle pain is rare in pregnant women following the use of succinylcholine, even without prior use of a nondepolarizing agent. (The editor's group does not administer nondepolarizing agents prior to administering succinylcholine to parturients.) Concerns regarding malignant hyperthermia remain the same as for the nonpregnant patient. In summary, succinylcholine remains the agent of choice for rapid-sequence induction for cesarean section, and the drug may be utilized with the same concerns and precautions as in the nonpregnant patient.

Nondepolarizing Muscle Relaxants

Nondepolarizing muscle relaxants produce neuromuscular blockade by competitive antagonism. All are large, ionized molecules with little placental transfer with clinical doses. Vecuronium and atracurium, agents of intermediate duration of action, have greatly reduced the use of D-tubocurarine (DTC) and pancuronium. Most obstetric procedures are short, and maternal safety is enhanced by easy reversal of muscle paralysis at the termination of procedure permitted with these drugs. Nevertheless, pancuronium and DTC provide reasonable alternatives when atracurium and vecuronium are unavailable.

Vecuronium is devoid of any significant cardiac or histamine-releasing effects in clinical doses. Atracurium does have the potential to release histamine (albeit much less than DTC), and the degree of release is related to the dose and speed of injection. Administering 0.5 mg/kg or less of atracurium minimizes these side effects. Vecuronium undergoes extensive liver metabolism and is excreted in the bile, whereas atracurium undergoes Hoffman elimination at physiologic pH and normal body temperature as well as ester hydrolysis. In theory, severe liver disease, as may occur in the HELLP (*h*emolysis, *el*evated *l*iver enzymes, *l*ow *p*latelets) syndrome, may make vecuronium the second choice. All nondepolarizing agents (with the exception of gallamine) cross the placenta to a very limited extent. In clinical doses, there are no adverse effects on neonatal outcome in terms of Apgar scores, umbilical cord acid-base status, or neurobehavioral scores. However, the effects of large bolus administration of any of these drugs, as might occur when used for rapid-sequence induction in patients in whom succinylcholine is contraindicated, are not reported. Finally, rocuronium, a short-acting nondepolarizing muscle relaxant, is not approved for rapid-sequence induction during pregnancy at the present time.

Drug Interactions

Magnesium sulfate, utilized for treatment of preeclampsia, eclampsia, and preterm labor, decreases the amount of acetylcholine released presynaptically, decreases the action of acetylcholine at the motor endplate, and reduces the amplitude of endplate potential and muscle fiber excitability. Thus, the action of nondepolarizing muscle relaxants is enhanced by magnesium sulfate administration. Although not intuitively apparent, some evidence exists that magnesium sulfate administration also potentiates succinylcholine's depolarizing action. Nevertheless, on a practical level, it is safer not to reduce the dose of succinylcholine during rapid-sequence induction. For maintenance, titrate nondepolarizing agents utilizing peripheral nerve stimulation for patients receiving magnesium sulfate therapy.

Aminoglycosides enhance neuromuscular blockade in either a prejunctional or a postjunctional manner similar to that of magnesium sulfate. Titration, rather than reduced dosage, enhances administration safety. In summary, depolarizing and nondepolarizing muscle relaxants incur the same potential side effects during pregnancy as in the nonpregnant state. Each drug may be used interchangeably, and titration of effects is the best method to avoid complications.

PARENTERAL OPIOID ANALGESICS

Indications for the administration of opioid analgesics in obstetrics include intrapartum pain relief and pain relief during and following operative procedures. Intrapartum administration confronts the obstetric anesthesiologist with the same dilemmas as those of general anesthesia. The desirable effect of pain reduction must be weighed against the potential direct drug depressant effects on the newborn as well as the systemic side effects that occur with each of the available analgesics.

Parenteral opioid analgesics exert their effects by interacting with specific receptors. At present, three receptors are generally recognized —μ, δ, κ. Agonist coupling to μ, δ receptors results in G protein–mediated reduction in intracellular cyclic adenosine monophosphate (cAMP) and increased potassium conductance, leading to membrane hyperpolarization. Agonist attachment to κ receptors results in G protein–mediated blockade of calcium channels. Opioid receptors are located strategically in the dorsal horn of the spinal cord, the periaqueductal gray matter, and the thalamus, all involved with processing of pain signals.

All systemically administered opioids produce some degree of undesirable effects on other organ systems. Euphoria, sedation, and nausea and vomiting relate to effects on the CNS. Indeed, the ability of opioids to cause euphoria is linked to the potential for abuse that these drugs possess. Occasionally, especially with the agonist-antagonists, dysphoria occurs. A dysphoric reaction may, if pronounced, outweigh the advantages of the desired effect of pain relief. In contrast, sedation may be a desirable quality, and it accompanies most therapeutic doses of opioids. Finally, nausea and vomiting, a central effect, are related to opioid-induced stimulation of the chemoreceptor trigger zone. Nausea and vomiting remain the most discomfiting of all the opioid side effects. Interestingly, at high doses, opioids depress the vomiting center. As with any drug, the potential for these undesirable side effects must be weighed against the indication for drug administration prior to administering the selected agent.

To a great degree, opioid administration produces hemodynamic stability, in both the presence and the absence of noxious stimuli. Their routine use during cardiac anesthesia emphasizes their ability to produce analgesia with minimal cardiac depression.

Opioids reduce sympathetic and increase parasympathetic tone and thus have the capability to produce hypotension. Furthermore, drugs such as morphine produce venodilatation and increase plasma histamine levels, which in turn produce arteriolar dilatation, further exacerbating hypotension. Opioids may also produce bradycardia, probably secondary to stimulation of the central vagal nucleus. Meperidine, in contrast to most opioids, causes tachycardia, probably related to its structural similarity to atropine. Prior to administration, the anesthesiologist must weigh the risks of hypotension or tachycardia-bradycardia, or both, when selecting the individual agents and must titrate the drug appropriately. Nevertheless, when used in analgesic doses, significant hemodynamic effects are rare.

All opioid agonists produce dose-dependent respiratory depression, mainly through an action on brain stem centers. Hypoventilation is usually accompanied by a marked decrease in respiratory rate and a decreased responsiveness of the brain stem centers to carbon dioxide. Partial agonists and agonist-antagonists have a maximal respiratory depressant effect. In fact, agents such as nalbuphine may reverse the respiratory depression of μ-receptor agonists such as morphine while maintaining some degree of analgesia. Finally, agonist-antagonist agents, although having a maximal respiratory depressant effect, may also have a maximal analgesic effect.

Not surprisingly, opioids depress upper airway and tracheal reflexes including the cough reflex. As sedation increases, the threat of aspiration increases. However, their antitussant effect is advantageous during general endotracheal anesthesia by decreasing the cough reflex stimulated by the endotracheal tube. Opioids also delay gastric emptying secondary to a central vagal effect and stimulation of opioid receptors in the myenteric plexus. Intrapartum administration of opioid analgesics thus reinforces the necessity of considering obstetric patients at high risk for aspiration of gastric contents.

Effects on other organ systems include reduction in urinary output, apparently secondary to an alteration in renal blood flow and glomerular filtration rate. Opioids also relax bladder smooth muscle, increasing the possibility of urinary retention, with morphine particularly likely to cause this effect. Large doses of opioids blunt the endocrine and metabolic responses to surgical stress, which serves as a major indication for opioid administration in some patients. Opioids can also produce pain mimicking angina through opioid-mediated spasm of the sphincter of Oddi. Gallbladder disease not infrequently accompanies pregnancy, and agents such as nalbuphine and butorphanol are less likely to produce this undesirable side effect.

Parenteral opioids, especially fentanyl and its analogues, in high doses, may produce chest wall rigidity sufficient to impair ventilation and require endotracheal intubation. Because obstetric anesthesiologists rarely administer large doses of any opioid prior to delivery of the infant, this should seldom be a problem in obstetric patients.

Finally, opioids can also affect the uterus and fetus. Although parenteral opioids probably have little effect on uterine activity, heavy sedation associates with prolongation of the latent phase of labor. Opioids possess little or no teratogenic potential. However, they rapidly cross the placenta and can result in significant fetal drug levels. Whether the fetus, and particularly the premature fetus, is more sensitive than an adult to the respiratory depressant effects of opioids is uncertain. However, since drug elimination of morphine and meperidine is delayed in the neonate, the wise anesthesiologist limits morphine and meperidine drug use intrapartum.

Individual Parenteral Agents: Pharmacodynamics and Pharmacokinetics

Compared with other opioids, morphine is relatively lipid insoluble. Nevertheless, morphine has a large volume of distribution, and clearance from the body is mainly a function of hepatic metabolism. Traditionally, morphine was assumed to depress neonatal respiration to a greater degree than meperidine. This assumption was strengthened by a study that demonstrated diminished respiratory response to carbon dioxide in infants between 12 and 60 hours of age.[23] However, this study included only four subjects in each group (morphine and meperidine). Furthermore, there were no controls and the study contained other methodologic flaws. However, an earlier animal study provided the rationale for this perceived sensitivity of the newborn to the respiratory depressive effects of morphine.[24] Thus, morphine utilization for labor analgesia fell into disfavor. Today, although it is unclear whether these early studies are valid, many anesthesiologists and obstetricians avoid morphine administration prior to delivery.

In contrast to morphine, meperidine is more lipid soluble and protein bound. Indeed, meperidine plasma levels correlate better with exhibited analgesia than morphine levels. However, hepatic metabolism of meperidine produces normeperidine and normeperidinic acid, which have inherent activity. Normeperidine is both an analgesic and a convulsant. Thus, maternal administration of meperidine can produce extended respiratory depression secondary to its active metabolite. Finally, meperidine, like morphine, can negatively influence the Apgar score and neurobehavioral examination.

Fentanyl's high lipid solubility accounts for its large volume of distribution. Fentanyl rapidly undergoes metabolism in the liver to what are believed to be inactive metabolites. Some concern exists regarding fentanyl's ability to depress ventilation following apparent recovery from its effects, perhaps secondary to recirculation of fentanyl from the skeletal muscle stores. The author's group rarely utilizes IV fentanyl for intrapartum analgesia and has never observed this phenomenon. However, IV fentanyl has been used by others to provide analgesia during labor (50–100 μg at hourly intervals) with minimal neonatal effects.[24] IV patient-controlled analgesia (25-μg bolus/10-min lockout, combined with a 25-μg/hr continuous infusion) has also been used as an alternative analgesic technique during labor in a patient with thrombocytopenia.[25] From a practical perspective, the author's group would consider fentanyl a reasonable alternative when other analgesic drugs or techniques are contraindicated.

Sufentanil is twice as lipid soluble as fentanyl. However, the smaller volume of distribution, high degree of plasma protein binding, and minimal tissue binding produce a shorter elimination half-life than that of fentanyl. Experience utilizing sufentanil intravenously for intrapartum analgesia is lacking.

Reports of alfentanil use during labor are scant. Alfentanil does have a lower lipid solubility than fentanyl and a smaller volume of distribution, making more of the drug available for metabolism and excretion. Thus, alfentanil has the desirable qualities of rapid onset and termination of effect. Alfentanil has been used during pregnancy in an attempt to ensure hemodynamic stability during induction of anesthesia in patients with severe pregnancy-induced hypertension or other cardiac disease.[26] Neonatal respiratory depression requiring naloxone reversal was associated with its use in this context.

Agonist-Antagonist Agents: Pharmacodynamics and Pharmacokinetics

Nalbuphine is an agonist at κ receptors and an antagonist at μ receptors. Analgesia, as well as respiratory depression, demonstrates a maximal ceiling effect, reportedly occurring at 30 mg/70-kg patient. Nalbuphine usage during labor associates with minimal deleterious neonatal effects.[27] Nalbuphine's μ-receptor antagonist properties have been utilized to reverse the adverse effects of neuraxial opioids including respiratory depression and pruritus. Nalbuphine is largely metabolized in the liver and excreted in the feces.

Butorphanol is a weak antagonist at μ receptors. However, it is five times more potent as an analgesic than morphine. Butorphanol's labor analgesia compares favorably with the analgesia provided with meperidine in terms of effects on the neonate.[28] Maternal drowsiness following administration can be significant and may even follow administration in the epidural space. Liver metabolism, followed by urinary and fecal excretion, terminates butorphanol's effect.

NEURAXIAL OPIOIDS

Following identification of opioid receptors in the spinal cord, morphine was proved to produce intense analgesia following epidural or intrathecal administration. Also identified were side effects including delayed respiratory depression, which is thought to occur with rostral spread in the cerebrospinal fluid. Subsequently, more lipid-soluble opioids were examined, hypothesizing that analgesia could be maintained and the side effects of rostral spread minimized. Unfortunately, this hypothesis has, for the most part, proved inaccurate. Potential side effects require monitoring and may require intervention.

Respiratory depression is by far the most dangerous side effect and, although associated most with morphine use, has been reported with other agents as well. The reported incidence is between 0.1 and 0.5% and appears to be related to rostral spread and consequent depression of brain stem respiratory centers. Epidural or subarachnoid narcotic administration dictates awareness of this potential complication, appropriate monitoring, and preparation for treatment. Treatment includes IV naloxone, in 0.1-mg increments, and if indicated, tracheal intubation and ventilatory support.

Pruritus is the most unpleasant side effect of neuraxial opioids and appears to be dose-related. Pruritus most commonly involves the face and trunk but may be generalized. Although not life-threatening, pruritus frequently requires treatment. Treatment consists of diphenhydramine (25–50 mg intramuscularly or intravenously) in mild cases; more refractory pruritus may require naloxone titration intravenously in 0.04-mg to 0.1-mg increments in an attempt to relieve itching without reversing analgesia. Occasionally, a naloxone infusion (0.4–0.6 mg/hr) is required to maintain the antipruritic effect. Some success has been reported with nalbuphine 5 to 10 mg for treating pruritus without analgesia reversal. Interestingly, propofol in 10 mg doses also treats pruritus.[28]

Nausea and vomiting occur with all neuraxial opioids but most commonly with morphine/meperidine, probably related to stimulation of the chemoreceptor trigger zone. Narcotic antagonists and antiemetics—including naloxone 0.1 to 0.2 mg IV, nalbuphine 5 to 10 mg IV, droperidol 0.625 to 1.25 mg IV, and prochlorperazine 10 to 20 mg IM—lessen nausea and vomiting.

Finally, although controversial, the use of neuraxial opioids has been associated with reactivation of herpes simplex lesions. The exact mechanism is unknown but could be related to pruritus and itching.

Morphine

Morphine has been the most widely used opioid in obstetrics both intrathecally and epidurally. Since morphine is more hydrophilic than other opioids, intrathecal morphine remains free in the cerebrospinal fluid longer with a greater potential for rostral spread to higher CNS centers. Intrathecal morphine (0.5–2 mg) has provided pain relief during labor. The time to maximal analgesia is 1 hour, but analgesia lasts several hours. Analgesia may be adequate for uterine contraction pain during the first stage of labor, but intrathecal morphine does not provide adequate pain relief for the second stage of labor and episiotomy repair. Furthermore, intrathecal morphine in this dose range associates with a high incidence of side effects including nausea, vomiting, and delayed respiratory depression. For analgesia following cesarean section, 0.2 to 0.3 mg administered in combination with fentanyl or sufentanil and the spinal local anesthetic can provide pain relief for up to 20 hours with few side effects. Smaller doses, 0.1 mg or less, may be equally effective with a reduction in dose-related side effects.[29]

Epidural morphine is the most widely used opioid for pain relief following cesarean section, with a dose range of 3 to 5 mg. Lower drug amounts associate with greater failure rates, and higher doses produce greater side effects. Some authors recommend a bolus administration followed by continuous infusion in an attempt to maximize analgesia while minimizing side effects. Regardless of the dosing method, meticulous nursing surveillance of the patient receiving epidural morphine has proved to be as effective as more sophisticated monitors in identifying respiratory depression. From a practical perspective, when considering intrathecal or epidural administration of morphine, weigh the indications for drug administration, the risks of respiratory depression in the patient, and finally, the reliability of monitoring by nursing staff.

Fentanyl

Fentanyl, a more highly lipid-soluble drug than morphine, administered intrathecally has a quicker onset and briefer duration of action. Twenty-five micrograms of fentanyl provides analgesia for approximately 80 minutes. Potential respiratory depression within 30 minutes of intrathecal administration associates with the high lipid solubility of fentanyl.

Epidural fentanyl enhances labor pain relief when combined with low concentrations of bupivacaine. The reduction in bupivacaine dose facilitated by fentanyl may reduce side effects and enhance bupivacaine safety. Importantly, epidural fentanyl is equipotent to IV fentanyl. One potential explanation for this phenomenon may be the high lipid solubility of fentanyl and rapid systemic absorption, leaving relatively smaller amounts receptor bound.

Sufentanil

Intrathecal sufentanil (3–15 μg) provides brief analgesia appropriate for the first stage of labor. When combined with epidural infusions of bupivacaine, sufentanil provides rapid onset of pain relief and comfort in advance of bupivacaine's onset. The author's group believes that 10 μg of intrathecal sufentanil administered in combination with local anesthetic for cesarean section may improve intraoperative analgesia, particularly during exteriorization of the uterus. Importantly, recent reports of blood pressure declines associated with 10 μg of sufentanil administered intrathecally without local anesthetic suggest that hemodynamic stability is not guaranteed when administered during labor.[30] The explanation for the blood pressure declines is unclear, but these may represent the effects of pain relief.

In contrast to fentanyl, sufentanil's high lipid solubility does not permit administering a lower epidural dose than that of the IV route. However, like fentanyl, when combined with bupivacaine, synergism exists, allowing a reduction in bupivacaine dosage.

Miscellaneous Agents

Meperidine, unlike other opioids, has an inherent local anesthetic property. Spinal meperidine has served as the sole anesthetic agent for cesarean section. Ten to 20 mg of intrathecal meperidine provides adequate pain relief of moderate duration for the first stage of labor but produces a high incidence of nausea and vomiting.[30] Not surprisingly, hypotension may occur. Finally, 50 mg of epidural meperidine provides short-lived analgesia following cesarean section.

Epidural alfentanil 25 μg/ml in combination with dilute solutions of bupivacaine provides improved pain relief when compared with dilute solutions of bupivacaine alone.

Epidural butorphanol 2 mg provides postoperative analgesia following cesarean section. Unfortunately, as discussed earlier, a high incidence of somnolence reduces its applicability in the obstetric population. Also, despite its widespread use, it is interesting to note that intrathecal butorphanol associates with histopathologic changes in the spinal cord of sheep.[31] This, combined with its tendency to produce sedation, makes it a less than optimal choice.

Finally, epidural *nalbuphine* with doses ranging from 5 to 20 mg has been used to provide analgesia following cesarean section with pain relief comparable to that of morphine.

COMMON NONANESTHETIC DRUGS

Antihypertensives

Antihypertensives are indicated during pregnancy to control chronic hypertensive states, to control antepartum and intrapartum blood pressure during severe preeclampsia, and to acutely reduce severe hypertension prior to the induction of general anesthesia in order to minimize the hypertensive response to tracheal intubation. Many drugs have been utilized, and indications for drug usage influence drug selection. This section addresses the agents most commonly used by anesthesiologists and obstetricians.

Hydralazine

Hydralazine may be the antihypertensive agent most extensively used during pregnancy. Hydralazine provides direct arteriolar smooth muscle relaxation, a portion of which may be endothelium-dependent and involve nitric oxide release. Not surprisingly, vasodilatation may lead to reflex tachycardia and increased cardiac output. Plasma renin activity increases. These compensatory effects partially mitigate hydralazine's antihypertensive effect. Hydralazine may work best when combined with some degree of β blockade. Widespread obstetric use is probably accounted for by hydralazine's suspected ability to improve uterine blood flow during preeclampsia. Side effects include headache, nausea, palpitations, angina, and rarely, immunologic reactions such as the lupus syndrome. Tachyphylaxis may occur. Finally, the hypotensive effect is unpredictable, and onset is delayed even when the drug is administered intravenously. Peak effect may occur as late as 40 minutes following IV injection. Therefore, wise administration includes 5- to 10-mg IV boluses and titration to effect, with 20 to 30 minutes between injections.

Methyldopa

Methyldopa has a proven safety record during pregnancy; children followed for up to 7 years whose mothers received methyldopa reveal normal development.[32] Thus, it offers an advantage for the control of chronic hypertension during pregnancy with its stated primary benefit of fetal safety. It reduces blood pressure by acting centrally in the brain. Metabolism of methyldopa to methylnorephrine, secondary stimulation of α_2-adrenergic receptors in the brain stem, and subsequent decreases in central sympathetic activity may account for much of its action. It may produce sedation, postural hypotension, parkinsonian symptoms, and depression. Less common but more serious side effects associated with chronic use include hemolytic anemia, leukopenia, thrombocytopenia, and hepatitis. Methyldopa is not useful for anesthetic purposes because even IV administration requires hours to reach peak effect. Methyldopa reduces MAC of potent inhalation agents.

β *Blockers*

β blockers are becoming increasingly popular antihypertensive agents in both the nonpregnant and the pregnant population. In pregnant women, early uncontrolled reports of its use during pregnancy indicated increased perinatal mortality and associated intrauterine growth retardation. However, subsequent prospective clinical trials did not substantiate these findings and validated the safety of atenolol and labetalol. Nevertheless, potential placenta crossage requires consideration. The mechanism of action of β blockers' antihypertensive effect is unknown. Reduced renin secretion, cardiac output, impaired baroreceptor function, altered prostaglandin synthesis, and effects on the CNS vasomotor centers may relate to the antihypertensive effect. However, since stereoisomers that lack β-adrenergic properties do not have an antihypertensive effect, it appears the β blockade is an essential aspect of their therapeutic antihypertensive effect. Labetalol is unique among β blockers in that it has both α-blocking and β-blocking properties. Labetalol is a combination of four isomers in equal proportion that bestow on the drug four different properties—selective α_1 blockade, blockade of β_1 and β_2 receptors, an agonist activity at β receptors, and finally, inhibition of neuronal uptake of norepinephrine. α_1 blockade (with some contribution of β_2-agonist effect) leads to vasodilatation, and β_1 blockade prevents reflex sympathetic activation of the heart.

β blockers also affect the cardiovascular system by influencing cardiac rhythm and automaticity by reducing sinus discharge rate, decreasing activity of ectopic pacemakers, slowing conduction in the atria and atrioventricular (AV) node, and lengthening the refractory period of the AV node. These properties make them effective antiarrhythmic agents.

Important effects exerted on systems other than the cardiovascular include blockade of β-adrenergic receptors on bronchial smooth muscle, which has little effect in normal individuals but can lead to life-threatening bronchoconstriction in patients with asthma or chronic obstructive pulmonary disease. β blockade influences the metabolism of carbohydrates and lipids and, importantly, may mask the tachycardia observed during hypoglycemic episodes. Regarding the fetus, β blockers cross the placenta, and propranolol, especially with chronic use, has been associated with intrauterine growth retardation, fetal hypoglycemia, and bradycardia.[33, 34] Atenolol[35] and labetalol[36] are not considered hazardous for the fetus. Esmolol, however, has been associated with undesirable effects on the fetus in animal studies.[37]

At present, labetalol is the most popular agent utilized by anesthesiologists intraoperatively in management of the obstetric patient. Preoperative reduction of blood pressure is accomplished by 5- to 10-mg boluses titrated to an end-point prior to the induction of general anesthesia. Esmolol, rapidly hydrolyzed by erythrocyte esterases, has a half-life of 8 minutes and is, theoretically, an ideal agent to blunt the hemodynamic consequences of laryngoscopy and intubation. However, its fetal safety has not yet been established.

Calcium Channel Blockers

Calcium channel blockers are a structurally heterogeneous group of compounds that share the ability to block L-type voltage-sensitive calcium channels. Calcium channel blockage has important effects on the heart, blood vessels, and smooth muscles including those of the uterus. Five agents are currently approved for clinical use in the United States—verapamil, diltiazem, nifedipine, nicardipine, and nimodipine. From a practical perspective, verapamil and diltiazem mainly influence the heart whereas the others exert their predominant effect on smooth muscle. Nifedipine is the only calcium channel blocker widely prescribed during pregnancy; it was first used to inhibit preterm labor and subsequently utilized to treat hypertensive disorders of pregnancy. Nifedipine's mechanism of action is smooth muscle relaxation, which occurs at concentrations significantly lower than those that influence cardiac function. Clinical studies confirm the safety of nifedipine and nicardipine when used to control hypertension during pregnancy.[38, 39]

Normally, depolarization results in the opening of voltage-sensitive calcium channels and the subsequent influx of calcium ions down an electrochemical gradient. Calcium ions then initiate contraction of smooth muscle subsequent to the influx. Nifedipine blocks these calcium channels and thus prevents the rise in intracellular calcium. In addition, it may also inhibit cyclic nucleotide phosphodiesterases, thus increasing cellular cyclic nucleotides. The combination of these two effects is believed to be the basis of its greater effect on vascular smooth muscle.

Pharmacokinetic studies reveal near-complete absorption following oral administration of these agents with high first-pass metabolism by the liver to innocuous metabolites that are excreted in the urine. There is some doubt as to whether sublingual absorption occurs.[40] Nifedipine's onset occurs in less than 20 minutes and the drug has a half-life of 2 to 3 hours.

When considering use during pregnancy, it is important that no adverse effects on uteroplacental perfusion have been reported.[41] Both animal and human studies demonstrate that nifedipine decreases uterine contractions. It easily crosses the placenta; however, clinical studies in humans have not identified adverse fetal or neonatal effects.[38] Headaches and hot flashes are the most common distressing side effects accompanying administration. However, excess dosages may produce hypotension.

When considering administration during anesthesia, nifedipine's effects on systemic vascular resistance may be enhanced by inhalation and narcotic anesthetic agents producing hypotension. Finally, calcium channel blockers are highly protein bound and, by displacing drugs such as lidocaine and bupivacaine, could in theory increase the incidence of toxic side effects.

Potent Intravenous Antihypertensive Agents

Nitroglycerin

Nitroglycerin, like all other organic nitrates, relaxes almost all smooth muscle. Of interest to the obstetric anesthesia care provider are its effects on vascular and uterine smooth muscle. Nitroglycerin leads to formation of nitric oxide, which in turn leads to dephosphorylation of light chains of myosin, producing smooth muscle relaxation. Although used as an antihypertensive agent, it is mainly a vasodilator, which may impair its effectiveness in well-hydrated patients. Nitroglycerin's advantages include a quick onset and a brief half-life of 1 to 3 minutes secondary to rapid liver metabolism. Tachyphylaxis is common when administered continuously; thus, its most effective use is to effect rapid, but short-term, control of hypertension.[42] When administered by continuous infusion, the usual concentration is 25 to 50 μg/ml and it is commonly infused at a rate of 5 to 100 μg/min and titrated to the desired effect. Historically, its main use is in the preoperative reduction in blood pressure in severe preeclampsia.

The other major indication in obstetrics is secondary to nitroglycerin's effect on uterine contractions. The relaxant effect is unpredictable; clinical reports indicate that 50 to 500 μg of nitroglycerin relaxes the uterus and can permit manual removal of placenta, fetal manipulation, and treatment of uterine version. Although these dose ranges reportedly produce minimal cardiovascular effects, there are no controlled studies confirming the safety and efficacy of nitroglycerin when used for these indications. In the author's practice, administration usually begins with 50 to 75 μg intravenously.

Nitroprusside

In contrast to nitroglycerin, nitroprusside dilates both arterioles and venules and is particularly useful for brief control of blood pressure and blunting the response to tracheal intubation in severe preeclamptic patients. Sodium nitroprusside releases nitric oxide when it contacts red blood cells, and nitric oxide in turn accounts for the vasodilatation. The hypotensive effects begin within 30 seconds of administration and the effects peak within 2 minutes; dissipation of effect occurs within 3 minutes of cessation of infusion. Nitroprusside almost always requires arterial line blood pressure monitoring because of the rapid and potent effects on blood pressure. Since nitroprusside is an unstable compound and decomposes on exposure to light, the administration set should be protected from light. The drug is usually administered 50 mg in 250 to 1000 ml of 5% dextrose and titrated to effect.

Fetal concerns center on nitroprusside metabolism, which leads to the formation of cyanide radicals that are eventually metabolized in the liver. Hence, the potential for fetal cyanide toxicity does exist. The current recommendations are to start at an initial rate of 0.5 μg/kg/min and titrate to effect.

Trimethaphan

Historically, trimethaphan was a popular agent for acute control of blood pressure during hypertensive crises. Advantages during pregnancy include no effect on intracranial pressure, although that is rarely a consideration. Disadvantages include the relatively slow onset and offset and the potential during chronic infusions to interfere with the metabolism of succinylcholine. Trimethaphan impairs transmission in autonomic ganglia by competing with acetylcholine at ganglionic cholinergic receptor sites. Consequently, trimethaphan's effects on the body are widespread and potentially affect all autonomic functions. Reduced blood pressure occurs secondary to autonomic blockade and decreased sympathetic discharge to arterioles and veins, resulting in hypotension. Diminished venous return reduces cardiac output. Trimethaphan is usually prepared as a 0.1% solution in 5% dextrose and titrated to effect. Tachyphylaxis frequently occurs. Regarding obstetric use, placental transfer is believed limited secondary to trimethaphan's large molecular weight.

Tocolytics

Magnesium Sulfate

Obstetric indications for magnesium sulfate are for the prevention of eclamptic convulsions in preeclampsia and as a tocolytic agent during premature labor. Magnesium acts as a calcium antagonist either at membrane calcium channels or intracellularly. Indeed, it has been suggested that the biologic evolution of life may have placed these two bivalent elements as natural antagonists in living cells.[43] Magnesium has the ability to relax vascular smooth muscle, which may be secondary to its ability to enhance the release of prostacyclin.[44] In preeclampsia, there is evidence that cerebral vasospasm occurs and may be the basis of cerebral ischemia leading to convulsions. Relief of cerebral vasospasm may thus be the basis for magnesium's ability to prevent and possibly treat eclamptic convulsions.[45] Magnesium sulfate also may act as an anticonvulsant by depressing neuronal transmission in the CNS. Unclear is the degree to which magnesium sulfate's ability to depress neuromuscular transmission contributes to its effectiveness as an anticonvulsant. Although considered to be a sedative, the certainty of this effect is unclear.

The observation that magnesium sulfate utilized in the treatment of preeclampsia/eclampsia associated with prolonged labor and the laboratory observation that magnesium relaxed isolated myometrial strips led to its utilization as a tocolytic agent. Despite its widespread use for this indication, the effectiveness in preventing preterm labor is not universally accepted.[46]

In most centers, the preferred route of magnesium administration is IV. Usually, an initial bolus of 4 gm is administered followed by an infusion of 1 to 3 gm/hr. Ideally, serum magnesium levels should be monitored at regular intervals and the infusion rate modified depending on the results. The therapeutic range is between 4 and 8 mEq/L. Table 5–5 summarizes the signs and symptoms associated with various magnesium levels. Of practical importance is the fact that a magnesium blood level of 10 mEq/L coincides with the disappearance of deep tendon reflexes. Greater serum levels associate with peripheral muscle weakness and respiratory insufficiency. Epidural analgesia interferes with assessment of deep tendon reflexes in the knees, and the biceps reflex should be used in this circumstance. Treatment of major toxicity is supportive, including intubation and ventilation if needed, and very rarely, cardiopulmonary resuscitation. Further measures of treatment may include cautious use of calcium as an antagonist and diuretics to aid elimination.

Side effects associated with magnesium therapy include chest pain and pulmonary edema. These are more likely to occur if magnesium is administered in combination with a β agonist. Although magnesium sulfate's vasodilating effects can lead to transient hypotension, it may possibly improve uteroplacental circulation. Although the author's group advises caution when initiating a major conduction block in the presence of therapeutic levels of magnesium, problems are rare in hydrated patients. As discussed previously, magnesium interferes with muscle relaxants. Finally, in the absence of maternal toxicity, magnesium has few effects on the newborn and does not significantly alter the biophysical profile of the healthy preterm fetus.[47]

β Agonists

β agonists are widely utilized as tocolytics for the prevention of preterm labor. However, while

TABLE 5–5
Signs and Symptoms Associated With Different Plasma Levels of Magnesium

Plasma Level (mEq/L)	Comment
1.5–2.0	Level in normal individuals
4.0–7.0	Therapeutic level
10	Loss of deep tendon reflexes
12	Respiratory arrest

β agonists inhibit uterine contractility, they also affect other organ systems, which may have an impact on anesthetic management.

β-adrenergic agents relax uterine smooth muscle by increasing intracellular cAMP. Increased intracellular cAMP in turn reduces intracellular calcium and myosin light chain phosphorylation, which leads to diminished actin-myosin interaction. Hypokalemia may occur as a side effect, since cAMP also affects the sodium potassium pump. However, total body potassium remains the same in almost all instances and does not require treatment, returning to normal within hours of cessation of therapy. *Remember,* ***severe*** *hyperventilation can worsen existing hypokalemia.* Ritodrine was specifically developed to treat preterm labor and is the only β agonist currently approved by the U.S. Food and Drug Administration for use as a tocolytic. Other agents—terbutaline, fenoteral, and albuterol—have also been utilized to attempt to inhibit uterine contractility. However, all possess similar side effects.

β agonists produce a dose-related tachycardia and an increase in cardiac output secondary to a direct cardiostimulation effect and reflexly in response to lower diastolic pressure. With vigorous IV hydration, pulmonary edema may occur with or without evidence of myocardial dysfunction. The incidence of arrhythmias is greater in patients receiving β agonists. In the author's group's experience, arrhythmias have not posed a clinical problem; however, the selection of either regional or general anesthesia and the extent of cardiovascular monitoring must be made on an individual basis. Primary theoretical concerns are the potential effect of superimposing further sympathetic blockade secondary to epidural or spinal anesthesia in the face of preexisting vasodilatation. In the author's group's experience, this is not a major problem. Phenylephrine, with its α-agonist effect, may be an appropriate choice for restoration of blood pressure when this is a concern. However, recent animal studies suggest that ephedrine is still the best choice for restoring uterine perfusion and improving fetal oxygenation.[48] In practical terms, consider allowing sufficient time for decay of drug blood levels but do not allow this to jeopardize care.

Finally, β agonists can cause marked maternal hyperglycemia. Persistent hyperglycemia results in elevated serum levels of glucose in the fetus and the potential for reactive hypoglycemia in the neonate following delivery.

Oxytocics

Drugs that stimulate myometrial contractions are indicated in obstetrics to induce abortions, facilitate induction of labor, and control postpartum bleeding. Oxytocin, methylergometrine, prostaglandins $F_{2\alpha}$ and E_2 are the currently available agents, each with its appropriate indication.

Oxytocin is a naturally occurring hormone synthesized in the supraoptic and paraventricular nuclei of the hypothalamus and released from secretory granules from the neurohypophysis. Although natural oxytocin was used at one time, commercially available oxytocin is completely synthetic and has replaced natural oxytocin in obstetric use.

Human myometrium has oxytocin receptors that progressively increase in number as pregnancy advances. The mechanism by which oxytocin binding to receptors leads to increased force and frequency of contractions is unknown, but it may involve activation of voltage-sensitive calcium channels or the release of prostaglandins. Although very high doses of oxytocin initiate contraction of the myometrium in early pregnancy, uterine responsiveness to oxytocin increases after the 20th week of gestation, with the greatest increase in sensitivity taking place during the last 9 weeks of pregnancy.

Oxytocin administration has anesthetic implications. Oxytocin causes a transient relaxation of vascular smooth muscle and inhibits preganglionic sympathetic neurones as well as neurones located in the medulla. Hence, oxytocin can cause hypotension when administered in high doses. Oxytocin is usually administered as an infusion containing 20 units of oxytocin in 1000 ml of lactated Ringer's. Regarding hypotension, from a practical perspective, it is exceedingly difficult to cause hypotension by rapid infusion rates of this solution. Drug administration should not be withheld in the face of hypotension secondary to bleeding for fear of causing vasodilatation. The hypotension accompanying bolus administration of oxytocin is brief and likely to be clinically relevant only in those patients in whom acute afterload reduction would be hazardous. Some practitioners will administer, in emergency circumstances, 5 to 10 mg as an IV bolus. Finally, older, nonsynthetic preparations of oxytocin administered in conjunction with 5% dextrose in water (D5W) were capable of producing water intoxication secondary to the administration of large amounts of free water and the antidiuretic effect inherent in the older properties of naturally occurring oxytocin. This does not appear to be a problem with the synthetic preparations when administered with lactated Ringer's.

Prostaglandins are a ubiquitous group of autocoids found in rising concentrations in late pregnancy and during labor in the amniotic fluid and umbilical arterial and maternal blood. Prostaglandins may have a role in initiating labor, since their concentrations in amniotic fluid rise during labor. Prostaglandins are more effective than oxytocin in inducing contractions in the early months of pregnancy. There are two commercially available prostaglandins. Prostaglandin E_2 and dinoprostone (Prostin E_2) are vaginal suppositories and primarily used to induce abortions. Prostaglandin $F_{2\alpha}$, carboprost tromethamine (Hemabate), is prepared at 0.25 mg/ml in injection form and utilized for the induction and abetment of abortions. Prostaglandin $F_{2\alpha}$ is also used to treat postpartum hemorrhage secondary to uterine atony.

The primary concerns and anesthetic implications for obstetric anesthesia care providers are the precipitous drops in maternal arterial oxygen saturations that may occur following intravenous or intramyometrial administration. Interestingly, the reports of falling maternal oxygen saturation occurred in women undergoing general anesthesia to correct preexisting uterine atony.[49] Pulse oximetry is indicated for women receiving this drug, especially for those with preexisting pulmonary disease.

Ergot Alkaloids

Ergot alkaloids increase the force and frequency of uterine contractions and, in high doses, cause sustained uterine contractures. This latter property and the propensity for causing uterine rupture in later gestation reserve their use for treating postpartum bleeding. Ergonovine and methylergonovine are less toxic and more active as uterine stimulants than older agents and have replaced all other ergot alkaloids for the treatment of uterine atony.

Cardiovascular effects pose the most significant considerations when ergot alkaloids are administered. These drugs constrict both arteries and veins owing to partial agonism at α-adrenergic receptors, and severe hypertension can follow administration. IV use should be avoided, since the hypertension may be life-threatening. In theory, these drugs potentiate the effects of subsequently administered vasopressors. The author's group has not observed this phenomenon when ergot alkaloids have been administered orally postdelivery. However, ergot alkaloids should be used with caution, if at all, in patients with pregnancy-related hypertension. Nausea and vomiting are common following the use of ergot alkaloids, and serious side effects, including direct coronary artery vasoconstriction, are possible.[50] In the author's institution these drugs are not administered intravenously because of the potential complications.

Ergonovine, methylergonovine, and methergine are available in 0.2 mg/ml preparation. The response to intramuscular injection is rapid and sustained, and again IV injection is ill-advised.

Antiepileptics

Between 0.3 and 0.6% of pregnant women experience epilepsy, and epileptic patients in turn experience a two- to threefold increase in the risk of congenital anomalies in their offspring. Whether this increased frequency of congenital anomalies is secondary to disease effects or medication, or the combination of both, is unclear. Phenytoin, phenobarbital, and carbamazepine are the primary antiepileptic drugs utilized during pregnancy. Phenytoin's mechanism of action is probably the stabilizing effect on excitable membranes largely due to inhibition of sodium currents. Regardless, pregnancy influences the pharmacokinetics of phenytoin. Absorption after oral ingestion is slow and erratic. Further, in pregnancy, nausea and vomiting may lead to poor maternal compliance. Phenytoin is extensively bound to albumin, and in theory, more unbound drug is available secondary to the decreased serum levels during pregnancy. However, since blood volume and total protein are probably increased during pregnancy, the significance of this effect is uncertain. Phenytoin is metabolized in the liver, and less than 5% is excreted unchanged in the urine. The increased metabolic capacity of the liver occurring during pregnancy may enhance excretion. Finally, during pregnancy, there is an increase in total body water, which may contribute to drug dilution and lower than expected serum levels. Overall, altered pharmacokinetics suggest increased dose requirements during pregnancy and plasma levels should be monitored closely.

Cerebellar and vestibular effects such as vertigo and severe nystagmus are manifestations of CNS toxicity. Other potential side effects secondary to phenytoin administration include gingival hyperplasia, osteomalacia, and megaloblastic anemia. Manifestations of drug allergy include serious side effects on the skin, bone marrow, and liver. Phenytoin administration during pregnancy has been associated with the "fetal hydantoin syndrome," characterized by growth deficiency, microcephaly, dysmorphic facies, and mental deficiency.[51] Neonates born to mothers who received phenytoin during pregnancy may also exhibit clotting abnormalities requiring treatment. Vitamin K is the usual treatment.

Phenobarbital, historically used to manage mild preeclampsia, is also indicated for the treatment of epilepsy during pregnancy. Phenobarbital resembles phenytoin in maternal side effects and toxicity. Up to 25% of the drug is excreted unchanged in the urine, whereas the remainder is metabolized into inactive metabolites in the liver. Phenobarbital also associates with a fetal syndrome. Importantly, maternal drug administration can result in neonatal coagulopathy. In contrast to phenytoin, neonatal depression and drug withdrawal symptoms may occur in the newborn.

Carbamazepine has complex pharmacokinetics. Its extensive metabolism includes transformation to an active metabolite. Untoward maternal effects include drowsiness, vertigo, and blurred vision. Serious adverse effects include hematologic toxicity and hypersensitivity. Implicated fetal effects include craniofacial defects, fingernail hypoplasia, and delayed development.[52]

Vasopressors

Vasopressors are essential drugs for the safe practice of anesthesia. Gravid women are more prone to develop hypotension following spinal and epidural blockade secondary to the potentially greater spread of local anesthetic, increased sensitivity of neurones to local anesthetic, impaired venous return associated with aortocaval compression, and a greater reliance on sympathetic tone to ensure adequate venous return. Hypotension is not prevented or completely reversed by IV fluid alone.[61] Importantly, the restoration of maternal blood pressure should not be at the expense of uterine blood flow. Therefore, ideally, the vasopressor should not have direct or indirect adverse fetal effects.

Catecholamines are indicated for maternal resuscitation during cardiac arrest or for severe life-threatening hypotension unresponsive to other therapies. Their use, however, is limited in most circumstances because they reduce uteroplacental perfusion and may not be appropriate in less acute situations. The most hazardous forms of these drugs are those that exert primarily α-adrenergic effect. Methoxamine, phenylephrine, and norepinephrine, in animal studies, diminish uterine perfusion and lead to fetal asphyxia. Therefore, indirectly acting agents such as ephedrine and mephetermine, which act both directly and indirectly by enhancing the release of norepinephrine at nerve terminals to restore blood pressure and maintain uterine perfusion, are usually the agents of first choice for treatment of hypotension during pregnancy.

Individual Agents

Ephedrine

Ephedrine has α- and β-adrenergic-agonist properties. It also acts indirectly by enhancing the release of norepinephrine from sympathetic neurons. β stimulation results in increased heart rate, increased cardiac output, and to a lesser extent, increased peripheral resistance. In most circumstances, ephedrine administration leads to a rise in blood pressure with preservation of uterine perfusion. Ephedrine may also work primarily by increasing venous return.

Ephedrine may be administered orally, intramuscularly, subcutaneously, or intravenously. Ephedrine is excreted in the urine, mainly unchanged, and has a half-life of 3 to 6 hours. Usual anesthetic administration is an IV bolus of 5 to 10 mg in conjunction with fluid administration. In rare circumstances, ephedrine may cause maternal hypertension and arrhythmias. Tachyphylaxis can occur, and intrapartum administration may result in alterations in fetal heart rate variability.

Phenylephrine

Phenylephrine is a selective α_1-adrenergic agonist. β-receptor stimulation occurs only at very high concentrations. The major cardiovascular effect following phenylephrine administration is increased blood pressure, mainly due to arterial vasoconstriction; however, reflex bradycardia can occur after large doses. In healthy women, small boluses of phenylephrine have been shown to restore blood pressure without deleterious fetal effects. The recommended dosage during pregnancy is 20- to 100-μg boluses. In practical terms, intrapartum administration of phenylephrine should be limited for specific indications, and ephedrine should be used first.

ABUSABLE DRUGS

Cocaine, the first clinically used local anesthetic, is utilized today more as a recreational drug than for therapeutic indications. Approximately 5 million people in the United States use it regularly, and abuse during child-bearing age is common. Cocaine usage during pregnancy has led to increased maternal and neonatal morbidity and mortality.

Like other local anesthetic agents, cocaine's mechanism of action is the reversible blockade of sodium channels and the subsequent prevention of the rapid influx of sodium ions necessary for the propagation of action potentials. Importantly, cocaine has significant autonomic effects secondary to the blockage of the reuptake of norepinephrine into the sympathetic nerve endings. Cocaine may also act postsynaptically by effecting a greater response from the target cell. These two effects form the basis of its sympathomimetic effects. Cocaine affects both axonal transmission and synaptic function in the neurons that involve norepinephrine, dopamine, serotonin, tryptophan, and acetylcholine. These effects form the basis for the euphoria and behavioral effects that contribute to its addictive properties. The site and mechanism of cocaine-induced seizures are unknown but may be related to the blockade of the inhibitory pathways, or alternatively, the focus may lie in subcortical areas and the modification of turnover of catecholamines and serotonin.

Obstetric complications secondary to maternal cocaine ingestion include preterm labor, premature rupture of membranes, abruptio placentae, spontaneous abortion, pregnancy-induced hypertension, cerebrovascular accidents, precipitous labor, stillbirth, and meconium-stained fluid. Seizures may also occur, resulting in maternal and fetal hypoxemia.

Fetal and neonatal complications may arise secondary to uterine vasoconstriction, which, in turn, leads to fetal hypoxemia. Low birth weight, lower gestational age at delivery, and congenital urogenital abnormalities are manifestations of cocaine abuse during pregnancy.

The anesthetic implications of cocaine abuse involve cardiovascular considerations. Acute intoxication is associated with tachycardia and hypertension and a propensity for ventricular arrhythmias. General anesthesia, utilizing a rapid-sequence induction, may increase risk secondary to the usual sympathetic discharge accompanying tracheal intubation. Nevertheless, little evidence exists to advocate any particular anesthetic drug or regimen. In theory, β blockers (e.g., labetalol) or calcium channel blockers (e.g., nifedipine) may be desirable agents to reduce exaggerated response to intubation. Further, avoiding halothane and its propensity for ventricular arrhythmias in the presence of increased sympathetic levels may minimize the risk of dangerous arrhythmias. Hypotension following spinal or epidural block may also pose a significant threat. Chronic depletion of catecholamines may render indirectly acting agents such as ephedrine ineffective. However, in practice, ephedrine is effective.[53] Phenylephrine may be used for patients unresponsive to ephedrine and in the presence of profound tachycardia. Finally, thrombocytopenia has been associated with cocaine abuse, and a platelet count is a wise laboratory test prior to initiating spinal or epidural blockade.

DRUG EXCRETION INTO BREAST MILK AND POTENTIAL NEONATAL EFFECTS

There is a paucity of human studies on which to base recommendations regarding breast milk and drug ingestion. Animal data may be difficult to interpret, as human milk differs in composition and pH from animal milk, and these differences may in turn affect drug elimination.

Human milk is a suspension of protein and fat globules in a carbohydrate- and mineral-containing solution. Hence, protein and lipid binding of drugs occur. Transfer of drugs into milk is similar to drug transfer across any membrane and is generally related to the concentration gradient, lipid solubility, degree of ionization, and degree of protein binding on both sides of the membrane. Studies often cite milk:plasma ratio of drugs. However, these may be based on single measurements, which may not reflect equilibrium or may not be sampled at the same time in relation to maternal dosing and the time and frequency of nursing. More accurate elimination studies using radioactive tracers obviously cannot be done. At the moment, the presence of a drug in milk cannot be quantitatively related to neonatal effects. It is known that neonatal handling of drugs, particularly in the premature neonate, is not as well developed as in adults. At present, the recommendations of the American Academy of Pediatrics (AAP) Committee on Drugs provide the following guidelines:[54] (1) decide whether the drug therapy is really necessary; (2) use the safest drug; (3) consider measuring the blood concentration of any drug that carries the possibility of causing harm in the infant; (4) and minimize exposing the infant to medication by allowing the mother to breast feed just before receiving medication.

Regarding anesthetic drugs, IV agents are potentially the most concerning. The following is a brief survey of the available information to utilize when considering drug selection. Following TPL usage during cesarean section, the amount of drug ingested by the infant from breast milk is negligible.[55] Despite the fact that the half-life of TPL is prolonged in infants, the absolute blood concentrations are so small that they cannot affect neonatal behavior.

Propofol, discussed earlier, may be harmful to the infant during prolonged exposure. However, the amount identified in breast milk following induction and maintenance of anesthesia for cesarean section is negligible compared with the amount of exposure through placental transfer.[15] Among inhalation agents, information is available only for halothane. Prolonged occupational exposure to halothane results in detectable halothane levels in breast milk. However, infant exposure has been considered insignificant.[56]

Opioids are administered intrapartum as well as postpartum for pain management. A recent study comparing the effects of morphine and meperidine in breast milk suggested morphine was more desirable because it produced less neurobehavioral depression in the breast-fed neonates than meperidine.[57] All of these patients were receiving opioids for pain relief following cesarean section. Neonates in the meperidine group were less alert and more poorly oriented compared with those in the morphine group. Accumulation of an active metabolite, normeperidine, in maternal plasma and ultimately breast milk when combined with prolonged neonatal half-lives of both meperidine and normeperidine may account for these findings. As a result, despite meperidine's long history of safe use, the AAP no longer includes meperidine in the list of drugs compatible with breast feeding.[54]

Fentanyl is considered compatible with breast feeding by the AAP.[54] Although this agent is secreted in breast milk following its use as an analgesic during labor, neurobehavioral depression does not occur.[58]

Little information is available regarding nonnarcotic analgesics. However, one breast-feeding infant whose mother was receiving acetaminophen developed a rash that resolved following cessation of maternal acetaminophen intake. No other untoward effect was reported.[59] Despite this report, the AAP considers this drug compatible with breast feeding.[54] Finally, the AAP considers ibuprofen and ketorolac compatible with breast feeding despite the paucity of clinical evidence.

TEN PRACTICAL POINTS

1. During cardiovascular arrest, unless restoration of the circulation is expected promptly,

cesarean delivery improves both neonatal and maternal survival.

2. Pregnancy reduces the minimal alveolar concentration (MAC) of all inhalational agents, including nitrous oxide. Monitor maternal level of consciousness carefully if using inhalational analgesia.

3. Keep potent inhalational agent concentrations less than 1 MAC to enable uterine response to oxytocin.

4. Plasma pseudocholinesterase concentrations are reduced during pregnancy; however, not enough to justify reducing the succinylcholine intubation dose.

5. Remember, women receiving magnesium sulfate have markedly increased sensitivity to nondepolarizing muscle relaxants, but require normal doses of succinylcholine.

6. The use of lipophilic opioids such as sufentanil or fentanyl via epidural/spinal routes does not avoid risks for respiratory depression.

7. Spinal or epidural opioids alone provide insufficient analgesia for second-stage labor pain.

8. Remember, hyperventilation may worsen the hypokalemia that often accompanies β-agonist infusions when used as tocolytics.

9. Remember to check the platelet count in women who abuse cocaine or, conversely, to add cocaine abuse to the differential diagnosis of thrombocytopenia.

10. Only meperidine, of common postoperative analgesics, given repeatedly or by patient-controlled analgesia may accumulate sufficiently in breast milk to influence infant behavior.

REFERENCES

1. Juchau MR, Chao ST, Omiecinski CJ: Drug metabolism by the human fetus. Clin Pharmacokinet 5:320–339, 1980.
2. Krauer B, Dayer P: Fetal drug metabolism and its possible clinical implications. Clin Pharmacokinet 21:70–80, 1991.
3. Briggs GG, Freeman RK, Jaffe SJ: Drugs in pregnancy and lactation, 4th ed. Baltimore, Williams & Wilkins, 1994, pp 267–271.
4. Butterworth JF IV, Strichartz GR: Molecular mechanisms of anesthesia: A review. Anesthesiology 72:711–734, 1990.
5. Albright GA: Cardiac arrest following regional anesthesia with etidocaine or bupivacaine. Anesthesiology 51:285–287, 1979.
6. Clarkson CW, Hondeghan LM: Mechanism for bupivacaine depression of cardiac conduction: Fast block of sodium channels during the action potential with slow recovery from block during diastole. Anesthesiology 62:396–405, 1985.
7. Thomas RD, Behbehani MM, Coyle DE, Denson DD: Cardiovascular toxicity of local anesthetics: An alternative hypothesis. Anesth Analg 65:444–450, 1986.
8. Morishima HO, Pederson H, Finster M, et al: Bupivacaine toxicity in pregnant and nonpregnant ewes. Anesthesiology 63:134–139, 1985.
9. Moller RA, Datta S, Fox J, et al: Effects of progesterone on the cardiac electrophysiologic action of bupivacaine and lidocaine. Anesthesiology 76:604–608, 1992.
10. Santos A, Pederson H, Harmon TW, et al: Does pregnancy alter the systemic toxicity of local anesthetics? Anesthesiology 70:991–995, 1989.
11. Davis NL, de Jong RH: Successful resuscitation following massive bupivacaine overdose. Anesth Analg 61:62–64, 1982.
12. Kasten GW, Martin ST: Bupivacaine cardiovascular toxicity: Comparison of treatment with bretylium and lidocaine. Anesth Analg 64:911–916, 1985.
13. Long WB, Rosenblum S, Grady IP: Successful resuscitation of bupivacaine-induced cardiac arrest using cardiopulmonary bypass. Anesth Analg 69:403–406, 1989.
14. de Jong RH: Last round for a heavyweight? [Editorial]. Anesth Analg 78:3–4, 1994.
15. Dailland P, Cockshott ID, Lirzin JD, et al: Intravenous propofol during cesarean section: Placental transfer, concentrations in breast milk, and neonatal effects. A preliminary study. Anesthesiology 71:827–834, 1989.
16. Abadir AR, Humayun SG, Calvello D, Gintautas J: Effects of isoflurane and oxytocin on gravid human uterus in vitro. Anesth Analg 66:S1–S191, 1987.
17. Moir DD: Anaesthesia for cesarean section. Br J Anaesth 42:136–142, 1970.
18. Warren TM, Datta S, Ostheimer GW, et al: Comparison of the maternal and neonatal effects of halothane, enflurane, and isoflurane for cesarean delivery. Anesth Analg 62:516–520, 1983.
19. Piggott SE, Bogod DG, Rosen M, et al: Isoflurane with either 100% oxygen or 50% nitrous oxide in oxygen for cesarean section. Br J Anaesth 65:325–329, 1990.
20. Finster M, Poppers PJ: Safety of thiopental used for induction of general anesthesia in elective cesarean section. Anesthesiology 29:190–191, 1968.
21. Stenger VG, Blechner JN, Prystowsky H: A study of prolongation of obstetric anesthesia. Am J Obstet Gynecol 103:901–907, 1969.

22. Marx GF, Joshi CW, Orkin LR: Placental transfer of nitrous oxide. Anesthesiology 32:429–432, 1970.
23. Way WL, Costley EC, Way EL: Respiratory sensitivity of the newborn infant to meperidine and morphine. Clin Pharmacol Ther 6:454–461, 1965.
24. Rayburn W, Rathke A, Leuschen P, et al: Fentanyl citrate analgesia during labor. Am J Obstet Gynecol 161:202–206, 1989.
25. Rosaeg OP, Kitts JB, Koren G, Byford LL: Maternal and fetal effects of intravenous patient-controlled fentanyl analgesia during labor in a thrombocytopenic parturient. Can J Anaesth 39:277–281, 1992.
26. Allen RW, James MFM, Uys PF: Attenuation of the pressor response to tracheal intubation in the hypertensive proteinuric pregnant patient by lignocaine, alfentanil, and magnesium sulfate. Br J Anaesth 66:216–223, 1991.
27. Wilson SJ, Errick JK, Balkon J: Pharmacokinetics of nalbuphine during parturition. Am J Obstet Gynecol 155:340–344, 1986.
28. Maduska AL, Hajghassemali M: A double-blind comparison of butorphanol and meperidine in labor: Maternal pain relief and effects on the newborn. Can Anaesth Soc J 25:398–404, 1978.
29. Palmer CM, Voulgarpoulos D, Emerson SS, Alves D: What is the optimal dose of subarachnoid morphine for postcesarean analgesia? A dose-response study [abstract]. Proceedings of the 26th Annual Meeting, Society for Obstetric Anesthesia and Perinatology, Philadelphia, 1994, p 48.
30. Cohen SE: Intrathecal sufentanil for labor analgesia—Sensory changes, side effects, and fetal heart rate changes. Anesth Analg 77:1155–1160, 1993.
31. Camann WR, Bader AM: Spinal anesthesia for cesarean delivery with meperidine as the sole agent. Int J Obstet Anesth 1:156–158, 1992.
32. Cockburn J, Moar VA, Ounsted M, Redman CWG: Final report of study on hypertension during pregnancy: The effects of specific treatment on the growth and development of the children. Lancet 1:647–649, 1982.
33. Pruyn SC, Phelan JP, Buchanan GC: Long-term propranolol therapy in pregnancy: Maternal and fetal outcome. Am J Obstet Gynecol 135:485–489, 1979.
34. Redmond GP: Propranolol and fetal growth retardation. Semin Perinatol 6:142–147, 1982.
35. Rubin PC, Clark DM, Sumner DJ: Placebo-controlled trial of atenolol in treatment of pregnancy-associated hypertension. Lancet 1:431–434, 1983.
36. Pickles CJ, Symonds EM, Pipkin FB: The fetal outcome in a randomized double-blind controlled trial of labetalol versus placebo in pregnancy-induced hypertension. Br J Obstet Gynaecol 96:38–43, 1989.
37. Eisenach JB, Castro MI: Maternally administered esmolol produces fetal beta-blockade and hypoxemia in sheep. Anesthesiology 71:718–722, 1989.
38. Childress CH, Katz VL: Nifedipine and its indications in obstetrics and gynecology. Obstet Gynecol 83:616–624, 1994.
39. Carbonne B, Jannet D, Touboul C, et al: Nicardipine treatment of hypertension during pregnancy. Obstet Gynecol 81:908–914, 1993.
40. Motwani JG, Lipworth BJ: Clinical pharmacokinetics of drugs administered buccally and sublingually. Clin Pharmacokinet 21:83–94, 1991.
41. Lindow SW, Davies N, Davey DA, Smith JA: The effect of sublingual nifedipine on uteroplacental blood flow in hypertensive pregnancy. Br J Obstet Gynaecol 96:1276–1281, 1988.
42. Hood DD, Dewan DM, James FM III, et al: The use of nitroglycerin in preventing the hypertensive response to tracheal intubation in severe preeclampsia. Anesthesiology 63:329–332, 1985.
43. Iseri LT, French JH: Magnesium: Nature's physiologic calcium blocker. Am Heart J 108:188–193, 1984.
44. Watson KW, Moldow CF, Ogburn PL, Jacob HS: Magnesium sulfate: Rationale for its use in preeclampsia. Proc Natl Acad Sci USA 83:1075–1078, 1986.
45. Sadeh M: Action of magnesium sulfate in the treatment of preeclampsia-eclampsia. Stroke 20: 1273–1275, 1989.
46. Higby K, Xenakis EM-J, Pauerstein CJ: Do tocolytic agents stop preterm labor? A critical and comprehensive review of efficacy and safety. Am J Obstet Gynecol 168:1247–1259, 1993.
47. Gray SE, Rodis JF, Lettieri L, et al: Effect of intravenous magnesium sulfate on the biophysical profile of the healthy preterm fetus. Am J Obstet Gynecol 170:1131–1135, 1994.
48. McGrath JM, Chestnut DH, Vincent RD, et al: Ephedrine remains the vasopressor of choice for treatment of hypotension during ritodrine infusion and epidural anesthesia. Anesthesiology 80:1073–1081, 1994.
49. Hankins GDV, Berryman GK, Scott RT Jr, Hood D: Maternal arterial desaturation with 15-methyl prostaglandin F_2 alpha for uterine atony. Obstet Gynecol 72:367–370, 1988.
50. Taylor GJ, Cohen B: Ergonovine-induced coronary artery spasm and myocardial infarction after normal delivery. Obstet Gynecol 66:821–822, 1985.
51. Krauer B, Dayer P: Fetal drug metabolism and its possible clinical implications. Clin Pharmacokinet 21:70–80, 1991.

52. Jones KL, Lacro RV, Johnson KV, Adams J: Pattern of malformations in the children of women treated with carbamazepine during pregnancy. N Engl J Med 320:1661–1666, 1989.
53. Kain ZN, Rimar S, Barash PG: Cocaine abuse in the parturient and effects on the fetus and neonate. Anesth Analg 77:835–845, 1993.
54. American Academy of Pediatrics, Committee on Drugs: The transfer of drugs and other chemicals into human milk. Pediatrics 93:137–150, 1994.
55. Andersen LW, Quist T, Hertz J, Mogensen F: Concentrations of thiopentone in mature breast milk and colostrum following an induction dose. Acta Anaesthesiol Scand 31:30–32, 1987.
56. Cote CJ, Kenepp NB, Reed SB, Strobel GE: Trace concentrations of halothane in breast milk. Br J Anaesth 48:541–543, 1976.
57. Wittels B, Scott DT, Sinatra RS: Exogenous opioids in human breast milk and acute neonatal neurobehavior: A preliminary study. Anesthesiology 73:864–869, 1990.
58. Leuschen MP, Wolf LJ, Rayburn WF: Fentanyl excretion in breast milk. Clin Pharmacol 9:336–337, 1990.
59. Briggs GG, Freeman RK, Yaffe SJ: Drugs in pregnancy and lactation, 4th ed. Baltimore, Williams & Wilkins, 1994, pp 2–7.
60. Ravindran RS, Bond VK, Tasch MD et al: Prolonged neural blockade following regional anesthesia with 2-chloroprocaine. Anesth Analg 59: 447–451, 1980.
61. Rout CC, Rocke DA, Levin J, et al: A reevaluation of the role of crystalloid preload in the prevention of hypotension associated with spinal anesthesia for elective cesarean section. Anesthesiology 79:262–269, 1993.

SIX

Analgesia for Labor

Theodore G. Cheek, M.D. *Brett B. Gutsche, M.D.*

Labor pain can be treated with an array of methods ranging from parenteral drugs to more effective regional anesthesia techniques, including the lumbar epidural injection of local anesthetics, narcotics, and α agonists. Spinal analgesia, utilizing either narcotics or local anesthetics, offers an alternative to the epidural approach, and more recently, combined spinal/epidural techniques have emerged as an alternative to traditional epidural analgesia. This chapter focuses on the practical and technical aspects of these methods, especially lumbar epidural block for labor and delivery.

RATIONALE AND BENEFITS OF ANALGESIA

The idea that a labor floor is the only part of the hospital where pain is "acceptable or necessary" is disappearing from modern obstetric practice. Research shows the pain of labor often produces unnecessary maternal suffering, sustained maternal hyperventilation, elevated oxygen demand, and increased mechanical work.[1–4] These "natural" maternal responses to labor pain may result in dramatically increased catecholamine production, intermittent hypoxemia, and hypocapnia, which, in turn, can lead to uterine hypoperfusion, fetal hypoxia, and acidosis.[5–7] Pain relief and especially epidural analgesia avoids or attenuates many of the adverse maternal and fetal responses to labor. Although many mothers can tolerate the stress of labor without adverse neonatal outcome, high-risk pregnancies associated with maternal disease, decreased maternal reserves, or fetal placental compromise benefit from stable maternal physiology accompanying complete labor pain relief. It follows that, whenever possible, analgesia should also be available to normal mothers undergoing routine labor. Although parenteral medications do not attenuate the pain and stress response to labor as effectively as neuraxial methods, intravenous (IV)/intramuscular (IM) narcotics have a role in the management of labor pain when regional techniques are not available.

NONPHARMACOLOGIC ANALGESIC TECHNIQUES

Hypnosis

Hypnosis, used rarely in childbirth, requires that the mother enter a trance, a state of focused attention and hypersuggestibility. Success usually necessitates intensive training over many weeks before parturition, and the depth of trance obtainable varies from allowing performance of a surgical procedure to providing little analgesia. Most individuals fall between the extremes; hence, the technique is neither popular nor widely applicable.[8]

Acupuncture

Acupuncture has not been used extensively for vaginal delivery even in the People's Republic of China. Although some pain relief can be provided by acupuncture, this is usually incomplete and requires considerable pharmacologic supplementation. Its role is limited.

NONREGIONAL TECHNIQUES

Parenteral/Patient-Controlled Analgesia

Drugs are often administered parenterally to lessen pain and anxiety in the first stage of labor. In uncomplicated labors in which episiotomy is not required, systemic medications alone may provide adequate analgesia throughout labor and delivery.[9] Although these drugs were commonly administered intramuscularly in the past, they are now more commonly administered in small, IV doses at more frequent intervals, since absorption and onset of action are more predictable following IV administration.

Opioids, such as morphine and meperidine, diminish the perception of and reaction to pain and have been widely used in labor. Since equal analgesic doses of opioids cause the same degree of maternal and newborn respiratory depression, the choice of opioid is dictated by preferred duration of action. However, long-acting opioids, such as morphine, have largely been abandoned because of the difficulty in predicting the time of delivery. Meperidine remains the most frequently used opioid in obstetrics. Meperidine (Demerol) 50 to 75 mg is often given when the mother requests analgesia, usually when the cervix is dilated 4 to 6 cm. Although some practitioners may repeat the dose later in labor, this practice risks the increased newborn depression associated with narcotics administered within 4 hours of delivery.[10] From a practical perspective, although early newborn tests reveal some decrement in neonatal neurobehavioral function following even small doses of opioids, deficiencies persist only for a day or two and do not appreciably affect subsequent neonatal feeding, weight gain, or development. Nevertheless, respiratory depression can occur. Fortunately, opioid-induced respiratory depression is rapidly antagonized by naloxone in both mother and newborn. Remember, naloxone given before delivery not only rapidly antagonizes maternal analgesia but may also cause nausea, vomiting, and extreme discomfort. Hence, unless the mother is extremely depressed from opioids, naloxone should not be given to the mother before delivery. Remember, also, newborns of mothers who take opioids on a chronic basis may have severe signs and symptoms of opioid withdrawal following naloxone administration. Finally, newborns requiring naloxone should be observed for signs of recurrent respiratory depression as naloxone's effects wane.

Agonist-antagonists such as butorphanol and nalbuphine are advocated by some practitioners because of the reported limited respiratory depression associated with these drugs. Unfortunately, in the authors' experience, effective analgesia is also limited with this class of agent, and attempts to increase the dosage result in somnolence and occasional respiratory depression.[11]

Patient-controlled analgesia (PCA) for labor has gained popularity in recent years. Suggested advantages include increased patient satisfaction and possibly less total narcotic administration. Other purported advantages include less placental drug transfer and fewer maternal side effects (respiratory depression, nausea). Little documentation exists to support these claims. Nalbuphine, meperidine, and fentanyl have all been used via PCA with satisfactory results. In one report, fentanyl PCA utilized a background infusion of 25 μg/hour, patient bolus of 25 μg, with a lockout interval of 10 minutes and a 4-hour maximal dose of 600 μg. Of note, in this labor lasting 12 hours, the total fentanyl dose was 1025 μg.[12] Although this was an anecdotal report, the delivered newborn was vigorous. In the authors' practice, narcotic IV PCA use is uncommon. It is the authors' impression that recommended infusion rates tend to provide less than adequate analgesia because of the crescendo-like nature of labor pain and the wide variation in patient response to narcotic analgesia. The authors most frequently use fentanyl or nalbuphine for our IV infusion analgesics. Suggested dosing guidelines can be found in Table 6–1. Although PCA is not commonly used for labor in the authors' hospital, it has a place on labor floors where regional block availability is limited and when patients prefer to have more influence over the delivery of their obstetric care. Close nursing care is advisable, and if available, pulse oximetry is desirable.

Tranquilizers, including the antihistamines, phenothiazines, benzodiazepines, and butyrophenones, have been coadministered with opioids to provide sedation, allay anxiety, and di-

TABLE 6–1
Guidelines for IV PCA Narcotic Infusion Analgesia for Labor

Drug	Loading Dose IV	Initial Infusion	Patient Bolus	Lockout Interval	Dose Limit
Fentanyl	25–50 μg	20 μg/hr	20 μg	5–10 min	400 μg*
Nalbuphine	1.5–3 mg	1.5 mg/hr	1 mg	10 min	Unknown
Meperidine	25 mg	15 mg/hr	10 mg	20 min	100 mg*

Abbreviations: IV = intravenous; PCA = patient-controlled analgesia.
*These figures are estimates for an average labor and are derived by anecdotal association with increased reported neonatal naloxone use.

minish nausea and vomiting. As with opioids, their use has declined as more women choose to be awake and alert for delivery. If considering these drugs, remember, in the presence of untreated pain, tranquilizers may lead to confusion and delirium. The phenothiazines and butyrophenones have a prolonged duration extending as long as 8 hours. In addition, tranquilizers rapidly cross the placenta, may depress neonatal muscle tone, respiration, and temperature regulation, and are, with the exception of benzodiazepines, without effective antagonists. Barbiturates and scopolamine, popular several decades ago for sedation and amnesia (twilight sleep), are rarely used in modern obstetrics.

Ketamine, a dissociative anesthetic, is a potent analgesic against somatic pain. Small IV doses of 0.25 mg/kg yield profound analgesia and amnesia lasting from 2 to 5 minutes; with such small doses, consciousness is retained while hallucinations and unpleasant dreams are uncommon. Although the compound is not employed in the first stage of labor, it is most useful in providing rapid analgesia for spontaneous vaginal delivery, vacuum extraction, or forceps delivery. Incremental doses should not exceed 1 mg/kg. Larger doses can cause loss of consciousness and diminish protective airway reflexes. Furthermore, ketamine rapidly crosses the placenta; total doses exceeding 1 mg/kg have been associated with neonatal respiratory depression, muscle rigidity, and elevated uterine tone. The authors do not advocate using ketamine analgesia except in the operative setting.

Paracervical/Pudendal

Paracervical Block

The principle of the paracervical block (PCB) is to interrupt the pain pathways to the cervix and the uterus by blocking the paracervical plexus (Frankenhäuser) located lateral to the cervix. When effective, PCB blocks pain from manipulation of the cervix and uterus as well as uterine contraction pain. PCB in the past was indicated in labor to block the pain of uterine contractions during the first stage of labor. Advantages of PCB include simplicity, ease of repetition, relatively painless injection, rapid onset (<5 min), reliability, no maternal hypotension, little chance for local anesthetic (LA) toxicity (even if uterine artery injection occurs), complete analgesia of cervix and uterus, no motor block, preservation of the "bearing down reflex" in the second stage of labor, and no effect on urination or defecation. However, sacral anesthesia is absent, sometimes necessitating a second analgesic technique for delivery.

Although PCB offers many advantages, numerous reports of fetal bradycardia, acidosis, and death have all but stopped its use in labor.[13] Increased uterine arterial and myometrial tone mediated by LA absorbed from the uterosacral plexus is the suggested mechanism for reported fetal-neonatal depression associated with PCB. In the rare instance in which PCB is considered indicated for labor analgesia, these complications can be decreased by using low concentrations of low-toxicity LAs (1% chloroprocaine, 1% prilocaine, 1% lidocaine), no epinephrine, minimal volumes of LAs (e.g., 7.0 ml per side), and superficial injection (<0.5 cm deep). Avoid bupivacaine, etidocaine, and mepivacaine. The clinician should wait 5 to 10 minutes after the first injection, and if fetal bradycardia develops, *should not* inject the other side.

Other indications for PCB in obstetrics are to provide analgesia for dilatation and curettage, therapeutic abortion (dilatation and evacuation), repair of cervical laceration, and intrauterine manipulation (e.g., removal of retained placenta, manual inspection of uterine cesarean section scar, or version extraction). Remember, PCB does not produce uterine relaxation. Block placement requires the lithotomy or "frog-leg" position and an Iowa trumpet or guide. In the presence of a viable fetus, the needle should protrude <0.5 cm (bead left on needle). Seven to 10 ml of LA is injected after aspiration at both 3 and 9 o'clock (the cervix as a clock) for PCB or 4 and 8 o'clock for a uterosacral block or 3.5 to 5 ml at 3, 4, 8, and 9 o'clock for an intense block.

Pudendal Block

Pudendal nerve block is usually performed by the obstetrician at delivery to produce analgesia of the central area of the perineum. Bilateral nerve blockade produces analgesia that extends to the anus, the vagina including the labia, and the clitoris. The pudendal nerve is made up of the ventral branches of sacral roots 2 to 4, which converge immediately posterior to the lateral aspect of the ischial spines, which provide palpable landmarks for needle placement. Indications for pudendal block include analgesia for the second stage of labor and episiotomy repair. Some obstetricians administer the block (particularly in the prima gravida) as the patient enters the second stage of labor, to improve patient comfort while minimally affecting the "urge to push." Pudendal block is also useful for providing analgesia for operative vaginal delivery (low forceps or vacuum delivery) and for episiotomy repair. Mid forceps and mid forceps rotation usually require additional supplementation such as narcotics, low-dose ketamine, nitrous oxide, other inhalation analgesia, or preferably major regional block.

INHALATIONAL ANALGESIA

Subanesthetic (analgesic) concentrations of inhaled vapors and gases have been used since the days of Simpson (1850s) to provide labor pain relief. Fifty percent nitrous oxide in oxygen (entonox) is still widely administered by nurse-midwives in the United Kingdom. *Self*-administered inhalation analgesia for the first stage of labor has largely been abandoned in the United States. Although the neurotoxicity associated with trichloroethylene and the adverse renal effects of methoxyflurane have resulted in the virtual disappearance of these drugs, nitrous oxide and low-dose enflurane or isoflurane are still given as analgesics during labor in this and other countries.[14] Advantages of inhalation analgesia include rapid onset, maintenance of protective airway reflexes, absence of significant maternal and neonatal depression regardless of duration of analgesia, frequent maternal amnesia, little effect on uterine activity or the urge to bear down, increased maternal inspired oxygen concentration, and rapid maternal recovery. Obviously, these advantages are derived only when the mother remains awake and responsive to command.

Drawbacks of inhalational analgesia include potential maternal delirium and excitement, indicating entrance into the second stage of anesthesia. Safe administration requires constant supervision to avoid producing unintentional unconsciousness (remember, pregnancy decreases minimal alveolar concentration [MAC]). Other disincentives include inadequate analgesia resulting in a moving target for the obstetrician, greater maternal stress response, and the remote possibility of aspiration if maternal loss of consciousness is accompanied by vomiting or regurgitation. Inhalational analgesia will not prevent a precipitous delivery and is often not sufficient for operative and instrumental vaginal delivery without simultaneous effective pudendal block.

Despite these problems, the authors believe there are indications for inhalational analgesia and continue to use the technique. It is appropriate in a rapidly progressing labor where there is not enough time for regional block or when regional block proves ineffective or is contraindicated. This is especially true if the mother urgently requires analgesia for low outlet forceps delivery. The authors believe this method is preferable to the emergency induction of general endotracheal anesthesia. Continuous administration of 30 to 50% nitrous oxide in high flows is usually effective for the latter part of labor, delivery, and postpartum examination. Forceps delivery is often possible with inhalation analgesia, possibly supplemented with small doses of ketamine (10–30 mg) and LA infiltration of the perineum or pudendal block. Inhalation analgesia is impractical in many new labor, delivery, and recovery units.

GENERAL ANESTHESIA

General anesthesia is not desirable and rarely required for vaginal delivery. Since general anesthesia obligatorily results in loss of maternal expulsive efforts, induction must be delayed until birth is imminent. In addition to its association with loss of maternal airway protective reflexes, pulmonary aspiration, a higher incidence of forceps or vacuum extraction deliveries, and an increased occurrence of newborn depression, general anesthesia also denies the mother the birth experience and delays bonding. More importantly, failure to intubate and maintain the maternal airway along with pulmonary aspiration accounts for more than half of obstetric anesthetic deaths. In the past, general anesthesia utilizing greater than 2 MAC of a potent inhalation agent (halothane 1.5–2%) was administered to inhibit uterine contractions, terminate tetanic contractions, or allow intrauterine fetal manipulation to facilitate vaginal delivery. Today, except for removal of a retained placenta, intrauterine manipulation is rarely employed in modern obstetrics. Uterine relaxation is now more rapidly and safely produced with IV tocolytics, such as IV β_2 agonists, nitroglycerin, or inhaled amyl nitrite. A rare but potentially valid indication for general anesthesia and vaginal delivery is when mothers become physically uncontrollable during delivery and risk significant maternal or fetal harm during delivery. When general anesthesia is administered, ideally with the mother in the supine position utilize a rapid-sequence induction (circumstances sometimes preclude changing from the lithotomy position). Because of the risk of aspiration, potentially difficult intubation, and rapid development of hypoxia, general anesthesia should be undertaken only by an experienced anesthetist with a competent assistant present. Except in the most unusual circumstances, general anesthesia in the gravid patient beyond the first trimester of gestation without intubation is not acceptable anesthesia practice today. Techniques should resemble that described for cesarean section.

REGIONAL TECHNIQUES

Epidural Block

Advantages of Epidural Block for Labor

Lumbar epidural analgesia remains the most effective and versatile approach for relief of pain during labor and delivery. Lumbar epidural analgesia has largely replaced other methods of labor analgesia because of the following advantages:

1. Continuous, effective analgesia from early labor through delivery avoids the need for narcotics, hypnotics, or inhalation drugs, which can depress both maternal and neonatal reflexes.
2. In contrast to heavy sedation techniques, the fully conscious mother maintains airway reflexes that protect her from aspiration of stomach contents unless severe hypotension or systemic reactions to LAs occur.
3. It is the authors' opinion that epidural analgesia for labor does not appreciably prolong or significantly interfere with the forces of labor. Recent, carefully conducted, prospective studies have shown little or no difference in second stage duration with and without epidural block.[15–22] Indeed, effective analgesia has been shown by some to shorten the first stage of labor by improving both the strength and the frequency of uterine contractions.[23]
4. During second stage labor, the awake and well-coached parturient utilizing epidural analgesia maintains intercostal, diaphragmatic, and abdominal motor function, allowing effective voluntary expulsion of the fetus despite perineal anesthesia. Conversely, the "bearing down" perineal pressure reflex is of little use if it hurts too much to push.
5. A most attractive prospect to the mother is that she remains awake, can watch the delivery, and is able to interact almost immediately with her newborn.
6. Should the obstetrician desire the mother not to push, thereby avoiding a precipitous delivery, or should she or he desire a controlled vacuum or forceps delivery, this can easily be accomplished by intensifying the sensory block and instructing the mother not to push. Premature infants may benefit from this approach.
7. Postpartum examination and episiotomy repair can be performed without patient discomfort.
8. Trial of labor after previous cesarean section can be safely conducted with epidural analgesia by using low concentrations of LAs that alleviate intermittent contraction pain but preserve the signs of imminent uterine rupture such as continuous suprapubic pain, change in labor pattern, or contraction configuration.[24]

9. Should cesarean section be required, the level and intensity of blockade can be rapidly increased, allowing for timely delivery in an awake, participating mother while avoiding the potential complications of general anesthesia.

10. If postpartum tubal ligation is planned, surgical anesthesia can be established immediately after delivery, thus avoiding a second block placement and prolonged hospitalization.

Indications for Epidural Block During Labor

Pain is by far the most common indication for epidural block in labor. In the unlikely event that epidural analgesia adversely affects early labor, as long as the obstetric plan is delivery, oxytocin can almost always be used to enhance effective uterine activity. In the authors' practice, private obstetricians commonly request epidural analgesia as soon as their patients experience painful labor regardless of cervical dilatation. Indeed, there is an array of obstetric conditions for which early epidural block is highly advised and provides significant advantages for the mother, fetus, and obstetric care providers. These conditions include trial of labor for any reason, but especially for women who have undergone a previous cesarean section and those with other high-risk conditions. The authors believe preeclampsia, diabetes, recent tocolytic therapy, preterm delivery, signs of fetal stress or nonreassuring fetal heart tracing, multiple gestation, malpresentation, small-for-gestational-age infants, placenta previa, and prolonged rupture of membranes all indicate epidural analgesia unless contraindications exist. Indeed, the authors' usual practice in the presence of high-risk labor is to encourage early regional block and maintain a *solid* T8 sensory level to cold throughout labor. This degree of blockade blunts the pain-induced physiologic demands on the mother and fetus, decreases maternal catecholamine production, lessens fetal acidosis, and increases total available oxygen. Perhaps of greatest benefit to the mother, should a sudden emergency delivery of the fetus be required, the abdomen is usually "surgery-ready," allowing preparation for cesarean delivery to proceed with dispatch, avoiding the well-known risks of "crash" induction of general anesthesia. Remember, preexisting solid blocks lessen the time to establish surgical anesthesia. Should vaginal delivery become likely, block density may be decreased.

Contraindications to Epidural Analgesia in Labor

True contraindications to epidural block for labor analgesia are rare. The authors identify fewer than 1 in 300 potential candidates for epidural block who require alternate forms of analgesia because of contraindications. As understanding increases and clinical experience grows, the number of "absolute" contraindications to epidural anesthesia lessens.

Conditions in Which Regional Block Is Strongly Discouraged

1. Patient refusal.
2. Personnel, monitoring equipment, and continuous obstetric care for parturient unavailable.
3. Infection.
   a. At or near site of epidural injection.
   b. Septicemia.
4. Coagulation abnormality (inherited, acquired disease, anticoagulant therapy, disseminated intravascular coagulation). However, much recent debate addresses what constitutes a severe enough coagulation abnormality to contraindicate regional block. Thrombocytopenia accompanying preeclampsia is the most common condition raising this question. Although the subject is discussed in greater detail elsewhere, if the partial thromboplastin time (PTT) and the prothrombin time (PT) are normal, if whole blood clots in a test tube, if the activated clotting time is less than 150 seconds, and if there are no signs of oozing from skin puncture sites or multiple petechiae, the authors usually proceed with epidural block. At the authors' institution, we do not use an arbitrary platelet count such as 100,000 as a cutoff and a contraindication to regional block. However, with counts less than 75,000, the authors proceed with caution. Remember, bleeding times correlate poorly with platelet function and are poor predictors of hemorrhage, epidural or otherwise.[25] Other institutions utilize different criteria, and ultimately, the decision becomes a risk-benefit judgment.

The authors' opinion is that the risks to the mother associated with emergency general anesthesia caused by withholding of regional block can exceed those of developing epidural or subdural hematoma. Therefore, in selected high-airway-risk patients with "borderline" coagulopathy, it may be rational to preferentially proceed with a "light" epidural block for labor or epidural anesthetic for cesarean section using a short-acting LA and monitor the patient closely postoperatively for signs of epidural hematoma rather than subjecting the patient to a potentially greater risk of airway loss during general anesthesia.

5. Anatomic abnormalities.
   a. Spina bifida or meningomyelocele (spina bifida occulta is not a contraindication if the site of the lesion is known).
   b. Fused spine—caudal approach or spinal anesthesia still possible.
   c. Arteriovenous malformation diagnosed in vertebral column in close proximity to the proposed puncture site.

Relative Contraindications to Epidural Block in Labor

1. Anatomic or technical difficulties such as surgical fusions in the lumbar area.

2. Uncooperative patient.

3. Uncorrected hypovolemia. If time permits, IV therapy can restore euvolemia. Frank shock associated with active bleeding requiring immediate surgery is not a time to initiate regional block.

4. Chronic low back pain or back surgery.[26] The authors' usual practice is to offer these patients regional block for labor.

5. Recurrent neurologic disease such as multiple sclerosis. The authors no longer withhold regional analgesia from patients with a history of spinal injury or neurologic disorders.

6. Cardiac disease involving right-to-left shunts may lessen the risk.

7. Sustained fetal bradycardia. Most forms of "fetal distress" and nonreassuring fetal heart rate are *not* a contraindication to using an existing epidural catheter.[27] If rapid fetal delivery is required and there is no functioning epidural catheter, spinal block is preferred.

Requirements for Epidural Analgesia (Table 6–2)

The apparent simplicity of placing an epidural block, its associated low complication rate, and a high patient demand for pain relief may occasionally tempt provision of anesthesia in less than safe circumstances. However, epidural

TABLE 6–2
Requirements for Epidural Block for Labor

Requirements Before Establishing Epidural Block

1. Thorough evaluation of maternal medical and pregnancy history and physical examination. Available qualified nurse to remain with patient.
2. Informed verbal or written consent prior to any medication and, when possible, before onset of painful contractions.
3. Instruments immediately available to establish and maintain an airway, resuscitation drugs and equipment, suction, high-flow oxygen, and materials necessary to allow administration of positive airway pressure.
4. Maternal vital signs (Dinamap).
5. Continuous printout of fetal heart rate and uterine contractions (electronic fetal monitoring).
6. Adequate intravenous fluid preload (~500 ml of a dextrose-free balanced salt solution in labor).

Requirements After Establishing Epidural Block

1. Continuous maintenance of uterine displacement (usually left) at all times. Not necessary to place mother completely supine to obtain bilateral epidural anesthetic spread.
2. Complete anesthetic record maintained.
3. Close observation of maternal blood pressure for at least 20 min after the first dose of local anesthetic and after future top-off doses if block has completely regressed. Ten min of monitoring for follow-up doses. Frequent maternal vital signs maintained throughout epidural course.
4. Significant decreases in maternal blood pressure (20% fall below normal systolic or absolute fall below 100 mmHg systolic) treated promptly with increments (5–10 mg) of ephedrine and further balanced salt solution infusion. Special attention paid to fetal heart rate during period of blood pressure adjustment. Any hypotension associated with fetal heart rate deceleration treated immediately.
5. Anesthesiologist and obstetrician readily available to delivery area at all times.
6. Delivery performed in environment with facilities available to safely induce general anesthesia.

analgesia for labor is a major anesthetic and requires the same precautions, preparation, and care provided to surgical patients. Care begins with a physician accustomed to the anesthetic management of the pregnant patient and available nursing staff trained in monitoring epidural analgesia during the entire labor and delivery process. A qualified anesthesia provider obtains a thorough history and physical examination from the parturient desiring labor analgesia. During this period, options for labor analgesia are explained and every effort is made to provide a clear description of risks and benefits of the numerous alternative techniques. Risks the authors routinely mention are those of hypotension, headache, and backache following delivery. It is the authors' practice to mention the remote risks of seizure, respiratory or cardiac arrest, and nerve injury. However, these statements are followed by a reassuring description of their extreme rarity and how they can be avoided.

In the authors' practice, we require only a hematocrit before proceeding with regional block and, in some emergent cases, will dispense with this test if a thorough history and physical examination have been done. Other institutions do not require a hematocrit following a normal examination. If the patient's condition indicates the risk of a bleeding disorder, we obtain, in addition to a complete blood count, a PT, a PTT, and a platelet count. The authors do not use the bleeding time. For most healthy women in normal labor, the authors require only an automated blood pressure monitor in addition to normal resuscitation equipment. Recently, many of the authors' institution's labor rooms have been equipped with pulse oximeters. Although the authors believe these monitors improve the quality of patient monitoring, especially maternal heart rate monitoring during epidural catheter testing and potentially aid the recognition of arrhythmias, we *do not* feel they are mandatory.

Electrocardiography and equipment for invasive cardiovascular monitoring are available and obtained when parturients with a medical condition or disease require intensive care. As a general policy, all candidates for regional block receive a nondextrose crystalloid, IV fluid infusion of no more than 500 ml prior to the initiation of epidural blockade. This policy is not absolute. Exceptions are made for well-hydrated patients or those who require fluid restriction dictated by their clinical condition. In contrast, dehydrated patients may receive larger volume infusions. Continuous fetal heart rate monitoring is desirable, especially if labor is augmented by oxytocin. Finally, a source of high-flow maternal oxygen and a suction apparatus are absolute requirements. A summary of recommended safety requirements for regional block is found in Table 6–2.

Following delivery, the authors monitor the patient in an adequately staffed room until vital signs remain normal and the block has satisfactorily regressed. Unless these basic conditions are met, epidural analgesia for labor is ill-advised. No pain relief is better than an unsafe anesthetic.

ANATOMIC CONSIDERATIONS

The pain of first stage labor (cervical effacement and dilatation) is conveyed largely through thin, afferent, visceral sympathetic fibers entering the spinal cord at thoracic and lumbar roots T10–L1. Second stage labor pain (stretching and tearing of perineum and the descent of the fetus) is conducted via thicker, somatic nerve fibers entering the spinal cord at sacral roots S2–4. Complete pain relief during the first stage of labor can be obtained by segmental epidural visceral sensory block with dilute anesthetic concentrations bathing the thinner, more easily blocked spinal roots T10–L1. In contrast, adequate analgesia for second stage labor requires extending the block to include the somatic nerve fibers in nerve roots S2–4. Adequate sacral anesthesia frequently requires a greater density of blockade and more concentrated LA solutions than are needed for early stage 1 analgesia.

TECHNIQUES FOR EPIDURAL ANALGESIA IN LABOR

Position and Interspace

Patient position (sitting or lateral) during block placement and drug injection is relatively unimportant. The sitting position has disadvantages including potential (vasovagal) episodes. Occasionally, accidental dural puncture and subsequent injection of air into the subarachnoid space will occur. The sitting position allows rapid migration of injected air to cerebral ventricles, causing immediate headache. However, these disadvantages are balanced by the greater simplicity of landmark location when patients sit, since the sitting patient may curl more effectively than a patient in the lateral position. The lateral position offers convenience of speedy patient positioning and less gravity effect on the presenting fetal part. This may be important when the fetal head is not engaged prior to membrane rupture and poses the threat of umbilical cord prolapse if the membranes rupture during block placement. During preterm labor, when cervical dilatation is advanced, the lateral position may avoid precipitous delivery. Although some investigators suggest aortocaval compression may be less in the sitting than in the lateral decubitus position,[28–30] these observations require more study. For the time being, physician and patient preference are the most important factors determining the preferable patient position. Finally, intervertebral spaces L2–3, L3–4, and L4–5 are the most appropriate for labor epidural analgesia. Among these three, simply select the "best" interspace for easy placement.

Air Versus Saline Solution

The content of the loss of resistance syringe, whether air or saline solution (with or without bubble), is unlikely to make an important difference as long as the operator's thumb can establish a "bounce" during needle advancement.[31] Advocates of fluid (usually saline) claim the epidural space is "opened" by fluid injection, allowing easier threading of a catheter and fewer "patchy" blocks secondary to air bubbles.[32] This argument has been seriously questioned by Bromage.[33] Advocates of an air-filled syringe espouse the advantages of simplicity, compressibility, and rapid recognition of dural puncture. More recently, using "air as an IV test dose" has been described.[34] However, excessive air injected into tissue (subcutaneous, fascial planes, epidural) by energetic clinicians unsure of epidural needle placement has been implicated as causing postepidural complaints of back, shoulder, and neck pain as well as headache. Furthermore, some syringes require additional moistening with small amounts (2–3 ml) of saline solution prior to use, obviating the simplicity of the air technique. Although almost any 5- to 10-ml syringe that holds a seal can be used, plastic siliconized plunger/syringes are replacing the classic ground glass syringe because they bind less and are lighter. Ultimately, skill is more important than type of syringe or syringe content.

Catheter Distance

The authors limit catheter threading to 2 to 4 cm into the epidural space. We hope this avoids the tip exiting a root foramen or entering the anterior epidural space, producing a patchy or incomplete block. Although threading lesser distances might improve blockade, a catheter lying only 1 cm in the epidural space is likely to work its way out during the course of a long labor. Remember, never adjust catheter insertion lengths while the needle remains in place. This may result in shearing the catheter on the sharp trailing edge of the needle orifice, leaving a portion of the catheter in the patient's body. If necessary, adjust catheter lengths *after* needle removal.

Test Dose

The authors' practice is to inject a test dose of LA before establishing epidural anesthesia with larger volumes of LAs and also use a test dose prior to every subsequent "top-up" dose. Test doses establish that the needle or catheter does not lie in either a vessel or the subarachnoid space. Although the authors test both needle and the subsequently placed catheter, some authors argue that a catheter test dose is sufficient because it is the only route for LA injection. Regardless, an adequate test dose prior to a therapeutic epidural LA injection is an essential component of safe epidural administration. However, what constitutes an effective dose remains controversial.

One approach to catheter testing is to administer a "double test dose," consisting of two separate injections. The first injection contains a sufficient quantity of LA to produce a clearly demonstrable but low spinal block within 3 to 4 minutes. The second injection contains sufficient LA to produce safe but definite signs of intravascular injection such as tinnitus, metallic taste, and change of patient affect (Table 6–3). The initial test dose includes one of the following: lidocaine 40 to 60 mg; bupivacaine 8 to 10 mg; and 2-chloroprocaine 40 to 60 mg. Wait 3

TABLE 6–3
Double Test Dose

Drug	Quantity (mg)	Volume (ml)
First Dose		
Lidocaine 1.5%	45	3
2-Chloroprocaine 2%	60	3
2-Chloroprocaine 3%	90	3
Bupivacaine 0.25%	7.5	3
Bupivacaine 0.5%	10	2
Second Dose		
Lidocaine 1.5%	100	7
2-Chloroprocaine 2%	150	7.5
2-Chloroprocaine 3%	150	5
Bupivacaine 0.25%*†	20	8
Bupivacaine 0.5%*	20	4

*Bupivacaine does not consistently produce mild signs of central nervous system toxicity before convulsions; thus, the double test dose is not reliable with this drug.

†A commercial test dose of 0.5% bupivacaine with 1:200,000 epinephrine is available. Unfortunately, using 2.0 ml would provide 10 μg of epinephrine, which might not be adequate to produce signs and symptoms of intravascular injection; whereas using 3.0 ml would give 15 mg of bupivacaine, which if placed in the subarachnoid space, could result in a high level of block, especially in the obstetric patient.

to 5 minutes for signs of subarachnoid injection to appear before proceeding with the intravenous test consisting of 100 mg of lidocaine or 150 mg of 2-chloroprocaine. Remember, IV LA produces modest, brief analgesia. Do not get fooled! Also remember, the subarachnoid test is of limited value in the presence of already dense block as might occur when reinjecting catheters during prolonged labor or during cesarean surgery.

In the authors' practice, a single test dose is used to test for both spinal and intravenous placement. Our test dose contains sufficient LA to identify spinal placement plus epinephrine 15 μg. Spinal placement is diagnosed as with the double test dose (Table 6–4). However, in this instance, the authors also measure the pulse rate for 1 to 2 minutes following injection, looking for epinephrine-induced tachycardia, indicating intravenous placement. In the absence of uterine contractions or severe pain-induced tachycardia, epinephrine should cause a transient 15-beat-per-minute rise in heart rate, suggesting intravascular placement. Remember, the epinephrine test dose is *less* reliable in the pregnant than in the nonpregnant patient.[35, 36] Should any test dose procedure prove positive, the authors avoid further doses, remove the needle, and select an alternative site for replacement. If tachycardia is thought to be caused by pain, the tests are repeated with caution. The authors avoid epinephrine in the first test dose in patients with severe preeclampsia, in those with hypertensive disorders, and in those with a history of supraventricular tachycardia or cardiac disorders associated with frequent dysrhythmia.

Despite negative catheter testing, the authors also gently aspirate the catheter before, during, and after each epidural injection; utilize slow drug injection (use a large syringe); and fractionate drug injections into nontoxic doses, waiting 2 minutes prior to the next fractional dose (e.g., lidocaine 1.5 mg/kg, bupivacaine 0.5 mg/kg, 2-chloroprocaine 2 mg/kg). Thus, therapeutic doses are injected slowly (1 ml/2–3 sec) and in small increments that will not cause toxicity if injected intravascularly. Not only is rapid injection of LA not necessary to establish adequate LA spread, but also slow injection of epidural LA produces a more even dermatomal distribution.

In the authors' practice, following needle testing as described previously and after successful catheter placement, we retest the catheter to ensure location in the epidural space by syringe aspiration, repeating the test doses described previously. As discussed earlier, other authors test only the catheter. The authors also test the catheter in the same manner prior to each subsequent therapeutic dose and never assume that the catheter lies safely in the epidural space, as both clinical experience and numerous reports show that during the course of labor, epidural catheters occasionally migrate intravenously as

TABLE 6–4
Single Test Dose

Drug	Quantity (mg)	Volume (ml)	Epinephrine
Bupivacaine 0.5%	10	2	1:100,000 (20 μg)
Bupivacaine 0.25%	7.5	3	1:200,000 (15 μg)
Lidocaine 1.5%	45	3	1:200,000 (15 μg)
2-Chloroprocaine 2%	60	3	1:200,000 (15 μg)
2-Chloroprocaine 3%	90	3	1:200,000 (15 μg)

well as spinally. When Millipore filters are used, catheter aspiration is problematic at best. Repeated disconnecting increases the risk of infection and is not routinely advisable. Remember, always fractionate LA injections.

Local Anesthetic Selection

Factors Determining the Dosage of Local Anesthetic

Age influences the spread of epidural anesthesia, and peak drug requirements occur at approximately 19 to 20 years of age. From 20 to 40 years of age, approximately 2.0 ml of 2% lidocaine is required for each dermatome blocked on nonpregnant patients. Height also influences the spread of epidural anesthesia. Bromage suggests increasing the dose of LA by 0.1 ml per segment for each 2 inches over 5 feet of height. Not surprisingly, site of injection also influences spread. For example, injection of LA in the caudal, lumbar, and thoracic areas requires 2.0, 1.2 to 1.5, and 1.0 ml of 2% lidocaine per blocked segment, respectively. Epinephrine, 1:200,000 to 1:400,000, increases the spread, quality, and duration of block. The position of the patient (sitting vs. supine) has little effect on the spread of the epidural anesthesia and subsequent level of block. However, injection with patients in the lateral position will slightly favor the dependent side for speed of onset and density. Obesity may slightly decrease the LA requirement when compared with the nonobese patient. Finally, pregnancy, even as early as 10 to 12 weeks' gestation, decreases LA requirements by 30%. However, slow fractionation of LA injections makes these factors of limited import in clinical practice.

There is some debate whether concentration of LA influences the efficacy of blockade. Bromage found that when motor blocks were produced with lidocaine, mass of drug, not volume, determined the level of block. In other words, 20 ml of 2% lidocaine (400 mg) produces the same level of block as 8 ml of 5% lidocaine (400 mg). However, when lower concentrations of LA are used preferentially to produce sensory block only, drug volume becomes more important; for example, 20 ml of 0.5% lidocaine (100 mg) gives a greater spread than 10 ml of 1.0% lidocaine (100 mg).[37] However, even dilute LA solutions will eventually provide dense sensory and motor blockade.

Guidelines for Safe, Effective Dosing

Although the authors fractionate LA injections, for incremental bolus injections we use 75% of the maximal recommended dose in milligrams per kilogram. As labor proceeds, the authors note all administered drugs and record in milligrams, *not* in milliliters, the cumulative dose. This encourages us to use the lowest effective concentration. In the presence of *excellent* epidural analgesia, the authors do not have a maximal cumulative dose when labors are prolonged but consider chloroprocaine with its rapid metabolism for cesarean section after prolonged amide use.

Alkalinization of Local Anesthetic Solutions

At the authors' institution, we alkalinize LA solutions, especially bupivacaine and lidocaine, to increase speed of block onset. Alkalinization shortens the latency of bupivacaine by 33%. A comparison of the onset, duration, and drug levels of 0.25% epidural bupivacaine with and without alkalinization can be seen in Table 6–5. A method for alkalinizing LAs is found in Table 6–6.

Epinephrine

Advantages of adding epinephrine to LA solutions include: lower LA blood levels, increased

TABLE 6–5
pH Adjustment of 0.25% Bupivacaine 8.4% $NaHCO_3$ 0.05 ml Added to Each 10 ml of 0.25% Bupivacaine

	pH Adjusted (30)	Plain (30)	p Value
pH	7.26 ± 0.34	5.65 ± 0.07	<.001
Latency (min)	3.2 ± 0.24	6.0 ± 0.53	<.001
Duration (min)	96.5 ± 5.24	79.4 ± 4.39	<.02
Peak effect (min)	14.2 ± 1.1	16.6 ± 1.6	NS
Drug level (μg/ml)	0.342 ± 0.08	0.344 ± 0.07	NS

From McMorland GH, Douglas MJ, Jeffrey WK, et al: Effect of pH-adjustment of bupivacaine on onset and duration of epidural analgesia in parturients. Can Anaesth Soc J 33:537–541, 1986.

TABLE 6–6
Recommended Volumes of 7.5% or 8.4% $NaHCO_3$ for Each 10 ml of Anesthetic Solution

Bupivacaine 0.05 ml/10 ml. Do *not* exceed amount or bupivacaine will precipitate
Lidocaine 0.25 ml/10 ml
2-Chloroprocaine 0.5 ml/10 ml

TABLE 6–8
Mixing Epinephrine*

1:200,000	0.050 ml (5.0 μg/ml)
1:300,000	0.033 ml (3.3 μg/ml)
1:400,000	0.025 ml (2.5 μg/ml)

*Use these amounts (ml) of 1:1000 1 mg/ml epinephrine to each 10 ml of local anesthetic solution. Measure epinephrine with a tuberculin syringe.

intensity of block, longer duration of block, faster block onset, and possible identification of intravascular injection. An example of epinephrine's effect on onset and latency of 0.25% bupivacaine with and without fentanyl is seen in Table 6–7. Recommended epinephrine concentrations for LAs used in labor are 1:200,000 to 1:400,000. A method for mixing epinephrine with LAs in a concentration of 1:200,000 can be found in Table 6–8. Commercial solutions containing epinephrine are buffered to a pH of less than 4.5 to allow a reasonable shelf life. Unfortunately, the lower pH slows onset and decreases effectiveness of LAs. For this reason, the authors usually freshly mix our own solutions. Although the maximal safe dose of epinephrine varies, the authors try not to exceed 50 μg per dose during labor to minimize β-agonist effects on uterine activity.

Remember, use epinephrine in LAs for labor with caution in the presence of hypertensive disorders, multiple sclerosis, and a history of supraventricular tachycardia or cardiac disorders associated with frequent dysrhythmias. In the past, epinephrine use in preeclampsia was discouraged. Although it is still controversial, some evidence shows that its use is safe once proper epidural placement is established.[38]

TABLE 6–7
Effects of Epinephrine 1:200,000 and Fentanyl 50 μg on 10 ml of 0.25% Bupivacaine for Labor Epidural

Drug Group	Duration (min)	Latency (min)
Bupivacaine	86	8.2
Bupivacaine + Epinephrine	115*	6.3
Bupivacaine + Fentanyl	137†	6.0‡
Bupivacaine + Epinephrine + Fentanyl	180†	3.0‡

From Grice SC, Eisenach JC, Dewan DM, Weiner J: Effect of epinephrine on the duration of analgesia with epidural bupivacaine and fentanyl. Anesthesiology 67:A440, 1987.
*$p < .004$.
†$p < .001$.
‡$p < .025$.

Epidural Narcotics

Adding 50 μg of fentanyl to the initial epidural LA solution shortens the latency of block onset, prolongs the duration of the block, and allows one to decrease the LA concentration (usually by half), preserving motor function without sacrificing analgesia. During the second stage of labor, the mother receiving dilute LA solutions containing fentanyl may have painless contractions and still "push" more effectively than when more concentrated LA solutions without fentanyl are used. However, a pitfall of adding narcotics to epidural LAs for relief of labor pain is that narcotics may mask a "patchy" block and delay recognition of the need to replace the block until emergency conditions arise. Do not use narcotics to improve a poor block!

Epidural narcotics, without LAs, do not produce effective labor analgesia. However, if one desires good, but less dense, analgesia, especially in early labor, the authors use a "fentanyl epidural" that contains 8 to 12 ml of dilute LA (0.0625% or 0.125% bupivacaine) with 50 μg fentanyl and epinephrine 1:300,000. Repeat injections are permissible utilizing the same concentrations of bupivacaine containing 25 μg of added fentanyl. This dilute LA solution decreases motor block, minimizes sympathetic blockade, and decreases the frequency of maternal hypotension. Late in labor and delivery, when greater block density is required for blocking sacral roots, analgesia may be inadequate using this technique and require greater LA concentration.

The authors also use the "fentanyl epidural" for patients who want to "feel their contractions" or do not want to be "paralyzed." This solution may also be appropriate when there is inadequate nursing staff to allow what we consider adequate patient supervision of "real epidurals" with LA because of the lessened sympathectomy and threat of hypotension. Although the maximal safe maternal dose of fentanyl during labor that will not produce newborn depression is unknown, the authors limit the total amount of fentanyl to 150 to 200 μg during an 8-hour labor. Fentanyl 75 μg does not appear to affect fetal heart rate beat-to-beat variability.[39] Although controversial, fentanyl and other narcotics may *not* significantly improve the quality of block obtained with 2-chloroprocaine.

Establishing the Epidural Block/ Assessment

Following initial needle and catheter testing, the authors establish analgesia by injecting a volume and concentration of LA sufficient to produce a satisfactory level and density of block for the planned procedure. For example, with an indwelling catheter placed at L3–4, 8 to 12 ml (includes test dose) of either 0.25% bupivacaine, 1.5% lidocaine, or 2% 2-chloroprocaine usually produces a T10 or higher level sensory block and relieves the pain of first stage labor. Although a dense block is not absolutely necessary, the authors prefer to err on the side of comfort during the initial block establishment. The authors believe a slightly higher dermatomal level or greater density of block is far preferable to not quite enough. In the long run, the authors believe this philosophy reduces total drug usage and lessens misdiagnosis of poor blocks, and certainly saves time. The authors also frequently reinject a quarter to half the initial dose used to establish the block 10 to 15 minutes after the first dose ("repaint the fence") if analgesia is less than adequate. In the authors' experience, additional drug intensifies the sensory block without significantly increasing the level of the block. Although, in theory, this can be repeated as required, if the second dose fails to produce adequate analgesia or only patchy block is confirmed by ice or alcohol dermatome testing, the catheter is improperly positioned. Remove and replace! Further drug injection into an improperly functioning epidural catheter usually does not significantly improve the block. More important, it subjects the patient to prolonged pain and increases the risk of LA toxicity.

Maintenance

Intermittent Injection

The authors usually maintain analgesia continuously until completion of delivery and episiotomy repair. Very rarely, the authors allow the sensory block to dissipate so the patient will "push." When attempting to ensure continued analgesia using the intermittent bolus injections, the authors reinject LA at specific time intervals and *do not* await the return of pain or receding sensory level. A recommended intermittent dosing schedule is found in Table 6–9. The "top up" is usually 75 to 100% of the initial dose, not including the "repaint the fence" dose. The authors frequently repeat the

TABLE 6–9
Intermittent Injection Technique for Labor and Delivery

	Labor			Delivery	
Drug	*Volume (ml)*	*%*	*Reinjection Interval*	*Volume (ml)*	*%*
2-Chloroprocaine	8–10	2	q 30 min	10–14	2–3
With epinephrine			q 45 min		
Lidocaine	8–10	1.0–1.5	q 60 min	10–14	1.5
With epinephrine			q 75 min		
Bupivacaine	10–12	0.25	q 75 min	10–14	0.25–0.5
With epinephrine			q 120 min		

same concentration and LA used to initiate the block but may switch to 0.25% bupivacaine as appropriate to decrease motor block. However, if the sensory level decreases by more than two dermatomes before the "top up," repeat the entire initial dosage.

At the time of delivery, 10 to 15 ml of LA injected with the patient in the sitting or 45-degrees head-up position usually provides adequate perineal analgesia for vaginal delivery. If sacral analgesia is poor during injection, administer additional LA of a greater concentration (10–20 ml 1.5% lidocaine or 3% 2-chloroprocaine). Alternatively, although the technique is not ideal, the obstetrician can administer a pudendal block and provide adequate analgesia for uncomplicated vaginal deliveries.

If longer-lasting analgesia is desirable, either during labor or for delivery, 10 ml of 0.25% bupivacaine containing 5 μg/ml of fentanyl and approximately 3.3 μg of epinephrine per ml provides analgesia lasting about 180 minutes.[40] Repeat injections of this solution may provide an alternative when continuous-infusion lumbar epidural (CILE) analgesia is not available (discussed subsequently).

Continuous-Infusion Lumbar Epidural Analgesia

CILE represents a rational and simple practice for efficiently providing continuous, prolonged pain control. CILE is indicated when providing analgesia for labors expected to last longer than 1½ to 2 hours and provides many advantages over intermittent injections. Once an effective epidural block is established, CILE maintains continuous pain relief, thereby avoiding block regression and painful maternal waiting periods for reinjections, which commonly occurs on busy wards when using intermittent injections. CILE also avoids the sudden swings in sympathetic tone accompanying block regression and reestablishment. CILE can also maintain satisfactory analgesia with more dilute LA solutions than is possible when managing labor pain with intermittent bolus injection, because CILE constantly bathes the nerve fibers. During the first 4 or 5 hours of CILE, motor block is minimized allowing good maternal movement and an unimpaired ability to push and expel the fetus during second stage labor. CILE also avoids tachyphylaxis, which can occur when sensory blocks are allowed to wear off and reestablish.

The authors' experience suggests that CILE decreases LA requirements during labor when compared with intermittent bolus injections. Furthermore, sudden toxic reactions secondary to unrecognized IV LA injections are less frequent, since the small amounts (15 mg/hour bupivacaine, 200 mg/hour chloroprocaine) infused with CILE are not usually associated with central nervous system toxicity. Therefore, if the epidural catheter migrates intravascularly during the course of the labor, the maternal response will be a *return of pain,* not a seizure or cardiovascular collapse. In the unlikely but possible event of subarachnoid migration of the catheter, excessively high spinal anesthesia is unlikely because the onset of dense motor block will be slow but obvious and limited to the lower extremities, allowing early diagnosis. Nevertheless, close monitoring is essential. CILE also decreases obligatory anesthesia attendance time for reinjections once effective infusion for labor is established. Hourly 5-minute checks of maternal anesthetic level and vital signs are still required, but are less than the prolonged periods of physician monitoring required following each full "top-up" dose. CILE analgesia for labor does *not,* however, decrease the need to continuously monitor the parturient and is not an excuse to leave the patient unmonitored for hours until called for delivery.

Infusion Pumps

A wide variety of reliable infusion pumps are available. Although many clinicians may employ the same type of infusion pumps utilized concomitantly for oxytocin infusions, employing a different proprietary brand of pump devoted only to epidural analgesia avoids potential confusion between IV and epidural infusions. Pump specifications should include: accurate infusion rates down to 1 ml/hour, positive-pressure drive (not gravity flow), back-up battery, and an automatic infusion shut-off should power be lost or the front of the pump accidentally opened. The authors routinely mix our infusion mixture in a 150-ml bag of normal saline solution use an IVAC/IMED or Abbott-type infusion pump. If a Harvard-type pump is chosen, a 50- or 60-ml syringe is used. Guidelines for syringe mixing are in Table 6–10.

TABLE 6–10
Preparation of Continuous-Infusion Solutions

To Prepare 150 ml for Infusion Pump, Add the Following to 150-ml Bag of Normal Saline Solution*

Drug	*Volume (ml)*	*%*	*To Produce*	*Infusion Rate (ml/hr)*
Bupivacaine	30	0.75	0.125% solution	8–12
Bupivacaine	50	0.75	0.187% solution	8–12
Lidocaine	50	2	0.5% solution	15–20
Lidocaine	90	2	0.75% solution	15–20
2-Chloroprocaine	30	3	0.5% solution	30–40†
2-Chloroprocaine	50	3	0.75% solution	30–40†

To Prepare 50 ml Syringe for Infusion Pump (e.g., Harvard), add

Drug	*Volume (ml)*	*%*	*To Produce*
Bupivacaine	25	0.25 + 25 ml normal saline	0.125% solution
Lidocaine	25	1 + 25 ml normal saline	0.5% solution
2-Chloroprocaine	12.5	2 + 37.5 ml normal saline	0.5% solution

*Remove 30 ml excess IV solution. A 150-ml bag of fluid contains about 170 ml, placed by the manufacturer to allow filling of IV tubing.

†This volume of 2-chloroprocaine was arrived at during infusion studies. Higher-volume infusions were required at these lower concentrations to maintain adequate analgesia. Some clinicians may prefer to infuse lower volumes, but this may result in less effective analgesia.

Continuous-Infusion Techniques Local Anesthetic Infusions

Prior to initiating a continuous infusion, epidural block is performed and the block established as discussed previously. If the initial block is unilateral or patchy after 15 to 20 minutes, do not begin the infusion; repeat the epidural. A solid, bilateral epidural block of adequate height and density is essential for successful CILE analgesia. Once the block is established, maintain the continuous infusion with a dilute LA solution as outlined in Table 6–11. The authors often include 1:400,000 epinephrine in the solution to provide a denser block for patients experiencing severe pain. Epinephrine, however, hastens the onset of motor blockade. Ideally, continuous infusions should only maintain the block, *not* elevate or intensify it. When using short-acting LAs such as 2-chloroprocaine, the infusion must begin immediately after the mother is positioned recumbent with uterine displacement because the anesthetic effect decays more rapidly than intermediate or long-acting LAs. As a general rule, the *concentration* of the infused LAs should be half that of the drug concentration used for block establishment. These concentrations are effective and reduce the amount of drug infused during labor. When employing a bupivacaine infusion after establishing the sensory block with 2-chloroprocaine the authors' clinical impression is that some patients may become "spoiled" by the initial dense block with 2-chloroprocaine and not be as happy with bupivacaine's analgesia. Other authors report decreased duration of block (30–40 min instead of 90–120 min) when epidural bupivacaine follows 2-chloroprocaine.[41] Others identified little effect on bupivacaine for labor following 2-chloroprocaine when bupivacaine contains bicarbonate.[42] Establishing sensory blocks with lidocaine avoids this controversy.

The infusion rates and LA concentrations adequate to maintain a T10–8 level required for satisfactory visceral analgesia during labor are as follows:

Bupivacaine: 10–12 ml/hour of 0.125–0.1875%
Lidocaine: 10–15 ml/hour of 0.75–1%
Chloroprocaine: 10–15 ml/hour of 0.5–1%

TABLE 6–11
Guidelines for Dosing Continuous-Infusion Analgesia for Labor

Drug	Initial Bolus and "Top-Up" Dose	Concentration (%)	Infusion Maintenance (ml/hr)
Bupivacaine	8–10 ml 0.25%	0.125–0.25	8–12
Lidocaine	8–10 ml 1.5%	0.75–1	12–16
2-Chloroprocaine	8–10 ml 2%	0.5–1	30–40*

*This volume of 2-chloroprocaine was arrived at during infusion studies. Higher-volume infusions were required at these lower concentrations to maintain adequate analgesia. Some clinicians may prefer to infuse lower volumes, but this may result in less effective analgesia.

The authors generally do not exceed 15 ml/hour. Greater requirements may be a sign of poor catheter placement, not inadequate volume. Evaluate the block before increasing the infusion rate.

Narcotic/Local Anesthetic Combinations for Labor Analgesia

Adding narcotics to bupivacaine or lidocaine epidural infusions is popular. Advantages of adding narcotics to LAs include: faster onset, longer duration of block, lower required concentration of LA, and less motor block. In second stage, good analgesia persists while the mother often senses perineal pressure and may appear to "push" better when LA/narcotic combinations are used. Fentanyl, morphine, meperidine, sufentanil, alfentanil, butorphanol, nalbuphine, buprenorphine, and hydromorphone are among the many narcotics reported effective when combined with bupivacaine.

The authors employ this method in approximately 20% of labor infusions, especially when patients desire less motor blockade or when initiating blocks in patients in early painful labor as a means to hopefully decrease total LA drug infused during labor.

Epidural Fentanyl and Bupivacaine: A Suggested Technique

When establishing epidural analgesia with fentanyl/bupivacaine solutions, the authors recommend using 8 to 12 ml/hour of 0.125 to 0.25% bupivacaine containing 50 μg fentanyl. "Top-up" doses, when required, consist of 10 ml 0.125% bupivacaine containing 25 μg fentanyl. The authors use an infusate of 0.0625% bupivacaine containing 1 to 2 μg/ml fentanyl, which is infused at a rate of 8 to 14 ml/hour (Table 6–12). To obtain a mixture of 0.0625% bupivacaine and 2 μg/ml fentanyl for infusion (IMED, IVAC, Abbott "plum"), remove 86.5 ml from a 150-ml normal saline solution bag, and add 4 ml of fentanyl (50 μg/ml) and 12.5 ml of 0.5% bupivacaine. This provides 100 ml of the appropriate concentration. Recent studies demonstrate the effectiveness of bupivacaine/fentanyl solution as well as other combinations of bupivacaine with meperidine and sufentanil.[43–45]

If the total dose of fentanyl infused does not exceed 150 to 200 μg or 25 to 50 μg/hour in an average labor, no ill effects are detectable in the neonate. As discussed earlier, a number of investigators have reported decreased narcotic efficacy when combined with 2-chloroprocaine, and the authors do not use this combination.

Patient-Controlled Epidural Analgesia

The use of patient-controlled infusions to provide labor analgesia is gradually increasing,

TABLE 6–12
Mixing of 0.0625% Bupivacaine With 2 μg/ml of Fentanyl*

0.5% Bupivacaine	12.5 ml
Fentanyl	4.0 ml (50 μg/ml)
Saline solution	83.5 ml
Total volume	100 ml

*Start infusion at 8–12 ml/hr.

particularly for patients who desire greater control over their analgesia. Patient-controlled epidural analgesia requires a programmable pump and some extra time for patient instruction. A number of published reports describe this method, its safety, effectiveness, and patient satisfaction.[46–50] Most authors recommend using a basal infusion of approximately 6 to 8 ml/hour of 0.125% or 0.0625% bupivacaine either with or without fentanyl or another suitable narcotic. Usual management includes a patient bolus of 4 to 6 ml (30-min lockout). In the authors' practice, we try to establish a block that requires few patient boluses. For this reason, we use a basal infusion of 10 to 12 ml/hour with a patient bolus of 10 ml (approximately ½-hr lockout) and do not allow the mother more than two patient injections in a 4-hour period. In the author's group's experience, more frequent injections usually indicate that the block is not adequate and may need to be repeated. Furthermore, there is at least one report that some mothers may anesthetize themselves to a T2 dermatome level! Overall, complication rates with this modified technique do not appear higher than physician-controlled methods as long as the patient is supervised by a qualified nurse. Remember, patient-controlled does not mean physician-free.

Troubleshooting Continuous Infusions

Unilateral Block

Unilateral sensory block occasionally manifests during the infusions because either the initial block was one-sided or gravity caused the slowly infused drug to pool in the dependent area of the epidural space when a patient remained in one position. If this occurs, turn the patient to the full lateral position with the poorly blocked side down, reinject a full test and loading dose, and restart the infusion at a slightly higher rate in milliliters per hour up to 15 ml/hour. If this is not successful or the block continues regressing or once more demonstrates unilaterality, replace the epidural catheter and begin the loading-infusion procedure again. Do not waste time and drugs on a poorly functioning catheter! This catheter will not provide adequate anesthesia for cesarean section.

Breakthrough Pain Despite Loss of Cold Sense

If breakthrough pain occurs despite an apparently adequate sensory level determined by loss of cold and pinprick sensation, repeat the loading dose of 8 to 10 ml 0.25% bupivacaine and increase the infusion concentration by a third (e.g., 0.125% bupivacaine to 0.1875%). If unsuccessful, replace the catheter, and inject a loading dose as described previously. Believe the patient when she says "I still hurt"!! Patients are more accurate than pins.

Receding Sensory Level

If the sensory level recedes during the course of labor, ensure that the catheter is not intravascular by syringe aspiration, looking for signs of blood, and then inject an adequate intravenous test dose as described previously. Next administer a "top-up" dose and increase the infusion rate by a quarter to a half (maximum 15–16 ml). If the catheter is intravascular or the block does not improve, repeat the epidural as described previously.

Rising Sensory Level

If the sensory level rises excessively during the infusion, check for an unrecognized subarachnoid catheter placement. First, aspirate the catheter, looking for cerebrospinal fluid. If it is negative and the degree of block permits, repeat the spinal test dose. If both are negative, decrease the infusion rate by 25%. If the catheter lies in the subarachnoid space, either repeat the block or manage as a continuous spinal. The authors' usual practice is to repeat the epidural.

Do Not Discontinue the Infusion

The authors believe continuing the epidural infusion without interruption throughout labor, including the second stage of labor, offers the benefits of stable maternal physiology, improves maternal bearing-down efforts, and avoids tachyphylaxis and increased drug requirements at the time of delivery. Discontinuing the epidural during the second stage often results in dramatic, severe maternal pain that frequently has not been previously experienced. This, combined with the psychological "letdown" of pain, produces a frightened, suffering, angry, and uncooperative woman who is unable or unwilling to participate effectively in the final stages of delivery. Although most women can "push" effectively whether they feel their contractions or not during the second stage, requests to turn off the epidural so the mother can "bear down" more effectively occur. However, unless the sensory level is excessively high, the degree of sensory/motor blockade should not interfere with the primary muscles of expulsion (intercostal, diaphragm, larynx, and upper abdominals). The cause of ineffective pushing is more likely ineffective coaching, maternal exhaustion, or loss of desire to cooperate. The authors' approach when this occurs is to improve coaching or decrease the LA concentration or infusion rate. Persuasive evidence from the literature indicates that epidural blockade is unlikely to be a direct cause of an excessively prolonged second stage labor. It is rare in the authors' practice to receive absolute insistence by an obstetrician to turn off the epidural in the second stage. If, however, the obstetrician is adamant, the patient is informed of the plan, its rationale, and the reason for the request. In the authors' experience, most patients accept the practice, following an adequate explanation.

Delivery Analgesia

At delivery, adequate perineal analgesia is achieved in 50 to 70% of parturients maintained with a CILE. If it is achieved, continue the infusion until perineal repair is accomplished. Remember, 2-chloroprocaine blocks last only 15 to 20 minutes after the infusion is discontinued, whereas bupivacaine blocks last about 1 hour after the infusion is stopped. If perineal analgesia is inadequate, discontinue the infusion and establish adequate sacral analgesia with one of the following doses (see also Table 6–6):

2-Chloroprocaine: 10 to 15 ml of 2 to 3%.
Lidocaine: 10 to 15 ml of 1.5 to 2%.
Bupivacaine: 10 to 15 ml of 0.25 to 0.375%.

Mid forceps deliveries generally require greater volumes and concentrations of LAs to provide adequate sensory analgesia. Fifteen to 20 ml of 3% 2-chloroprocaine provides excellent analgesia and has the added benefit of providing near-surgical anesthesia for urgent delivery should cesarean section become necessary.

If cesarean section becomes necessary during continuous-infusion epidural analgesia, discontinue the infusion, repeat the test dose, and administer sufficient LA to establish cesarean section anesthesia (approximately 18–25 ml of 3% 2-chloroprocaine, 1.5% lidocaine, or 0.5% bupivacaine).

Helpful Hints

Initiate infusions with a slightly higher rate than you anticipate will provide adequate block maintenance. Taper the volume infused as the block duration increases. However, this practice means you must come back! Otherwise, increased block heights develop. Do not rely on the infusion to raise or intensify the block. If you wish to alter the intensity or level, rebolus with the appropriate drug and increase the infusion rate to maintain or increase the desired level of block. Increase the LA concentration if you wish to increase or maintain the density of the block.

Safety Precautions

Check the patient twice during the first hour after starting the continuous infusion and with hourly checks thereafter. Use preservative-free LAs and dilute as desired with IV solutions (normal saline solution). Tape all injection ports thoroughly and label the pump clearly as an "epidural infusion." Use pump-to-patient tubing without IV ports. Nothing but the prescribed anesthetic should find its way into the epidural space! Finally, check the infusion rate and the patient frequently.

Subarachnoid Analgesia Techniques

Local Anesthetics

In the past, subarachnoid block was rarely used to provide labor analgesia because of the limited duration of analgesia of single-shot subarachnoid block, the unpredictable length of labor, and the unavoidable risk of dural puncture headache in the young population of parturients. Subarachnoid block was reserved primarily to provide anesthesia for delivery and operative obstetrics.

However, continuous subarachnoid analgesia during labor becomes an option following accidental dural puncture during attempted epidural block. This approach is more appealing if epidural catheter placement is particularly difficult or when the anatomy of the epidural space is distorted, as may be the case following vertebral disk surgery, Harrington rod placement, or secondary to structural changes associated with severe scoliosis. In these circumstances, the authors occasionally electively choose to thread a 20-gauge epidural catheter into the subarachnoid space and proceed with continuous spinal analgesia. If selecting continuous spinal analgesia, all involved personnel must be fully aware of the spinal catheter, maintain absolute sterility, and double-check medication before injection. Remember, confusion between epidural and spinal catheters is a real possibility on a busy labor epidural service. Label the catheter as well as the chart!

Another condition in which the authors may choose spinal block during labor include tumultuous painful late first stage labor in a multipara when delivery is imminent and rapid analgesia is desirable. Even though spinal analgesia meets these conditions, there remains the risk that analgesia requirements will outlive the duration of block and necessitate another anesthetic. Thus, drug selection is important. The choice of LA depends on the anticipated length of labor or anticipated procedure and the desired duration of block. Drugs must be preservative-free spinal preparations, and at the authors' institution the most commonly used drugs are hyperbaric lidocaine 15 to 30 mg or hyperbaric bupivacaine 1 to 3 mg. We select hyperbaric solutions because isobaric solutions tend to produce higher dermatomal blocks and spare sacral segments. Dosages are repeated when analgesia regresses and always following gentle catheter aspiration to document free flow of spinal fluid. There is debate over the maximal advised dose of continuous spinal LA. Recent reports suggest that dosages of hyperbaric lidocaine exceeding 150 mg associate with increased risk of direct neurotoxicity and cauda equina syndrome.[51, 52] This association has been observed with large-bore and small-bore spinal catheters. The mechanism, although not fully understood, may involve poor spread of the anesthetic with "pooling" of high osmolar solution over sensitive nerve roots of the cauda equina with subsequent swelling and tissue inflammation. At present, when using continuous spinal block, the authors limit the total dose during labor to 125 mg of lidocaine and 15 mg of bupivacaine.

Spinal catheters must not be confused with epidural catheters. Remember, fine-gauge continuous spinal catheters are at present proscribed by the U.S. Food and Drug Administration. Perhaps controlled outcome studies currently under way may lead to their return in the future.

Spinal Narcotics

In contrast to subarachnoid LAs, intrathecal narcotics have proved popular in recent years because they provide highly effective analgesia without some of the most troublesome side effects of LAs such as sympatholysis, dense motor blockade, and potential systemic toxicity. Other advantages of spinal narcotics include specific pain receptor blockade, little depression of consciousness, and possible ambulation. Side effects of intraspinal narcotics include urinary retention, most commonly seen with morphine. Pruritus occurs in more than 50% of patients receiving morphine but is considerably less frequent or severe following fentanyl and sufentanil administration. Nausea and vomiting are uncommon with short-acting narcotics and are best treated with antiemetics (e.g., 10 mg prochlorperazine IM). Naloxone is not very effective for prophylaxis or therapy for nausea and vomiting, and its role is unclear in the treatment of urinary retention, nausea, and vomiting. Remember, nausea and vomiting and severe pruritus may herald delayed respiratory depression. Respiratory depression, extremely rare with short-acting spinal narcotics such as fentanyl and sufentanil, is rapidly reversed by 0.4 mg naloxone IV.[53] Sedation and lethargy occur more often with agonist-antagonist analgesics such as butorphanol and can also be treated with small doses of naloxone. The authors' treatment regimens are listed in Table 6–13.

Headache remains a potential complication of spinal injection irrespective of drug selection. However, Sprotte "cone" point and Whitacre spinal needles decrease the incidence of postspinal headache. However, despite a reported incidence of less than 0.5%,[54] the authors' incidence of headache after more than

TABLE 6–13
Side Effects of Intrathecal Opioids and Their Treatment

Problem	Treatment	Comments
Itching	Diphenhydramine 25 mg IV, nalbuphine 5–10 mg IV, propofol 10 mg IV, naloxone 40 μg IV (last resort) Naltrexone 25 mg p.o. (after delivery, morphine only)	Itching, usually mild and of limited duration; morphine can cause severe, prolonged itching
Nausea and vomiting	Metoclopramide 5–10 mg IV, nalbuphine 5–10 mg IV, propofol 10 mg IV, naloxone 40 μg IV (last resort) Naltrexone 25 mg p.o. (after delivery, morphine only)	Nausea after intrathecal meperidine is usually self-limited and resolves without treatment; morphine can cause significant nausea both during and after delivery
Hypotension	IV fluids, ephedrine	Minor decreases in blood pressure are common with all intrathecal opioids; significant hypotension (systolic BP < 90 mmHg) is rare, but may occur
Urinary retention	Catheterization, naloxone 400 μg IV (may have to repeat)	Occasionally a problem after delivery with morphine

Abbreviations: IV = intravenous; BP = blood pressure.

2000 Sprotte 24-gauge spinals is approximately 3%. Fortunately, in the authors' experience, these headaches are usually mild and short-lived. Another disadvantage of the single-shot spinal technique is the duration of the analgesia, which is determined by the type and dose of drug. An unsuccessful attempt to design a long-lasting subarachnoid analgesic cocktail intended for the duration of labor,[55] consisting of 25 μg fentanyl and 0.25 mg morphine, resulted in an unacceptable incidence of nausea and itching that required naloxone or naltrexone reversal in a high number of subjects. Short-acting, preservative-free spinal narcotics such as 25 μg fentanyl, 15 mg meperidine, and 10 μg sufentanil have proved to be highly effective first stage labor analgesics with a lower incidence and intensity of nausea and itching.[56–58] Unfortunately, labor often lasts longer than the analgesia provided by these short-acting compounds (1–2.5 hours), even when combined with 0.25% bupivacaine, leading to efforts to find alternative techniques. The safety of repeat spinal narcotic injections is unclear.

Despite the apparent safety of this technique, Cohen and coworkers[53] reported demonstrable blood pressure and sensory changes after subarachnoid sufentanil administration to laboring women. In their view, possible mechanisms for the sensory/motor blockade included LA effect, hypobaricity causing wider than expected spread of the drug (their subjects were sitting and had pinprick sensation loss from T4 to L4), direct sympathetic blockade at preganglionic receptors, and a decrease of pain associated with circulating catecholamines. These findings do not contraindicate allowing these patients to ambulate, but emphasize the importance of examining each patient for a response to spinal narcotics before the patient gets out of bed. Although subarachnoid meperidine has also been used, doses exceeding 15 to 20 mg act like a subarachnoid LA, producing sympathetic and motor blockade.[56]

Use of Combined Spinal/Epidural Techniques

The recent Food and Drug Administration proscription against continuous spinal techniques with ultra-small-bore catheters has left combined spinal/epidural techniques as the only effective alternative that provides the advantages of rapid labor analgesia with minimal side effects of spinal narcotics combined with the long-term benefits of an indwelling epidural catheter. First popularized by Carrie and O'Sullivan,[59] the major attraction of this technique is the remarkably rapid relief (30 sec–2 min) experienced by the parturient following spinal fentanyl 25 μg or sufentanil 10 μg. Analgesia lasts 60 to 120 minutes; can be initiated early in labor; does not cause motor blockade, thus allowing ambulation in selected patients; and decreases the amount of LA used during subsequent labor epidural analgesia. The technique involves first entering the epidural space as usual with a 17- or 18-gauge Tuohy-type needle. The subarachnoid space is then entered with a 4.5-inch 24-gauge pencil-point needle through the larger epidural needle (used as an introducer). Be sure to check the compatibility of needles before starting! Subarachnoid fentanyl 25 μg in 1 to 1.5 ml of preservative-free saline solution is injected, the spinal needle removed, and a 20-gauge epidural catheter threaded into the epidural space. The catheter is aspirated for spinal fluid, and a spinal test dose is given. The epidural catheter rarely enters the spinal space (approximately 4 in 1650 patients in the authors' hands) and such an event is usually recognized immediately on administration of a test dose. Patients receiving spinal narcotics rapidly develop intense analgesia without sympathetic or motor block, but often report mild facial itching. Rarely, itching requires treatment with 0.2 mg IV naloxone; this treatment does not reverse analgesia. The authors no longer administer subarachnoid morphine during labor because of the more intense side effects of itching, nausea, and urinary retention and the required prolonged respiratory monitoring. The authors allow patients to walk ½ hour after subarachnoid narcotic injection, after examining them in the sitting position to ensure that no postural changes in blood pressure occur and ruling out possible motor blockade. The patient always walks with a support person. In over 2000 cases of subarachnoid fentanyl, the authors have had 1 patient who received spinal fentanyl 50 μg and experienced sudden respiratory arrest 15 minutes after injection and required ventilatory support until the effects of the narcotic were reversed. There were no other complications. Clearly, monitoring is important.

The indwelling epidural catheter, after a test dose, provides analgesia when the narcotic effect wanes, labor pain becomes more severe, or operative delivery or cesarean section is required. In theory, because of the presence of a hole in the dura, the dose of LA might need to be reduced. An argument against this is that a pressure gradient exists from the subdural to the epidural space and is unlikely to be overcome during slow epidural injection. Nevertheless, inject slowly!! In practice, epidural dose requirements appear to be similar whether a double-needle technique is used or not. Remember, failed epidural blocks occur despite successful spinal placement.

To extend the duration of narcotic analgesia, Morgan and colleagues[60, 61] suggest adding 2.5 mg bupivacaine (hyperbaric) to 25 μg of spinal fentanyl. Bupivacaine prolongs the analgesic activity often beyond 2 hours without significant motor block. A large number of their patients ambulated with this combination receive an average of one to two "top-up" doses of 10 to 12 ml epidural 0.1% bupivacaine for the entire labor. The authors have begun to use this method and find it appeals to women who desire more personal control over the conduct of their labor and analgesia.

The presence of a known dural puncture does not alter epidural drug selection. Although 2-chloroprocaine containing bisulfite preservative was avoided in the past in the presence of a dural puncture, the authors' will now use 2-chloroprocaine with citrate preservative, when indicated, in the presence of a dural puncture.

COMPLICATIONS OF REGIONAL BLOCK FOR LABOR

Failed or Incomplete Block

Incomplete epidural block frustrates both patients and physicians. Even in experienced hands, block failure occurs 5 to 10% of the time, perhaps secondary to catheter advancement too far into the anterior epidural space or passage of the catheter out a nerve root foramen. Rarely, stenosis of the epidural space or vertebral disk disease partially occludes the continuity of the epidural space and contributes to failure.[62] The incidence of partial block can be decreased by careful midline entry into the epidural space and threading catheters only 3 to 4 cm beyond the needle tip. Catheters that do not thread easily often associate with placement outside the epidural space. In the authors' opinion, forcing the catheter or using stylets increases the chance of exiting the epidural space or puncturing a vessel. Although pulling the catheter back and reinjecting can result in a successful block, this maneuver often prolongs suffering and increases maternal drug levels secondary to multiple drug injections. The authors' recommended management of incomplete block is to repeat the procedure at the same or another interspace. In our experience, failed block rarely occurs in repeat blocks.

Unilateral Block

Unilateral epidural block is usually caused by a catheter lying in the anterior epidural space or, rarely, the existence of an epidural-dural adhesion. The cause, similar to that of spotty block, is advancing the catheter too far into the epidural space or side entry into the epidural space. In contrast to incomplete blocks, withdrawing the catheter 1 to 2 cm, rebolusing with the initial dose, and placing the patient with the unblocked side down may result in an effective block. Further doses should be repeated with the patient in this position. However, if this therapy does not work after one attempt, the block should be completely repeated without apologies. Delay of block replacement results in unnecessary extra drug administration and an unhappy patient.

Maternal Hypotension

Maternal hypotension, defined as a systolic blood pressure less than 100 mmHg or a maternal blood pressure decrease of 25 to 30% below the preblock average, is the most common side effect associated with an effective epidural block. Although in the vast majority of cases, the blood pressure decrease is transient and of little importance for the mother or fetus, significant hypotension, if ignored, can result in significant maternal or fetal morbidity and possibly mortality. The placenta, an organ that lacks significant autoregulation, depends on normal maternal blood pressure to maintain intervillous blood flow. If placental dysfunction exists as in placental insufficiency, preeclampsia, or diabetes, the fetus may not tolerate even a 15 to 20% fall in maternal blood pressure. For high-risk patients, continuous electronic fetal heart rate monitoring is the most reliable guide for judging fetal response to decreased maternal blood pressure. The authors recommend continuous fetal heart rate monitoring throughout labor and believe late decelerations following block establishment indicate blood pressure treatment even when the classic definition of hypotension is not met. Despite these concerns, if maternal hypotension is rapidly treated, fetal asphyxia rarely occurs. Hence, fetal stress or a nonreassuring heart tracing is not a contraindication to epidural analgesia or catheter reinjection. Remember, severe maternal hypotension, untreated, can also cause loss of maternal consciousness, predisposing the mother to vomiting and pulmonary aspiration. For details on fetal stress, see Chapter 8.

Avoiding hypotension is superior to treatment. Clinically significant hypotension is minimized by ensuring adequate maternal volume preload with approximately 500 ml of IV non–dextrose-containing balanced salt solution and continuous left uterine displacement after the block placement. Although some advocate ephedrine prophylaxis prior to starting the block, this is rarely necessary following IV hydration and applying strict left uterine displacement. If hypotension occurs despite these precautions, administer further IV fluid, ensure complete lateral position with legs elevated, and administer IV ephedrine 10 to 15 mg. Allow 1 minute for ephedrine effects before repeating a blood pressure measurement. If fetal heart rate abnormalities occur, continue this therapy and administer high-flow maternal oxygen by face mask.

Intravascular Injection of Local Anesthetic

Pregnancy-induced dilated epidural veins are frequently cannulated during epidural block placement because either the catheter is forced during placement or, rarely, the tip migrates intravascularly during the course of labor. This potential disaster is diagnosed by careful catheter testing prior to therapeutic dosing, gentle aspiration on the catheter prior to and during injection, and having a high index of suspicion when the block fails. Unfortunately, catheter aspiration may be unreliable secondary to collapse of the vein. Therefore, failed blocks are IV cannulations until proved otherwise. Opening the hub to air and lowering it below the level of the back may allow blood flow back by gravity drainage and, along with aspiration, should be part of catheter testing. If blood returns briskly through the catheter, there are two choices. Replacing the catheter, either at the same or at a different interspace, is the authors' first choice. If the initial catheter placement was somewhat difficult, the catheter can be withdrawn a centimeter or two until blood flow ceases and then can be retested as discussed earlier in this chapter. Most importantly, the clinician avoids the serious consequences of accidental IV LA by limiting LA injection to increments of no more than 0.75 mg/kg bupivacaine, 2.5 mg/kg 2-chloroprocaine, or 2 mg/kg lidocaine and waiting 1 minute between injections. Inject LAs slowly (3–5 sec/ml) while questioning and observing the patient for signs of toxicity. It is impossible to overstate the importance of strict, slow, incremental administration of epidural LAs with constant patient surveillance in order to avoid the life-threatening results of unrecognized intravascular injection of large boluses of LA.

Treatment of Local Anesthetic Toxicity

If, during injection of LA, the patient exhibits mild signs of anesthetic toxicity such as tinnitus, metallic taste, visual or sensory changes, or alterations of consciousness, including dizziness, immediately cease injection and observe the patient for further changes and prepare to treat a major toxic reaction. If the patient begins to twitch or convulse, protect the airway by placing the patient in a lateral position with head down. Administer a high inspired concentration of oxygen by mask. In most cases, intubation will not be necessary unless repeated convulsions or cardiac arrest occurs as a result of bupivacaine toxicity. If the patient continues convulsing, prevent or terminate convulsions with a *small IV dose of a rapid-acting anticonvulsant* such as thiopental 25 to 50 mg, diazepam 2.5 mg, or midazolam 1.0 mg. Do not make the treatment riskier than the convulsion! With cessation of the convulsion, a short period of hypertension is likely. If, following the convulsion, the patient is not breathing, attempt gentle ventilation with 100% oxygen using mask and bag. Do not give a muscle relaxant unless all necessary equipment is available and ready, oxygen and suction are available, and adequate assistance is present to intubate the patient. Muscle relaxants do *not* stop the pathophysiology of convulsions but will provide conditions that allow intubation and, when necessary, ventilation. Somnolence, unconsciousness, or unresponsiveness may occur following large infusions of LAs, regardless of route. If this occurs, support the cardiovascular system by uterine displacement, elevation of the legs, rapid IV infusion, and appropriate IV vasoactive drugs, for example, IV ephedrine 10 to 15 mg. Recovery is usually rapid, provided no further LAs or other depressant drugs are given. In the event of cardiac depression or cardiac arrest following accidental IV injection of bupivacaine, only immediate aggressive and proper therapy allow the mother and fetus to recover. Treatment of bupivacaine-induced cardiac arrest may be prolonged. The following recommendations for treatment of bupivacaine-induced cardiac arrest differ from standard advanced cardiac life support protocols and are based on pregnant animal experiments.[63, 64]

If bupivacaine-related cardiac arrest occurs, initiate full cardiopulmonary resuscitation at once. Severe hypoxia develops in previously well-oxygenated dogs within 90 seconds of bupivacaine-induced cardiac arrest; therefore, rapid control of the airway and ventilation with 100% oxygen are absolutely necessary.[64] Aortocaval compression by the gravid uterus impairs venous return to the heart, making external cardiac compression ineffective. If adequate blood pressure and sinus cardiac rhythm are not immediately restored (5 min) with treatment, consider emergency cesarean section to facilitate cardiopulmonary resuscitation. In one case report of bupivacaine-induced cardiac arrest, the patient could not be resuscitated, despite uterine displacement, until emergency cesarean section was performed.[65]

Ventricular arrhythmias are common during bupivacaine toxicity. If ventricular tachycardia occurs, treat with IV bretylium (not lidocaine) 2.5 to 5 mg/kg every 30 seconds up to a maximum of 30 mg/kg and, if the patient is pulseless or severely hypotensive, direct current cardioversion. Ventricular fibrillation should be treated with bretylium as discussed previously, plus 1 to 2 mg epinephrine and direct current cardioversion. Torsades de pointes ventricular tachycardia has been induced by bupivacaine overdose in animals and may require isoproterenol or atrial pacing in addition to bretylium. Because the resuscitation may be prolonged and because severe acidosis/hypoxia is common in bupivacaine-induced cardiac arrest, treatment of acidosis may be necessary with IV bicarbonate.

Bradycardia with electromechanical dissociation or asystole may also develop. In this situation, animals require massive doses of epinephrine and atropine intravenously to be resuscitated. Administer epinephrine 1 mg and atropine 0.8 mg IV, followed by epinephrine 0.5 mg and atropine 0.4 mg every 30 to 60 seconds until adequate blood pressure and pulse return.

Accidental Dural Puncture or "Wet Tap"

The reported incidence of accidental dural puncture during attempted epidural analgesia ranges from 0.5 to 2%. More than 50% of patients experiencing a dural puncture with an 18-gauge needle develop postdural puncture headache. Careful attention to technique such as a firm needle grip, slow needle advancement, and careful plunger resistance testing lessens the chance of dural puncture. Whenever there is doubt as to whether the needle has reached an excessive depth, the wise anesthesiologist repositions and redirects the needle before possibly encountering cerebrospinal fluid. Tissue plugs also may obscure the sense of loss of resistance, and replacing the stylet periodically during placement may occasionally prevent an accidental dural puncture. If dural puncture occurs, the authors recommend withdrawing the needle, marking the first entry site with a small scratch should future epidural blood patch be required, and siting the block at another interspace. Patients experiencing a pain-free labor accept dural puncture headache better than those without analgesia. The catheter also serves as a route for later blood or saline solution headache prophylaxis. At the authors' institution, we perform prophylactic epidural blood patch, if a demonstrated wet tap occurs,[66] after the therapeutic block has worn off, provided the patient is afebrile. The authors obtain 15 to 20 ml of autologous drug sterilely in four 5-ml syringes and inject them into the indwelling epidural catheter at approximately 1 ml/sec. The authors try to inject a minimal volume of 15 ml and a maximal volume of 20 ml. However, if the patient complains of back pain or radiating limb discomfort, the injection is stopped and the catheter removed. Following injection, the patient remains recumbent for about an hour. Thereafter, we allow ambulation but also encourage avoidance of straining or exertion for a few days. Other institutions prefer delaying blood patch for 24 to 48 hours. Potential spontaneous headache resolution and concerns regarding infection from a contaminated epidural catheter or delivery-associated bacteremia are their primary considerations. Fever remains a contraindication to blood patch. More conservative treatment measures include infusing up to an 80-ml bolus of saline solution into the epidural space, and then gravity-infusing further normal saline solution at approximately 100 ml/hour for 24 hours. If the patient refuses blood patch, the authors apply a tight abdominal binder and administer IV or oral fluids, or both, from 3000 to 3500 ml/day for 1 to 2 days. However, the effectiveness of forced oral fluids has been questioned.[67] Analgesic treatments include aspirin or acetaminophen containing narcotics. Intravenous caffeine (500 mg) infused over ½ hour has been recommended as effective for 24 hours, but the authors have had mixed results following large-bore dural punctures and rarely use it.

Prior to discharge, a final evaluation of the patient's condition and severity of headache is made. If no *prophylactic* blood patch was performed and the headache persists and interferes with the mother's ability to care for herself or her infant, epidural blood patch is strongly recommended. After consent is obtained, identify the epidural space and administer 15 to 20 ml of sterile autologous blood to an endpoint sensation of lower back pressure. If a previous blood patch or prophylactic injection fails, the authors repeat the process in 24 hours. If two blood patches fail, the patient's condition is reassessed and consideration for 24-hour epidural saline infusion is made. This has been necessary only twice in 10 years. If the patient refuses this therapy, allowance is made for a return visit and outpatient blood patch, should she change her mind. In the authors' combined experience of over 50 prophylactic blood patches, 95% of the patients have not required further treatment. Three have required a repeat blood patch. Measures to prevent headache that are not effective include confining the patient to bed rest in the absence of headache and numerous drugs such as ergot and pitressin.

Accidental Subarachnoid Injection of Local Anesthetic

For equivalent level of block, epidural anesthesia requires five times the mass of drug compared with subarachnoid anesthesia. Hence, if LA is injected into the subarachnoid space, the volume and concentration required for epidural labor analgesia are sufficient to produce a high or total spinal block. Accidental subarachnoid anesthesia is most frequently caused by unrecognized dural puncture or forcing a styleted catheter through the dura. Only rarely do epidural catheters migrate to the subarachnoid space during labor. Although syringe aspiration for cerebrospinal fluid prior to drug injection may avoid accidental subarachnoid injection, careful administration of a drug test dose prior to injecting larger volumes is essential. As discussed previously, an adequate LA test dose for determining subarachnoid placement contains no preservative and is sufficient to render a rapid but safe block of the lower extremities. Forty to 60 mg lidocaine, 5 to 10 mg bupivacaine, or 50 to 100 mg 2-chloroprocaine serves this purpose. A high or total spinal block should not endanger the life of either the mother or the fetus if managed properly. Should total spinal block occur, ensure ventilation with a patent, protected airway by rapidly performing endotracheal intubation and manual or mechanical ventilation. Do not forget to have all necessary equipment available. Despite apnea, muscle relaxant anesthetics may be necessary! Maintain adequate perfusion pressure with appropriate left uterine displacement, rapid IV fluid infusion, and if necessary, ephedrine or similar pressor drug. Do not elevate the head in an attempt to stop cephalad progression of the block. This will not prevent the upward spread of the drug and may result in disastrous postural hypotension. If 2-chloroprocaine was administered, the authors no longer attempt to drain the cerebrospinal fluid because the present formulation is felt to be no more toxic than other LAs. Proper management of a total spinal should not significantly increase either maternal or neonatal morbidity and mortality. Once the mother with a total spinal block is stabilized, there is no reason to delay the obstetric procedure for which the block was administered. If the patient is intubated, the delivery is carried out under light general anesthesia. If the spinal block is high but the patient is conscious and comfortable, the authors usually proceed using continuous spinal anesthesia, supplementing as necessary with 50-mg doses of hyperbaric lidocaine, not exceeding 150 mg total dose.

Body Temperature and Epidural Block

Epidural anesthesia associates with little net change in core temperature during labor.[68] Most observations documenting heat loss have been made during cesarean section, where large IV volumes of room temperature fluids, extensive body surface exposure, and surgical site evaporative heat loss all contributed to the mild hypothermia.[69] In contrast to this setting, Marx and Loew[68] found that during labor, metabolic and skeletal energy expenditure occurred with lessened perspiration secondary to an epidural-induced sympathectomy. Decreased perspiration could theoretically lead to an increase in body temperature,[65] and a number of studies associate mild maternal hyperthermia when epidural anesthesia lasts 5 hours or longer.[70, 71] However, these laboring women were confined at a room temperature of 75° to 82°F. Camann and associates[72] found similar increases when epidural drug solutions included narcotics.

Importantly, no patients in any of the studies had signs of infection, chorioamnionitis, or sepsis, and the number of vaginal examinations, a potential infectious source, did not differ between groups. Most importantly, a 0.5° to 1° C change in maternal core temperature did not adversely affect the intrauterine environment or result in fetal compromise in the absence of signs of infection and is thus of little clinical import.

Backache and Epidural Block

Back pain occurs in more than 40% of women[73] during and after pregnancy and is attributed to a wide array of causes that include lordosis of pregnancy, mechanical strain during labor, and familial tendency to back pain. Epidural block in labor also associates with postpartum back pain, with a reported incidence ranging from 3 to 45%,[74] and MacArthur and coworkers suggest that labor epidural analgesia increases the risk of postpartum back pain.[75] However, their study suffered from a low sampling rate of the total deliveries (only 11,701 of 30,000 deliveries) and recall bias (subjects asked to recall events 1 to 9 years previously). A more carefully designed study examined more than 88% of 1042 deliveries within 2 months of delivery.[76] The incidence of back pain was 44%. Predisposing factors included younger age, greater weight, and shorter stature (new-onset pain). Epidural anesthesia did not associate with increased back pain 1 to 2 months postpartum. In summary, proper labor analgesia management should attempt to elicit any maternal history of back pain and related disorders and follow with a clear discussion of the risks of postpartum back pain. During the anesthetic course, regardless of history, maternal positioning should minimize factors such as excessive torso torque or sacral "overhang" in the lithotomy position, which may contribute to postpartum back pain.

Urinary Retention

Urinary retention may occur during labor with or without epidural anesthesia, and regional block may decrease the maternal sensation or ability to void. Since large fluid IV infusions may increase diuresis, hourly evaluation of bladder fullness should be performed by the nurse and the patient encouraged to void as needed. Bladder catheterization may be necessary during the course of labor to prevent bladder distention, which may lead to postdelivery urinary retention. Other factors contributing to urinary retention include pain, perineal edema, hematoma, and trauma.

Fetal Effects

When properly administered, epidural analgesia produces no deleterious effect on the fetus. Indeed, Apgar scores following epidural analgesia for labor are no different from those obtained following a drug-free childbirth. Early epidural neurobehavioral scores comparing infants born of mothers with and without epidural analgesia indicated a small but statistically significant decrease in neonatal muscle tone following maternal epidural analgesia with lidocaine or mepivacaine. Today, most practitioners think that this decreased muscle tone, if present, is evanescent and of no clinical significance. Rarely, an association has been noted between epidural lidocaine during labor and a decrease in long-term fetal heart rate variability. This association is probably of no clinical significance and has not been observed following epidural bupivacaine or 2-chloroprocaine. Finally, high maternal LA levels following accidental intravascular injection are associated with uterine hypertonus lasting 4 to 7 minutes with in utero placental blood flow lowered markedly. Recovery should be uneventful. These indirect causes of fetal depression can be consistently avoided by following the guidelines for safe practice described previously.

LABOR IN HIGH-RISK PREGNANCY: AN INDICATION FOR EPIDURAL ANALGESIA

As the protective advantages of epidural block for labor have become better understood and the availability of anesthetists more widespread, the criteria for maternal and fetal conditions considered contraindications to epidural block have changed. Today, certain maternal and fetal conditions are considered indications for epidural analgesia. For the premature fetus, epidural analgesia offers the advantage of allowing a controlled delivery and preventing precipitous expulsion caused by reflex painful bearing down during the second stage. In the premature or small-for-gestational-age fetus, epidural analgesia is preferred in labor, as it avoids central neonatal depression associated with narcotics and other systemic medication used to control pain. When significant compromise of the fetal environment exists, epidural block is indicated, since it provides a less stressful labor, reducing maternal oxygen consumption, ventilation, and catecholamine production, and lessens adverse changes in acid-base balance. These beneficial effects optimize fetal oxygen exchange. In maternal disease states such as preeclampsia or diabetes, epidural block improves fetal oxygen transport and minimizes maternal metabolic and cardiovascular demands, lessens the required time for surgical anesthesia, and makes epidural anesthesia the "ideal" form of pain relief for high-risk pregnancy.

The concept of a "prophylactic" epidural in the high-risk parturient as an insurance policy against a later emergency need to "crash" the patient has much merit. As a rule, the authors do not place epidural catheters in women who are not in labor, who are not expected to deliver within the day, or who are not in pain. However, in some circumstances, especially on a busy day, the authors will place epidural catheters early in labor before the parturients are defined as "active" if membranes are ruptured, delivery is planned, or they are receiving oxytocin but pain is not present. This is especially true in trial of labor, obesity, preeclampsia, diabetes, prematurity, small for gestational age, or postmaturity, or if there are signs of fetal stress. The authors believe this practice has considerably reduced the need for emergency induction of general anesthesia on our labor floor. Acting is preferable to reacting.

In summary, lumbar epidural block provides an array of advantages for both mother and fetus that make it an ideal form of pain relief for labor and vaginal delivery. For the best results, the technique must be tailored to specific requirements of the mother, fetus, and labor. The laboring woman must not be treated as a second-class patient merely because she is apparently normal. Epidural block for labor provides a safe, high-quality form of analgesia equivalent to that routinely provided for patients undergoing surgery. It allows a pain-free, alert, and cooperative mother to interact early with her new baby. Perhaps most important, she can experience a happier childbirth with a minimum of fear and pain.

TEN PRACTICAL POINTS

1. Beware of using epidural narcotics to improve a poor block.

2. Catheter location, not drug choice, is the most common reason for failed epidural analgesia.

3. Initiate blocks early in a high-risk patient undergoing a trial of labor. Maintain a higher, more dense block.

4. Do not waste time correcting a patchy, one-sided, or otherwise unsatisfactory block. Repeat at once at another interspace.

5. Aim for a T9–S5 sensory level for vaginal delivery and a T2–S5 level for cesarean section. Err slightly on the high side of the dose of local anesthetic administered.

6. Use 1:300,000 to 1:400,000 freshly mixed epinephrine in the local anesthetic solutions and alkalinize with sodium bicarbonate immediately prior to injection to improve onset and density of analgesia.

7. Pain, a commitment to deliver, and an obstetric willingness to use oxytocin are sufficient indications for epidural analgesia.

8. Appropriate catheter testing, fractionalization of local anesthetic solutions, and patient monitoring are keys to safe anesthesia.

9. For block evaluation, the patient is smarter than your pin.

10. Devise a system that reliably identifies IV, epidural, and continuous spinal catheters. Confusion is deadly!

REFERENCES

1. Camann WR, Ostheimer GW: Physiological adaptations during pregnancy. Int Anesthesiol Clin 28:2–10, 1990.
2. Huch R: Maternal hyperventilation and the fetus. J Perinat Med 14:3–17, 1986.
3. Hagerdal M, Morgan CW, Sumner AE, Gutsche BB: Minute ventilation and oxygen consumption during labor with epidural analgesia. Anesthesiology 59:425–427, 1983.
4. Sangoul F, Fox GS, Houle CL: Effect of regional anesthesia on maternal oxygen consumption during the first stage of labor. Am J Obstet Gynecol 191:1080–1083, 1975.
5. Shnider SM, Abboud TK, Artal R, et al: Maternal catecholamines decrease during labor after lumbar epidural anesthesia. Am J Obstet Gynecol 147:13–15, 1983.
6. Shnider SM, Wright RG, Levinson G: Uterine blood flow and plasma norepinephrine changes during maternal stress in the pregnant ewe. Anesthesiology 50:524–527, 1979.
7. Zador G, Nilsson BA: Low-dose intermittent epidural anaesthesia in labour. II. Influence on labour and fetal acid-base status. Acta Obstet Gynecol Scand (Suppl) 34:17, 1974.
8. Jenkins MW, Pritchard MH: Hypnosis: Practical applications and theoretical considerations in normal labour. Br J Obstet Gynaecol 100:221–226, 1993.
9. Hawkins JL, Gibbs CP, Orleans M, Schmid K: Obstetric anesthesia manpower survey: 1992 versus 1981 [Abstract 12]. Soc Obstet Anesthes Perinatol 1994.
10. Shnider SM, Moya F: Effects of meperidine on the newborn infant. Am J Obstet Gynecol 89:1009–1015, 1964.

11. Podlas J, Breland BD: Patient-controlled analgesia with nalbuphine during labor. Obstet Gynecol 70:202–204, 1987.
12. Rosaeg OP, Kitts JB, Koren G, Byford LJ: Maternal and fetal effects of intravenous patient-controlled fentanyl analgesia during labour in a thrombocytopenic parturient. Can J Anaesth 39:277–281, 1992.
13. Baxi LV, Petrie RH, James LS: Human fetal oxygenation following paracervical block. Am J Obstet Gynecol 135:1109–1112, 1979.
14. Wee MYK, Hasan MA, Thomas TA: Isoflurane in labour. Anaesthesia 48:369–372, 1993.
15. Phillips KC, Thomas TA: Second stage of labour with or without extradural analgesia. Anaesthesia 38:972–976, 1983.
16. Chestnut DH, Bates JN, Choi WW: Continuous infusion epidural analgesia with lidocaine: Efficacy and influence during the second stage of labor. Obstet Gynecol 69:323–327, 1987.
17. Chestnut DH, Vandewalker GE, Owen CL, et al: The influence of continuous epidural bupivacaine analgesia on the second stage of labor and method of delivery in nulliparous women. Anesthesiology 66:774–780, 1987.
18. Chestnut DH, Laszewski LJ, Pollack KL, et al: Continuous epidural infusion of 0.0625% bupivacaine–0.0002% fentanyl during the second stage of labor. Anesthesiology 72:613–618, 1990.
19. Vertommen JD, Vandermeulen E, VanAken H, et al: The effects of the addition of sufentanil to 0.125% bupivacaine on the quality of analgesia during labor and on the incidence of instrumental deliveries. Anesthesiology 74:809–814, 1991.
20. Dewan DM, Cohen SM: Epidural analgesia and the incidence of cesarean section. Anesthesiology 80:1189–1192, 1994.
21. Chestnut DH, Vincent RD, McGrath JM, et al: Does early administration of epidural analgesia affect obstetric outcome in nulliparous women who are receiving intravenous oxytocin? Anesthesiology 80:1193–1200, 1994.
22. Chestnut DH, McGrath JM, Vincent RD, et al: Does early administration of epidural analgesia affect obstetric outcome in nulliparous women who are in spontaneous labor? Anesthesiology 80:1201–1208, 1994.
23. Moir D, Willocks J: Management of incoordinate uterine action under continuous epidural analgesia. Br Med J 3:396–400, 1967.
24. Rudick V, Niv D, Hetman-Peri M, et al: Epidural analgesia for planned vaginal delivery following previous cesarean section. Obstet Gynecol 64:621–623, 1984.
25. Rodgers RPC, Levin J: A critical reappraisal of the bleeding time. Semin Thromb Hemost 16:1–20, 1990.
26. Daley MD, Rolbin SH, Hew EM, et al: Epidural anesthesia for obstetrics after spinal surgery. Reg Anesth 15:280–284, 1990.
27. Committee on Obstetrics: Maternal and Fetal Medicine: Anesthesia for Emergency Deliveries. ACOG Committee Opinion No. 104, March 1992. Washington, DC: The American College of Obstetricians and Gynecologists, 1992.
28. Andrews PJD, Ackerman WE III, Juneja MM: Aortocaval compression in the sitting and lateral decubitus positions during extradural catheter placement in the parturient. Can J Anaesth 40:320–324, 1993.
29. Preston R, Crosby ET, Kotarba D, et al: Maternal positioning affects fetal heart rate changes after epidural analgesia for labour. Can J Anaesth 40:1136–1141, 1993.
30. Chadwick IS, Eddleston JM, Candelier CK, Pollard BJ: Haemodynamic effects of the position chosen for the insertion of an epidural catheter. Int J Obstet Anesth 2:197–201, 1993.
31. Bromage PR: Epidural Analgesia. Philadelphia, WB Saunders, 1978, pp 666–667.
32. Dalens B, Bazin JE, Haberer JP: Epidural bubbles as a cause of incomplete analgesia during epidural anesthesia. Anesth Analg 66:679–683, 1987.
33. Bromage PR. Epidural air bubbles and frothy syllogisms. Anesth Analg 67:91–94, 1989.
34. Leighton BL, Gross JB: Air: An effective indicator of intravenously located epidural catheters. Anesthesiology 71:848–851, 1989.
35. Cartwright PD, McCarroll SM, Antzaka C: Maternal heart rate changes with a plain epidural test dose. Anesthesiology 65:226–228, 1986.
36. Leighton BL, Norris MC, Sosis M, et al: Limitations of epinephrine as a marker of intravascular injection in laboring women. Anesthesiology 66:688–691, 1987.
37. Cheek TG, Kenepp NB, Schantz BB, et al: Lidocaine: Continuous infusion epidural analgesia for labor. Anesthesiology 63:A451, 1985.
38. Dror A, Abboud TK, Moore J, et al: Maternal hemodynamic responses to epinephrine-containing solutions in mild preeclampsia. Reg Anesth 13:107–111, 1988.
39. Viscomi CM, Hood DD, Melone PJ, Eisenach JC: Fetal heart rate variability after epidural fentanyl during labor. Anesth Analg 71:679–683, 1990.
40. Grice SC, Eisenach JC, Dewan DM: Labor analgesia with epidural bupivacaine plus fentanyl: Enhancement with epinephrine and inhibition with 2-chloroprocaine. Anesthesiology 72:623–628, 1990.
41. Corke BC, Carlson CG, Dettbarn WD: The influence of 2-chloroprocaine on the subsequent analgesic potency of bupivacaine. Anesthesiology 60:25–27, 1984.
42. Chestnut DH, Geiger M, Bates JN, Choi WW: The influence of pH-adjusted 2-chloroprocaine

on the quality and duration of subsequent epidural bupivacaine analgesia during labor: A randomized, double-blind study. Anesthesiology 70: 437–441, 1989.

43. Chestnut DH, Owen CL, Bates JN, et al: Continuous infusion epidural analgesia during labor: A randomized, double-blind comparison of 0.0625% bupivacaine/0.0002% fentanyl versus 0.125% bupivacaine. Anesthesiology 68:754–759, 1988.
44. Brownridge P, Plummer J, Mitchell J, Marshall P: An evaluation of epidural bupivacaine with and without meperidine in labor. Reg Anesth 17:15–21, 1992.
45. Steinberg RB, Dunn SM, Dixon DE, et al: Comparison of sufentanil, bupivacaine, and their combination for epidural analgesia in obstetrics. Reg Anesth 17:131–138, 1992.
46. Lysak SZ, Eisenach JC, Dobson CE 2d: Patient-controlled epidural analgesia during labor: A comparison of three solutions with a continuous infusion control. Anesthesiology 72:44–49, 1990. [See comments in: Anesthesiology 73:789–790, 1990.]
47. Viscomi C, Eisenach JC: Patient-controlled epidural analgesia during labor. Obstet Gynecol 77:348–351, 1991.
48. Ferrante FM, Lu L, Jamison SB, Datta S: Patient-controlled epidural analgesia: Demand dosing. Anesth Analg 73:547–552, 1991.
49. Fontenot RJ, Price RL, Henry A, et al: Double-blind evaluation of patient-controlled epidural analgesia during labor. Int J Obstet Anesth 2:73–77, 1993.
50. Gambling DR, Huber CJ, Berkowitz J, et al: Patient-controlled epidural analgesia in labour: Varying bolus dose and lockout interval. Can J Anaesth 40:211–217, 1993.
51. Rigler ML, Drasner K, Krejcie TC, et al: Cauda equina syndrome after continuous spinal anesthesia. Anesth Analg 72:275–281, 1991.
52. Lambert DH, Hurley RJ: Cauda equina syndrome and continuous spinal anesthesia. Anesth Analg 72:817–819, 1991.
53. Cohen SE, Cherry CM, Holbrook H Jr, et al: Intrathecal sufentanil for labor analgesia—Sensory changes, side effects, and fetal heart rate changes. Anesth Analg 77:1155–1160, 1993.
54. Cesarini M, Torrielli R, Lahaye F, et al: Sprotte needle for intrathecal anaesthesia for caesarean section: Incidence of postdural puncture headache. Anaesthesia 45:656–658, 1990.
55. Leighton BL, DeSimone CA, Norris MC, Ben-David B: Intrathecal narcotics for labor revisited: The combination of fentanyl and morphine intrathecally provides rapid onset of profound, prolonged analgesia. Anesth Analg 69:122–125, 1989.
56. Honet JE, Arkoosh VA, Norris MC, et al: Comparison among intrathecal fentanyl, meperidine, and sufentanil for labor analgesia. Anesth Analg 75:734–739, 1992.
57. Camann WR, Minzter BH, Denney RA, Datta S: Intrathecal sufentanil for labor analgesia. Anesthesiology 78:870–874, 1993.
58. Grieco WM, Norris MC, Leighton BL, et al: Intrathecal sufentanil labor analgesia: The effects of adding morphine or epinephrine. Anesth Analg 77:1149–1154, 1993.
59. Carrie LE, O'Sullivan G: Subarachnoid bupivacaine 0.5% for caesarean section. Eur J Anaesthesiol 1:275–283, 1984.
60. Stacey RGW, Watt S, Kadim MY, Morgan BM: Single-space combined spinal-extradural technique for analgesia in labour. Br J Anaesth 71:449–502, 1993.
61. Morgan BM: Ambulation and anesthesia: Are they compatible? [Abstract]. Soc Obstet Anesth Perinatol May 1994, pp 21–23.
62. Husemeyer RP, White DC: Topography of the lumbar epidural space. Anaesthesia 35:7–11, 1980.
63. Kasten GW, Martin ST: Successful cardiovascular resuscitation after massive intravenous bupivacaine overdosage in anesthetized dogs. Anesth Analg 64:491–497, 1985.
64. Kasten GW, Martin ST: Comparison of resuscitation of sheep and dogs after bupivacaine-induced cardiovascular collapse. Anesth Analg 65:1029–1032, 1986.
65. DePace NL, Betesh JS, Kotler MN: "Postmortem" cesarean section with recovery of both mother and offspring. JAMA 248:971–973, 1982.
66. Cheek TG, Banner R, Sauter J, Gutsche BB: Prophylactic epidural blood patch is effective. Br J Anaesth 61:340–342, 1988.
67. Dieterich M, Brandt T: Incidence of post-lumbar puncture headache is independent of daily fluid intake. Eur Arch Psychiatry Neurol Sci 237:194–196, 1988.
68. Marx GF, Loew DA: Tympanic temperature during labour and parturition. Br J Obstet Gynaecol 47:600–602, 1975.
69. Chan VS, Morley-Forster PK, Vosu HA: Temperature changes and shivering after epidural anesthesia for cesarean section. Reg Anesth 14:48–52, 1989.
70. Fusi L, Steer PJ, Maresh MJA, et al: Maternal pyrexia associated with the use of epidural analgesia in labor. Lancet 1:1250–1252, 1989.
71. Macaulay JH, Randall NR, Bond K, Steer PJ: Continuous monitoring of fetal temperature by noninvasive probe and its relationship to maternal temperature, fetal heart rate, and cord arterial oxygen and pH. Obstet Gynecol 79:469–474, 1992.

72. Camann WR, Hortvet LA, Hughes N, et al: Maternal temperature regulation during extradural analgesia for labour. Br J Anaesth 67:565–568, 1991.
73. Grove LH: Backache, headache and bladder dysfunction after delivery. Br J Anaesth 45:1147–1149, 1973.
74. Crawford JS: The second thousand epidural blocks in an obstetric hospital practice. Br J Anaesth 44:1277–1287, 1972.
75. MacArthur C, Lewis M, Knox EG: Investigation of long-term problems after obstetric epidural anesthesia. Br Med J 304:1279–1282, 1992.
76. Breen TW, Ransil BJ, Groves PA, Oriol NE: Factors associated with back pain after childbirth. Anesthesiology 81:29–34, 1994.

SEVEN

Anesthesia for Cesarean Section

Deborah L. Holden, M.D.

The incidence of cesarean delivery approximates 25% of all live births in the United States, close to one million operative deliveries annually. Uterine dystocia and elective repeat cesarean section are the most common indications (Table 7–1). Operative deliveries pose higher maternal risks than do vaginal deliveries. Although neonatal morbidity and mortality rates are generally low, the incidence of fatal maternal complications increases fourfold for cesarean deliveries performed emergently. Although many factors play a role, Gibb attributes the increased mortality in this setting to "lack of preparation and the stressed situation,"[1] emphasizing the importance of communication and a thorough understanding of maternal physiologic changes and pathophysiologic states. Ultimately, the selected anesthetic technique will depend on the indication for surgery, the degree of urgency, maternal and fetal conditions, and the anesthetist's expertise.

TABLE 7–1
Indications for Cesarean Delivery

Previous cesarean section
Cephalopelvic disproportion
Failure to progress
Breech
Multiple gestation; abnormal lie
Fetal macrosomia
Maternal disease, hemorrhage, previa, preeclampsia, herpes genitalia
Fetal distress

This chapter describes the most frequently employed techniques of general and regional (spinal and epidural) anesthesia.

PREOPERATIVE CONSIDERATIONS

Regardless of anesthetic technique, a comprehensive evaluation of the patient's airway is essential (see "Difficult Airway," later in this chapter). Airway complications are the most common cause of maternal death; these include hypoxia, difficult tracheal intubation, impossible mask ventilation, and aspiration. Pregnancy-associated increases in anterior and posterior chest diameter, increased breast size, and weight gain may impede manipulation of the head and neck during airway management and intubation. Furthermore, capillary engorgement contributes to airway edema and friable oropharyngeal mucosa, increasing the chance of airway injury and bleeding and complicating intubation attempts. Not only may intubation be difficult but also hypoxia develops more rapidly during apnea in the pregnant patient secondary to decreased functional residual capacity (FRC) and increased oxygen consumption. Additionally, pregnancy, especially during difficult intubation, is associated with increased risk for aspiration of gastric contents. In theory, pregnancy-induced hormonal changes decrease lower esophageal sphincter tone and the enlarging uterus displaces the stomach, contributing to an increased likelihood of gastroesophageal reflux. Regardless of the mechanism, a recent

American Society of Anesthesiologists Closed Claims Survey documented a fourfold increase in aspiration in pregnant patients when compared with that in nonpregnant patients.[2]

Aortocaval compression by the gravid uterus decreases venous return, reduces uterine blood flow and placental perfusion pressure, and possibly causes fetal compromise. Since aortic compression can occur independently of venocaval compression, brachial blood pressure measurements may not accurately reflect uterine artery pressure because the aortic compression occurs distal to the upper extremity arterial supply. In the presence of regional anesthesia, maternal hypotension almost invariably accompanies aortocaval compression. Aortocaval compression should be avoided by effecting left uterine displacement (LUD) in the patient. Placing a wedge under the patient's right hip or tilting the operating table 15 degrees to the left is usually sufficient. A small proportion of patients may demonstrate fetal heart rate signs of stress following LUD but not right uterine displacement (RUD). Presumably, this is a case of exacerbating aortic compression, reducing uterine blood flow. Therefore, try RUD if fetal heart rate monitoring indicates increased stress following LUD. Finally, pregnancy reduces anesthetic requirements for most commonly used agents, including local anesthetics, predominantly owing to hormonal changes and changes in acid-base status. In the sheep model, minimal alveolar concentration (MAC) for halothane, isoflurane, or methoxyflurane is 25 to 40% lower in pregnant animals when compared with that for nonpregnant animals. Decreased FRC and increased minute ventilation result in a faster rate of equilibration between inspired and alveolar gas tension, which allows rapid changes in anesthetic depth during general anesthesia. In practice, the potent inhalation agents and local anesthetics should be titrated to effect.

GENERAL ANESTHESIA

General anesthesia offers distinct advantages. It provides rapid, reliable anesthesia with little risk of hypotension in the healthy patient (Table 7–2). Usual indications for general anesthesia include severe fetal or maternal stress requiring emergent delivery, active bleeding, severe hypovolemia, coagulopathy, and some types of cardiovascular disease. Risks or disadvantages of general anesthesia include potential difficult airway management, possible aspiration, a hypertensive response to laryngoscopy and tracheal intubation, fetal drug exposure, potential stress-related decrease in uterine blood flow, and possible maternal intraoperative awareness or recall.

TABLE 7–2
General Anesthesia: Advantages and Disadvantages

Advantages
Rapid, reliable induction of anesthesia
Excellent surgical conditions
Administration possible in the presence of coagulopathy, hemorrhage, sepsis (contraindications to regional anesthesia)
Anesthetist's familiarity with technique
Disadvantages
Unconscious patient
Potential for difficult or failed intubation
Aspiration
Fetal effects

The technique the author's group recommends is presented in Table 7–3. A large-bore intravenous catheter should be inserted prior to the administration of any anesthetic technique. The author's group commonly uses an 18-gauge catheter; however, they prefer a 16-gauge catheter when increased risks for hemorrhage are anticipated. Aspiration prophylaxis is accomplished with the administration of an oral nonparticulate antacid, such as sodium citrate, within 30 minutes of anesthetic induction. Sodium citrate (30 ml of 0.3 molar) significantly raises gastric pH within 5 to 6 minutes of administration and lasts 75 minutes.[3] Since longer operating times may outlast the duration of the effect of sodium citrate, other options include intravenous administration of an H_2 blocker (1 hour before) to increase the pH of gastric secretions and metoclopramide to facilitate gastric emptying, thus providing a safety margin for tracheal extubation.

Routine monitoring should include precordial stethoscope, blood pressure measurement, electrocardiogram, pulse oximeter, end-tidal carbon dioxide, temperature probe, and peripheral nerve stimulator. LUD is maintained until delivery of the infant despite the apparent adequacy of maternal blood pressure. Remem-

TABLE 7–3
Technique for General Anesthesia for Cesarean Delivery

1. Large-bore IV; crystalloid infusion
2. Aspiration prophylaxis
3. Left uterine displacement
4. Monitors: BP, ECG, pulse oximeter, end-tidal CO_2, temperature, precordial stethoscope, peripheral nerve stimulator
5. Preoxygenation 100% O_2, surgical mask: four vital capacity breaths or 5 min tidal volume breathing (preferred)

Induction

6. Rapid sequence induction: cricoid pressure, thiopental 3–4 mg/kg or ketamine 0.5–1.0 mg/kg, succinylcholine 1–1.5 mg/kg, endotracheal tube 6.5–7.0 mm

Maintenance

7. Before delivery: 50% N_2O, 0.75 MAC volatile anesthesia, muscle relaxant
   After delivery: 70% N_2O, $\leq$0.5 MAC, narcotic, muscle relaxant, possible sedative hypnotic
8. *Extubate* after patient awake and responsive

Abbreviations: IV = intravenous; BP = blood pressure; ECG = electrocardiogram; MAC = minimal alveolar concentration.

ber, brachial blood pressure is not the same as uterine blood flow.

Preoxygenation and denitrogenation precede rapid-sequence induction and endotracheal intubation. Increased oxygen consumption and decreased FRC contribute to the *rapid* development of maternal hypoxemia during periods of apnea. Pregnant patients experience a three times more rapid fall in arterial oxygen compared with nonpregnant patients following a 1-minute period of apnea.[4] The author's group usually preoxygenates by having the patient breathe 100% oxygen by tight-fitting mask for 3 to 4 minutes. However, having the patient take four vital capacity breaths in 30 seconds provides equivalent oxygenation to 3 to 5 minutes of tidal volume breathing of 100% oxygen and may be used for emergent situations.[5] Nevertheless, the author's group prefers the 3- to 5-minute technique if time permits because it provides additional safety during longer periods of apnea that might accompany difficult intubation.[6] Although the fetal oxygen saturation equilibrates with maternal oxygen saturation during the 5 minutes of preoxygenation, following induction of general anesthesia the fetus equilibrates with the delivered FI_{O_2} which is usually 50%.

Neonatal depression occurs more frequently with general anesthesia than with regional and is related to the duration of anesthesia. Neonatal depression is reflected in lower Apgar scores, especially at 1 minute, and is probably due to sedation rather than asphyxia.[7, 8] Since all anesthetic agents cross the placenta to varying degrees, minimizing the time from anesthesia induction to delivery reduces fetal drug exposure. Intervals of less than 10 minutes do not result in neonatal depression. Thiopental rapidly crosses the placenta and peaks in the fetal circulation in 1 to 2 minutes. However, significant neonatal effects are not seen with doses less than 4 mg/kg because of rapid drug redistribution in mother and fetus and fetal liver uptake. When higher concentrations of inspired oxygen and lower concentrations of nitrous oxide (50%) are used and when delivery is expeditious (less than 10 to 15 minutes from induction of general anesthesia to delivery), the transient neonatal sedation is probably not significant. In addition, if maternal blood pressure and oxygenation are maintained, fetal acid-base status remains normal despite prolonged general anesthesia.[9] To minimize the length of fetal anesthetic exposure, the patient's abdomen can be prepared and draped and the surgeon ready to start before the induction of general anesthesia.

Regardless of anesthetic technique, a uterine incision–to–delivery time of greater than 3 minutes has been associated with lower umbilical pH and lower 1-minute Apgar scores.[10–12]

General anesthesia induction is accomplished by the administration of thiopental, 3 to 4 mg/kg, and succinylcholine, 1 to 1.5 mg/kg, intravenously, with a concurrent Sellick maneuver (cricoid pressure), followed by expeditious intubation of the trachea once muscle relaxation is achieved. Ketamine, 1 mg/kg, may be the drug of choice for actively bleeding or hypovolemic patients. After proper placement of the endotracheal tube is confirmed by the presence of a carbon dioxide waveform on the capnograph and by auscultation of both sides of the chest and abdomen, the surgery may proceed.

Since airway mishap is a leading cause of anesthetic morbidity and mortality in the obstetric population, one should always be prepared for this occurrence and should have a difficult airway protocol and emergency intubating equipment readily available.[13] This is discussed later.

Anesthesia is maintained prior to delivery with nitrous oxide 50% in oxygen and low concentrations of any of the volatile anesthetics (0.75 MAC). Muscle relaxants should be used as necessary to prevent maternal coughing and to allow adequate mechanical ventilation (remembering that pregnancy has already relaxed the abdominal wall). After delivery, the inspired concentration of nitrous oxide may be increased to 70%, intravenous narcotics may be administered for analgesia, and the concentration of volatile anesthetic may be decreased to less than 0.5% MAC or discontinued. Sedative hypnotics such as midazolam or diazepam also prevent maternal recall and can be utilized.

Succinylcholine is the drug of choice for intubation owing to its reliably rapid onset and rapid metabolism by plasma pseudocholinesterases. Although it rapidly crosses the placenta, clinically insignificant amounts reach the fetus because maternal plasma half-life ($t_{½}$) is only 21 seconds (in the absence of pseudocholinesterase deficiency). Remember, if the mother has a pseudocholinesterase deficiency, the newborn may also be affected. Normally, what does reach the fetus is rapidly hydrolyzed by fetal cholinesterases ($t_{½}$ = 43 sec). Pregnancy-associated reductions in maternal pseudocholinesterase prolong the duration of neuromuscular block only slightly following an intubating dose. For surgeries of short duration, succinylcholine may be used in small boluses of 10 to 20 mg or as an infusion to maintain muscle relaxation during the procedure; but the author's group prefers nondepolarizing muscle relaxants, thus avoiding possible maternal bradycardia from repeated doses of succinylcholine or the development of phase II neuromuscular block. Minimal amounts of nondepolarizing muscle relaxants cross the placenta owing to their high degree of ionization and large molecular weight. Nitrous oxide crosses the placenta, and prolonged administration of high concentrations may delay the time to sustained respiration in the neonate. However, this effect disappears in 1 to 3 minutes following administration of oxygen to the fetus. Minimal adverse effects are seen when nitrous oxide concentrations less than 50% are maintained, or when induction-to-delivery intervals are short.

Low concentrations of volatile anesthetics provide good maternal intraoperative amnesia when administered in approximately 50% MAC concentrations. These concentrations result in minimal or no neonatal depression, minimal effect on intraoperative blood loss, and no effect on uterine tone provided oxytocin is utilized.

Significant newborn depression is rare following general anesthesia, provided other causes of depression are not present. Potential sources of non–drug-related neonatal depression include maternal hypoxia, extreme prolonged maternal hyperventilation, maternal hypotension, concealed aortocaval impression, preexisting fetal compromise, and prolonged uterine incision–to–delivery times resulting in decreased uterine blood flow.

Recalling that the parturient requires full stomach precautions, at the completion of the surgical procedure, residual muscle relaxation should be fully reversed and the patient fully awake, ventilating adequately and responsive to commands prior to extubation.

In summary, although general anesthesia poses little risk to the fetus, significant maternal risk is present owing primarily to difficulties in airway management. The author's group reserves general anesthesia for situations that preclude the safe administration of regional anesthesia. Maternal outcome is improved with good preoperative assessment of the patient's airway and preparation with aspiration prophylaxis, LUD, preoxygenation, and rapid-sequence induction with concurrent cricoid pressure and tracheal intubation.

REGIONAL ANESTHESIA

Regional anesthesia offers significant advantages for the pregnant patient (Table 7–4). The

TABLE 7–4
Regional Anesthesia: Advantages and Disadvantages

Advantages
Awake patient
Avoidance of airway manipulation
Minimal fetal effects

Disadvantages
Potential for inadequate block → emergent, intraoperative, general anesthesia
High/total spinal; intravenous administration → possible seizures and cardiac arrest
Hypotension
Postdural puncture headache
Neurologic sequelae

patient is awake for the birth of her infant, airway manipulation is avoided, and fetal drug exposure is minimized. Potential disadvantages include inadequate or high block necessitating emergent, intraoperative general anesthesia; local anesthetic toxicity; and although this is rare, permanent neurologic sequelae. Absolute contraindications include severe coagulopathy, infection at the site of insertion, and patient refusal. Relative contraindications include severe hypovolemia, active bleeding, sepsis, and severe fetal distress when there is insufficient time for block establishment (Table 7–5). Spinal and epidural anesthesia, each with its own advantages and disadvantages, are the most common regional anesthetic techniques.

Preparation for either epidural or spinal anesthesia includes aspiration prophylaxis, insertion of a large-bore intravenous catheter, and infusion of 1500 to 2000 ml of a dextrose-free crystalloid solution immediately before induction of anesthesia. However, lack of time for volume loading should not preclude regional anesthesia in the presence of fetal distress when regional is the preferred anesthetic technique. Monitors include blood pressure, electrocardiogram, and pulse oximeter. Fetal heart tones should be periodically auscultated during regional anesthesia induction and this should be continued until abdominal preparation begins. This practice will document fetal well-being during induction of regional anesthesia or provide the impetus for consideration of an alternate anesthetic technique should fetal stress develop. Maternal oxygen should be administered by either face mask or nasal prongs, and LUD should be maintained until the infant is delivered. Ephedrine should be readily available to treat maternal hypotension.

TABLE 7–5
Contraindications to Regional Anesthesia

Coagulopathy
Sepsis
Local infection
Patient refusal

A sensory block from T4 to S4 bilaterally provides good anesthesia for abdominal surgery, peritoneal traction, and bladder manipulation. The author's group finds the greatest patient comfort during regional anesthesia for cesarean section occurs following dense blockade of both the sacral and the high thoracic nerve roots. Despite the purported reduction in local anesthetic requirements in pregnant patients, the group has not observed a problem with the use of standard doses.

Hypotension, the most frequent complication of regional anesthesia, often defined as a decrease in systolic blood pressure of 20% or to less than 100 mmHg, occurs in as many as 75% of patients despite intravenous preload and uterine displacement. The sympathetic blockade produces vasodilatation, venous pooling in the lower extremities, and decreased venous return to the heart. Aortocaval compression exacerbates this process. Decreased maternal cerebral perfusion pressure may result in nausea and vomiting, and decreased uterine perfusion may lead to potential fetal compromise. Although moderate maternal hypotension of short duration may be tolerated by the healthy fetus, prolonged (greater than 2 min), severe hypotension has been shown to produce fetal acidosis, lower Apgar scores, and prolonged time to sustained respiration. Since fetal monitoring is not used in this setting, vasopressor therapy is warranted.

Ephedrine, the vasopressor of choice, is predominantly β sympathetic and preserves or improves uterine, while raising maternal, blood pressure. Early aggressive treatment of developing maternal hypotension with ephedrine lowers the incidence of maternal nausea and vomiting and improves neonatal outcome.[14] The author's group usually starts administering intravenous ephedrine as soon as developing hypotension is recognized. The group does not necessarily wait for arbitrary reductions in systolic blood pressure before treating.

Pure α agonists such as phenylephrine or methoxamine, although they are potent vasopressors, may decrease uterine blood flow by direct vasoconstriction despite improved maternal blood pressure.[15] However, recent clinical studies have demonstrated no adverse effects when phenylephrine was used for treating maternal hypotension during epidural and spinal anesthesia for cesarean section.[16] Nevertheless, this was in healthy patients undergoing elective cesarean in whom moderate decreases in uterine blood flow may be well tolerated. The author's group limits α agents to situations in which the β effects of ephedrine may be contraindicated and uses fetal monitoring when possible.

Shivering is another common and annoying side effect that may be partially ameliorated by infusing warmed intravenous fluids or intrathecal opioids or by the administration of low-dose intravenous meperidine after the cord is clamped.

Maternal nausea and vomiting occur in as many as 50% of patients undergoing cesarean delivery. The incidence is dramatically reduced (to 15%) when maternal hypotension is avoided. Peritoneal traction inducing a vagal response has also been implicated. Small doses of droperidol (0.25 to 0.625 mg) or metoclopramide (5 to 10 mg) may further decrease the incidence.

At the author's institution, the incidence of postdural puncture headache requiring blood patch is similar following either spinal or epidural anesthesia. This low incidence may be ascribed to the use of either small-gauge needles (27- or 29-gauge Quincke) with the bevels oriented parallel to the longitudinal axis of the dural fibers or the blunt-tipped Whitacre (25- to 27-gauge) and Sprotte (24-gauge) needles.

Total spinal block from accidental subarachnoid injection of large amounts of local anesthetic is a rare complication. Routine testing of epidural catheters for spinal placement should minimize risk. Significant morbidity may be avoided by immediate recognition and treatment, with control of the airway, prevention of aspiration by tracheal intubation, ventilatory support, and maintenance of blood pressure.

Spinal Anesthesia

Spinal anesthesia provides rapid, reliable, intense anesthesia with minimal fetal drug exposure (Table 7–6). Although one disadvantage of spinal anesthesia is its finite duration, the duration and density of block are highly predictable. Correct placement of the needle is ensured by cerebrospinal fluid return. The author's group believes that easy aspiration is also key. Even with 27-gauge needles, cerebrospinal fluid should flow freely and easily during aspiration. The failure rate is as low as 1 to 5% and is sometimes attributable to use of a low interspace.[17] The author's group prefers to use L2–3 and L3–4. Contraindications to spinal anesthesia include severe, untreated hypertensive disease, hypovolemia, sepsis, and certain cardiac lesions where an acute decrease in systemic vascular resistance may be catastrophic.

A recommended technique is shown in Table 7–7. After blood pressure, electrocardiogram, and pulse oximeter monitors are applied, the patient is placed in either the sitting or the lateral decubitus position. Sprague recommends placing the patient in the right lateral decubitus position for initiation of block, then changing to the left semilateral position before surgery to allow bilateral spread of the local anesthetic.[18] However, at the author's institution where the lateral positioning of the patient is determined by operating room limitations, problems with unilateral block have not been encountered. In obese patients or those with spinal deformities, the sitting position may allow better identification of anatomic landmarks.

The spinal needle should be placed at the L2–3 or L3–4 interspace, thus avoiding the spinal cord above and preventing the deposition of local anesthetic below the lumbar lordosis.

TABLE 7–6
Spinal Anesthesia: Advantages and Disadvantages

Advantages	Disadvantages
Usually rapidly and easily performed	Finite duration
Reliable, intense anesthesia	Postdural puncture headache
Minimal fetal drug exposure	Greater risk for hypotension

TABLE 7–7
Technique for Spinal Anesthesia for Cesarean Delivery

1. Large-bore IV, crystalloid infusion
2. Aspiration prophylaxis, sodium citrate 30 ml
3. Routine monitors, O_2
4. Lateral decubitus or sitting positions
5. L2–3 or L3–4 intervertebral space
6. 27- or 29-g Quincke, 24-g Sprotte, 25- or 27-g Whitacre needles
7. Left uterine displacement
8. BP q 1–2 min until delivery, q 3–5 min thereafter
9. Check block, need T4
10. IV sedation following delivery if needed
    Early IV ephedrine treatment with 10-mg increments

Abbreviations: IV = intravenous; BP = blood pressure.

Once the patient is placed supine with LUD, the level of sensory block is determined. If the level fails to rise to T4 within 3 to 4 minutes, maneuvers such as lifting the patient's legs or flexing the knees to reduce the lumbar lordosis or positioning the operating room table in slight Trendelenburg position may improve cephalad spread of local anesthetic. This may be of particular importance in patients who were sitting when the spinal anesthesia was administered.

The local anesthetics commonly used for spinal anesthesia for cesarean delivery are listed in Table 7–8. However, the author's group almost exclusively uses hyperbaric 0.75% bupivacaine. In the group's experience, the dose requirements, onset, density, extent of spread, and duration have all been exceptionally predictable for women within the normal range of height.[19] Lidocaine, 5%, has been used for more rapid onset of a block of shorter duration and tetracaine, 1%, for longer-duration surgery. At the author's institution, surgery almost invariably lasts less than 60 minutes and usually 40 to 45 minutes. Thus, the group does not have a need for tetracaine and, in fact, does not even stock it. Combinations of tetracaine and procaine have been used, but the group believes these do not provide advantages over bupivacaine alone. Epinephrine improves the quality and duration of spinal block for lidocaine and tetracaine but not significantly for bupivacaine. Alternatively, opioids may be added for additional intraoperative and postoperative analgesia. Commonly used opioids include fentanyl (10 to 20 μg), which may provide early postoperative pain relief, and morphine (0.1 to 0.2 mg), which provides 18 to 24 hours of pain relief. The author's group rarely uses intrathecal opioids because patient-controlled analgesia (PCA) is widely used and very well accepted by the patient population.

Epidural Anesthesia

The advantage of using epidural anesthesia is the ability to control speed of onset, depth, and duration of anesthesia (Table 7–9). As with spinal anesthesia, fetal drug exposure is minimal. Maternal hypotension occurs less frequently than during spinal anesthesia, probably secondary to the slower onset of conduction blockade. Thus, some patients, in whom spinal anesthesia is contraindicated, may still be candidates for epidural anesthesia. However, if large doses of rapid-acting local anesthetics such as 2-chloroprocaine are used to initiate the block, the incidence of hypotension may approach that of spinal anesthesia. Epidural anesthesia is a more difficult and time-consuming technique

TABLE 7–8
Dosages of Spinal Anesthetics for Cesarean Delivery

Local Anesthetic	Dose (mg)	Onset (min)	Duration (min)
Lidocaine 5%/D 7.5%	60–80	4–5	60–90
Bupivacaine 0.75%/D 8.25%	12–15	4–8	90–120
Tetracaine 1%/D 10%	7–11	4–15	120–180

Abbreviation: D = dextrose.

TABLE 7–9
Epidural Anesthesia: Advantages and Disadvantages

Advantages	Disadvantages
Slower onset; titratability	Length of time required for placement/dosing
Ability to maintain analgesia/anesthesia with repeat dosing	Inadequate, failed block
Less hypotension	

than that of spinal anesthesia and requires meticulous catheter testing to ensure correct placement. Unintentional intravenous or subarachnoid administration of the required large local anesthetic doses poses a significant maternal risk. A technique for epidural anesthesia is listed in Table 7–10.

Following insertion of a large-bore intravenous catheter and infusion of a crystalloid solution, the patient is placed in either the lateral decubitus or the sitting position. The patient's back is cleaned with iodine or alcohol solution and sterilely draped. After local infiltration with 1% lidocaine, an epidural needle (16-, 17-, or 18-gauge) is inserted at L2–3, L3–4, or L4–5, and the epidural space is identified by loss of resistance to air or normal saline. A catheter is then passed 2 to 6 cm through the needle into the epidural space, and the needle is removed. Catheter distances depend on (1) patient size, (2) ease of placement, and (3) estimated time of use. Paresthesias are common with placement of the catheter, but these should be mild and transient. The needle and catheter should be withdrawn if a paresthesia persists.

If no blood or cerebrospinal fluid return is noted passively or with aspiration, catheter testing may begin. At Wake Forest University, the author's group utilizes local anesthetics to test the epidural catheter. First, a subarachnoid test dose of 2 to 3 ml of local anesthetic, usually 2% lidocaine, is administered. If no sign of spinal block is observed after 5 minutes, an intravenous test dose of 5 ml of lidocaine, 2%, is administered, and the patient is observed and questioned regarding systemic symptoms of circumoral paresthesias, tinnitus or ringing in the ears, tunnel vision, and jitteriness. Intravenous testing with bupivacaine is avoided, since this drug does not reliably elicit central nervous system symptoms and may result in a false-negative test dose. Two percent 2-chloroprocaine offers an alternative to 2% lidocaine for intravenous testing. Alternatively, the subarachnoid and intravenous test doses may be administered concomitantly, utilizing 3 ml of lidocaine 1.5 to 2% containing 15 μg of epinephrine. If no block develops in 5 minutes and the maternal heart rate does not increase by 15 beats per minute within 60 seconds, routine dosing may proceed. Remember, pain and contractions may mask the increased heart rate. Intravenous administration of even 15 μg of epinephrine may reduce uterine blood flow, so, as always, the correct placement of the epidural catheter must be ensured prior to dosing large volumes. Most importantly, the absence of a block is assumed to be a misplaced catheter (e.g., an intravenous catheter) until proved otherwise.

2-Chloroprocaine, lidocaine, and bupivacaine are all appropriate choices for block establishment. The choice of local anesthetic is gov-

TABLE 7–10
Technique for Epidural Anesthesia for Cesarean Delivery

1. Large-bore IV; crystalloid infusion.
2. Aspiration prophylaxis, sodum citrate 30 ml.
3. Routine monitors, O_2 by face mask.
4. Lateral decubitus or sitting position; after catheter taped in place, turn supine with LUD.
5. L2–3 or L3–4 intervertebral space, 16-g–18-g epidural needle; epidural space indicated by loss of resistance to air or saline.
6. Catheter threaded 2–6 cm into space. Paresthesia noted/recorded.
7. Subarachnoid test dose: 2 ml of lidocaine 2% or 2-chloroprocaine 2%. Wait 5 min. If no block:
8. Intravenous test dose: 5 ml lidocaine 2% or 2-chloroprocaine 2%.
9. Test doses may be combined by adding epinephrine 5 μg/ml to 3 ml of local anesthetic and continuously monitoring maternal heart rate for increases secondary to epinephrine.
10. Dosing should proceed in 5-ml increments up to recommended volumes.
11. BP q 3 min until delivery, then q 5 min.
12. Check block to pinprick; fentanyl (50 μg) may be added to lidocaine or bupivacaine for additional analgesia.
13. IV sedation postdelivery if needed.
14. Maintain blood pressure at baseline with 10 mg IV boluses of ephedrine.

Abbreviations: IV = intravenous; LUD = left uterine displacement; BP = blood pressure.

erned by the clinical situation and maternal and neonatal conditions. 2-Chloroprocaine and lidocaine provide rapid onset of analgesia with relatively short duration, whereas bupivacaine allows a slower onset of block and longer duration. Typical concentrations and volumes used for cesarean delivery are listed in Table 7–11. 2-Chloroprocaine (3%) is an excellent drug for cesarean delivery especially in emergent conditions or when fetal stress is present. It provides quick onset of dense sensory and motor block. 2-Chloroprocaine is rapidly hydrolyzed by maternal and fetal plasma cholinesterases, reducing maternal systemic and fetal toxicity. However, large intravenous doses of all local anesthetics including 2-chloroprocaine can result in significant central nervous system toxicity, so patients should be carefully monitored during injection for symptoms of toxicity. The author recommends administering all epidural local anesthetics in 5-ml aliquots, and waiting at least 1 minute before administering subsequent aliquots.

Subarachnoid injection of large doses of 2-chloroprocaine has been associated with neurotoxicity. Since the drug formulation has been changed to reduce the metabisulfite content and to increase the pH, to the author's group's knowledge no permanent neurologic deficits have been reported. Nonetheless, the group tries to avoid 2-chloroprocaine when dural puncture has occurred.

Lidocaine has a slightly slower onset and longer duration than 2-chloroprocaine. Sodium bicarbonate speeds onset and may increase the block density. There is significant systemic uptake of lidocaine from the epidural space, and toxic doses may be reached during routine administration for cesarean delivery. For this reason, the author's group adds epinephrine to the lidocaine (in concentrations of 1:200,000 to 1:400,000) when dosing for cesarean section. Epinephrine reduces vascular absorption of lidocaine and improves the quality and duration of block. Lower maternal plasma levels result in decreased fetal plasma levels.

TABLE 7–11
Dosages of Epidural Anesthetics for Cesarean Delivery

Local Anesthetic	Dose (ml)	Duration (min)
2-Chloroprocaine 3%	20–40	40–50
Lidocaine 2% with epinephrine 1:300,000 and bicarbonate 1 mg/10 ml	20–30	75–90
Bupivacaine 0.5%	20–25	90–120

Bupivacaine has the slowest onset but provides the longest duration of sensory block. Bupivacaine's slow onset precludes its use in emergent situations, but encourages its use in conditions for which rapid onset of block is undesirable—for example, in preeclamptic patients or when the start of surgery is expected to be delayed or the duration prolonged. Unintentional intravenous administration of bupivacaine has been associated with cardiovascular toxicity and collapse refractory to therapy, leading to the removal of the 0.75% preparation from obstetric use. Although lower concentrations have been deemed safe, concern over bupivacaine toxicity persists and dosing should be slow and cautious.

Epidural opioids may improve the quality of intraoperative analgesia and provide postoperative pain relief. Fentanyl, 50 to 100 μg, has a fairly rapid onset and may provide 2 to 4 hours of pain relief with minimal side effects. Epidural morphine (3 to 5 mg) provides up to 24 hours of pain relief but results in a high incidence of pruritus, vomiting, and urinary retention. Respiratory depression is an infrequent but serious side effect that mandates postoperative monitoring with frequent observation of respiratory rate or pulse oximetry. Intrathecal narcotics also cause a high incidence of annoying complications such as nausea and vomiting, pruritus, and urinary retention. Epidural or spinal narcotics are not routinely used for postoperative pain management at the author's institution where PCA is readily available. The group's patients prefer PCA, which offers a lower incidence of side effects and the ability to titrate their own drug dosing.

Spinal Versus Epidural

Spinal anesthesia is an excellent choice for most patients who are undergoing either elective or urgent cesarean delivery. Its administration is usually rapid, relatively painless, and reliable. The author's group utilizes it for our busy service because it is an efficient technique.

When rapid blockade is contraindicated—for example, in hypovolemic or hemorrhaging patients—epidural anesthesia may be a good alternative. The local anesthetic may be administered slowly, producing slower sympathetic blockade and, optimally, less hypotension. Epidural anesthesia also provides control over duration and density of blockade should surgery be prolonged. Obstetric conditions that may require longer durations of anesthesia include multiple-gestation pregnancy; obesity; placental abnormalities such as placenta accreta that may require cesarean hysterectomy; and preeclampsia.

Safe regional anesthesia can be performed if caution is used during the administration of block and the patient is closely observed for any untoward effects.

CESAREAN HYSTERECTOMY

Anesthetic management of cesarean hysterectomy depends largely on the indication for the procedure. Common indications are listed in Table 7–12 and may be classified into three groups: emergency procedures, indicated nonemergency cases, and purely elective procedures.[20] Obstetric hemorrhage resulting from uterine atony or placental disorders and uterine rupture are the most common indications for emergent peripartum hysterectomy. Uterine fibroids and cervical neoplasias are common indications for nonemergent, indicated cesarean hysterectomy.

Emergency hysterectomy associated with hemorrhage, sepsis, hypovolemia, or emergency cesarean section for fetal distress may mandate general anesthesia. All the usual considerations for cesarean section apply for cesarean hysterectomy. Large-bore intravenous access must be instituted, and LUD and oxygenation maintained. The author's group usually prefers general anesthesia for this emergency surgery. When a patient is hypotensive, ketamine, 1 to 1.5 mg/kg, may be preferable for induction.

For elective cesarean hysterectomy, a regional anesthetic may be an acceptable technique, especially if the parturient prefers to be awake for the delivery of the infant. Excessive blood loss and hypotension occur less frequently during elective cesarean hysterectomy; however, operative time for elective cesarean hysterectomy is almost twice that of cesarean alone, and intraperitoneal manipulation and traction may be greater and may result in pain, nausea, and retching.

Although a high incidence of patients (22 to 28%) with an initially satisfactory regional technique required intraoperative induction of general anesthesia, in the majority of patients, regional anesthesia was adequate throughout the surgery.[21, 22] Hemodynamic instability was not a problem. However, when a patient requires excessive supplemental analgesia to maintain comfort or adequate relaxation, rapid-sequence induction of general anesthesia with tracheal intubation should be performed for airway protection.

DIFFICULT AIRWAY

Difficulty in airway management is the leading cause of anesthesia-related maternal mortality and contributes significant morbidity to the parturient undergoing cesarean delivery. Hypoxia and aspiration, following difficult intubation, are the two main causes of maternal death.

Whenever anesthesia induction is performed

TABLE 7–12
Indications for Cesarean Hysterectomy

Emergencies	Indicated Nonemergencies	Elective
Hemorrhage	Uterine fibroids	Previous gynecologic disorders
Uterine rupture	Defective uterine scar	Uterine prolapse
Placenta previa	Neoplasias	
Abruptio placentae	Menorrhagia	
Placenta accreta		
Uterine atony		
Severe uterine infection		

on the obstetric patient, but especially when general anesthesia is planned, a complete evaluation of the airway and a plan for management of the difficult airway are essential.

The author assesses both the oropharyngeal structures (OP) and the mentum–to–thyroid cartilage distance (MT) as recommended by Lewis and colleagues.[23] Table 7–13 illustrates a standardized method for grading OP. To increase the likelihood of successfully predicting difficult intubation, the distance from the inside of the mentum to the thyroid cartilage should be measured with the patient's neck in full extension and the mouth open. Clinically, the author uses her fingers to measure MT; 3 finger breadths (FB) are approximately 5.3 cm. The predicted and actual risks of difficult intubation for patients of OP class 3 or 4 and 3-FB MT are illustrated in Table 7–14. Note that 25% of patients with an OP class 3 and 3-FB MT distance are predicted to have a difficult intubation, but only 55% of these patients actually do. In contrast, a patient with the more extreme example of an OP class 4 and 3-FB MT is predicted to have a 70% chance of difficult intubation; 95% of these patients will subsequently have difficult intubations. Other anatomic structures such as prominent upper teeth and significant overbite may further increase risks for difficult intubation.

TABLE 7–13
Method for Grading Oropharyngeal Structures and Measuring Mentum–to–Thyroid Cartilage Distance

Patient Positioning
1. Sitting
2. Full neck extension
3. Tongue out
4. Phonating
5. Mouth open

Visual Grading of Oropharyngeal Structures
Class 1: Soft palate, fauces, uvula, anterior and posterior tonsillar pillars
Class 2: Soft palate, fauces, uvula
Class 3: Soft palate, base of uvula
Class 4: Soft palate only (uvula not visible)

Mentum–to–Thyroid Cartilage Distance (MT)
Measure from inside of mentum to top of thyroid cartilage

Modified from Lewis M, Keramati S, Benumof JL, Berry CC: What is the best way to determine oropharyngeal classification and mandibular space length to predict difficult laryngoscopy? Anesthesiology 81:69–75, 1994.

TABLE 7–14
Predicting Difficult Intubation: Approximate Risk of Difficulty*

Difficult intubation	OP 3† 3-FB MT	OP 4† 3-FB MT
Predicted	25%	70%
Percentage‡	55%	95%

Abbreviations: OP = oropharyngeal structures; FB = finger breadths; MT = mentum–to–thyroid cartilage distance.

*Difficult intubation: visualizing only epiglottis and soft palate or only soft palate.

†OP class 3 or 4.

‡Percentage of patients with predicted difficulty who actually had difficulty.

Modified from Lewis M, Keramati S, Benumof JL, Berry CC: What is the best way to determine oropharyngeal classification and mandibular space length to predict difficult laryngoscopy? Anesthesiology 81:69–75, 1994.

If a difficult airway is suspected, awake laryngoscopy should be performed. If the glottic opening is visualized, intubation can usually be accomplished in the standard fashion. If the glottis cannot be visualized, one should consider the use of regional anesthesia or awake intubation.

Whichever technique is chosen for awake intubation, it is a time-consuming procedure, and the patient, her family, and her surgeon should be advised of this. The extent to which the airway is anesthetized prior to intubation is controversial. Since the pregnant patient is considered to have a "full stomach," loss of protective reflexes should be avoided. The author routinely uses a dollop of topical lidocaine 5% ointment on a tongue depressor, which can be applied to the back of the tongue. Significant upper airway anesthesia can be accomplished with this method, but onset is very slow (20 min). In this way, superior laryngeal nerve function and tracheal cough reflex are preserved and airway trauma is minimized. For most patients, topical anesthesia and gentle airway manipulation are adequate for visualization and placement of an endotracheal tube. If more anesthesia is required, bilateral superior laryngeal nerve blocks may be performed. The author avoids transtracheal block and preserves the cough reflex.

Fiberoptic intubation may be a good option

if it is available and if personnel are trained in its use. However, in the author's experience, successful bronchoscopic intubation of the trachea requires both vocal cord and upper trachea anesthesia. This requirement necessarily blocks the glottic reflexes and may increase risks for aspiration of gastric contents. Still, bronchoscopic tracheal intubation may be the only method of protecting the patient's airway, short of surgical intervention.

Unanticipated airway emergencies occur despite careful preoperative preparation. A protocol for management of airway emergency is described in Figure 7–1.[13] If failed intubation occurs following rapid-sequence induction, mask ventilation should be attempted with cricoid pressure to maintain maternal oxygenation. If the surgery is emergent or fetal distress is present, another attempt at tracheal intubation should be made using ancillary techniques while maintaining maternal oxygen saturation. If this is unsuccessful, consider completing surgery using mask ventilation if severe, life-threatening maternal or fetal conditions exist. If mask ventilation is adequate, anesthesia is maintained with potent inhalational agents with concentrations of 1 to 2 MAC in 100% oxygen. If possible, paralysis of the patient should be avoided to allow return of spontaneous respirations, which may be assisted by the anesthetist. Once the infant is delivered, the concentration of agent should be reduced to 0.5 to 0.75 MAC, and anesthesia should be supplemented by intravenous agents, as discussed earlier. If mask ventilation is possible but surgery is not emergent, allow the patient to awaken and consider regional anesthesia or awake intubation. If mask ventilation following failed intubation is not possible, emergency procedures such as cricothyroid catheter placement or tracheal intubation via cricothyroidotomy must be performed. The cricothyroid ring should be palpated prior to the start of surgery.

In summary, with careful preoperative evaluation and the use of regional anesthesia, most airway mishaps can be avoided. However, unanticipated airway emergencies may occur and protocol for management of these emergencies must be in place.

TEN PRACTICAL POINTS

1. Conduct early preanesthetic evaluation of parturients.
2. Carefully evaluate the airway for possible difficult intubation.
3. Maintain LUD at all times.
4. Monitor blood pressure frequently after institution of regional anesthesia and treat developing hypotension immediately with ephedrine.
5. Test epidural catheter for subarachnoid and intravenous placement prior to administering total dose.

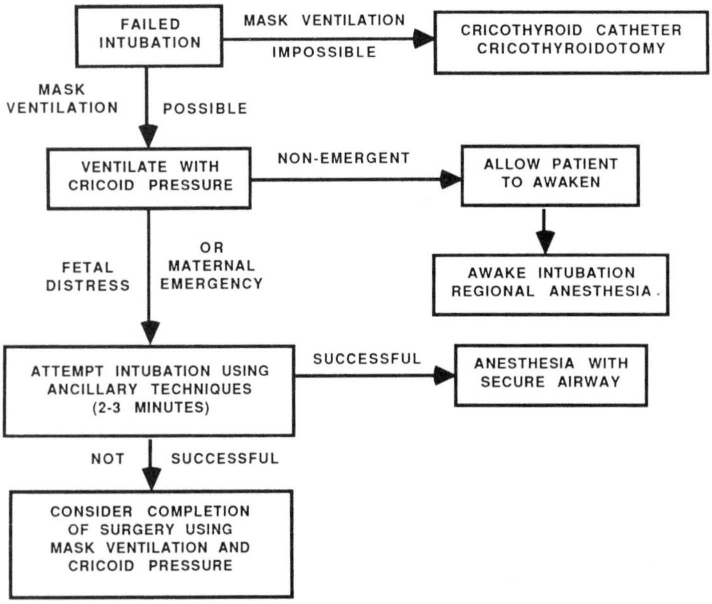

Figure 7–1. Sample protocol for failed intubation. (From Malan TP, Johnson MD: The difficult airway in obstetric anesthesia: Techniques for airway management and the role of regional anesthesia. J Clin Anesth 1:104–111, 1988. With permission from the publisher, Butterworth-Heinemann.)

6. Dose epidural catheters with incremental boluses of no more than 5 ml.

7. Monitor block levels frequently.

8. Never use 0.75% bupivacaine for epidurals.

9. Administer a non–dextrose-containing crystalloid fluid bolus prior to administration of regional anesthesia.

10. Use epidural anesthesia if regional anesthesia is desired for cesarean hysterectomy.

REFERENCES

1. Gibb D: Commentaries: Confidential enquiry into maternal death. Br J Obstet Gynaecol 97:97–101, 1990.
2. Chadwick HS, Posner K, Caplan RA, et al: A comparison of obstetric and nonobstetric anesthesia malpractice claims. Anesthesiology 74:242–249, 1991.
3. Dewan DM, Floyd HM, Thistlewood JM, et al: Sodium citrate pretreatment in elective cesarean section patients. Anesth Analg 64:34–37, 1985.
4. Archer GW, Marx GF: Arterial oxygen tension during apnea in parturient women. Br J Anaesth 46:358–360, 1974.
5. Norris MC, Dewan DM: Preoxygenation for cesarean section: A comparison of two techniques. Anesthesiology 62:827–829, 1985.
6. Gambee AM, Hertzka RE, Fisher DM: Preoxygenation techniques: Comparison of three minutes and four breaths. Anesth Analg 66:468–470, 1987.
7. Benson RC, Shubeck F, Clarke WM, et al: Fetal compromise during elective cesarean section. Am J Obstet Gynecol 91:645–651, 1965.
8. Ong BY, Cohen MM, Palahniuk RJ: Anesthesia for cesarean section: Effects on neonates. Anesth Analg 68:270–275, 1989.
9. Stenger VG, Blechner JN, Prystowsky H: A study of prolongation of obstetric anesthesia. Am J Obstet Gynecol 103:901–907, 1969.
10. Marx GF, Cosmi EV, Wollman SB: Biochemical status and clinical condition of mother and infant at cesarean section. Anesth Analg 48:986–993, 1969.
11. James FM, Crawford JS, Hopkinson R, et al: A comparison of general anesthesia and lumbar epidural analgesia for elective cesarean section. Anesth Analg 56:228–235, 1977.
12. Datta S, Ostheimer GW, Weiss JB, et al: Neonatal effect of prolonged anesthetic induction for cesarean section. Obstet Gynecol 75:600–603, 1990.
13. Malan TP, Johnson MD: The difficult airway in obstetric anesthesia: Techniques for airway management and the role of regional anesthesia. J Clin Anesth 1:104–111, 1988.
14. Datta S, Alper MH, Ostheimer GW: Method of ephedrine administration and nausea and hypotension during spinal anesthesia for cesarean section. Anesthesiology 56:68–70, 1982.
15. Ralston DH, Shnider SM, deLorimier AA: Effects of equipotent doses of ephedrine, metaraminol, mephentermine and methoxamine on uterine blood flow in the pregnant ewe. Anesthesiology 70:354–370, 1974.
16. Moran DH, Perillo M, LaPorta RF, et al: Phenylephrine in the treatment of hypotension following spinal anesthesia for cesarean delivery. J Clin Anesth 3:301–305, 1991.
17. Tarkkila PJ: Incidence and causes of failed spinal anesthetics in a university hospital: A prospective study. Reg Anesth 16:48–51, 1991.
18. Sprague DH: Effects of position and uterine displacement on spinal anesthesia for cesarean section. Anesthesiology 44:164–166, 1976.
19. Norris MC: Height, weight, and the spread of subarachnoid bupivacaine in the term parturient. Anesth Analg 67:555–558, 1988.
20. Plauché WC: Peripartal hysterectomy. Obstet Gynecol Clin North Am 15:783–795, 1988.
21. Chestnut DH, Dewan DM, Redick LF, et al: Anesthetic management for obstetric hysterectomy: A multi-institutional study. Anesthesiology 70:607–610, 1989.
22. Chestnut DH, Redick LF: Continuous epidural anesthesia for elective cesarean hysterectomy. South Med J 78:1168–1173, 1988.
23. Lewis M, Keramati S, Benumof JL, Berry CC: What is the best way to determine oropharyngeal classification and mandibular space length to predict difficult laryngoscopy? Anesthesiology 81:69–75, 1994.

E I G H T

Complicated Obstetrics—Management Considerations: Fetal Stress, Premature Fetus, Breech/Twins

BettyLou Koffel, M.D.   Andrew M. Malinow, M.D.

The topics of this chapter interrelate extensively. Breech presentation and twins often associate with each other. Additionally, both frequently present in women with preterm labor. Breech presentation, twins, and preterm labor predispose to fetal stress and distress. This chapter reviews fetal stress and its importance before exploring the anesthetic implications and considerations for prematurity, breech presentations, and multiple gestations.

FETAL STRESS

Fetal oxygen deprivation produces fetal physiologic and biochemical adaptations (Table 8–1), some of which can be detected by various methods of fetal surveillance. The extent and duration of oxygen deprivation determine the degree of fetal response and distinguish between fetal stress and fetal distress. Fetal stress may exist as a chronic state not requiring immediate intervention. In contrast, fetal distress represents severe oxygen deprivation and dictates urgent delivery. Importantly, fetal distress may occur simultaneously with fetal stress, requiring immediate action. Occasionally, perinatologists may modify the fetal environment and prevent the onset of fetal distress that requires immediate delivery. For example, fetal stress may arise from a variety of conditions (Table 8–2). Some, but not all, of these conditions may be modified by specific maternal therapeutic measures.

TABLE 8–1
Fetal Responses to Stress

Fetal respiratory acidosis followed by fetal metabolic acidosis
Increased vagal activity (bradycardia)
Systemic hypertension
Redistribution of blood flow to the heart, brain, adrenal glands
Decrease in fetal breathing movements
Gasping movements
Increased circulatory catecholamines

TABLE 8–2
Causative Factors for Fetal Stress

Fetal congenital anomaly
Inadequate maternal nutrition (e.g., alcohol or narcotic addiction)
Inadequate maternal oxygenation (e.g., asthma)
Inadequate delivery of oxygen to the placenta (e.g., maternal anemia, hypertension, diabetes, heart disease, cigarette smoking)
Inadequate transfer of oxygen across the placenta (e.g., placenta previa, placental abruption)
Inadequate fetal circulation of hemoglobin and oxygen (e.g., fetal tachyarrhythmia, hemolytic disease)

TABLE 8–3
Antepartum Assessment for Fetal Stress

Fetal movement counts
Nonstress test
Contraction stress test
Biophysical profile
Umbilical artery flow velocity waveform analysis
Fetal echocardiography
Percutaneous umbilical cord blood sampling
Fetal acoustic stimulation

Obstetricians use various methods to detect fetal stress (Tables 8–3 and 8–4). (For a complete discussion of fetal monitoring, see Chapter 2.) Something as simple as fetal movement may offer useful information, since a change in fetal movement often signifies the need for further antepartum fetal assessment. A nonstress test (NST) monitors fetal heart rate (FHR), looking for two FHR accelerations of at least 15 beats per minute for at least 15 seconds' duration within 20 minutes. If these are found, the test is "reactive" and normal. A more sensitive test of fetal well-being is the contraction stress test (CST) or oxytocin challenge test (OCT). Dilute oxytocin is administered (or its secretion increased by nipple stimulation), and FHR is assessed for the presence of late decelerations associated with contractions. Late decelerations define a "positive" test and suggest further evaluation or delivery. A negative CST suggests a low risk of fetal death within the next week.

Obstetricians also utilize the fetal biophysical profile (BPP) for antepartum fetal evaluation. The BPP is scored similarly to the Apgar score and assigns 2 points for the presence of and no points for the absence of

1. Reactive NST
2. Normal amniotic fluid volume
3. Gross fetal movement
4. Fetal tone
5. Fetal respiratory movement

TABLE 8–4
Intrapartum Assessment for Fetal Stress

Assessment of amniotic fluid for meconium
Electronic fetal heart rate monitoring
Fetal scalp capillary blood sampling
Scalp stimulation test

A score of less than 4 to 6 (or a decreasing score in a given patient) raises concern. The BPP score that requires immediate delivery has not been accurately documented.

Fetal evaluation continues intrapartum. The presence of meconium-stained amniotic fluid implies at least one episode of fetal stress causing decreased perfusion of the intestine and increased peristaltic activity and suggests increased fetal risk. FHR abnormalities can also suggest acute fetal distress. Decreased beat-to-beat or long-term variability, or both, and either tachycardia (>160 bpm) or bradycardia (<100 bpm) may develop. Good short-term variability may be the most important indicator of fetal well-being. Early, late, and variable decelerations are discussed elsewhere and have their own importance.

Fetal scalp sampling provides additional useful information in laboring patients. The fetal scalp capillary pH is generally greater than 7.25, and a pH less than 7.20 signifies fetal acidosis and usually indicates immediate delivery by the appropriate obstetric route.

Acute distress often occurs because of decreased uteroplacental perfusion. Premature placenta separation, placental infarcts, and calcifications or cord compression can evoke distress and may be diagnosed after delivery and examination of the placenta. Umbilical cord blood gases may provide additional information.

Analgesia for Labor

Chronic fetal stress does not preclude labor or labor analgesia but does require meticulous attention to detail. Continuous lumbar epidural anesthesia may offer the best choice in this situation. Epidural bupivacaine provides excellent analgesia with minimal fetal effects. Because limited data exist regarding the use of epidural (or systemic) narcotics in the marginally compensated fetus, one may choose to avoid these drugs that alter, albeit transiently and not uniformly, FHR variability. An additional advantage of epidural anesthesia is its flexibility. The ability to rapidly obtain surgical anesthesia for an instrumental or abdominal delivery may prevent the need for induction of general anesthesia and the risks for maternal airway disasters when distress dictates immediate operative delivery. To speed rapid attainment of surgical anesthesia, the authors often choose a "more concentrated" bupivacaine (0.125 to 0.5%) for labor analgesia, as dense labor blocks shorten the time to establish surgical anesthesia. Continuing supplemental maternal oxygen may be desirable during transport to the operating room.

Anesthesia for Vaginal Delivery

The unanesthetized patient presenting for immediate vaginal delivery of a stressed fetus requires a rapidly and reliably administered anesthetic. Although general anesthesia is rapid and reliable, it has additional maternal risks that make regional anesthesia preferable. For these reasons, the authors choose "single-shot" spinal anesthesia with a relatively small dose of hyperbaric local anesthetic, bupivacaine 7.5% (7.5 mg) or lidocaine (20 to 30 mg of 1.5% or 2% solutions), for operative vaginal delivery and strive for sensory anesthesia to the T10 dermatome. Although a "saddle block" limited to the sacral dermatomes will provide adequate anesthesia for low forceps delivery, it may not be sufficient for mid forceps delivery, subsequent repair of cervical lacerations, or manual removal of the placenta. The added benefits of a T10 spinal anesthetic (compared with those of a true saddle block) may be obtained without added maternal or fetal risks accompanying low thoracic sensory anesthesia, and all patients should receive a rapid non–dextrose-containing fluid infusion of about 1 L. Even though the limited sympathetic blockade during low subarachnoid block rarely causes hypotension, the use of a pressure infusor should be considered to rapidly infuse this fluid during preparations for and administration of spinal anesthesia. Supplemental oxygen and fetal monitoring should be continued during anesthetic induction. If the spinal proves difficult and time-consuming for an experienced anesthesiologist, the use of alternative techniques should be considered.

Alternatively, obstetricians may use pudendal anesthesia. Even if pudendal anesthesia is used, the prudent obstetrician may request the presence of an anesthesiologist in case the operative delivery fails in this emergency situation. The authors do not administer inhalational (30 to 50% nitrous oxide) analgesia because of its potential to obtund protective airway reflexes in the parturient with a physiologically decreased anesthesia requirement or minimal alveolar concentration (MAC). Techniques of inhalational or intravenous (ketamine 0.25 mg/kg) analgesia have been used safely by some and are described elsewhere (see Chapter 5).[1] Irrespective of the choice of anesthesia, the anesthesiologist should recheck equipment and drugs for the administration of emergency general anesthesia if called to attend such a delivery.

Regardless of the selected anesthetic technique, standard aspiration prophylaxis, left uterine displacement, and supplemental oxygen should be provided. The patient with existing epidural analgesia may require complete sensory blockade for an instrumental delivery. In the face of possible fetal stress or distress, the authors choose 2-chloroprocaine (2 or 3%) because of its rapid onset and because it is rapidly hydrolyzed even by the acidotic fetus. This prevents accumulation ("ion trapping") of local anesthetic in the acidotic fetus, which may occur with amide local anesthetics. Ion trapping occurs when decreased fetal pH increases the concentration of ionized drug (a weak base) in the fetus, preventing diffusion across the placenta back to the mother. Placental transfer of nonionized drug continues with subsequent trapping of ionized drug. Thus, when fetal pH decreases, local anesthetics can accumulate in the fetus.

Anesthesia for Cesarean Delivery

The best anesthesia for the patient with evidence of chronic fetal stress or acute fetal distress is unclear. Theoretical reasons support both regional and general anesthesia. The critical factors to be considered when contemplating regional versus general anesthesia in cesarean section indicated for fetal stress/distress are: (1) What is the degree of fetal stress/distress? (2) In what time frame can regional anesthesia be instituted? (3) What are the relative risks of the two anesthetic techniques? The American College of Obstetricians and Gynecologists (ACOG) recently published ACOG Committee Opinion No. 104: Anesthesia for Emergency Deliveries, which noted that a diagnosis of "fetal distress" does not necessarily preclude the safe use of regional anesthesia.[2]

The degree of fetal stress/distress may range from chronic stress with superimposed intermittent decelerations to severe, sustained, fetal bradycardia. The degree of fetal stress influences the sense of urgency and possibly the anesthetic choice. The fetus evidencing mild distress probably has more reserve than the fetus with agonal bradycardia.

The time frame in which regional anesthesia can be accomplished is also important. Epidural analgesia can rapidly be extended to cesarean section anesthesia. Ramanathan and associates[3] converted labor epidurals for use in cesarean sections with fetal distress and reported that epidural injection–to–delivery times were 10.4 to 16.0 minutes. The present authors commonly extend labor epidurals while moving the patient to the operating room. Injection-to-delivery times of less than 10 minutes are not uncommon when using 3% 2-chloroprocaine (20 to 25 ml).

Marx and coworkers[4] allowed the mother to select the anesthetic method (either regional or general anesthesia). If the mother selected regional anesthesia, she received a spinal anesthetic, or if she had a functioning labor epidural, the epidural was rapidly extended to cesarean section levels. All cesarean sections started within 20 minutes of the decision to operate.

Obviously, it is possible to rapidly institute either epidural or spinal anesthesia for cesarean section; however, placing a spinal necessitates additional uncertainty. The individual anesthesiologist's skills, patient anatomy, and urgency all influence the decision to proceed with spinal anesthesia. In addition, the obstetrician ideally should concur with the anesthetic method.

The relative maternal and fetal risks of regional versus general anesthesia become a deciding factor for many. Three pertinent maternal mortality risk factors appear repeatedly in the literature. (1) The vast majority of fatal maternal anesthetic outcomes are due to airway complications.[5] (2) *Unanticipated* failed tracheal intubations are more common in obstetric compared with nonobstetric patients.[6] (3) Emergency cesarean sections are several times more likely to result in fatal maternal anesthetic complications.[7] In the emergency situation, general anesthesia for cesarean section has greater maternal mortality risk than regional anesthesia.

Potential fetal risks of regional anesthesia involve delay in delivery and sustained maternal hypotension, either of which may worsen fetal stress. However, the incidence of maternal hypotension following cesarean section regional anesthesia induction is reduced for laboring patients compared with elective, fasting patients.[8] In Marx and coworkers' study, no patient (out of 55) with fetal distress suffered reductions in systolic blood pressure to less than 100 mmHg following cesarean section regional anesthesia induction.[4] Similarly, in Ramanathan and associates' study, labor epidurals that were rapidly extended to cesarean section levels produced comparable hypotension when compared with general anesthesia.[3] Importantly, transient, treated maternal hypotension has minimal if any associated neonatal compromise, even in the case of fetal distress.[8] Fetal outcome may indeed be better with regional anesthesia (Table 8–5), at least when measured by Apgar score.

Ultimately, the best anesthetic choice for a particular patient with fetal distress will most likely vary with practitioner and institution. An attempt to extend existing epidural anesthesia should be made in most, if not all, cases. In those patients without existing epidural anesthesia, the authors usually choose general anesthesia in the face of severe fetal distress. The editors, in their practice and institution, may initiate spinal anesthesia for similar patients. Table 8–6 details important points regarding anesthesia for cesarean section for fetal distress. Ultimately, the individual practitioner's judgment and skill are most important when deciding the "best" anesthetic method for fetal distress cesarean sections.

The usual induction of general anesthesia

TABLE 8–5
Fetal Outcome After Regional Versus General Anesthesia for Cesarean Section

	Apgar Scores <8 (%)	
	1 min	*5 min*
General (n = 71)	49	15
Spinal (n = 33)	21	3
Epidural (n = 22)	23	0

From Marx GF, Luykx WM, Cohen S: Fetal-neonatal status following caesarean section for fetal distress. Br J Anaesth 56:1009–1013, 1984.

TABLE 8–6
Cesarean Section Anesthesia for Fetal Distress

1. Open intravenous fluids immediately, consider pressure-bag to speed infusion
2. For functioning, tested, labor epidurals
   a. Maintain uterine displacement, fetal heart rate monitoring, and maternal supplemental oxygen
   b. Rapidly administer 20–25 ml 3% 2-chloroprocaine before or during transport to the operating room
3. Spinal anesthesia
   a. Agree in advance to minimize spinal attempts/time
   b. If possible, have an assistant prepare supplies and drugs in the operating room
   c. Have the most experienced anesthesiologist administer the spinal block
   d. Maximize the likelihood of success (needle choice, patient position)
   e. Denitrogenate with 100% oxygen during spinal placement
   f. Abandon spinal anesthesia after two or three attempts
4. General anesthesia
   a. *Always* thoroughly evaluate the patient's airway
   b. *Never* initiate general anesthesia unless confident that the patient's airway can be managed safely
   c. *Never* gamble with the mother's life out of a sense of urgency based on presumed fetal distress

may require modification in the face of fetal distress. Some advocate intravenous ketamine 1 mg/kg as the anesthetic induction drug of choice for cesarean delivery of the distressed fetus. In animals, ketamine maintains uteroplacental blood flow without deleteriously affecting fetal cerebral or myocardial blood flow or acid-base measurements. Induction of anesthesia with ketamine better preserves fetal blood pressure and cerebral blood flow as compared with thiopental.[9] Since the clinical significance of this is not known, the authors generally use thiopental 4 mg/kg as the induction agent of choice, reserving ketamine for those gravidae with decreased intravascular volume secondary to hemorrhage. In these situations, the authors use 0.5 to 1.0 mg/kg of intravenous ketamine.

There is little information about the effects of volatile anesthetic agents on fetal environment during acute fetal distress. An acidotic fetus compensates for decreased cardiac output by cerebral vasodilatation and decreased cerebral metabolic oxygen consumption. Maternal administration of low-dose halothane maintains cerebral blood flow and cerebral oxygen supply and lowers cerebral metabolic oxygen consumption during the first 15 minutes of asphyxia.[10] In periods of experimental fetal asphyxia, halogenated agents sometimes decrease fetal cerebral blood flow, worsening fetal acid-base status. In the clinical situation of general anesthesia for cesarean delivery of the distressed fetus, maternal administration of ⅔ MAC isoflurane or halothane in 50% nitrous oxide/oxygen does not alter neonatal outcome as measured by Apgar score or umbilical cord blood acid-base analysis.[11]

There is little neonatal benefit to increasing inspired maternal oxygen concentrations above 50 to 60%. In addition, 100% inspired maternal oxygen delivery increases the incidence of maternal awareness.

Good communication among obstetricians, anesthesiologists, and neonatologists maximizes maternal and fetal outcome when fetal stress occurs. The obstetric anesthesiologist's vigilance and meticulous care play a major role in providing optimal outcome with minimal maternal and fetal risk.

PREMATURE FETUS

Prematurity remains a leading cause of perinatal morbidity and mortality in the United States, accounting for as many as 85% of the neonatal deaths occurring in otherwise normal infants. Premature infants commonly develop problems associated with respiratory distress syndrome, intraventricular hemorrhage, patent ductus arteriosus, and necrotizing enterocolitis. Surviving premature infants may demonstrate permanent handicaps, such as learning disabilities, chronic pulmonary disease, visual defects, lower IQ scores, and a higher incidence of neurologic abnormalities.

Definitions and Incidence

Regular uterine contractions that produce cervical change (dilatation or effacement) prior to 37 completed weeks of gestation define pre-

TABLE 8–7
Prematurity Risks: Maternal Characteristics

<15 years old or >40 years old and nulliparous
Black
Underweight for height (esp. prepregnancy weight <50 kg)
Use of
Nicotine (especially >20 cigarettes/day)
Cocaine
Ethanol (controversial)
Narcotics (controversial)
Under stress
Work related
Psychosocial
Sexually active (coitus) after 20 weeks' gestational age

term labor. Definitions utilizing birth weight (usually 500 to 2499 gm) to define prematurity may unfortunately include many term infants with growth retardation and exclude preterm infants who are large for gestational age. These infants may experience different medical complications.

The incidence of preterm birth varies among countries, communities, and hospitals. In the United States, 7 to 9% of deliveries occur preterm. Because early preterm labor is sometimes difficult to diagnose and does not uniformly result in preterm birth, preterm labor rates are unavailable, although they are undoubtedly greater than those for preterm birth. Patients who are not truly in preterm labor may sometimes receive tocolytic agents as a precautionary measure. Although multiple studies support utilizing tocolytic agents to reduce preterm birth, demonstrating improved perinatal mortality is difficult. Patients in preterm labor often require transfer, after tocolysis, to perinatal centers to provide optimal maternal and neonatal care.

Fetal membrane rupture occurring between 20 and 37 completed weeks of gestation defines preterm rupture of membranes. Uterine contractions may or may not be present. Thirty percent of preterm deliveries directly follow preterm membrane rupture.

Risk Factors

Although the cause of preterm labor is only partially understood, four groups of risk factors have been identified: maternal characteristics (Table 8–7), socioeconomic factors (Table 8–8), reproductive history (Table 8–9), and current pregnancy complications including infections (Table 8–10). Although prompt diagnosis with aggressive obstetric management may prevent preterm birth, pharmacologic therapy complicates anesthetic management. Communication among the perinatologists, neonatologists, and anesthesiologists provides opportunity for joint, efficient care of the gravida and her baby.

TABLE 8–8
Prematurity Risks: Socioeconomic Factors

Public clinic patients
Limited antenatal care
Employment in physically demanding jobs (e.g., laborers)
Single mothers (esp. white women)

Anesthetic Management of Preterm Labor and Delivery

Appropriate anesthetic technique and agents may decrease maternal and fetal intrapartum complications. Regional anesthesia benefits the gravida in preterm labor in several ways. Continuous lumbar epidural anesthesia provides excellent analgesia for operative vaginal or abdomi-

TABLE 8–9
Prematurity Risks: Reproductive History

Preterm Birth
One previous preterm birth—up to 35% chance of preterm *labor*
Two or more previous preterm births—up to 70% chance of preterm *labor*
Abortion
Second trimester spontaneous abortions (but not first trimester therapeutic abortion)
Uterine Abnormalities
Uterine malformation or septum
Diethylstilbestrol exposure
Intramural or submucosal leiomyomata
Asherman syndrome
Cervical incompetence
Bleeding
Previous placenta previa or placental abruption

TABLE 8–10
Prematurity Risks: Current Pregnancy Complications

Uterine Distention
Multiple gestation—increasing risk with each additional fetus
Monozygous twins > dizygous twins
Polyhydramnios—30–40% incidence

Fetal Abnormalities
Congenital anomalies (genetic or environmental)
Growth retardation

Antepartum Hemorrhage
Placenta previa
Placental abruption

Maternal Illness
Severe maternal disease or trauma
Coexisting maternal illness including
- Asthma
- Collagen vascular disease
- Coronary, hepatobiliary, or endocrine disease
- Surgical abdomen
- Systemic infections
- Asymptomatic bacteriuria (±)

Genital Tract Infections
Cervicovaginal infections
Transplacental infections (bacterial, viral)
Amniotic fluid infection

nal delivery, often needed for fetal distress. Inadequate placental perfusion (and subsequent fetal distress) often occurs perhaps because placental dysfunction plays a role in initiating preterm labor. Epidural anesthesia also obviates the need to induce general anesthesia with its increased maternal risks should cesarean delivery become necessary. Additionally, obstetric analgesia for labor can be an integral part of intrauterine resuscitation of the stressed fetus. Intravenous hydration, maternal pain relief, and subsequent decrease in circulating catecholamines may improve uteroplacental perfusion.

Anesthetic management must include consideration of associated medical, obstetric, and social conditions (see Tables 8–7 and 8–10) as well as possible drug interactions between anesthetics and maternal drug therapy (Table 8–11). Personnel trained in neonatal resuscitation should be present at the delivery with all necessary equipment ready for immediate use. This may require transfer to a Level III perinatal center prior to delivery.

FETAL CONSIDERATIONS

Prematurity reduces FHR variability, complicating interpretation of FHR tracings. In addition, baseline FHR may be higher. Heart rates exceeding 170 beats per minute require investigation. Fetal scalp blood sampling provides useful information when FHR tracings suggest compromise. Interpretation of these results has been discussed under "Fetal Stress," earlier in this chapter.

Should variable FHR decelerations occur, a saline amnioinfusion abolishes this pattern by restoring fluid volume and relieving cord compression. Amnioinfusion should be done with warm fluids. Obstetricians at the authors' institution find a blood warmer ideal for warming the fluids.

Anesthetic Implications of Preterm Labor Pharmacologic Treatment

Ethanol

Thankfully, the use of intravenous ethanol as a tocolytic agent has essentially disappeared. Maternal alterations in mental status, respiratory depression, lactic acidosis, hyper- or hypothyroidism, hypertension, and increased gastric volume and acidity complicate the care of intoxicated patients. Aspiration risk increases in such patients. Alcohol intoxication decreases MAC, and additive depressant effects of ethanol with anesthetic agents must be expected. As with any intoxicated patient, disturbances in fluid and electrolyte balance should be corrected prior to induction of anesthesia.

TABLE 8–11
Treatment of Preterm Labor: Pharmacologic Agents

Tocolytic Agents
β-Adrenergic agonists
- Terbutaline
- Ritodrine

Magnesium sulfate
Prostaglandin synthetase inhibitors
Calcium channel blockers

Steroids

β-Adrenergic Agonists

β-adrenergic agonists relax smooth muscle through their interaction with β_2-receptor sites on the outer membrane of myometrial cells, thereby increasing the intracellular concentration of cyclic adenosine monophosphate (cAMP). Intracellular calcium decreases and prevents the actin-myosin interaction necessary for smooth muscle contraction.

All β-adrenergic agonists have both β_1 and β_2 effects. Maternal side effects of β-adrenergic agonists are extensive owing to the widespread distribution of β-adrenergic receptors (Table 8–12). Although ritodrine is the only β agonist approved for parenteral use in preterm labor, a large body of literature supports terbutaline safety and efficacy, and in many institutions, it remains the agent of choice.

The inherent β_1 activity of all β-adrenergic agonists produces direct cardiac effects. Cardiac arrhythmias occur, primarily premature ventricular and atrial contractions. Patients receiving ritodrine often complain of chest pain. Electrocardiogram (ECG) changes such as ST segment depression, T wave flattening or inversion, and prolongation of the QT interval suggest myocardial ischemia. Myocardial ischemia does indeed occur in this population and ECG findings should not be ignored. Chest pain with *or* without ECG changes may require a change to another class of tocolytic agents.

Although early reports cite pulmonary edema occurring in up to 5% of women treated with intravenous therapy, an ensuing decade of experience has decreased the incidence of pulmonary edema and identified risk factors for its development. Multiple gestation, fluid overload, anemia, and prolonged duration of maternal tachycardia increase the risk of pulmonary edema. Importantly, arterial hypoxemia may be severe and out of proportion to the radiographic picture during β agonist–induced pulmonary edema. Respiratory distress requires early evaluation and perhaps a change in tocolytic agents. Pulse oximetry may provide useful information.

β-adrenergic stimulation of aldosterone, renin, and antidiuretic hormone potentiates fluid and sodium retention. β-adrenergic agonist therapy decreases serum albumin and protein concentrations, decreasing the colloid oncotic pressure–hydrostatic pressure gradient. β-adrenergic stimulation may decrease pulmonary vascular permeability. The common finding of low or normal pulmonary capillary wedge pressure pulmonary edema in these patients suggests a role of increased pulmonary vascular permeability in pulmonary edema.[12] Although most patients do not manifest left ventricular failure, intravenous hydration may decompensate an already fragile, hyperdynamic cardiac state. Invasive hemodynamic monitoring may be beneficial (or may even be required) for patients with severe tachycardia or pulmonary edema, irrespective of anesthetic technique. Hypotension associated with severe maternal tachycardia may best be treated with dilute intravenous phenylephrine boluses (25 to 100 μg).

Anemia develops as the patient placed at bed rest mobilizes third space fluid into the intravascular space. Intravenous hydration stimulates the renin-angiotensin-aldosterone system and results in further volume expansion. Hematocrit decreases an average of 15%. Oxygen-carrying capacity should not change in the absence of blood loss.

β-adrenergic-receptor stimulation induces hyperglycemia and increased insulin levels. Glucose peaks 3 to 6 hours after the initiation of therapy, returning to baseline within 24 hours of therapy cessation. Exogenous insulin is usually unnecessary. However, insulin-dependent diabetics require special attention. Transient hypokalemia occurs as potassium redistributes from the extracellular to the intracellular compartment. Levels commonly fall to a nadir of 2.7 mEq/L, but total body potassium remains unchanged. Potassium levels also return to normal without therapy within 24 hours. The authors have not found it necessary to treat hypokalemia in any patient, although the symp-

TABLE 8–12
Maternal Side Effects of β-Adrenergic Tocolytic Therapy

Anemia	Nausea
Arrhythmias	Palpitations
Chest pain	Paralytic ileus
Elevated hepatic transaminase levels	Pulmonary edema
	Rash
Glucose intolerance	Restlessness, agitation
Hypokalemia	Tremor
Myocardial ischemia	

tomatic patient with arrhythmias may require judicious potassium infusion. If replacement therapy is necessary, exercise extreme caution and prevent rapid infusion of concentrated potassium solutions.

Abnormal serum glucose, potassium, and hematocrit generally do not require pharmacologic or transfusion therapy prior to anesthetic induction. Many patients will benefit from an ECG to detect arrhythmias or to evaluate symptomatic chest pain. Symptomatic patients may require pharmacologic therapy with a different agent.

Although preload reduction occurring with the sympathectomy accompanying regional anesthesia may be beneficial to the parturient with pulmonary edema, empirical prophylactic intravenous hydration prior to regional anesthesia may increase risks of inducing or worsening pulmonary edema. Tachycardia or pulmonary edema may necessitate invasive monitoring of right-sided or bilateral cardiac filling pressures to estimate intravascular volume status before anesthetic induction. Generally, the authors invasively monitor patients who are unresponsive to initial therapy or who require anesthesia while their pulmonary status is unstable. The autotransfusion occurring after delivery due to uterine involution makes the immediate postpartum period a time of potential danger.

Continuous epidural or spinal anesthesia (as opposed to single-shot spinal anesthesia) for abdominal delivery may provide the smoothest anesthesia in these parturients by avoiding sudden vasodilatation or large, arbitrary intravenous infusions that could produce hemodynamic compromise. In theory, even incremental intravenous ephedrine titration might worsen cardiac output in the presence of severe maternal tachycardia. In the case of extreme hypotension, *dilute* intravenous phenylephrine infusion may prove beneficial, minimizing tachycardia and arrhythmias. However, neosynephrine safety has not been proved in the high-risk patient, and the practitioner must weigh the risks of potential decreases of uterine blood flow versus the risks of maternal tachycardia and hypotension.

Fetal considerations often necessitate emergency abdominal delivery and therefore general anesthesia. General anesthesia may be required for its reliability and rapidity of induction, as well as for its safety in the face of maternal hemorrhage. Sympathomimetic agents such as ketamine should be avoided during severe maternal tachycardia. Atropine, glycopyrrolate, and pancuronium should be used with caution. Small doses of barbiturates or ketamine may be necessary in the hypotensive, tachycardic patient. Halothane, by sensitizing the myocardium to catecholamines, may lead to arrhythmias and is best avoided. Enflurane or isoflurane provides relative safety when given at less than ⅔ MAC. The tachycardia and hypertension accompanying laryngoscopy and intubation may require adjuncts such as intravenous low-dose narcotics (fentanyl 50 to 100 μg), lidocaine (50 to 100 mg), or low doses of β-adrenergic-blocking agents, especially in the parturient with preeclampsia. Labetalol[13] (incremental doses of 5 to 10 mg up to 1 mg/kg) may be preferable to esmolol owing to fetal hypoxemia seen with esmolol in animals.[14] Potential fetal effects preclude routinely using these agents. The resuscitation and neonatal care personnel should be notified when these drugs are used.

Magnesium Sulfate

Magnesium competes with calcium for entry into the cell during depolarization and also increases cAMP levels, both of which reduce intracellular calcium. In addition, magnesium indirectly promotes calcium uptake into the sarcoplasmic reticulum by stimulating calcium-dependent adenosine triphosphatase (ATPase). Increased urinary excretion of calcium also decreases its availability. The end result is that less intracellular free calcium is available for actin-myosin interaction of smooth muscle contraction. Magnesium also acts at the neuromuscular junction, decreasing acetylcholine release and the postjunctional membrane potentials generated by acetylcholine-receptor interaction.

Magnesium potentiates depolarizing and nondepolarizing neuromuscular relaxants. Even the small doses used for "precurarization" may lead to respiratory difficulty. The dose of succinylcholine needed for intubation should *not* be decreased, since the extent of magnesium sulfate potentiation is variable and optimal conditions for intubation are essential. During maintenance of anesthesia, the need for additional neuromuscular relaxation should be guided by a neuromuscular blockade monitor.

Normal serum magnesium level during pregnancy is 1.8 to 3.0 mg/dl. Inhibition of uterine activity requires magnesium levels of 5 to 8 mg/dl, but levels as high as 11 mg/dl do not guarantee labor inhibition. Compared with ritodrine and terbutaline, magnesium is equally effective and produces fewer side effects. Although combination therapy with magnesium sulfate and a β-adrenergic agent may produce better results than using either agent alone, combination therapy increases side effects.

Magnesium sulfate causes peripheral vasodilatation (Table 8–13). Nausea, headache, and lethargy are not uncommon. Dizziness, chest tightness, palpitations, and visual symptoms secondary to ocular muscle paresis can occur. Although cardiovascular side effects are minimal, transient maternal tachycardia and reduced mean arterial pressure may be associated with the initial intravenous dose.[15] Therapeutic maternal serum levels of magnesium are also associated with maternal ECG changes such as a widened QRS complex and prolonged PR interval at serum levels of approximately 10 mg/dl. If these changes are seen, the magnesium sulfate infusion should be slowed. Estimating the required volume of prophylactic intravenous hydration prior to regional anesthesia is complicated in parturients on magnesium therapy for reasons similar to those previously discussed with β-adrenergic-agonist therapy. In a gravid ewe model, magnesium potentiates hypotension after hemorrhage. Thus, the possibility of hypotension during abdominal delivery should be anticipated by the placement of large-bore intravenous access.

Several investigators, although not all, observe decreased FHR variability and baseline FHR without evidence of neonatal compromise in patients receiving magnesium for the treatment of preeclampsia or preterm labor. These changes are probably the result of pharmacologic depression of the fetal central nervous system.

In the majority of neonates, there is no significant alteration in neurologic state or Apgar score. However, neonatal depression manifested as flaccidity, hyporeflexia, respiratory depression requiring assisted ventilation, and a weak or absent cry may follow prolonged high-dose intravenous magnesium therapy proximate to delivery. These infants clinically improve within 24 to 36 hours.

TABLE 8–13
Maternal Side Effects of Magnesium Sulfate Therapy

Warmth, flushing, headache
Nausea, dizziness
Transient hypotension
Electrocardiographic changes
Widened QRS
Increased PR interval
Depressed deep tendon reflexes
Muscle weakness
Respiratory depression
Cardiac arrest

Prostaglandin Synthetase Inhibitors

Prostaglandins are integral to the final pathway of smooth muscle contraction. Prostaglandin $F_{2\alpha}$ ($PGF_{2\alpha}$) stimulates entry of calcium into the cell and its release from the sarcoplasmic reticulum. At the same time prostaglandin E_2 (PGE_2) induces biochemical changes in collagen that facilitate cervical dilatation.

Indomethacin, when administered orally or rectally, specifically and reversibly inhibits the cyclooxygenase enzyme necessary to convert arachidonic acid to prostaglandin. Indomethacin abolishes spontaneous contractions when added to human myometrial strips.

Although indomethacin inhibits the synthesis of all classes of prostanoids including prostaglandins, prostacyclins, and thromboxanes, few maternal side effects have been reported with its use for tocolysis. Decreased thromboxane A_2 inhibits platelet aggregation with a more transient effect on platelets than the antiplatelet effect of aspirin. A bleeding time to test platelet function might be prudent before induction of regional anesthesia, given the theoretical (albeit unlikely) possibility of epidural hematoma. Postpartum hemorrhage may be exacerbated owing to inhibition of myometrial contraction and platelet inactivation.

Calcium Channel Blockers

Calcium channel blockers inhibit calcium ion influx through voltage-dependent, calcium-selective, cell membrane channels. The reduction of cytoplasm-free calcium inhibits smooth muscle contractility. Most research in preterm labor reports nifedipine use. Calcium channel blockers have a wide variety of anesthetic interactions. Although tocolytic doses of nifedipine rarely impair atrioventricular conduction, they can cause vasodilatation, hypotension, and reflex tachycardia.[16] Exaggerated hypotension should be anticipated with a volatile anesthetic or regional anesthesia in the parturient receiving nifedipine.

Residual nifedipine in the postpartum period may adversely affect postpartum uterine contraction. A variety of uterine stimulants including oxytocin, methylergonovine maleate, 15-methyl-$PGF_{2\alpha}$, and calcium chloride should be immediately available for use. The availability of compatible blood products and large-bore intravenous access should be ensured prior to delivery.

Antibiotics

Many institutions initiate antibiotic therapy, especially in parturients with premature rupture of membranes delivered abdominally. Most antibiotic regimens use ampicillin or a cephalosporin; all of these antibiotics are devoid of neuromuscular blocking potential. Other antibiotics with possible neuromuscular relaxant potentiation, especially in the parturient on magnesium sulfate, require the use of a neuromuscular blockade monitor to safely manage administration of neuromuscular paralysis during general anesthesia. The use of regional anesthesia in the febrile parturient raises the question of possible hematogenous contamination of the epidural or subarachnoid space. However, most, if not all, parturients with a diagnosis of chorioamnionitis are treated with intravenous antibiotics prior to the consideration of regional anesthesia. The authors' practice is to offer epidural or spinal anesthesia to parturients with diagnosed chorioamnionitis who are not overtly septic and who are without other contraindications to regional anesthesia. Fever alone, especially if antibiotics have been given, does not contraindicate regional anesthesia. If the patient is obviously ill or has shaking chills or hypotension, regional anesthesia is deferred until antibiotic therapy or resuscitation has been started with resolution of the signs and symptoms of sepsis.

Anesthetic Considerations

Appropriate selection of anesthetic technique and agents may potentially benefit the preterm fetus.

Labor and Vaginal Delivery

Particularly in preterm labor, epidural analgesia may be superior to the use of sedatives or narcotics. The preterm fetus exhibits increased drug sensitivity compared with the term fetus. Less protein-binding capacity increases circulating free drug concentrations. Drug metabolism and excretion proceed less efficiently in the preterm infant. The preterm blood-brain barrier demonstrates increased drug permeability. The preterm fetus is especially sensitive to decreased uteroplacental perfusion and may quickly evidence fetal asphyxia. Asphyxia increases cerebral blood flow and central nervous system exposure to maternally administered drug. Epidural analgesia benefits uteroplacental perfusion by decreasing maternal stress, provided maternal arterial pressure is maintained. Epidural analgesia for labor that provides excellent perineal anesthesia or low spinal anesthesia at delivery facilitates atraumatic delivery by allowing generous episiotomy, often used to decrease extracranial pressure and to better control delivery. Restricting the rapid infusion of non–dextrose-containing fluid to about 500 ml for labor and titrating incremental anesthetic doses limit risks for hemodynamic compromise with the epidural anesthesia induction. Hypotension is treated with increased intravenous fluids and incremental doses of ephedrine. If maternal tachycardia contraindicates ephedrine use, incremental doses of phenylephrine (25 to 100 μg) are used to maintain blood pressure.

Local Anesthetic

Local anesthetic choice for epidural anesthesia may influence fetal outcome. Gestational age does not alter fetal pharmacokinetics or pharmacodynamics of lidocaine. However, the asphyxiated preterm fetus is more sensitive to lidocaine depressant effects than is the asphyxiated term fetus. 2-Chloroprocaine, rapidly hydrolyzed in maternal and fetal plasma, exposes the acidotic fetus to less local anesthetic. Therefore, the authors prefer 2-chloroprocaine to intensify or extend epidural anesthesia for operative vaginal or abdominal delivery of distressed preterm fetuses. The small amount of local anesthetic needed for single-shot spinal anesthesia for vaginal delivery allows the choice of spinal local anesthetic to be made independent of fetal considerations.

Cesarean Delivery

Regional Anesthesia

The choice of local anesthetic for epidural anesthesia in the nondistressed fetus is not an issue. Although a significant percentage of parturients receiving spinal anesthesia experience hypotensive episodes after induction, prompt treatment of maternal hypotension renders these episodes inconsequential to fetal outcome in the term fetus. However, this may not be the case during abdominal delivery of the distressed preterm fetus. Therefore, meticulous attention should be paid to hydration as well as to pharmacologic support of maternal blood pressure. Vast experience with spinal anesthesia for abdominal delivery of the preterm fetus, with successful outcome, has shown it to be an excellent method of surgical anesthesia.

General Anesthesia

Drugs used for general anesthesia induction and maintenance can potentially anesthetize the preterm infant. Therefore, the induction-to-delivery, as well as the uterine incision–to–delivery times (as always) should be minimized. Newborn sensitivity to general anesthetics may manifest as low Apgar scores. Immediate neonatal ventilation and oxygenation and concomitant elimination of inhaled anesthetics should significantly improve the 5-minute Apgar scores. Although important in the resuscitation of all "depressed" neonates, these techniques are vital in the resuscitation of the depressed preterm neonate.

Intravenous ketamine 1 mg/kg is an acceptable alternative induction agent to thiopental 4 mg/kg except in the parturient with preeclampsia, coexisting neurologic or cardiac disease, or severe tachycardia. In the distressed fetal lamb, ketamine better maintains perfusion of the central nervous system. "Light" anesthesia should be avoided. Increased maternal catecholamine production may decrease uteroplacental perfusion. Maternal inspired oxygen concentration should be at least 50%. Hyperventilation should be avoided, since respiratory alkalosis increases maternal oxygen-hemoglobin affinity, potentially decreasing oxygen transfer to the fetus. In addition, intermittent positive-pressure ventilation decreases uteroplacental blood flow. The net result is decreased maternal oxygen presentation to the fetoplacental unit. Following delivery, the pharmacologic implications of tocolytic therapy previously discussed predominate.

Summary

Early induction of epidural analgesia is the authors' technique of choice for providing labor analgesia. Anesthesia for vaginal or abdominal delivery can then be readily accomplished, using 3% 2-chloroprocaine if the fetus manifests distress. Spinal anesthesia is an excellent alternative to epidural anesthesia for elective or urgent cesarean delivery, as long as maternal hypotension is prevented or promptly treated. General anesthesia can be safely achieved for abdominal delivery of a distressed fetus. Previously informed pediatric staff should be present at delivery and available for immediate evaluation and resuscitation of any preterm fetus.

BREECH PRESENTATION

Obstetric management of breech presentation remains controversial; thus, the anesthesiologist must adapt a specific anesthetic to one or several possible scenarios. An elective abdominal delivery requires an anesthetic different from that used for anesthesia for a trial of labor, yet the trial of labor may rapidly turn into an emergency abdominal delivery. Because of the higher incidence of obstetric complications, analgesia for a laboring patient with breech presentation differs from analgesia for a routine patient with vertex presentation.

TABLE 8–14
Types of Breech Presentation

Frank Breech
Lower extremities flexed at the hips and extended at the knees (60% of breech presentations)

Complete Breech
Lower extremities flexed at both the hips and the knees (10% of breech presentations)

Incomplete Breech
One or both extremities extended and one or both feet present in the vagina (30% of breech presentations)

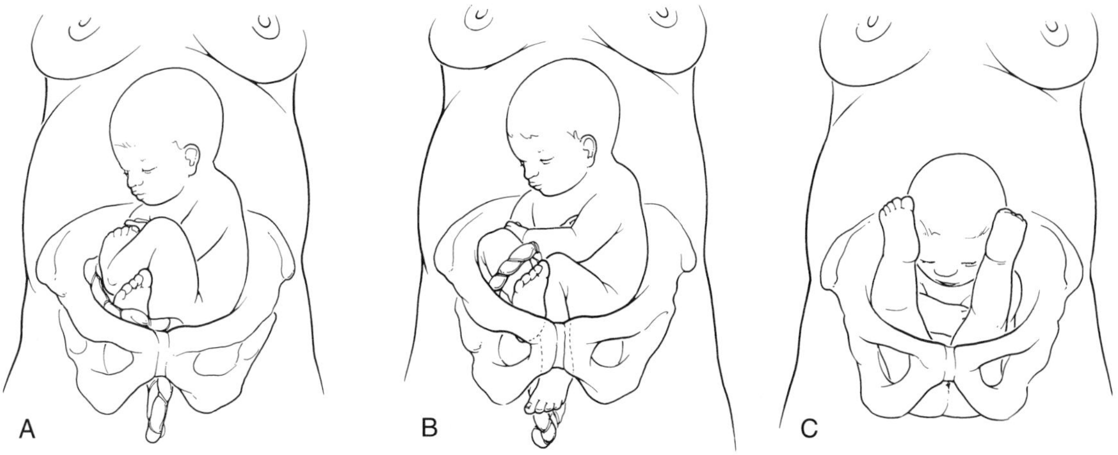

Figure 8–1. Three possible breech presentations. *A,* The complete breech demonstrates flexion of both the hips and the knees. *B,* The incomplete breech demonstrates intermediate reflexion of one hip and one knee. *C,* The frank breech demonstrates flexion of the hips and extension of both knees. Prolapsed cord is shown for both complete and incomplete breech. (Redrawn from Seeds JW: Malpresentations. *In* Gabbe SG, Niebyl JR, Simpson JL [eds]: Obstetrics: Normal and Problem Pregnancies, 2nd ed. Churchill Livingstone, New York, 1991, p 539.)

Definitions, Incidence, and Obstetric Considerations

Three types of breech presentation are described (Table 8–14 and Fig. 8–1). Since the highest incidence of successful vaginal delivery occurs with frank breech presentations, the obstetrician must accurately assess position when deciding for or against a trial of labor. Although about 7% of term infants present in breech position, up to 33% of infants present as breech in *preterm* labor. Factors predisposing to breech presentation (Table 8–15) interfere with the normal process of fetal head accommodation in the uterine cavity and maternal pelvis.[17]

Frightening obstetric complications may occur during breech labor and vaginal delivery (Table 8–16). Head entrapment, whereby the fetal head is lodged above the incompletely dilated cervix, may occur in any vaginal breech delivery (Fig. 8–2). However, premature infants with their relatively large head–to–body size ratio and frequent incomplete breech presentations are particularly predisposed to head entrapment. The frightening emergency of head entrapment rapidly leads to fetal demise owing to asphyxia. Preterm labor should heighten awareness of possible entrapment of an aftercoming head. Abdominal delivery does not necessarily lower the incidence of these complications.[18]

At the present time in the United States, ap-

TABLE 8–15
Factors Predisposing to Breech Presentation

Prematurity	Fetal anencephaly
Multiparity	Previous breech delivery
Multiple gestation	Uterine anomalies
Hydramnios	Uterine tumors
Oligohydramnios	Cornual fundal implantation
Fetal hydrocephalus	

TABLE 8–16
Incidence of Complications Seen With Breech Presentation

Complication	Approximate Incidence
Intrapartum fetal death	Increased 16-fold*
Intrapartum asphyxia	Increased 4-fold*
Cord prolapse	0–20%
Birth trauma	Increased 13-fold*
Arrest of aftercoming head	5–10%
Major congenital anomalies	5–20%
Prematurity	
Hyperextension of head	
Intracranial hemorrhage	

*As compared with vertex presentation.

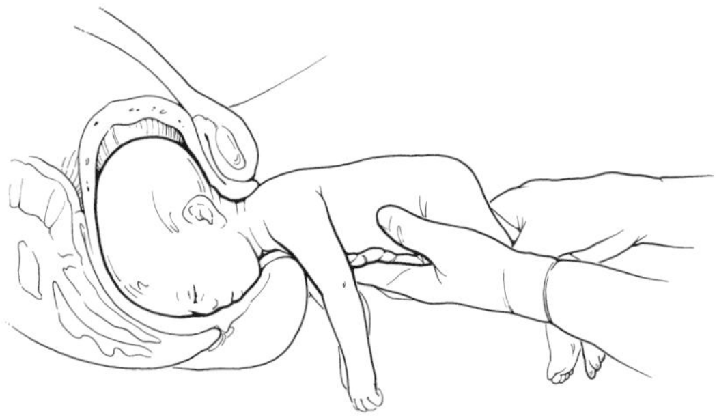

Figure 8–2. Aftercoming head entrapment.

proximately 80% of breech term infants deliver abdominally. Historically, vaginal breech delivery, compared with vertex, had increased maternal morbidity owing to increased incidence of cervical, uterine, or perineal lacerations as well as an increased incidence of infection. Currently, however, vaginal breech delivery occurs successfully in 70 to 84% of selected term patients without increased fetal or maternal morbidity and mortality compared with breech abdominal delivery. Nevertheless, experienced obstetricians, obstetric anesthesiologists, and personnel skilled in neonatal resuscitation are required when vaginal breech delivery is attempted.

External cephalic version attempts conversion of a breech to a vertex presentation. When performed after 37 weeks' gestation in nonlaboring patients, success rates of external cephalic version approximate 50 to 70%. Vaginal delivery after successful version is about 75%. Although anesthesia is not required for external cephalic version, immediate availability of an anesthesiologist is wise during attempted external version. Fetomaternal hemorrhage, placental abruption, or umbilical cord compression may require immediate delivery. Some anesthesiologists and obstetricians believe that regional anesthesia (usually continuous lumbar epidural) may increase the success rate of attempted versions. This is not well documented.

Anesthesia for Labor and Vaginal Delivery

Owing to possible rapid change in fetal status with breech presentation, it is more important than ever to have a reliable large-bore indwelling intravenous catheter placed soon after the gravida's arrival in the labor and delivery suite. Anesthetic equipment and drugs must be immediately available for the induction of general anesthesia. In the authors' institution, this includes the items specified in Table 8–17. At delivery, the gravida should breathe 100% oxygen to facilitate rapid denitrogenation in the event general anesthesia becomes necessary.

Continuous lumbar epidural analgesia offers major advantages and few disadvantages in the laboring patient with breech presentation. Epidural analgesia does not prolong the first stage of labor or increase the need for breech extraction.[19, 20] It provides a comfortable patient who can cooperate for a controlled delivery. A reduced bearing down reflex accompanying regional anesthesia may improve uteroplacental blood flow with subsequent improved fetal condition as evidenced by improved fetal pH during the second stage and Apgar scores of the neonate delivered with maternal epidural anesthesia. Epidural analgesia provides pelvic muscle relaxation and lessens pressure on the fetal head and possibly decreases the likelihood of fetal trauma. The extent of relaxation desired may vary with the institution and specific obstetric anesthesia team. Most importantly, epidural surgical anesthesia can rapidly and safely be obtained in the event of obstetric complication (or fetal distress), avoiding general anesthesia induction risks. For

TABLE 8–17
Anesthesia Equipment and Drugs Prepared in Each Delivery Room

Anesthesia machine with disposable circuit
Face masks (sizes 3, 4, 5, 6)
Short-handled laryngoscope with MacIntosh 3 blade (extra laryngoscope handle and Miller 3 blade also available)
Endotracheal tubes with cuffs checked (sizes 5.5, 6.5, 7.0 inside diameter)
Oral airways
Syringes of
- Thiopental 750 mg or equivalent short-acting barbiturate
- Succinylcholine 100–120 mg

Monitors
- Neuromuscular blockade monitor
- Continuous noninvasive blood pressure
- Electrocardiogram
- Pulse oximeter
- Capnography

Nonparticulate antacid

these reasons, epidural anesthesia plays a role in increasing vaginal breech delivery safety.[21]

The authors usually induce continuous lumbar epidural anesthesia with bupivacaine (0.25%). The addition of a lipid-soluble narcotic (fentanyl 25 to 50 μg, sufentanil 5 to 15 μg, or butorphanol 1 to 2 mg) to the local anesthetic may relieve the profound "rectal pressure" frequently noted by patients with a breech fetus. Dilute bupivacaine infusions (0.0625 to 0.125%) containing fentanyl (1 to 2 μg/ml), sufentanil (0.5 to 1.0 μg/ml), or butorphanol (0.1 to 0.2 mg/ml) may be used to provide continuous analgesia. However, these narcotic dosages all have significant side effects if they are administered into the subarachnoid space. Importantly, butorphanol, in animals, may be toxic if administered in the subarachnoid space. The *epidural* placement of a catheter should be confirmed prior to narcotic drug administration. Use narcotics with caution in the gravida with a premature infant owing to the premature fetus's increased sensitivity to narcotic respiratory depression. Epidural narcotics may transiently alter the FHR tracing by decreasing variability or providing a sinusoidal tracing. Concentrated bupivacaine solutions (0.375 to 0.5%) effectively alleviate rectal pressure but increase perineal muscle motor blockade. Some anesthesiologists advocate delay in "blocking" sacral segments, thus minimizing motor blockade while maintaining effective maternal expulsive efforts. At the authors' institution, it has been found that sacral analgesia with bupivacaine 0.25% or less does not significantly inhibit maternal expulsive efforts yet provides maternal comfort. Carbonated (or pH-adjusted) lidocaine or 2-chloroprocaine may then be used to rapidly produce epidural anesthesia for breech delivery or extraction if necessary.

Spinal anesthesia provides excellent anesthesia for breech extraction. Spinal anesthesia offers the advantages of rapid onset, good perineal relaxation, and minimal fetal drug exposure. Since the U.S. Food and Drug Administration limits microcatheter use to approved investigational protocols, continuous spinal anesthesia for labor requires the use of the larger "epidural" catheters (and the subsequent postdural puncture headache risk). During continuous spinal anesthesia, profound motor block may be a disadvantage, although narcotics can provide analgesia without motor blockade.

Emergency Uterine Relaxation

Full breech extraction requires general anesthesia and uterine relaxation even with adequate "anesthesia" using a regional technique. Profound and complete regional anesthesia does not relax the uterus. Although induction of general anesthesia with the patient in the lithotomy position may increase the risk of maternal aspiration, the emergent nature of the situation may require this technique. Aspiration prophylaxis measures, cricoid pressure, proper patient positioning, and the use of a short-handled laryngoscope are mandatory in this emergency situation. After tracheal intubation, uterine relaxation is obtained with a volatile anesthetic agent (up to 2 MAC as needed). An experienced resuscitation team will support neonatal ventilation, allowing pulmonary elimination of anesthetic gases. Following delivery, the volatile agent should be discontinued and anesthesia maintained with intravenous narcotics and nitrous oxide permitting efficient oxytocin-induced uterine contraction. A succinylcholine infusion (0.1%) or a short-acting nondepolarizing agent will provide appropriate muscle relaxation. Alternative techniques of uterine relaxation such as the use of intravenous nitroglycerin or terbutaline or amyl nitrate inhalation require further investigation before routine use is advocated.

Severe maternal hemorrhage may occur if Dührssen's incisions (multiple radial incisions of the cervix) are made to relieve head entrapment. These incisions often bleed intra-abdominally more than vaginally, producing occult blood loss. Blood for transfusion should be prepared as quickly as possible. Blood replacement should be guided by maternal hemodynamic status or laboratory measurement of maternal hematocrit. Transfusion may require uncrossmatched type-specific or even O-negative universal donor blood.

Anesthesia for Cesarean Delivery

Regional or general anesthesia may be indicated by maternal preference or fetal-maternal well-being. The techniques resemble those for other abdominal deliveries. Meticulous attention to intravenous fluid administration, aspiration prophylaxis, and maintenance of left uterine displacement helps ensure an optimal outcome. The patient with regional anesthesia should breathe 100% oxygen before hysterotomy. Encountering difficulty in delivering the fetus through the uterine incision may require general anesthesia induction (a rare occurrence) to provide uterine relaxation.

MULTIPLE GESTATION

Definitions and Incidence

Twin gestations occur in about 1% of all pregnancies, triplets in 0.01%. Monozygotic fetuses result when a single fertilized ovum splits after a variable number of divisions. The fetuses may or may not have separate amniotic sacs and placentas. Multizygotic fetuses develop from separate fertilized ova; each fetus develops with a separate placenta. Dizygotic multiple gestation is becoming more common with assisted reproductive technology.

Morbidity and Mortality

Offspring of multiple gestations account for 10% of all perinatal mortality, usually secondary to prematurity. Preterm labor occurs in 50% of gravidas with multiple gestation and approximately 35% deliver before 37 weeks of gestation.

Multiple gestation increases maternal morbidity and mortality owing to increased incidence of complications (Table 8–18). Preeclampsia/eclampsia is more severe and occurs earlier in gestation and may occur in multiparas without a hypertensive history. Primary abdominal delivery may occur in as many as 50% of multiple gestations.[22]

Twin pregnancies experience four to six times greater perinatal mortality rates than singleton pregnancies. Fetal and neonatal complications occur more frequently in multiple gestations (Table 8–19). Antepartum death of one twin occurs in 0.5 to 6.8% of twin pregnancies. Subsequent disseminated intravascular coagulation may develop in the gravida or the surviving fetus. Unless the death involved complete placental abruption, disseminated intravascular coagulation usually does not develop in less than a week's time. Recent work[22] contradicts the previously reported greater incidence of acidosis or higher mortality in the second twin (Twin B). The time interval between vaginal delivery of Twin A and that of Twin B does not influence neonatal status. The acid-base status between twins and among triplets is similar.

Mode of delivery is an obstetric decision based primarily on gestational age and presentation. Vaginal delivery is more likely if Twin A is in vertex position. The position of Twin B bears less relevance to the decision about mode of delivery, as external version frequently succeeds when performed after the delivery of Twin A. Although many obstetricians will deliver twins vaginally, few obstetricians deliver three or more infants vaginally.

TABLE 8–18
Obstetric Complications of Multiple Gestations

Premature rupture of membranes
Preterm labor
Prolonged labor
Preeclampsia/eclampsia
Placental abruption
Operative delivery (forceps and abdominal)
Uterine atony
Obstetric trauma
Antepartum or postpartum hemorrhage, or both

TABLE 8–19
Fetal/Neonatal Complications of Multiple Gestations

Congenital anomalies	Intrauterine growth retardation
Hydramnios	Twin-twin transfusion
Cord entanglement	Malpresentation
Umbilical cord prolapse	

Physiologic Implications of Multiple Gestation

Multiple gestation exaggerates the physiologic changes of singleton pregnancy. The increased size of the uterus and its contents, especially near term, further decreases total lung capacity, functional residual capacity, expiratory reserve volume and residual volume. Decreased functional residual capacity allows hypoxemia to develop more rapidly, particularly in the supine parturient.

There is an increased tendency to relative or actual anemia. Maternal blood volume increases about 500 ml more with each additional infant. Cardiovascular changes occur earlier and to a slightly greater extent during multiple gestation. Greater cardiac output increases limit cardiac reserve. The greater combined fetal weight and larger amount of amniotic fluid predispose to aortocaval compression and supine hypotensive syndrome. The larger uterine size may add to lower esophageal sphincter dysfunction, making aspiration pneumonitis a greater hazard. Placental gastrin production increases gastric volume and acidity.

The larger uterine size also predisposes to uterine atony. Postpartum hemorrhage occurs with greater frequency. Large-bore intravenous access is essential. Crossmatched blood for transfusion should be readily available. In the authors' institution a "type and screen" is performed on all patients, allowing crossmatched blood to be available in 20 minutes. The bleeding atonic uterus may require a more concentrated oxytocin solution, methylergonovine maleate, or $PGF_{2\alpha}$, to achieve hemostasis. Since preterm labor is common, many patients requesting labor analgesia or presenting for abdominal delivery will have received tocolytic agents within the previous 12 hours. The implications of tocolytic therapy have already been discussed.

Anesthetic Management of Labor

Epidural anesthesia offers clear benefits. The biochemical status of both twins delivered under epidural anesthesia is superior to that of neonates delivered without epidural anesthesia, especially if the maternal bearing-down reflex is obtunded.[23] Five-minute Apgar scores, need for resuscitation, neonatal death, cerebral irritability, jaundice, and intensive care unit admission are similar between twins delivered with and without epidural anesthesia. The perineal relaxation and maternal cooperation with epidural anesthesia decrease fetal and maternal trauma. Meticulous attention to hydration (500 to 1000 ml immediately prior to regional anesthesia), uterine displacement, and intravenous ephedrine, as necessary, will support uteroplacental perfusion. The authors generally prefer bupivacaine 0.25% to obtain analgesia.

Vaginal Delivery

A resuscitation team for *each* fetus should be informed during labor and immediately available for delivery. Adequate resuscitation equipment must be available for *each* fetus. The anesthesiologist must be alert and prepared. The time between delivery of Twin A and that of Twin B is most likely to present changing obstetric and, therefore, anesthetic needs.

When less concentrated local anesthetic solutions are chosen for labor, a "top-up" with a higher concentration is advisable prior to delivery because of the frequent need for operative delivery. *Abdominal delivery of the second twin is necessary in 4 to 8% of gravidas in whom the first twin was delivered vaginally.* If this occurs, surgical anesthesia can be rapidly obtained in a patient with established epidural analgesia.

Oxygen should be administered to the parturient throughout delivery to maximize fetal well-being and speed denitrogenation, should the induction of general anesthesia become required. As with breech presentations, the relaxed abdominal muscles during epidural analgesia may facilitate external version. However, the upper dermatomal level during epidural anesthesia that produces adequate analgesia and facilitates internal manipulation of the second twin (i.e., version and full breech extraction) does *not* produce uterine relaxation. Thus, internal podalic version followed by a total breech extraction may require induction of general anesthesia despite adequate epidural anesthetic sensory level. Following rapid sequence induction and endotracheal intubation, a potent halogenated inhalational agent effects maximal uterine relaxation. Following delivery, the volatile agent should be discontinued, as hypotension may ensue owing to vasodilatation and blood loss from an atonic uterus. Alternative techniques for uterine relaxation as already discussed under "Emergency Uterine Relaxation" may be considered.

Abdominal Delivery

In this situation, neither regional nor general anesthesia is clearly superior for mother or baby. Improved uterine relaxation with general anesthesia may benefit intrauterine manipulation for delivery of premature fetuses or abnormal presentations. However, a well-conducted spinal or epidural anesthetic, with appropriate measures to prevent or immediately treat hypotension, results in good neonatal outcome at delivery. Elective abdominal delivery may be performed under the anesthetic of choice, considering the patient's desires and medical condition. Epidural anesthesia is perhaps preferable to spinal anesthesia because of the decreased risk of hypotension (slower onset of sympathetic blockade) in the gravida particularly susceptible to aortocaval compression. This becomes more important as the number of infants (and, thus, uterine size) increases. Simultaneous popliteal and brachial blood pressure measurement will allow detection of occult supine hypotension (decreased uterine perfusion owing to aortic compression in the presence of normal maternal brachial blood pressure). The authors usually document the similarity of popliteal and blood pressures at least once before abdominal delivery. Occult supine hypotension becomes more common with three or more fetuses in utero. Particular attention should be paid to administration of oxygen and aspiration prophylaxis in light of the decreased functional residual capacity and increased production of gastrin with multiple gestation. Hypoxemia develops even more rapidly than in the gravida with a single fetus. Epidural, spinal, or general anesthesia induction is otherwise similar to that for the gravida with a singleton gestation.

CONCLUSION

Recognition of the anesthetic considerations in complicated obstetrics allows the anesthesiologist to communicate his or her concerns to the rest of the perinatal care team. Such communication and early preparation help to provide optimal obstetric and anesthetic care of the patient and her infant(s). In addition, advance planning alleviates much of the stress associated with difficult cases.

TEN PRACTICAL POINTS

1. Do not sacrifice maternal safety in the face of "fetal distress."
2. "Fetal distress" does not necessarily preclude regional anesthesia.
3. Utilizing 2-chloroprocaine limits fetal accumulation of local anesthetic.
4. Carefully consider the hazards of large-volume intravenous infusions in patients receiving β-adrenergic agonists.
5. Arterial hypoxemia may be out of proportion to the x-ray changes observed during β agonist–induced pulmonary edema.
6. Intravenous magnesium sulfate potentiates all neuromuscular blocking agents.
7. Prematurity predisposes to head entrapment through an incompletely dilated cervix during attempted vaginal breech delivery.
8. Regional anesthesia does not provide uterine relaxation.
9. During twin vaginal delivery, be prepared for possible emergency abdominal delivery, including performing cesarean section for the second twin.
10. Multiple gestation increases the frequency and severity of aortocaval compression.

References

1. Cohen SE: Inhalation analgesia and anesthesia for vaginal delivery. *In* Shnider SM, Levinson G (eds): Anesthesia for Obstetrics, 2nd ed. Baltimore, Williams & Wilkins, 1987, pp 142–156.
2. American College of Obstetricians and Gynecologists, Committee on Obstetrics: Maternal and Fetal Medicine Opinion No. 104: Anesthesia for Emergency Deliveries. Washington, DC, ACOG, March 1992.
3. Ramanathan J, Ricca DM, Sibai BM, Angel JJ: Epidural vs. general anesthesia in fetal distress with various abnormal fetal heart rate patterns. Anesth Analg 67:S180, 1988.
4. Marx GF, Luykx WM, Cohen S: Fetal-neonatal status following caesarean section for fetal distress. Br J Anaesth 56:1009–1013, 1984.
5. Turnball AC, Tindall VR, Beard RW, et al: Report on confidential enquiries into maternal deaths in England and Wales 1982–1984. Department of Health and Social Security, Reports on Health and Social Subjects #34. London, Her Majesty's Stationery Office, 1989.
6. Samsoon GL, Young JR: Difficult tracheal intubation: A retrospective study. Anaesthesia 42:487–490, 1987.
7. Tomkinson J, Turnball AC, Robson G, et al: Report on confidential enquiries into maternal deaths in England and Wales 1976–1978. London, Her Majesty's Stationery Office, 1982, p 1.
8. Brizgys RV, Dailey PA, Shnider SM, et al: The incidence and neonatal effects of maternal hypotension during epidural anesthesia for cesarean section. Anesthesiology 67:782–786, 1987.
9. Pickering BG, Palahniuk RJ, Cote J, et al: Cerebral vascular response to ketamine and thiopentone during foetal acidosis. Can Anaesth Soc J 29:463–467, 1982.
10. Cheek DBC, Hughes SC, Dailey PA, et al: Effect of halothane on regional cerebral blood flow and cerebral metabolic oxygen consumption in the fetal lamb in utero. Anesthesiology 67:361–366, 1987.

11. Mokriski BLK, Malinow AM: Neonatal acid-base status following general anesthesia with halothane or isoflurane for emergent abdominal delivery. J Clin Anesth 4:97–100, 1992.
12. Pisani J, Rosenow EC: Pulmonary edema associated with tocolytic therapy. Ann Intern Med 110:714–718, 1989.
13. Ramanathan J, Sibai BM, Mabie WC, et al: The use of labetalol for attenuation of the hypertensive response to endotracheal intubation in preeclampsia. Am J Obstet Gynecol 159:650–654, 1988.
14. Eisenach JC, Castro MI: Maternally administered esmolol produces beta-adrenergic blockade and hypoxemia in sheep. Anesthesiology 71:718–722, 1989.
15. Cotton DB, Gonik B, Dorman KF: Cardiovascular alterations in severe pregnancy-induced hypertension: Acute effects of intravenous magnesium sulfate. Am J Obstet Gynecol 148:162–165, 1984.
16. Reves JG, Kissin I, Lell WA, et al: Calcium entry blockers: Uses and implications for anesthesiologists. Anesthesiology 57:504–518, 1982.
17. Dystocia due to abnormalities in presentation, position, or development of the fetus. *In* Cunningham FG, MacDonald PC, Gant NF (eds): Williams Obstetrics, 18th ed. Norwalk, CT: Appleton & Lange, 1988.
18. Seeds JW: Malpresentations. *In* Gabbe SG, Niebyl JR, Simpson JL (eds): Obstetrics: Normal and Problem Pregnancies. Edinburgh, Churchill Livingstone, 1986, p 473.
19. Breeson AJ, Kovacs GT, Pickles BG, Hill JG: Extradural analgesia—The preferred method of analgesia for vaginal breech delivery. Br J Anaesth 50:1227–1230, 1978.
20. Confino E, Ismajovich B, Rudick V, David MP: Extradural analgesia in the management of singleton breech delivery. Br J Anaesth 57:892–895, 1985.
21. Bingham P, Hird V, Lilford RJ: Management of the mature selected breech presentation: An analysis based on the intended method of delivery. Br J Obstet Gynaecol 94:746–752, 1987.
22. Redick LF: Anesthesia for twin delivery. Clin Perinatol 15:107–122, 1988.
23. Crawford JS: A prospective study of 200 consecutive twin deliveries. Anaesthesia 42:33–43, 1987.

NINE

Anesthesia for the Bleeding Obstetric Patient

Medge D. Owen, M.D.

Hemorrhage remains an important obstetric problem despite dramatic decreases in maternal mortality over the last several decades.[1-3] In the United States, bleeding is the leading reported cause of maternal death following ectopic pregnancy and abortion. In live births, bleeding represents the third most common reported cause of death (1.3 deaths per 100,000 live births).[1] Significant bleeding accompanies 3% of pregnancies[4] and occurs more commonly in older parturients, in members of racial minorities, and in patients who are in the third trimester.[1-3] In hospitals performing 300 or fewer annual deliveries,[2] hemorrhage-related maternal deaths are more frequent, perhaps because blood banks at smaller hospitals are not as well equipped to manage severe hemorrhage.[3]

This chapter provides an overview for treating hemorrhage, identifies the major causes of obstetric hemorrhage (Table 9–1), and discusses appropriate anesthetic management.

PHYSIOLOGIC CHANGES IN THE BLEEDING PARTURIENT

Pregnancy-related bleeding arises from the placental implantation site, from disrupted blood vessels in the uterus and birth canal, or secondary to inadequate surgical hemostasis. Uterine involution usually controls bleeding from the placental site. Bleeding normally initiates a series of reactions that leads to stable fibrin clot formation and bleeding cessation. Most coagulation factors increase during pregnancy, offering some protection against hemorrhage (Table 9–2). In fact, fibrinogen levels within the normal nonpregnant range represent a disease state in pregnancy. The platelet count is unaltered in normal pregnancy, remaining between 150,000 and 300,000/mm^3. Values for coagulation tests also remain unchanged compared with those of nonpregnant women.

Many pregnancy-related physiologic changes help prepare the parturient for blood loss at delivery. The 35 to 50% increase in blood volume and the 500-ml "autotransfusion" from uterine involution following placental expulsion easily compensate for the reported 500- to 1000-ml blood loss accompanying vaginal birth and

TABLE 9–1
Causes of Obstetric Hemorrhage

Incomplete or missed abortion
Advanced ectopic pregnancy
Placenta previa
Abruptio placentae
Placenta accreta/increta/percreta
Uterine rupture
Uterine atony
Cervical or vaginal lacerations
Retained placenta
Uterine inversion
Coagulopathy

TABLE 9-2
Coagulation Factors and Inhibitors During Normal Pregnancy

Factor	Nonpregnant	Late Pregnancy
Factor I (Fibrinogen)	200–450 mg/dl	400–650 mg/dl
Factor II (Prothrombin)	75–125%	100–125%
Factor V	75–125%	100–150%
Factor VII	75–125%	150–250%
Factor VIII	75–150%	200–500%
Factor IX	75–125%	100–150%
Factor X	75–125%	150–250%
Factor XI	75–125%	50–100%
Factor XII	75–125%	100–200%
Factor XIII	75–125%	35–75%
Antithrombin III	85–110%	75–100%
Antifactor Xa	85–110%	75–100%

From Hathaway WE, Bonnar J: Coagulation in pregnancy. *In* Hathaway WE, Bonnar J (eds): Perinatal Coagulation. New York, Grune & Stratton, 1978.

cesarean section.[5, 6] During bleeding, increased renin, antidiuretic hormone, and catecholamines also help maintain plasma volume, cardiac output, and perfusion pressure.[7] In pregnancy, therefore, vital signs may appear stable despite blood loss that would be symptomatic in nonpregnant patients. Hypotension and tachycardia are usually late indicators of blood loss in healthy parturients. Furthermore, bleeding can be concealed within the uterus, making estimation difficult.[8] Enlarging uterine size may be the only clue to continuing blood loss. When acute losses approach 30 to 50% (1500 to 2500 ml), clinical signs of bleeding appear (pallor, decreased urine output, hypotension, tachycardia), and untreated losses exceeding 50% of blood volume can lead to irreversible shock and death.[9] One must, therefore, have a high index of suspicion for bleeding and a low threshold for fluid resuscitation prior to clinical deterioration. It is easier to prevent hypovolemic shock than to treat it.

The safe limit for anemia in pregnancy is unknown. Historically, a hemoglobin below 10 gm/dl (hematocrit below 30%) indicated the need for blood transfusion in surgical patients. With the growing risk of hepatitis and acquired immunodeficiency syndrome (AIDS), transfusion practices have become more conservative, even in the obstetric population. Between 1976 and 1986, Klapholz documented a decrease in obstetric transfusion rates, from 4.6 to 1.9%.[10] Healthy, nonpregnant patients with normal cardiac function tolerate hematocrits of 20% or below if volume resuscitation is adequate.[11, 12] The safe limit for anemia in pregnancy, however, may differ from that in nonpregnancy for several reasons. Pregnant patients have increased metabolic demands (oxygen-consuming placenta/fetus) and a decreased oxygen content ("anemia" of pregnancy), but compensatory mechanisms help offset the risks of tissue oxygen deprivation. For instance, hyperventilation in pregnancy results in arterial oxygen tensions averaging 103 mmHg. Increased cardiac output, vasodilatation, and hemodilution increase blood flow to target organs. Furthermore, the maternal oxyhemoglobin dissociation curve is shifted right, increasing tissue oxygen availability.[5] Because the lowest safe hemoglobin concentration in pregnancy is unknown and may vary with individual circumstances, one must transfuse according to good clinical judgment. For example, if the patient demonstrates signs of hypovolemia despite volume resuscitation, or the fetus displays evidence of uteroplacental insufficiency in the face of ongoing bleeding, transfusion is probably warranted. With adequate hemostasis, however, low hemoglobins may be well tolerated without transfusion, especially in the postpartum period as the physiologic stresses of pregnancy subside. Postoperative hemoglobins in the 6 to 8 mg/dl range appear safe for patients without cardiovascular disease.[13]

TREATMENT MODALITIES

Fluid Replacement

Infusion Techniques

If a patient demonstrates signs of hypovolemia and is facing further significant blood losses, aggressive intravenous fluid resuscitation is imperative to maintain tissue perfusion and oxygenation. Rapid fluid infusion is more important than the choice of fluid or immediate hemodynamic monitoring.[14] Obstetric patients do not die from receiving the wrong fluid, but they do die because they do not receive enough of any fluid to prevent irreversible shock and organ damage. Every parturient should routinely have a 16- to 18-gauge intravenous catheter placed. A larger or additional cannula should be inserted if known risks for hemorrhage are present. Intravenous cannula size greatly affects the rate of fluid administration (Fig. 9–1).

Infusion Solutions

Blood is initially replaced with crystalloid or colloid until losses approach 30% (approximately 1500 ml). Blood administration should be considered if the patient or fetus becomes symptomatic or bleeding is likely to continue. The author's group does not routinely transfuse anemic parturients if they are isovolemic and lack signs of fetal stress. Debate continues as to whether colloids or crystalloids are better for maintaining intravascular volume prior to red cell replacement. Because crystalloids redistribute extravascularly, the infused amount should be three times the volume lost. However, redistribution is not immediate, and appropriate resuscitative volumes of crystalloid probably do not increase the likelihood of pulmonary edema in healthy patients owing to the diuresis that normally follows delivery.[15] Furthermore, hemorrhage creates an extracellular fluid deficit by shifting interstitial fluid into the depleted blood vessels, making crystalloid replacement important. It probably makes little difference which solution is initiated, provided quick action is taken to establish fluid replacement.

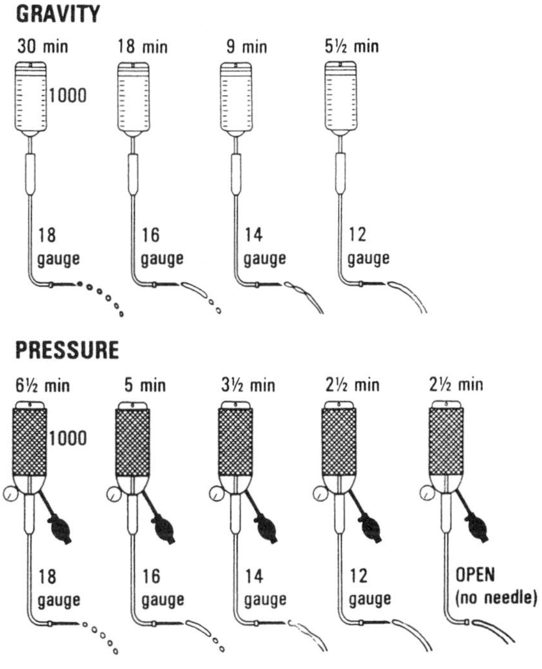

Figure 9–1. Intravenous cannula size affects the rate of fluid administration. The approximate times to infuse 1 L of fluid through various cannulas are shown. The fluids in the upper group infuse by gravity alone; the fluids in the lower group infuse under 300 mmHg constant pressure. Internal diameters of cannulas vary among manufacturers, even for identical gauge; the infusion rate rises with larger diameter and falls with longer length. (From Plumer MH: Bleeding problems. *In* James FM, Wheeler AS, Dewan DM [eds]: Obstetric Anesthesia: The Complicated Patient, 2nd ed. Philadelphia, FA Davis, 1988, pp 309–344.)

Crystalloid Solutions

Crystalloids, or balanced salt solutions, are composed of water and salts that approximate the composition of body fluids. Crystalloids are inexpensive, easy to store, sterile, and noninfectious, but they readily leave the vascular space and do not provide oxygen-carrying or hemostatic capacity. Both lactated Ringer's and normal saline solution are used for resuscitation. Normal saline solution is recommended for administration with blood products because lactated Ringer's solution, containing calcium, chelates the anticoagulant citrate preservative in stored blood, causing clot formation.

Colloid Solutions

Colloids are large molecules that pass poorly through undamaged capillaries, and although they lack hemostatic and oxygen-carrying capacity, they increase colloidal osmotic pressure and pull interstitial fluid into the intravascular compartment. Colloids, like crystalloids, are sterile, easy to store, and noninfectious, but they cost more than crystalloids. Albumin and hydroxyethyl starch are the most widely used colloid solutions.

Albumin. Albumin, available in a 5% or 25% solution, is prepared from pooled human plasma. Heat treatment eliminates the risk of infectious disease. Albumin 25% expands intravascular volume less effectively than albumin 5% since it contains less fluid volume than the more dilute solution. Furthermore, fluid drawn from the interstitial space by the concentrated

25% solution may worsen an extracellular volume deficit.[14]

Hydroxyethyl Starch. Six percent hydroxyethyl starch (hetastarch, Hespan) is a synthetic molecule resembling glycogen. Hetastarch replaces blood in a 1:1 ratio and functions as effectively as albumin for volume expansion, but it costs less and lasts longer than albumin. If hetastarch infusions exceed 20 mg/kg/24 hours, coagulopathy can occur from hemodilution, poor platelet adhesion, and decreased Factor VIII.[16, 17] Hetastarch also interferes with blood typing if blood samples contain more than 30% starch.[18] It is prudent to limit hetastarch administration to 1000 to 1500 ml in an acute setting and thereafter transfuse crystalloids or blood products if warranted.

Blood and Component Therapy

Conditions most often associated with blood transfusion are uterine atony, placenta previa, retained placental tissue, abruptio placentae, and coagulopathy secondary to hemolysis, elevated liver enzymes, and low platelets (HELLP) syndrome.[19] Procedures most associated with transfusion include emergency cesarean hysterectomy, vacuum extraction, and forceps delivery. In one study, even uncomplicated cesarean and vaginal deliveries required blood transfusions in 1.4% and 0.4% of cases, respectively.[19] Although preexisting antepartum conditions predict less than 25% of patients requiring blood products,[19] obtaining a type and screen routinely on *all* parturients is probably not cost-effective. A type and screen is appropriate for patients undergoing cesarean section. Patients with higher transfusion risks (planned cesarean hysterectomy, cesarean section for placenta previa after previous cesarean delivery) require a crossmatch.

When a transfusion is required, type-specific, crossmatched blood should be administered. Even in an emergency when crossmatched blood is not yet available, it is better to give type-specific uncrossmatched blood than O-negative blood. Patients needing immediate transfusion can usually be stabilized with crystalloid or colloid solutions while typing (ABO and Rh) is performed. If O-negative blood is needed (rare), packed red blood cells (PRBCs) are preferable to whole blood because PRBCs contain less plasma and therefore fewer anti-A and anti-B antibodies that may be detrimental to a patient with A, B, or AB blood (55% of the population). Once two units of O-negative blood are transfused to a patient with non–group O blood, hemolysis can result from subsequent administration of type-specific blood.[20] The blood bank should determine when the transfused anti-A and anti-B antibody titers have fallen, allowing safe administration of type-specific blood.

Whole Blood

Although whole blood is expensive and capable of transmitting diseases, it is indispensable in treating acute massive hemorrhage. The American Association of Blood Banks recommends whole blood administration for acute 25% or greater blood volume loss.[20] Only whole blood replaces all the functions of lost blood because it possesses both oxygen-carrying and hemostatic capacity. Five hundred milliliters of whole blood has a 35 to 40% hematocrit and, initially, normal levels of clotting factors and platelets. Clotting Factors V and VIII, the "labile factors," may decrease by 50% within 1 week of storage, but routine transfusion rarely results in coagulopathy because less than 30% of these factors are needed for hemostasis.[20] Whole blood also lacks functioning platelets after 48 hours of storage, but as discussed later in this chapter, this is *not* an indication to routinely coadminister platelets during massive transfusion. Always administer blood through a standard blood filter and blood warmer.

Blood Component Therapy

Using blood components improves blood product availability, decreases the amount of plasma transfused (containing antigens or antibodies), and allows patients to receive specifically what they lack. Blood components, however, can be used inappropriately. For example, platelets and fresh frozen plasma (FFP) are often transfused prophylactically during massive hemorrhage, but this practice *does not* reduce subsequent transfusion and does increase cost and doubles the infection risk.[21] Acutely bleeding patients, irrespective of the amount of blood transfused, should not receive hemostatic components unless generalized bleeding from nonsurgical sites (microvascular bleeding) develops.

Packed Red Blood Cells

When plasma (containing platelets and coagulation factors) is separated from whole blood, PRBCs remain. PRBCs treat anemia unassociated with severe hemorrhage (when plasma volume is normal), with the goal of increasing oxygen-carrying capacity, not volume. However, when whole blood is indicated but not available, PRBC and crystalloid coadministration are equally efficacious for volume replacement. One 250- to 300-ml unit of PRBCs with a 70 to 80% hematocrit increases hemoglobin by 1 gm/dl and hematocrit by 3% in adults. Diluting PRBCs with normal saline solution facilitates infusion and minimizes hemolysis.

Platelets

Platelets are indicated for acute thrombocytopenia associated *with* microvascular bleeding. A patient with a platelet count higher than $50{,}000/mm^3$ will probably not benefit from a platelet transfusion, if thrombocytopenia is the sole abnormality.[22] Although dilutional thrombocytopenia is the most frequent cause of transfusion-related coagulopathy, platelets should not be given to treat laboratory abnormalities unless bleeding is present.[20] The majority of patients who receive rapid one to two blood volume transfusions *do not* develop microvascular bleeding and therefore should not receive prophylactic platelets.[22] One unit of platelets (50 ml) increases the platelet count by 7000 to $10{,}000/mm^3$. Platelets may be ABO compatible but often come from multiple donors and are not type-specific. Type-specific platelets minimize the risk of immune-mediated transfusion reactions if red cells are present. Transfusion risks include antigen-antibody reactions and infectious disease.

Fresh Frozen Plasma

FFP is the fluid (minus the platelets and blood cells) from a unit of whole blood frozen within 6 hours of collection that contains all coagulation factors. Transfusion risks include infectious disease transmission and allergic reactions. FFP, 10 to 15 ml/kg, is indicated during massive transfusion when uncontrolled surgical bleeding exists with a prolonged partial thromboplastin time (PTT) and a platelet count *above* $70{,}000/mm^3$.[23] FFP also treats isolated coagulation factor deficiencies and coumarin-induced coagulopathies prior to emergency surgery (unlikely in the obstetric population, since coumarin may cause birth defects). Again, prophylactic FFP administration does not reduce blood transfusion requirements and is rarely indicated.

Cryoprecipitate

Cryoprecipitate is the fraction of plasma that precipitates when FFP is thawed and contains high quantities of Factor VIII and fibrinogen. Cryoprecipitate is reserved to treat hemophilia A and Factor VIII deficiency when commercial preparations are unavailable; it is rarely indicated in obstetric anesthesia.

Pharmacologic Control of Hemorrhage

Oxytocin

Oxytocin, a uterine smooth muscle constrictor, is widely used to induce or augment labor and to control postpartum uterine bleeding. Other properties include vascular dilatation, which increases renal, coronary, and cerebral blood flow. Oxytocin's inherent antidiuretic effect may cause water intoxication and convulsions, but only if large doses (40 to 50 mU/minute) are inappropriately infused over time in combination with free water.[24] Oxytocin, administered by intramuscular or continuous infusion (the plasma half-life is only 3 to 5 minutes), produces prompt uterine contraction. Large, undiluted intravenous boluses may cause transient hypotension and reflex tachycardia, but oxytocin, in the usual dosage, should never be withheld for this concern even if rapid infusions are required. The usual dose is 10 to 20 units (1 to 2 ml) in 1000 ml of crystalloid, but more (up to 80 units in 1000 ml) may be given in extreme circumstances.

Methylergonovine

Methylergonovine (Methergine) treats postpartum and postabortion hemorrhage refractory to oxytocin. As a potent constrictor of uterine and vascular smooth muscle, methylergonovine produces uterine contraction and elevates blood pressure. When given methylergonovine, preeclamptic or hypertensive patients are predisposed to headache, arrhythmias, seizures, and cerebrovascular accidents (although these complications may occur in any patient). Nausea and vomiting are also common. Methylergonovine is usually administered intramuscularly; however, up to 60% may be absorbed after oral administration.[24] Undiluted, intravenous injection produces intense vasoconstriction, potentially causing peripheral ischemia, gangrene, and coronary ischemia. For this reason, the author's group does not administer intravenous methylergonovine. The intramuscular dose is 0.2 mg (1 ml), which may be repeated every 2 to 4 hours up to five doses. Effects usually occur within 2 to 5 minutes.

Prostaglandin $F_{2\alpha}$

Prostaglandin $F_{2\alpha}$ ($PGF_{2\alpha}$; Hemabate) is used to induce second trimester abortion and to control severe postpartum hemorrhage. Synthesized by the gravid uterus, $PGF_{2\alpha}$ may help initiate normal labor. $PGF_{2\alpha}$ constricts uterine, vascular, gastrointestinal, and bronchial smooth muscle, producing uterine contraction, hypertension, nausea, vomiting, diarrhea, and bronchoconstriction. Therefore, extreme caution must govern administration in asthmatic and hypertensive patients. Transient fever also occurs, which may be confused with postpartum infection. $PGF_{2\alpha}$ 0.25 mg (1 ml) is given by intramuscular or interuterine injection. Intrauterine administration has produced sudden, marked ventilation-perfusion mismatch and severe hypoxemia in women undergoing cesarean section with general anesthesia.[25] Although the hypoxemia is transient, intubation and ventilatory support may be required postoperatively. The drug may be readministered every 90 minutes, not to exceed eight doses (2.0 mg), but one dose often suffices.

Surgical Control of Hemorrhage

Delivery

Mild antepartum or intrapartum bleeding associated with normal labor, marginal placenta previa, or abruptio placentae is often treated by vaginal delivery rather than cesarean section or drug therapy. The rate of bleeding relative to the progress of labor often determines the route of delivery.

Hypogastric Artery Ligation

If pharmacologic measures fail to control postpartum hemorrhage, hypogastric artery ligation may be attempted. Hypogastric (internal iliac) artery ligation reduces pulsatile blood flow to the uterus and vagina allowing hemostasis, provided an intact clotting mechanism exists. Alternatively, uterine artery ligation stops uterine but not vaginal hemorrhage. Although these procedures are useful to attempt, success is limited. In one series, none of 19 attempted bilateral uterine artery and none of 9 attempted bilateral hypogastric artery ligations were successful, and hysterectomy was ultimately performed to control hemorrhage.[26]

Cesarean Hysterectomy

Hysterectomy definitively treats postpartum hemorrhage refractory to more conservative measures. Placenta previa and accreta are the most common conditions necessitating emergency obstetric hysterectomy. Uterine atony and rupture are other common indications.[27] Elective obstetric hysterectomies occur for carcinoma, uterine myomata, and dysmenorrheal menorrhagia.

Significant differences exist between planned and emergency obstetric hysterectomies. Women receiving emergency hysterectomy experience greater intraoperative blood losses and crystalloid replacement and are more likely to develop intraoperative hypotension and receive donor blood than women undergoing elective surgery.[27] In emergencies, the mean estimated blood loss is 2000 to 5000 ml and 86 to 96% of patients will require blood transfusions.[26, 27]

ANESTHETIC APPROACH TO THE BLEEDING OBSTETRIC PATIENT

Monitored Anesthesia Care

Vaginal or cervical lacerations and retained placenta commonly obligate exploration of the birth canal and uterus. Nitrous oxide or intravenous sedation, or both, facilitate examination, but these should be administered judiciously only in the presence of emergency airway equipment, since anesthesia requirements, already reduced in pregnancy, may be further lowered if bleeding and hypovolemia coexist. Nitrous oxide, 50 to 70% in oxygen, can be administered by mask for analgesia. Hemodynamic depression is unlikely during this technique, but patients need close observation for excess sedation, which, fortunately, is rapidly reversed by increasing the inhaled oxygen concentration. Small intravenous doses of midazolam (1 to 2 mg), ketamine (10 to 20 mg; maximum 1 mg/kg in divided doses), fentanyl (50 to 100 μg), or morphine (5 to 10 mg) may also be slowly titrated to the desired effect. The goal is light sedation and analgesia without loss of consciousness or airway reflexes. Remember, sedation does not produce anesthesia; therefore, local infiltration or pudendal block may be necessary for birth canal exploration or repair.

Regional Anesthesia

The use of regional anesthesia in bleeding patients is controversial. If hypovolemia exists, regional anesthesia is contraindicated because the associated sympathectomy can produce severe, intractable hypotension. With minimal bleeding, regional anesthesia may be safely conducted, provided normovolemia exists prior to block establishment. Normovolemic patients at risk for bleeding (placenta previa, previous cesarean section) may receive regional anesthesia in preparation for either vaginal or operative delivery, provided the anesthesia caregiver is adequately prepared to treat ongoing blood losses. In this situation, the quality of intravenous access is more important than the choice of anesthesia. If an epidural has been used for labor or cesarean section, the catheter should always remain in place until the patient is discharged from the labor floor or recovery room. When a postpartum condition warrants operative intervention, a preexisting catheter may be redosed quickly to provide surgical anesthesia.

General Anesthesia

For uncontrolled antepartum hemorrhage, the anesthetic approach is similar regardless of the cause of the bleeding (Table 9–3). Emergency cesarean section with general anesthesia is usually indicated for hypovolemic, hemodynamically unstable patients. A brief history quickly determines drug allergies, medications, and medical or previous anesthetic problems. The physical examination should focus on vital signs, evaluation of the airway, and blood loss. Laboratory test results should not delay surgery. As soon as possible, however, hemoglobin, hematocrit, platelets, prothrombin time (PT), PTT, fibrinogen, fibrin degradation products (FDP), and type and crossmatch should be obtained.

Aggressive intravenous fluid resuscitation is key in preventing hypovolemic shock. If intravenous access is not present, at least two large-bore (14- or 16-gauge) catheters should be established quickly. Central venous pressure catheters and arterial lines can help guide intraoperative and postoperative fluid management, but placement should not delay surgery. In the author's practice, a pulmonary artery catheter is rarely indicated. Vasopressors should be titrated to maintain blood pressure and adequate organ and uterine perfusion. Although ephedrine is the vasopressor of choice in the pregnant patient, phenylephrine or epinephrine should not be withheld if warranted, despite the fetal risks.

As with all cesarean sections, preparation for general anesthesia induction includes a nonparticulate oral antacid, maintenance of left uterine displacement, and denitrogenation with oxygen. If the airway appears suitable for uncomplicated endotracheal intubation, a rapid-sequence induction with cricoid pressure should be performed. If difficult endotracheal intubation is predicted, an awake intubation should be conducted regardless of bleeding or fetal distress.

The most appropriate induction agent depends on the clinical situation. Thiopental 3 to 4 mg/kg, the induction agent most commonly used in obstetrics, can potentiate hypotension and produce myocardial depression. Ketamine 0.5 to 1.0 mg/kg may be preferable in the bleeding patient, as it increases blood pressure, heart rate, and cardiac output by catecholamine release. In patients with maximal sympathetic nervous system stress and catecholamine depletion, even ketamine can cause hypotension by direct myocardial depression. Etomidate 0.2 mg/kg is another alternative that produces min-

TABLE 9–3
General Anesthesia for Emergency Laparotomy in the Bleeding Parturient

Preoperative
Brief history and physical examination
Intravenous fluid resuscitation—two large-bore IV catheters (14-g–16-g)
Laboratory studies—CBC, type and crossmatch, coagulation studies, DIC profile
Preinduction
Nonparticulate oral antacid
Left uterine displacement
Preoxygenation/denitrogenation
Induction
Rapid-sequence induction and intubation with cricoid pressure
Induction agents
Thiopental up to 3–4 mg/kg + succinylcholine 1–2 mg/kg
Ketamine 0.5–1 mg/kg + succinylcholine 1–2 mg/kg
Etomidate 0.2 mg/kg + succinylcholine 1–2 mg/kg
Maintenance
Predelivery
100% O_2
Muscle relaxant as needed
Volatile anesthetic as tolerated
Postdelivery
Nitrous/narcotic or volatile anesthetic
Muscle relaxant as needed
Emergence
Extubate awake after gastric suctioning and 100% O_2
Consider intubation/mechanical ventilation if major surgery with multiple transfusion

Abbreviations: IV = intravenous; CBC = complete blood count; DIC = disseminated intravascular coagulation.

imal hemodynamic change. Disadvantages include myoclonus, transient burning at the injection site, and adrenocortical suppression, but these do not contraindicate using etomidate in an unstable patient. Unconscious patients (rare) require only muscle relaxation. Succinylcholine 1 to 2 mg/kg is the preferred muscle relaxant to facilitate endotracheal intubation. After the endotracheal tube is correctly placed, 100% oxygen should be continued and low concentrations of halogenated agents should be titrated as tolerated. After delivery, a nitrous/narcotic technique may be employed. Following massive blood transfusion and fluid administration, consider leaving the patient intubated postoperatively until she is hemodynamically stable.

In contrast to antepartum bleeding, general anesthesia for postpartum bleeding varies with the cause of the bleeding. General anesthesia for laceration repair or retained placenta is usually of short duration in patients who have had only mild to moderate blood losses and adequate fluid resuscitation. Women requiring laparotomy for ruptured ectopic pregnancy, uterine artery ligation, or repair or removal of a ruptured or atonic uterus usually have significant hemorrhage and may be hemodynamically unstable. Expect longer surgical duration and continued intraoperative blood losses. The intravascular fluids and anesthetic agents must be tailored to each clinical situation.

ANTEPARTUM AND INTRAPARTUM HEMORRHAGE

Incomplete Abortion

Ten percent or more of pregnancies end in spontaneous abortion.[28] Fetal and placental abnormalities most commonly cause fetal death, but maternal systemic disease and reproductive tract deformities are other contributing factors.[28] With bleeding or retained fetal products, the uterus is surgically emptied by cervical dilatation and curettage (D&C), usually an outpatient procedure. Complications include uterine perforation, cervical lacerations, hemorrhage, incomplete tissue removal, and infection.[29]

Preoperative laboratory tests including hemoglobin, hematocrit, and type and screen are *not* required at the author's institution unless the patient is actively bleeding. Coagulation studies are performed if clinical signs of coagulopathy exist and for gestations beyond the second trimester (especially if fetal demise exceeds 2 weeks).[30, 31] Bleeding quantification is often by patient report, making appropriate preoperative fluid replacement difficult. Hemodynamically stable patients usually receive up to 1 L of crystalloid solution preoperatively and tolerate surgery well. Premedicating with fentanyl (50 to 100 μg) or midazolam (1 to 2 mg) may help reduce pain and anxiety, and as with all pregnant patients, intravenous metoclopramide or oral nonparticulate antacids should be administered within 30 minutes of surgery.

D&C may be performed utilizing paracervical block, regional anesthesia, or general anesthesia. Mask general anesthesia may be conducted, but for gestations beyond 12 weeks, recent oral intake, or obesity, this technique is inadvisable and endotracheal intubation should be employed. Oxytocin (10 to 20 U), administered by continuous intravenous infusion, reduces bleeding after tissue removal. For regional techniques, short-acting spinal (1.5 to 5% lidocaine) or epidural agents (3% chloroprocaine) are appropriate but may prolong recovery room time because patients should demonstrate full motor and sensory function before discharge.

Ectopic Pregnancy

Since the mid 1970s, the number of reported ectopic pregnancies has quadrupled from 17,800 to approximately 88,000.[32] This dramatic increase is probably due to improved treatment of pelvic inflammatory disease (which would have rendered patients sterile in the past), failed elective sterilization, and intrauterine device usage.[33] Ectopic pregnancy, or nonuterine ovum implantation, usually occurs in the fallopian tube.[34] Abdominal pain, a consistent finding, is often without vaginal bleeding. If vaginal bleeding occurs, the diagnosis may be confused with spontaneous abortion. Tubal rupture, a surgical emergency, produces intra-abdominal bleeding, distention, and shock. Diagnostic aids include pregnancy tests, ultrasound, culdocentesis, laparoscopy, and laparotomy.

Ruptured tubal pregnancies mandate fluid resuscitation and immediate surgery. Some surgeons initially attempt laparoscopy, but bleeding often impedes visualization, necessitating laparotomy. Regional anesthesia is contraindicated with hypovolemia; therefore, general anesthesia is usually performed, adhering to the guidelines mentioned previously.

Diagnostic laparoscopy is often conducted in hemodynamically stable patients having suspected, but nonruptured, ectopic pregnancies. Regional anesthesia is possible for laparoscopy, but the pneumoperitoneum, steep Trendelenburg position, and prolonged surgical length may be intolerable despite adequate anesthetic levels. Pneumoperitoneum, produced by insufflating carbon dioxide (the most frequently used gas), can also irritate the peritoneum and cause hypercarbia, since carbon dioxide is rapidly absorbed from the peritoneal cavity. Controlled ventilation and end-tidal carbon dioxide monitoring may help prevent hypercarbia, which can trigger endogenous catecholamine release, hypertension, and cardiac arrhythmias. With pneumoperitoneum, intra-abdominal pressures exceeding 20 cmH_2O decrease cardiac output and functional residual capacity; consequently, hypotension, ventilation-perfusion mismatching, and hypoxia may result.[29] Other complications include gas embolism, tension pneumothorax, pneumomediastinum, visceral perforation, and hemorrhage.

When diagnostic laparoscopy is performed with regional anesthesia, the author's group insufflates nitrous oxide instead of carbon dioxide to facilitate patient comfort. Because nitrous oxide is combustible, a bipolar cautery electrode must be utilized to prevent intra-abdominal nitrous oxide ignition, which may occur with a unipolar electrode.

Laparoscopy is frequently an outpatient procedure; therefore, administration of barbiturates, benzodiazepines, and narcotics should be minimized. Patients should not exhibit severe pain, nausea, or sedation on discharge.

Placenta Previa

Once in 200 pregnancies,[4] placental implantation occurs in the lower uterine segment, partially or completely covering the cervical os (Fig. 9–2). The painless vaginal bleeding, maternal in origin, results from placental separation during cervical dilatation and lower uterine segment lengthening in late pregnancy. Risk factors include increased maternal age, parity, and uterine scarring. After four or more cesarean sections, 1 in 10 women subsequently has placenta previa![35] Third trimester ultrasound, safe and highly diagnostic, now replaces the "double setup" cervical examination, which occasionally produced uncontrolled vaginal bleeding requiring emergency cesarean section.

Management depends on the previa type and bleeding. Total or significant partial placenta previa mandates cesarean section, since vaginal delivery guarantees hemorrhage. In marginal placenta previa, vaginal birth is possible at the obstetrician's discretion. Regardless of which previa type is present, antepartum bleeding is unpredictable during pregnancy. If bleeding resolves, the patient is volume resuscitated and usually remains at hospital bed rest until fetal lung maturity develops. Regional anesthesia may then safely accompany vaginal or cesarean delivery, given limited bleeding and stable maternal hemodynamics. Subarachnoid or continuous epidural anesthesia is appropriate for primary cesarean section in the hemodynamically stable patient. For repeat cesarean section combined with placenta previa, the chance of placenta accreta and cesarean hysterectomy increases, making epidural anesthesia preferable (catheter is present for redosing). In contrast, for severe uncontrolled hemorrhage, regardless of gestational age, emergency cesarean section under general anesthesia is the best treatment.

During uterine incision, a surgically lacerated anterior placenta may bleed briskly prior to delivery, which, if prolonged, may compromise the fetus. Placental bleeding stops with uteroplacental separation, but uterine bleeding may continue because the lower uterine segment has little smooth muscle and, therefore, poor contractile capacity.

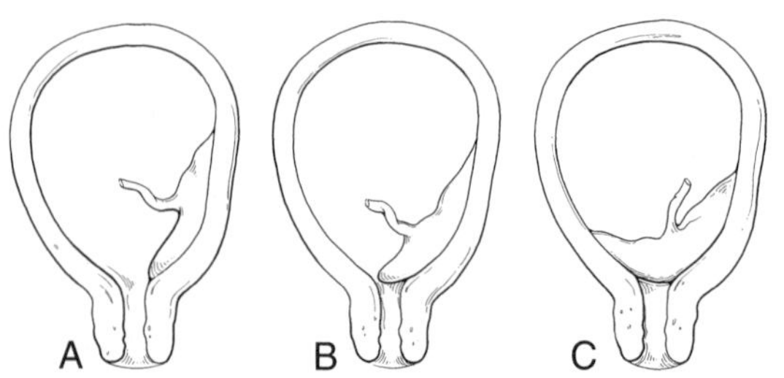

Figure 9–2. Placenta previa. *A*, Marginal. *B*, Partial. *C*, Total.

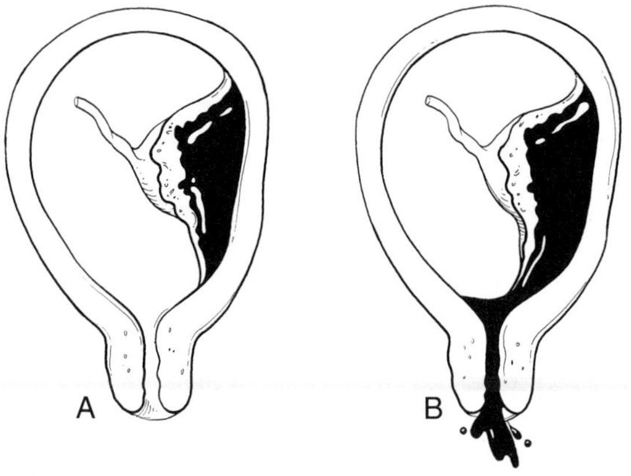

Figure 9–3. Abruptio placentae. *A*, Internal or concealed hemorrhage. *B*, External hemorrhage. (Redrawn from Bonica JJ, Johnson WL: Placenta praevia, abruptio placentae or rupture of the uterus. *In* Bonica JJ [ed]: Principles and Practice of Obstetric Analgesia and Anesthesia, Vol 2. Philadelphia, FA Davis, 1969, p 1166.)

Abruptio Placentae

Abruptio placentae, accompanying 1 or 2 in 100 pregnancies,[4, 36] is premature uteroplacental separation that occurs antepartum or intrapartum (Fig. 9–3). Ninety percent of abruptios are mild to moderate and 10% are severe.[4] In severe cases, when placental detachments exceed 50%, maternal mortality is 1 to 3%, and fetal mortality approaches 50%, making rapid action imperative.[4, 36] Classically, patients have severe abdominal pain, hypertension, uterine hypertonus, and fetal distress, with or without vaginal bleeding. Severe abruptios may lead to hypotension, shock, renal failure, and disseminated intravascular coagulation (DIC). In contrast to placenta previa, bleeding from abruptio may be concealed within the uterus (up to 6 L) and is often underestimated.[36] Risk factors include hypertension, smoking, cocaine abuse, multiparity, advanced maternal age, uterine abnormalities, previous abruptio, abdominal trauma, and premature rupture of membranes.

Treatment varies with abruptio size, gestational age, fetal distress, cervical dilatation, hemodynamic status, and coagulopathy. Ultrasound examination can detect the abruptio location and size, but retroplacental clots may be missed. Mild abruptios are managed expectantly until fetal lung maturity or distress develops. Vaginal delivery, guided by continuous fetal monitoring, may occur rapidly because increased uterine tone accompanies abruptio placentae. Epidural labor analgesia is safe provided maternal hypovolemia and coagulopathy are absent. Platelet counts below 100,000/mm^3 or prolonged PT/PTT contraindicate regional anesthesia. Beware of performing regional anesthesia for cesarean section in patients with severe abruptio placentae. Patients initially having hypertension, tetanic uterine contractions, and pain may suddenly bleed and decompensate following uterine incision because the uterine tamponade is released. Abruptio is also associated with uterine atony and postpartum hemorrhage. If elevated fibrin degradation products (FDP) exist, bleeding may be exacerbated because FDP cause uterine relaxation and can inhibit the action of oxytocin.[36]

Severe abruptios, regardless of fetal viability, are obstetric emergencies that often require cesarean section under general anesthesia. Laboratory work (complete blood count, type and crossmatch, PT, PTT, fibrinogen, FDP) should not delay surgery, but should be obtained as soon as possible. A bedside clot tube (red top) may detect a coagulopathy if blood does not clot within 6 minutes or is lysed within 1 hour of collection.[37]

Placenta Accreta/Increta/Percreta

Placenta accreta, increta, and percreta are conditions of abnormal placentation that make normal uteroplacental separation virtually impossible. In placenta accreta (Fig. 9–4), the placenta incorrectly adheres to the myometrium, whereas in placenta increta, myometrial invasion occurs. Placenta percreta penetrates the uterus into the surrounding abdominal cavity. The abnormal attachment may involve part or all of the placenta. Risk factors include placenta previa and previous cesarean section. Clark and coworkers found a 24% chance of placenta accreta in patients with placenta previa and one previous cesarean section.[35] This likelihood increased to 67% with the diagnosis of placenta previa and four or more previous cesarean sections. With the increasing numbers of cesarean

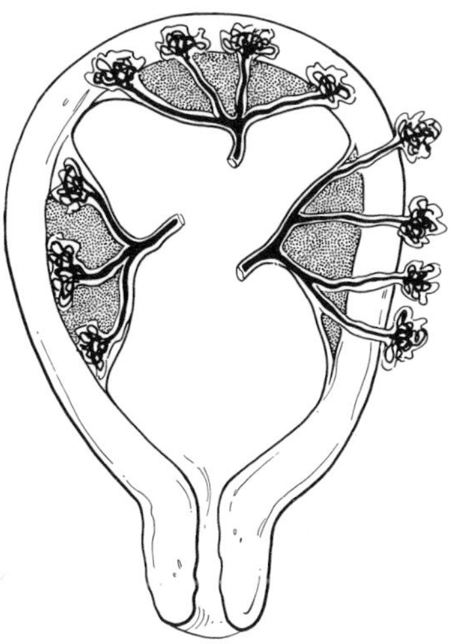

Figure 9–4. Classification of abnormal placentation by degree of myometrial penetration. (Redrawn from Kamani AAS, Gambling DR, Christilaw J, Flanagan ML: Anaesthetic management of patients with placenta accreta. Can J Anaesth 34:613–617, 1987.)

sections performed, placenta previa/accreta is now the leading cause of emergency obstetric hysterectomy, replacing uterine atony.[27] Diagnosis usually occurs during cesarean placental delivery, but abnormal placentation must also be considered in patients having retained placenta following vaginal birth after cesarean section. With known risk factors, an ultrasound-guided diagnosis can sometimes precede delivery.

Because uterine blood flow is 700 ml/minute at term, profuse bleeding follows the dysfunctional uterine contraction associated with placenta accreta, percreta, and increta. Once this is detected, additional intravenous access should be established quickly and supplemental oxygen should be continued. Immediately send for blood and perhaps additional anesthesia personnel. Regional anesthesia can be continued for cesarean hysterectomy, provided the patient remains comfortable and hemodynamically stable. Patients may become nauseated from peritoneal manipulation and restless if the procedure is prolonged. In a recent multi-institutional study, none of the continuous epidurals for emergency hysterectomy needed conversion to general anesthesia.[27] However, if the patient becomes hemodynamically unstable, proceed with general anesthesia for airway protection.

In patients at risk for placenta accreta, regional anesthesia is not contraindicated, but epidural anesthesia provides longer duration (redose indwelling catheter) than subarachnoid anesthesia,[27] should a cesarean hysterectomy become necessary.

Uterine Rupture

Uterine rupture may occur antepartum, intrapartum, or postpartum, but fortunately, it is relatively uncommon (0.08 to 0.1%) in the general obstetric population.[36] With a previous uterine scar, the incidence of rupture during labor increases to 0.5% with a low transverse and to 2.0% with a classic (vertical) incision.[4] For this reason, patients who have had previous classic incisions are rarely allowed attempted vaginal birth after cesarean section (see Chapter 10).

Reported maternal mortality rates vary widely (between 0.1 and 60%) depending on the type of rupture.[38, 39] Uterine scars may develop small areas of dehiscence, which are often insignificant and undetected until the time of cesarean section or postpartum tubal ligation. Traumatic or spontaneous ruptures result in higher maternal and fetal mortality. Sudden intense abdominal pain, prolonged fetal bradycardia, hypotension, and shock usually accompany complete traumatic ruptures. Partial ruptures may exhibit only mild abdominal pain, shoulder discomfort (from subdiaphragmatic irritation), or vaginal bleeding, which can lead to hypotension and shock (especially if unrecognized postpartum). Current evidence suggests that labor epidural analgesia does not prevent the recognition of uterine rupture.[40–42] Risk factors are listed in Table 9–4.

TABLE 9–4
Risk Factors for Uterine Rupture

Rapid tumultuous labor
Prolonged labor with oxytocin stimulation
Uterine scar—previous cesarean section or myomectomy
Uterine distention—multiparity, multiple gestation, polyhydramnios
Uterine manipulation/instrumentation—external version, forceps delivery
Placenta accreta
Trophoblast invasion
Prostaglandin $F_{2\alpha}$
Trauma

Complete antepartum uterine rupture is usually managed by emergency cesarean section under general anesthesia. Blood loss may be massive. In incomplete ruptures, a functioning epidural catheter may be utilized for surgical anesthesia if the patient remains comfortable and hemodynamically stable. The anesthesiologist should remember that the associated sympathetic block may exacerbate hypotension.

POSTPARTUM HEMORRHAGE

Uterine Atony

In 2 to 5% of vaginal births, uterine involution fails following placental delivery, making uterine atony the most common cause of postpartum hemorrhage.[43] With poor uterine contractility, bleeding continues from the myometrial arterioles and decidual veins that once supplied and drained the placental intervillous spaces. Normally, uterine contracture tamponades this bleeding. The classic presentation, painless vaginal bleeding with a rising uterine fundus, may occur immediately or several hours after delivery. Risk factors are listed in Table 9–5.

Management includes volume resuscitation, vigorous uterine massage, and pharmacologic intervention with intravenous oxytocin or intramuscular methylergonovine or $PGF_{2\alpha}$. Surgery is considered when all else fails.

TABLE 9–5
Risk Factors for Uterine Atony

Multiparity	Precipitous or prolonged labor
Multiple gestation	Oxytocin use during labor
Macrosomia	Chorioamnionitis
Polyhydramnios	Retained placenta

Cervical or Vaginal Lacerations

Cervical or vaginal lacerations, common after precipitous, macrosomic, or instrumental (forceps or vacuum extractor) vaginal deliveries, should be suspected if bleeding continues in the postpartum period without evidence of uterine atony. Lacerations are the second most common cause of intrapartum and postpartum bleeding but are massive only when large vessels are involved.

Postpartum bleeding from vaginal or cervical lacerations may require exploration of the birth canal. The anesthesia care provider must be flexible in approaching this situation; a gentle surgeon and a cooperative patient may require minimal analgesia. A labor epidural, maintained at T8–10, is usually adequate for exploration and repair. Without an epidural in place, the obstetrician may alternatively use local anesthetic infiltration or a pudendal block (S2–4) to provide perineal analgesia. If these measures fail and the patient is uncooperative or uncomfortable, it is best to move to the operating room for further sedation or regional or general anesthesia.

Retained Placenta

Retained placenta, the third most common cause of postpartum bleeding, occurs after 1% of vaginal deliveries[38] when the uterine fundus contracts around the placenta, preventing complete separation. Uterine relaxation, manual exploration, or a D&C may be required for detachment; therefore, patient comfort and cooperation are needed. Rarely, placenta accreta is diagnosed, necessitating abdominal surgery.

Anesthetic management varies with clinical judgment and experience. A labor epidural, maintained at T8–10, is usually adequate for exploration. In the absence of hypotension and hypovolemia, spinal anesthesia is also appropriate, using 30 to 50 mg of 1.5 to 5.0% lidocaine. General anesthesia, if required, should include rapid-sequence induction and endotracheal intubation. Uterine relaxation can be rapidly obtained with 1.5 to 2.0 times the minimal alveolar concentration of halothane, enflurane, or isoflurane.[44] Theoretically, isoflurane may be most desirable because its low solubility allows the quickest concentration changes; however, these cases are usually brief, making drug selection relatively unimportant. Sedation with nitrous oxide, midazolam, or ketamine must be carefully titrated, as these patients risk gastric content aspiration. Sublingual and intravenous nitroglycerin 50 to 100 μg reportedly produces uterine relaxation 30 to 40 seconds after administration and restoration of uterine tone within several minutes. Potential side effects including headache (from cerebral vasodilatation), nausea, and hypotension have not been demonstrated in obstetric patients.[45, 46] Nonanesthetic tocolytics, such as ritodrine and terbutaline, produce rapid but persistent uterine relaxation, an unacceptable condition when immediate uterine contracture is needed following placenta removal. Likewise, magnesium sulfate, although an important agent of antepartum tocolysis, acts too slowly and persists too long for emergency postpartum use.[14] In addition, magnesium sulfate may further decrease the parturient's ability to vasoconstrict if hypovolemia ensues during regional anesthesia.

Uterine Inversion

Uterine inversion is rare, occurring once in 2000 pregnancies.[47] Following delivery, an atonic uterus and open cervix permit the uterus to "turn inside out" through the birth canal, usually from fundal pressure or inappropriate traction on the umbilical cord to hasten placental delivery. Risk factors include primiparity, fundal placental implantation, antepartum magnesium sulfate administration, uterine atony, and uterine malformation.

If uterine inversion occurs, the obstetrician should immediately replace the uterus before placenta removal to minimize blood loss. Oxytocin should not be given prior to uterine replacement, as the resulting uterine contracture can prevent replacement. Peritoneal traction, elicited by uterine inversion, can produce a profound vasovagal response resulting in vasodilatation and increased bleeding. Blood loss can be massive, and shock may rapidly ensue. Intravenous narcotics and nitroglycerin may be initially attempted for uterine replacement, but general anesthesia is usually necessary for profound analgesia and uterine relaxation (via potent inhalational agents) in the absence of preexisting labor epidural anesthesia.

ACQUIRED COAGULATION DEFECTS

Coagulopathies may arise antepartum, intrapartum, or postpartum, making obstetric bleeding even more difficult to treat. Acquired coagulation defects during pregnancy include dilutional thrombocytopenia after massive transfusion (discussed earlier), hemolytic transfusion reactions, DIC, and preeclampsia.

Hemolytic Transfusion Reactions

Hemolytic transfusion reactions most commonly result from patients accidentally receiving incompatible blood.[48] Intravascular hemolysis results from the recipient's antibodies and complements directly attacking the foreign donor blood. Substances released by the hemolyzed cells result in DIC and acute renal failure. As little as 20 ml of blood can initiate a potentially life-threatening reaction.[13]

Classic signs and symptoms include fever, chills, nausea, hypotension, and chest and flank pain. During general anesthesia, unexplained hypotension, hemoglobinuria, and bleeding may be the only signs present.[13]

Treatment is directed toward correcting the coagulopathy and preventing renal failure. When an acute reaction is suspected, the transfusion should be stopped immediately and the blood bank notified for retesting of all crossmatched units. The circulation and urine output must be maintained with intravenous fluids, vasopressors, and diuretics, if necessary.

Disseminated Intravascular Coagulation

DIC usually results from conditions producing poor regional and hepatic blood flow, such as hemorrhagic shock. In pregnancy, however, severe abruptio placentae is the commonest cause of DIC, with up to 30% of patients developing coagulopathy[49] from placental thromboplastic material entering the open maternal venous sinuses. DIC may also occur following retained intrauterine fetal demise because fetal or placental degradation products enter the maternal circulation.[4, 49]

Whatever the initiating event, DIC converts a normally localized coagulation process into a generalized one. Subsequently, widespread fibrin deposition consumes coagulation factors and platelets, rendering the blood unclottable. Fibrin thrombi also clog the microcirculation, leading to organ ischemia. Plasmin, normally a protective fibrinolytic agent, contributes to bleeding as FDP (anticoagulants) are generated. Although some patients are asymptomatic, most will display signs of either excessive bleeding or intravascular thrombosis, depending on the balance between the production of thrombin and that of plasmin.[14]

Clinical suspicion usually prompts laboratory testing. Findings consistent with DIC include decreased fibrinogen levels, decreased platelet counts, increased FDP, and a prolonged thrombin time. Treating obstetric DIC involves maintaining circulatory volume while eliminating the triggering event. Restoring the circulation improves regional and hepatic blood flow, which removes activated clotting factors for hepatic clearance. Administration of heparin, fibrinogen, or α-aminocaproic acid may worsen bleeding or thrombosis and is not recommended.

Preeclampsia

Preeclamptic patients may develop coagulopathy secondary to thrombocytopenia, which is especially prominent in the preeclamptic variant, HELLP syndrome. Fibrinogen levels, PT, and PTT are usually normal, and FDP are absent in contrast to DIC. Coagulopathy results from platelet dysfunction and increased platelet turnover as platelets adhere to damaged vascular endothelium.[50] Treatment consists of platelet transfusions for clinically apparent bleeding and expedient delivery.

CONCLUSION

Hemorrhage in the obstetric patient is often unexpected and may lead to death within minutes. Although modern medical care and blood transfusion availability have led to dramatic decreases in maternal mortality over the years, each individual death is no less a tragedy. Aggressive fluid resuscitation is the most important response to obstetric bleeding, followed by interventions to stop the bleeding. The anesthesia care provider must be prepared to manage hemorrhage, recognize patients at increased bleeding risk, and make the appropriate anesthetic choices to help ensure both maternal and fetal well-being.

TEN PRACTICAL POINTS

1. Blood loss is usually underestimated, not overestimated.
2. Intravascular volume is more important than hemoglobin/hematocrit when planning the anesthetic.
3. In a bleeding parturient, *rapid* fluid infusion is more important than the type of fluid or immediate hemodynamic monitoring.

4. *Type-specific* uncrossmatched blood is preferable to O-negative blood for emergency transfusion.

5. Prophylactic transfusion of platelets and fresh frozen plasma during massive hemorrhage is not indicated. Administer hemostatic components only if microvascular bleeding develops.

6. Do not give methylergonovine or prostaglandin $F_{2\alpha}$ intravenously.

7. If the parturient is bleeding severely, do not delay surgery for laboratory tests.

8. When placenta previa and previous cesarean section coexist, beware of placenta accreta.

9. Cesarean hysterectomy does not contraindicate regional anesthesia. Just be prepared for bleeding.

10. Do not hesitate to call for help!

REFERENCES

1. Atrash HK, Koonin LM, Lawson HW, et al: Maternal mortality in the United States, 1979–1986. Obstet Gynecol 76:1055–1060, 1990.
2. Kaunitz AM, Hughes JM, Grimes DA, et al: Causes of maternal mortality in the United States. Obstet Gynecol 65:605–612, 1985.
3. Schaffner W, Federspiel CF, Fulton ML, et al: Maternal mortality in Michigan: An epidemiologic analysis, 1950–1971. Am J Public Health 67:821–829, 1977.
4. Chantigian RC: Antepartum hemorrhage. *In* Datta S, Ostheimer GW (eds): Common Problems in Obstetric Anesthesia. Chicago, Year Book Medical, 1987, pp 236–244.
5. Cheek TG, Gutsche BB: Maternal physiologic alterations during pregnancy. *In* Shnider SM, Levinson G (eds): Anesthesia for Obstetrics, 2nd ed. Baltimore, Williams & Wilkins, 1987, pp 3–13.
6. Ueland K: Maternal cardiovascular dynamics. VII. Intrapartum blood volume changes. Am J Obstet Gynecol 126:671–677, 1976.
7. Priano LL: Trauma. *In* Barash PG, Cullen BF, Stoelting RK (eds): Clinical Anesthesia. Philadelphia, JB Lippincott, 1989, pp 1365–1377.
8. McLennan CE, Sandberg EC: Abruptio placentae and placenta previa. *In* McLennan CE, Sandberg EC (eds): Synopsis of Obstetrics, 9th ed. St. Louis, CV Mosby, 1974, pp 250–266.
9. Moore SB: Management of transfusion in the massively bleeding patient. Hum Pathol 14:267–270, 1983.
10. Klapholz H: Blood transfusion in contemporary obstetric practice. Obstet Gynecol 75:940–943, 1990.
11. Singbartle G, Becker M, Frankenberger C, et al: Intraoperative on-line ST-segment analysis with extreme normovolemic hemodilution. Anesth Analg 74:S295, 1992.
12. Consensus Conference: Perioperative red blood cell transfusion. JAMA 260:2700–2703, 1988.
13. American Society of Anesthesiologists: Questions and Answers About Transfusion Practices, 2nd ed. Park Ridge, IL, American Society of Anesthesiologists, Inc., 1992.
14. Plumer MH: Bleeding problems. *In* James FM, Wheeler AS, Dewan DM (eds): Obstetric Anesthesia: The Complicated Patient, 2nd ed. Philadelphia, FA Davis, 1988, pp 309–344.
15. Gallagher J, Banner MJ, Barnes PA: Large-volume crystalloid resuscitation does not increase extravascular lung water. Anesth Analg 64:323–326, 1985.
16. Strauss RG: Review of the effects of hydroxyethyl starch on the blood coagulation system. Transfusion 21:299–302, 1981.
17. Strauss RG, Stansfield C, Henriksen RA, Villhauer PJ: Pentastarch may cause fewer effects on coagulation than hetastarch. Transfusion 28:257–260, 1988.
18. Daniels MJ, Strauss RG, Smith-Floss AM: Effects of hydroxyethyl starch on erythrocyte typing and blood crossmatching. Transfusion 22:226–228, 1982.
19. Sherman SJ, Greenspoon JS, Nelson JM, Paul RH: Obstetric hemorrhage and blood utilization. J Reprod Med 38:929–934, 1993.
20. Miller RD: Transfusion therapy. *In* Miller RD (ed): Anesthesia, 4th ed, Vol 2. New York, Churchill Livingstone, 1994, pp 1619–1646.
21. Reed RL II, Ciavarella D, Heimbach DM, et al: Prophylactic platelet administration during massive transfusion. Ann Surg 203:40–48, 1986.
22. Consensus Conference: Platelet transfusion therapy. JAMA 257:1777–1780, 1987.
23. National Institutes of Health: Fresh Frozen Plasma: Indications and Risks. Consensus Development Conference Statement. Bethesda, MD, National Institutes of Health, 1984.
24. American Hospital Formulary Service: Ergonovine maleate. *In* AHFS Drug Information. Bethesda, MD, American Society of Health-System Pharmacists, 1993, pp 2037–2041.
25. Hankins GDV, Berryman GK, Scott RT Jr, Hood D: Maternal arterial desaturation with 15-methyl prostaglandin $F_{2\alpha}$ for uterine atony. Obstet Gynecol 72:367–370, 1988.
26. Clark SL, Yeh S-Y, Phelan JP, et al: Emergency hysterectomy for obstetric hemorrhage. Obstet Gynecol 64:376–380, 1984.
27. Chestnut DH, Dewan DM, Redick LF, et al: Anesthetic management for obstetric hysterectomy: A multi-institutional study. Anesthesiology 70:607–610, 1989.

28. Pritchard JA, MacDonald PC, Gant NF: Abortion. *In* Pritchard JA, MacDonald PC, Gant NF (eds): Williams Obstetrics, 17th ed. Norwalk, CT, Appleton & Lange, 1985, pp 467–490.
29. Mandell GL: Problems of early pregnancy. *In* James FM, Wheeler AS, Dewan DM (eds): Obstetric Anesthesia: The Complicated Patient, 2nd ed. Philadelphia, FA Davis, 1988, pp 77–88.
30. Pritchard JA, MacDonald PC, Gant NF: Obstetric hemorrhage. *In* Pritchard JA, MacDonald PC, Gant NF (eds): Williams Obstetrics, 17th ed. Norwalk, CT, Appleton & Lange, 1985, pp 389–421.
31. Pritchard JA: Haematological problems associated with delivery, placental abruption, retained dead fetus and amniotic fluid embolism. Clin Haematol 2:563–586, 1973.
32. Centers for Disease Control: Ectopic Pregnancy—United States, 1987. MMWR 39:401–404, 1990.
33. DeCherney AH, Maheux R: Modern Management of Tubal Pregnancy. Chicago, Year Book Medical, 1983, pp 4–38.
34. DeCherney AH, Seifer DB: Ectopic pregnancy. *In* Gabbe SG, Niebyl JR, Simpson JL (eds): Obstetrics. Normal and Problem Pregnancies, 2nd ed. New York, Churchill Livingstone, 1991, pp 809–827.
35. Clark SL, Koonings PP, Phelan JP: Placenta previa/accreta and prior cesarean section. Obstet Gynecol 66:89–92, 1985.
36. Gatt SP: Anaesthetic management of the obstetric patient with antepartum or intrapartum haemorrhage. Clin Anaesthesiol 4:373–388, 1986.
37. Varner M: Postpartum hemorrhage. Crit Care Clin 7:883–897, 1991.
38. Biehl DR: Antepartum and postpartum hemorrhage. *In* Shnider SM, Levinson G (eds): Anesthesia for Obstetrics, 3rd ed. Baltimore, Williams & Wilkins, 1993, pp 385–394.
39. Ware HH Jr: Rupture of the uterus. Clin Obstet Gynecol 3:637–645, 1960.
40. Meier PR, Porreco RP: Catastrophic uterine rupture. Obstet Gynecol 66:296, 1985.
41. Chestnut DH: Uterine rupture and epidural anesthesia. Obstet Gynecol 66:295, 1985.
42. Leung AS, Farmer RM, Leung EK, et al: Risk factors associated with uterine rupture during trial of labor after cesarean delivery: A case-control study. Am J Obstet Gynecol 168:1358–1363, 1993.
43. Herbert WNP, Cefalo RC: Management of postpartum hemorrhage. Clin Obstet Gynecol 27:139–147, 1984.
44. Miller AC, DeVore JS, Eisler EA: Effects of anesthesia on uterine activity and labor. *In* Shnider SM, Levinson G (eds): Anesthesia for Obstetrics, 3rd ed. Baltimore, Williams & Wilkins, 1993, pp 53–69.
45. Redick LF, Livingston E: A new preparation of nitroglycerin for uterine relaxation. Int J Obstet Anesth 4:14–16, 1995.
46. DeSimone CA, Norris MC, Leighton BL: Intravenous nitroglycerin aids manual extraction of a retained placenta. Anesthesiology 73:787, 1990.
47. Watson P, Besch N, Bowes WA Jr: Management of acute and subacute puerperal inversion of the uterus. Obstet Gynecol 55:12–16, 1980.
48. Sazama K: Reports of 355 transfusion-associated deaths: 1976 through 1985. Transfusion 30:583–590, 1990.
49. Naumann RO, Weinstein L: Disseminated intravascular coagulation: The clinician's dilemma. Obstet Gynecol Surv 40:487–492, 1985.
50. Kelton JG, Hunter DJS, Neame PB: A platelet function defect in preeclampsia. Obstet Gynecol 65:107–109, 1985.

TEN

Anesthesia for Vaginal Delivery Following Cesarean Section

Brenda L. Berkebile, M.D.

Between 1965 and 1986, the cesarean birth rate increased from 4.5 to 24.1% and, since 1986, has stabilized, with a rate of 23.5% reported in 1990. In 1987, the nearly one million cesarean sections performed made this procedure the most common major surgery in America. Of the estimated 982,000 cesarean sections in 1990, 630,000 were primary cesarean sections and 352,000 were repeat cesarean sections.[1] The common indications for this frequent surgery are listed in Table 10–1.

RATIONALE

Not surprisingly, cesarean section has come under close scrutiny regarding its impact on health care costs and as a possible opportunity for cost containment. For example, the average cost of an uncomplicated vaginal delivery at the author's institution is $2750 versus $3555 for an uncomplicated cesarean section. Extended hospital stay accounts for the majority of the cost differential. Nationwide, the cost impact of cesarean sections is astounding. In 1979, Shy and colleagues, using a technique of decision analysis, investigated hypothetical cohorts of 10,000 pregnant women with previous low transverse cesarean incisions and calculated hospital, physician, anesthesiologist, and neonatal intensive care costs for the expected number of cesarean and vaginal births. For these 10,000 patients, *direct* costs were $5 million greater in the repeat cesarean section cohort.[2] Certainly, these costs have risen since Shy and colleagues' study and represent a potential major area for cost containment.

TABLE 10–1
Common Indications for Cesarean Section

History of prior cesarean section
Failure to progress
Cephalopelvic disproportion
Fetal distress
Breech or other malpresentation
Multiple gestation
Placenta previa
Abruptio placentae
Maternal medical history

However, when considering reducing the number of cesarean sections by performing fewer repeat cesarean sections, maternal and fetal safety, as well as patient preference, must be examined. For example, would decreasing the repeat cesarean section rate influence maternal safety? According to Hood and Dewan, there is a five- to sixfold increased risk of maternal death directly attributable to cesarean section,[3] and according to Flamm and associates, the corrected relative risk of a mother's death is from 2 to 11 times greater with a cesarean section than with a vaginal birth.[4] Thus, at first glance, it appears that cesarean sections pose greater maternal risk than vaginal delivery and that performing fewer cesarean sections should improve maternal safety. However, attempted vaginal delivery in a scarred uterus may pose new maternal and fetal risks.

OBSTETRIC CONSIDERATIONS

When considering the safety of labor in a scarred uterus, one challenges the historical philosophy of "Once a cesarean section, always a cesarean section" and the fear of uterine rupture. "Is vaginal birth after cesarean section (VBAC) safe for the mother and baby?" and "How successful is it?"

The Uterine Scar

The type of uterine scar is the prime determinant regarding suitability of candidates for a trial of labor or VBAC and potential for uterine rupture. Scars are either classic (vertical in the uterine fundus), low transverse, low (vertical within the lower uterine segment), or occasionally unknown (Fig. 10–1). Unknown scars are usually considered classic vertical. Importantly, the abdominal scar does not necessarily reflect the direction of the uterine scar, although a vertical skin incision is more likely associated with a vertical uterine scar, since both vertical abdominal and uterine incisions provide more room for delivery. Importantly, regardless of the type of incision, both uterine ruptures and uterine dehiscences can occur.[4, 5] "Uterine dehiscences" (Fig. 10–2) are nontraumatic separations of the uterine scar, usually without bleeding or extrusion of the fetus through the wound. In contrast, "uterine ruptures" involve traumatic scar separation or separation of an intact uterus, with bleeding, hematoma formation, and potential extrusion of the fetus. The ramifications of each are obvious.

Most reviews identify a greater incidence of uterine rupture associated with classic or vertical incisions (2%) than with low transverse incisions (0.5%).[1, 6] Indeed, uterine rupture and dehiscence rates associated with *low transverse* scars during a trial of labor do not differ significantly from the rupture rate occurring in women planning elective repeat cesarean section.[7] The information regarding low vertical incisions is less clear. The concern with low vertical scars, which by definition should be in the lower uterine segment, is accurate determination of the exact extent of the lower uterine segment that develops during labor. Ineffective labor may not produce a definable lower uterine segment and precludes making a "low" incision. Indeed, the subsequent development of the lower uterine segment during vaginal delivery trials indicated that some scars from previous cesarean sections thought to be in the lower segment extended into the uterine *fundus.* Fundal incisions increase the likelihood of rupture, since the lower uterine segment is more fibrous and heals more completely than the muscular tissue of the fundus. Thus, low vertical incisions can in reality be fundal incisions, and trials of labor for patients with low vertical incisions await definitive study. In conclusion, low transverse scars enhance safety when considering VBAC.

Outcome

Multiple studies exist evaluating the success *and* safety of VBAC with low transverse incisions. Success rates for vaginal delivery vary from 60 to 90%.[8–10] Surprisingly, even women whose prior cesarean section was performed for cephalopelvic disproportion may have success rates approaching 70%.[1] However, even if VBACs have a high success rate, they must also be safe. Lavin reviewed 32 years of English obstetric literature and identified 5200 VBACs and noted a 0.7% incidence of uterine rupture and a 0.9% perina-

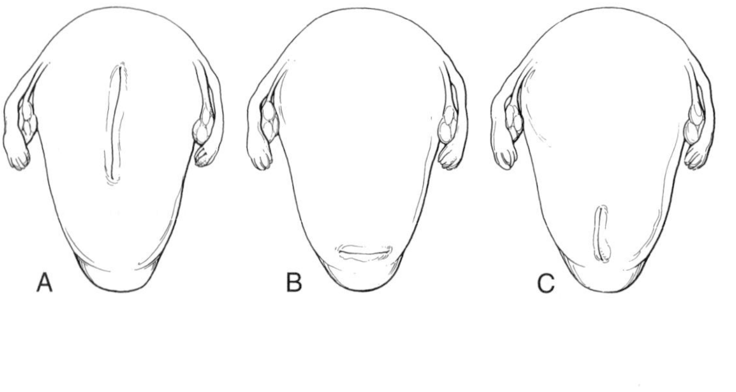

Figure 10–1. Types of uterine scars from cesarean section. *A,* Classic. *B,* Low transverse. *C,* Low vertical.

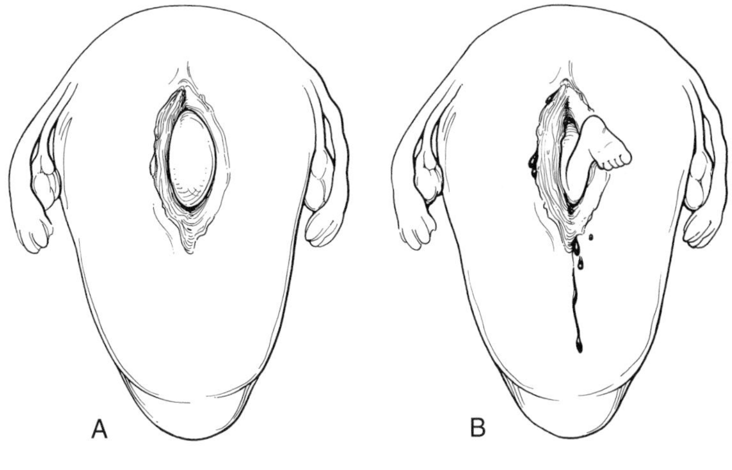

Figure 10–2. Examples of uterine scar dehiscence without overt rupture *(A)* and uterine scar rupture with extrusion of fetal leg *(B)*.

tal mortality rate. Importantly, no maternal deaths occurred secondary to uterine rupture.[6] Surprisingly, truly emergent cesarean section rates were similar (less than 2%) to those occurring in patients without a previous cesarean, and fetal distress occurred with equal frequencies.[11, 12] Finally, uterine scar *dehiscence* rates are similar regardless of whether the patient delivers vaginally or has an elective cesarean section.

Special Considerations

Time and experience have liberalized the criteria for suitability for a trial of labor. Many criteria, previously believed to be absolute contraindications to VBAC, are now being reexamined and are addressed in the 1995 *American College of Obstetricians and Gynecologists (ACOG) Practice Patterns.*[29] Multiple gestation was once considered a contraindication for VBAC because of concerns that greater uterine size and the potential need for intrauterine fetal manipulation could increase the risk of uterine rupture. In 1988, Strong and coworkers evaluated the outcome of 25 women with twin gestations attempting VBAC. Seventy-two percent delivered vaginally, and the dehiscence rate was 4%, compared with 2% in singleton pregnancies. However, no significant differences occurred in either maternal or neonatal mortality rates, and the authors concluded that attempted vaginal delivery should be considered, provided the usual safeguards for trial of labor in twin gestation are followed.[5]

Similarly, women with more than one previous cesarean section do not experience increased risk for uterine scar dehiscence or rupture when compared with those women having only one previous cesarean section. Novas and colleagues' study "strongly suggests that patients with more than one previous cesarean section may undergo a trial of vaginal delivery under similar guidelines proposed by ACOG for patients with only one previous cesarean section."[13]

Fetal weight was examined as a possible risk factor, and most studies identified either no effect or effects that became apparent with fetal weights greater than 3720 to 4000 grams. Greater weights decreased the likelihood of successful trial of labor.[8, 14] However, a prior history of successful vaginal delivery increased the likelihood of a successful vaginal delivery of a macrosomic infant in a scarred uterus.[4, 15]

What about oxytocin inductions or augmentations of labor? Lavin and associates discouraged the use of oxytocin in these patients for fear of increasing the risk of uterine rupture.[16] More recent series challenge this opinion and note improved success rates in women receiving oxytocin for induction or augmentation without increased maternal or fetal mortality.[15, 17]

Based on this data, the October 1988 ACOG Committee opinion on *Guidelines for Vaginal Delivery After a Previous Cesarean Birth*[30] remains a valid overview:

> In 1980, the National Institute of Child Health and Human Development Conference on Childbirth concluded that vaginal delivery after cesarean birth is an appropriate option. Current data show that a trial of labor was successful in 50 to 80% of patients who had low transverse uterine

incisions from previous deliveries and who were selected candidates for vaginal birth in subsequent pregnancies. Moreover, a trial of labor was successful in this selected group in up to 70% of women for whom the indication for cesarean delivery was "failure to progress in labor." The data also indicate that maternal and perinatal mortality rates for subsequent attempted vaginal delivery are lower than those for repeat cesarean births. Although uterine rupture can occur, it is rarely catastrophic with modern obstetric care. The benefits of a successful vaginal delivery include elimination of operative and postoperative complications and shortened hospital stay.

Patient Preference

Finally, patient preference is another force deserving consideration when examining cesarean section. Possible psychological benefits associate with successful vaginal delivery. Lavin states that women who delivered by cesarean section have more negative psychological responses involving self-image, sense of failure, and maternal attitudes toward their infants than women who delivered vaginally.[6] This contrasts with the positive effects associated with family involvement and support through labor and vaginal delivery. Indeed, patients with a history of a prior vaginal delivery were more likely to consent to a trial of labor than women who never experienced a successful vaginal delivery.[15] Overall patient acceptance rates for trial of labor range from 22 to 92%.[11, 18]

DIAGNOSIS OF UTERINE RUPTURE

Accurate and early diagnosis of uterine rupture is vital for optimal maternal and fetal outcome. Felmus and coworkers noted that maternal death risk directly relates to the interval between diagnosis and arrest of hemorrhage.[19] Although uterine rupture is uncommon, it is a potentially catastrophic obstetric complication that must be dealt with swiftly. Uterine *rupture* occurs in approximately 1 in 1250 of all births and accounts for 5% of maternal deaths.[1, 12] Remember, rupture may occur at any stage of pregnancy or labor and can occur postpartum. Causes of uterine rupture are listed in Table 10–2.

TABLE 10–2
Causes of Uterine Rupture

Separation of a previous uterine scar
Rupture of myomectomy scar
Previous difficult deliveries
Precipitous labor
Prolonged labor with excessive oxytocin use or cephalopelvic disproportion
Weak or stretched uterine muscle secondary to multiple gestation
High parity
Polyhydramnios
Traumatic rupture secondary to intrauterine manipulation
Difficult forceps delivery
Excessive suprafundal pressure

Signs and Symptoms

The signs and symptoms associated with uterine rupture depend on the size and location of the rupture (Table 10–3). The lower uterine segment tends to be less vascular and thus bleeds less. Ruptures of the fundus bleed more and are more likely to cause maternal cardiovascular decompensation and fetal distress, especially when the rupture includes the area of placental implantation. Major uterine rupture can be deceptively difficult to diagnose and can be confused with appendicitis, intestinal obstruction, or abruptio placentae. Therefore, a high level of suspicion for uterine rupture should be held in any stage of labor or postpartum when known predisposing factors exist. Uterine rupture is more common and more often devastating in multiparous women. The most common factors associated with ruptures

TABLE 10–3
Signs and Symptoms of Uterine Rupture

Vaginal bleeding
Severe uterine or abdominal pain—sharp/unremitting
Shoulder pain (referred from hemoperitoneum)
Tender uterine scar
Fetal distress
Loss of fetal heart tones
Severe maternal hypotension or shock
Recession of the presenting fetal part
Fetal death

are cephalopelvic disproportion and neglected transverse lie.[20] Rupture of an *unscarred* uterus, especially in the fundus, usually causes severe complications with excessive bleeding, hypotension, and shock. Patients experiencing primary ruptures in the fundus may require multiple transfusions and commonly need partial or total hysterectomy for definitive management. Maternal mortality associated with spontaneous rupture approaches 26% and may be as high as 66% when secondary to trauma.[17, 21] Death is usually secondary to diagnosis delay, inadequate blood transfusion, and delayed laparotomy. Fetal mortality with rupture of the unscarred uterus is 44%.[22]

In contrast to primary ruptures, either asymptomatic dehiscence or overt rupture may occur via a uterine scar. Although no maternal deaths have been reported secondary to uterine rupture through a scar, fetal mortality may reach 30% in this situation.[22] *Remember,* ruptures may occur remote from the previous uterine scar and cause more severe complications with increased maternal and fetal mortality.

Recommendations for the management of a woman undergoing a trial of labor are listed in Table 10–4. Recommendations requiring intrauterine pressure measurement have recently been questioned. Intrauterine pressure catheters provide quantitative measurements of uterine resting tone as well as of the duration and intensity of contractions. Reputedly, decreased intrauterine pressure and cessation of labor are classic signs of uterine rupture and suggest a role for intrauterine pressure catheters in the diagnosis of uterine rupture. However, a retrospective chart review of patients experiencing uterine rupture at the Los Angeles University of Southern California Women's Hospital from 1979 to 1988 could not reliably identify loss of uterine tone or cessation of labor in women monitored by either external or intrauterine pressure monitors. Indeed, the most common sign of uterine rupture was *fetal distress,* which occurred in 78% of cases and *preceded* pain and hemorrhage. Ten percent of patients actually had an increase in baseline uterine tone from 15 to 35 mmHg. Importantly, in this series, maternal and fetal morbidity and mortality showed no significant differences between women with external uterine monitoring and those with internal monitoring. However, in a small study by Beckley and colleagues, a "clipping" off of intrauterine pressure peaks was noted to occur *prior* to a decrease in fetal heart rate in 4 of 10 women studied. This was speculated to be secondary to a decrease in wall tension by the yielding scar.[23] In summary, a lack of changing uterine pressure should not rule out the diagnosis of uterine rupture, and internal pressure monitors are not mandatory for laboring women with prior cesarean section.

ANESTHETIC CONSIDERATIONS

Monitored Anesthesia Care

Anesthesia options for the patient attempting a VBAC resemble those for women without a uterine scar. Prepared childbirth and intravenous sedation are reasonable options if the patient desires. As with any delivery, both techniques may require supplementation with a pudendal block or saddle block if forceps assistance becomes necessary during the second stage of labor. The presence of the anesthesia provider may improve safety and decrease delay time for treatment should uterine rupture occur.

TABLE 10–4
Recommendations for Trial of Labor After Cesarean Section

No additional indication for cesarean section in the current pregnancy
Documentation of a low vertical or transverse uterine scar
Careful monitoring by an obstetrician who is physically present
Continuous fetal heart tone monitoring
Continuous uterine tonometry (external or internal)
24-hour blood bank availability
2 units of packed red blood cells typed and screened (or crossmatched) and available for use at all times
Access to operative intervention within 15 minutes
Evaluation of the uterine scar after delivery

Epidural Anesthesia Concerns

Initial experience with VBACs antedated electronic fetal monitoring and the recognition of fetal stress as a sign of uterine rupture. In this setting, the cardinal signs and symptoms of uterine rupture were considered to be maternal abdominal pain, tachycardia, and hypotension all of which could potentially be masked by epidural analgesia. Recent trials of labor raise three important points when considering the validity of this concern. First, as discussed, continuous fetal heart monitoring identified fetal distress as the usual first sign of uterine rupture. Maternal pain with associated tachycardia and hypotension from excessive blood loss *followed* changes in fetal heart rate. Second, *painless* uterine rupture occurs with and *without* epidural analgesia.[17, 24] Thus, pain is not a reliable diagnostic sign. In fact, complete fetal expulsion has occurred without severe pain even without epidural anesthesia.[25] Third, epidural analgesia may not eliminate the pain of uterine rupture. Pain associated with uterine rupture may "break through" a previously adequate epidural block. A similar breakthrough pain is seen commonly with bladder distention and bladder rupture during transurethral resections of the prostate. This breakthrough pain was referred to by Crawford as the "epidural sieve."[24] Breakthrough pain is often described as sharp and unremitting, not associated with contractions, and sometimes abnormally located in the upper abdominal quadrants, shoulders, arms, or neck. The pain may not be relieved with additional epidural local anesthetic administration. Rudick and associates found that breakthrough pain of uterine rupture was not relieved by 0.35% epidural bupivacaine, but was removed when 0.5% bupivacaine was utilized to establish surgical anesthesia for cesarean section.[26] Therefore, the onset of pain in the presence of a previously functioning epidural that persists despite additional local anesthetic deserves investigation. At the author's institution, there was a case of a small, hemodynamically stable uterine rupture that, despite surgical anesthesia with 3% chloroprocaine, produced unremitting pain. Epidural narcotics may also delay the diagnosis of uterine rupture (discussed later in this chapter).

The sitting position for the placement of an epidural in women with a uterine scar has also been questioned as a possible risk factor. Plauché and coworkers reported a series of 23 uterine ruptures in which 2 ruptures were associated with extreme anteflexion during epidural placement in the sitting position. They postulated that anteflexion increased amniotic fluid pressure, causing rupture of the uterine scar.[22] Golan and colleagues also reported 5 cases of uterine scar rupture attributed to anteflexion for epidural placement.[27] At the author's institution, intrauterine amniotic fluid pressure was measured in a series of women sitting anteflexed for epidural placement. No increases in amniotic pressure related to positioning occurred. The author's group doubts that the sitting anteflexed position is a cause of uterine rupture and believes this position should be used at the discretion of the anesthesiologist to ease epidural placement.

Advantages of Epidural Anesthesia

Advantages of epidural analgesia for a trial of labor include: (1) As with all patients, patient comfort during labor and delivery may decrease circulating catecholamines and potentially improve uteroplacental perfusion. (2) Excellent analgesia and relaxation of the perineum is helpful when *forceps-assisted delivery* is necessary. (3) Postpartum digital examination of a lower uterine segment when searching for rupture is better tolerated in the presence of epidural anesthesia. (4) If repeat cesarean section is necessary, the epidural may be utilized, avoiding the need for general anesthesia.

Management

Presently at the author's institution, epidural pain control is offered to laboring women with low transverse scars. The author's group's usual drug regimen entails establishing the block with 2% lidocaine and utilizing 0.125 to 0.25% continuous infusions of bupivacaine for maintenance analgesia. Although epidural narcotics are not contraindicated, a case report documented that adding fentanyl to 0.25% bupivacaine obliterated the breakthrough pain of uterine rupture.[28] Beware!

In summary, VBAC is no longer considered a full or even relative contraindication to epidural anesthesia. Indeed, the *ACOG Practice Patterns* guidelines suggest that more women may consent to VBAC if epidural analgesia is available, and candidates should be advised about its availability.[29] Recommendations for epidural analgesia during trial of labor are: (1) continue fetal monitoring throughout labor, (2) administer the lowest concentration of local anesthetic that *relieves* uterine contractile pain, and (3) maintain a high index of suspicion of uterine rupture at all times.

TEN PRACTICAL POINTS

1. Trials of labor after a previous cesarean section with a low transverse incision are safe for mother and fetus.
2. No additional monitoring is necessary beyond the usual for laboring women.
3. Be vigilant for signs of uterine dehiscence or rupture (i.e., fetal stress, unusual unrelenting pain, hypotension, vaginal bleeding).
4. Fetal distress is often the first sign of uterine rupture.
5. Uterine rupture may be painless.
6. Act quickly if uterine rupture is suspected. Most maternal mortality is secondary to delay of diagnosis and treatment of rupture.
7. Epidurals are safe and effective means of pain control for labor and delivery after cesarean section.
8. Utilize the lowest concentration of local anesthetic that *maintains* maternal comfort.
9. Beware of epidural narcotics.
10. Unrelenting and severe pain in an unusual location for labor, despite usually adequate doses of local anesthetic, should raise the question of uterine rupture, especially with a previously functioning epidural anesthetic.

REFERENCES

1. Taffel SM, Placek PJ, Kosary CL: U.S. cesarean section rates 1990: An update. Birth 19:21–22, 1993.
2. Shy K, LoGerfo J, Karp L: Evaluation of elective repeat cesarean section as standard of care: An application of decision analysis. Am J Obstet Gynecol 139:123–129, 1981.
3. Hood DD, Dewan DM: Obstetric anesthesia. *In* Brown DL (ed): Risk and Outcome in Anesthesia, 2nd ed. Philadelphia, JB Lippincott, 1992, pp 356–413.
4. Flamm BL, Lim OW, Jones C, et al: Vaginal birth after cesarean section: Results of a multicenter study. Am J Obstet Gynecol 158:1079–1084, 1988.
5. Strong TH, Phelan JP, Ahn MO, et al: Vaginal birth after cesarean delivery in the twin gestation. Am J Obstet Gynecol 161:29–32, 1989.
6. Lavin JP: Vaginal delivery after cesarean birth: Frequently asked questions. Clin Perinatol 10:439–453, 1983.
7. Phelan JP, Clark SL, Diaz F, Paul RH: Vaginal birth after cesarean. Am J Obstet Gynecol 157:1510–1515, 1987.
8. Yetman TJ, Nolan TE: Vaginal birth after cesarean section: A reappraisal of risk. Am J Obstet Gynecol 161:1119–1123, 1989.
9. Chazotte C, Cohen WR: Catastrophic complications of previous cesarean section. Am J Obstet Gynecol 163:738–742, 1990.
10. Meier PR, Porreco RP: Trial of labor following cesarean section: A two-year experience. Am J Obstet Gynecol 144:671–678, 1982.
11. Paul RH, Phelan JP, Yeh S: Trial of labor in the patient with a prior cesarean birth. Am J Obstet Gynecol 151:297–304, 1985.
12. Finley BE, Gibbs CE: Emergent cesarean delivery in patients undergoing a trial of labor with a transverse lower-segment scar. Am J Obstet Gynecol 155:936–939, 1986.
13. Novas J, Myers SA, Gleicher N: Obstetric outcome of patients with more than one previous cesarean section. Am J Obstet Gynecol 160:364–368, 1989.
14. Flamm BL, Goings JR: Vaginal birth after cesarean section: Is suspected fetal macrosomia a contraindication? Obstet Gynecol 74:694–697, 1989.
15. Silver RK, Gibbs RS: Predictors of vaginal delivery in patients with a previous cesarean section, who require oxytocin. Am J Obstet Gynecol 156:57–60, 1987.
16. Lavin JP, Stephens RJ, Miodomik M, Barden TP: Vaginal delivery in patients with a prior cesarean section. Obstet Gynecol 59:135, 1982.
17. Flamm BL, Dunnett C, Fischermann E, Quilligam EJ: Vaginal delivery following cesarean section: Use of oxytocin augmentation and epidural anesthesia with internal tocodynamic and internal fetal monitoring. Am J Obstet Gynecol 148:759–763, 1984.
18. Martin J, Harris BA Jr, Huddleston JF, et al: Vaginal delivery following previous cesarean birth. Am J Obstet Gynecol 146:255–263, 1983.
19. Felmus LB, Pedomitz P, Nassberg S: Spontaneous rupture of the apparently normal uterus during pregnancy: A review. Obstet Gynecol Surv 8:155–172, 1953.
20. Boulle P, Crichton D: Rupture of the unscarred uterus. Lancet 1:360–363, 1964.
21. Adams DM, Druzin ML, Cederqvist LL: Intrapartum uterine rupture. Obstet Gynecol 73:471–473, 1989.

22. Plauché WC, Von Almen W, Muller R: Catastrophic uterine rupture. Obstet Gynecol 64:792–797, 1984.
23. Beckley S, Gee H, Newton JR: Scar rupture in labour after previous lower uterine segment caesarean section: The role of uterine activity measurement. Br J Obstet Gynaecol 98:265–269, 1991.
24. Crawford JS: Epidural analgesia and uterine rupture. Lancet 1:361, 1974.
25. Myerscough PR: Munro Kerr's Operative Obstetrics, 9th ed. London, Bailliere-Tindall, 1977.
26. Rudick V, Niv D, Hetman-Peri M, et al: Epidural analgesia for planned vaginal delivery following previous cesarean section. Obstet Gynecol 64:621–623, 1984.
27. Golan A, Sandbank O, Rubin A: Rupture of the pregnant uterus. Obstet Gynecol 56:549, 1980.
28. Tehan B: Abolition of the extradural sieve by addition of fentanyl to extradural bupivacaine. Br J Anaesth 69:520–521, 1992.
29. American College of Obstetricians and Gynecologists, ACOG Practice Patterns: Vaginal delivery after previous cesarean birth. Washington, DC, American College of Obstetricians and Gynecologists, August 1995.
30. American College of Obstetricians and Gynecologists: Guidelines for vaginal delivery after a previous cesarean birth. Washington, DC, American College of Obstetricians and Gynecologists, October 1988.

ELEVEN

Anesthesia for Forceps Deliveries

Robert D'Angelo, M.D.

Obstetric forceps were first used over 300 years ago, and nearly 900 varieties now exist. Despite this variety, all obstetric forceps have the same component parts and perform two primary functions—traction and rotation. Unfortunately, traction and rotation generate forces that can potentially compress the fetal head and increase fetal morbidity and mortality.[1, 2] Traction and rotation may also produce maternal injury.[3] Increased fetal and maternal risk are the heart of the controversy surrounding forceps deliveries. Consequently, forceps deliveries have steadily declined over the past three decades as the number of cesarean deliveries increased.[4–6] Nevertheless, forceps deliveries are still commonplace, and the anesthesiologist involved with the management of obstetric patients must be able to safely administer anesthesia for this procedure.

CLASSIFICATION

In 1988, forceps deliveries were reclassified according to station and rotation by the American College of Obstetricians and Gynecologists (ACOG).[7] Forceps deliveries are subdivided into outlet, low, mid, and high forceps. "Outlet forceps deliveries" occur when forceps are applied after the fetal head has reached the pelvic floor and the fetal scalp is visible at the introitus without separating the labia. Additionally, the sagittal suture of the fetal skull is in the anteroposterior diameter of the pelvis with fetal head rotation not exceeding 45 degrees prior to delivery. "Low forceps deliveries" occur when forceps are applied while the apex of the fetal skull is stationed 2 cm or more below the maternal ischial spine, but not on the pelvic floor. Low forceps deliveries are subdivided into type A and type B. "Type A" is defined as fetal head rotation of 45 degrees or less prior to forceps placement, and "type B" is defined as fetal head rotation exceeding 45 degrees prior to forceps placement. "Mid forceps deliveries" occur when forceps are applied while the apex of the fetal skull is engaged and the apex is less than 2 cm below the maternal ischial spine. ("Engagement" is the descent of the fetal head biparietal diameter below the plane of the pelvic inlet.) "High forceps deliveries" were not included in the 1988 reclassification because they are virtually never justifiable, but these occur when forceps are applied prior to engagement of the fetal skull.

INDICATIONS AND STATUS

Indications for forceps deliveries may be maternal or fetal. Maternal indications include: maternal exhaustion, debilitating disease limiting maternal physical reserve, and conditions that increase risk during maternal expulsive efforts—that is, cardiac or cerebrovascular disease. Fetal indications include fetal distress, arrested rotation, abnormal fetal position, and head entrapment during breech deliveries. Safe forceps application also requires meeting the prerequisites listed in Table 11–1.[8, 9] Unless

TABLE 11–1
Prerequisites for Forceps Delivery

Membranes are ruptured
Cervix is fully dilated
Fetal head is engaged
Exact position and station of the fetal head are known
Maternal pelvis is of adequate capacity for the fetus
Adequate anesthesia is present
Obstetrician is familiar with forceps delivery
Bladder and rectum are empty

these criteria are met, alternative approaches for delivery are required, including expectant labor, oxytocin (Pitocin) augmentation, and possibly cesarean delivery.

Table 11–2 lists fetal and maternal complications associated with obstetric forceps.[9–11] All complications can occur irrespective of the type of forceps delivery. However, one would expect that the greater the force required to deliver the fetus, the greater the likelihood of fetal or maternal injury. In fact, older studies indicated that mid forceps deliveries are associated with greater maternal and fetal injury compared with outlet forceps deliveries because the obstetrician must first rotate the fetal head into the anteroposterior diameter of the maternal pelvis and then must pull harder to deliver the fetus from the higher station.[1–3, 10, 12, 13] This increased risk leads opponents of mid forceps deliveries to argue that they should be abandoned in favor of cesarean delivery,[11–13] especially when the fetus weighs less than 2500 gm or more than 4500 gm[13] and the risk of maternal or fetal injury is increased.

TABLE 11–2
Fetal and Maternal Complications Associated with the Use of Obstetric Forceps

Fetal	Maternal
Cephalhematoma	Perineal laceration
Skull fracture	Uterine rupture
Interventricular hemorrhage	Uterine atony
Facial or brachial nerve palsy	Severe hemorrhage
Shoulder dystocia	Sacral plexus injury
Cord compression	Rectal laceration
Asphyxia	Rectovaginal fistula
Death	

Unfortunately, these older studies were generally uncontrolled and performed prior to the use of continuous electronic fetal monitoring. More recent, well-controlled studies fail to substantiate these findings. In fact, no significant differences have been found in Apgar scores, fetal acidosis, or long-term outcome when comparing indicated outlet forceps, indicated mid forceps, and cesarean deliveries.[14, 15] The only significant findings were an increased incidence of maternal perineal lacerations and decreased maternal postdelivery hematocrits associated with mid forceps deliveries compared with spontaneous vaginal deliveries. These studies have led to a reexamination of the issues surrounding mid forceps deliveries, and the debate continues.

As discussed previously, high forceps deliveries have been universally abandoned because the risk of fetal and maternal injury is so great.[8, 9] High forceps deliveries are virtually never justifiable.

ANESTHETIC CONSIDERATIONS

Anesthetic management varies with the anticipated type of forceps delivery. However, subtle differences defined in the ACOG classification have little bearing on anesthetic management. For practical purposes, the discussion addresses only outlet and mid forceps deliveries.

Analgesic requirements vary throughout the course of labor and delivery. Pain associated with cervical dilatation (stage 1 labor) is transmitted along small sympathetic fibers that enter the spinal cord at T10, T11, and T12 and L1. In contrast, pain associated with delivery of the fetus and placenta (stages 2 and 3 labor) is transmitted via the large pudendal nerve entering the spinal cord at S2, S3, and S4 and is somatic pain (Fig. 11–1).[9, 16, 17] This has significant anesthetic implications because epidural analgesia may be adequate for stage 1 but inadequate for stage 2 labor because of the required greater distribution and density of sensory and motor blockade during stage 2 labor.

Outlet forceps deliveries require relatively little analgesia when compared with mid forceps deliveries because the greater forces generated during mid forceps deliveries are associated with greater maternal discomfort. Pudendal nerve blockade or perineal infiltration with local anesthetic may suffice. When these tech-

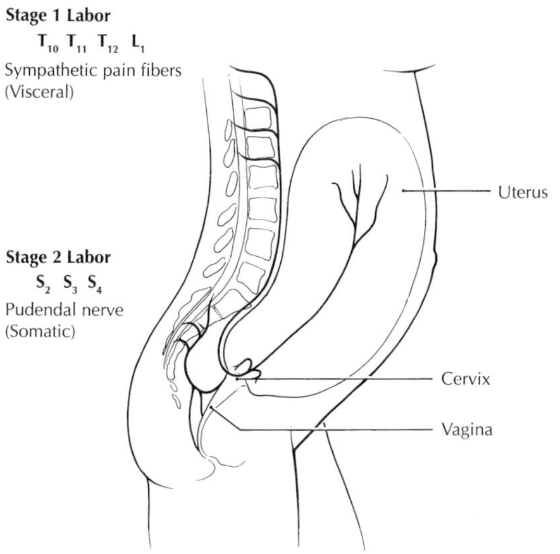

Figure 11–1. Pain transmission during stage 1 and stage 2 labor.

niques are insufficient, short-acting intravenous narcotics, inhalational analgesia (50% nitrous oxide, 0.5% isoflurane, or 0.8% ethrane), or low-dose intravenous ketamine (0.25 mg/kg) provide alternative methods of supplementation. A dense T10–S4 sensory blockade achieved with either epidural or spinal anesthesia can provide adequate anesthesia for outlet forceps deliveries. In contrast, mid forceps deliveries potentially pose greater maternal and fetal risk than outlet forceps deliveries and can lead to emergency cesarean section. Importantly, profound perineal and pelvic muscle relaxation reduce the amount of force required to deliver the fetus and may reduce the incidence of maternal and fetal injury.[2, 10] Unfortunately, local anesthesia, intravenous narcotic, inhalational analgesia, low-dose ketamine, and pudendal blockade rarely meet the requirements for mid forceps delivery. Consequently, mid forceps deliveries need either major regional or, rarely, general anesthesia to meet the requirements of analgesia and pelvic muscle relaxation. Regional anesthesia is preferred.

Forceps deliveries may injure the sacral plexus, especially rotational mid forceps delivery that involves rotation of the forceps and fetal skull over the nerves in the maternal pelvis. Regional anesthesia will not inhibit muscle contraction from a directly stimulated nerve but will mask pain associated with the stimuli. In other words, occasionally during forceps deliveries under spinal or epidural anesthesia, a maternal leg will "jump" during rotation of the fetal skull but have no associated pain. This occurrence should be noted in the patient's permanent record because the risk of postoperative nerve injury exists.

REGIONAL ANESTHESIA

Regional anesthesia for labor and delivery is commonplace in modern obstetric practice. Regional anesthesia offers the advantages of providing maternal pain relief, without altering maternal awareness, while producing minimal adverse effects on the fetus or course of labor. Despite relative safety, complications associated with spinal and epidural anesthesia occur (Table 11–3).[18, 19] The American Society of Anesthesiologists' guidelines for conduction anesthesia in obstetrics attempt to improve patient safety when instituting major regional anesthesia in the obstetric suite (see "Obstetric Anesthesia Guidelines," in Chapter 3).

Continuous lumbar analgesia placed during stage 1 labor offers the advantage of titratable analgesia that can readily be augmented for forceps or cesarean delivery. With this in mind, no epidural placed for stage 1 labor should be considered acceptable unless a bilateral T10–L2 sensory blockade has been demonstrated by pin-

TABLE 11–3
Complications Associated with Spinal and Epidural Anesthesia

Spinal	Epidural
Backache	Backache
Hypotension	Hypotension
Nausea/vomiting	Nausea/vomiting
Postdural puncture headache	Accidental spinal
High spinal placement	Intravascular injection → seizure or cardiovascular collapse
Meningitis	Postdural puncture headache
Cauda equina syndrome	Epidural hematoma
Nerve injury or paralysis	Epidural abscess
Death	Sheared catheter tip
	Nerve injury or paralysis
	Death

prick or temperature change. Additionally, some degree of motor block usually occurs, and most importantly, the patient should experience excellent pain relief. Although sacral analgesia is usually unnecessary during stage 1 labor, establishing adequate sacral anesthesia for forceps delivery may be difficult or impossible unless the conditions discussed earlier are met. Although adding fentanyl to an inadequate epidural may provide sufficient analgesia for stage 1 labor, this practice may mask an epidural that will be insufficient for mid forceps delivery. Therefore, the author recommends aggressively replacing epidural catheters that do not clearly meet these criteria.

Although, as previously mentioned, outlet forceps deliveries can be performed with various anesthetic techniques. Epidural and spinal anesthesia can provide a dense T10–S4 sensory blockade, assuring patient comfort. Local anesthetic agents and recommended dosages for spinal and epidural anesthesia are listed in Table 11–4.[19-21] Outlet forceps deliveries can be performed in the labor room using an existing epidural catheter. However, at the author's institution, spinal anesthesia for outlet forceps is performed in a delivery room equipped with appropriate monitors and resuscitation equipment. The patient may sit or lie in the lateral decubitus position, depending on the anesthesiologist's preference. The author recommends a 27-gauge Quinke, a 24-gauge Sprotte, or a 25- to 27-gauge Whitacre needle to minimize the risk of postdural puncture headache. Interspaces below L2 minimize the likelihood of inadvertent spinal cord trauma. Although theoretical concern exists for higher sensory and motor levels following injection of local anesthetics during uterine contraction, the author does not believe this to be clinically significant; and during urgent spinal placement, the author recommends quickly proceeding with the injection. Following injection, the blood pressure should be monitored every 1 to 2 minutes for at least the first 10 minutes, and treated if a 20% decrease in systolic blood pressure is noted (assurance of left uterine displacement, oxygen administration, elevating the patient's legs, additional intravenous fluids, and ephedrine 5 to 10 mg intermittent intravenous boluses).

One indication for outlet forceps delivery is fetal distress. Severe persistent fetal distress (fetal heart rate less than 60 beats per minute) potentially limits the use of spinal anesthesia because of time constraints and may indicate using alternative forms of anesthesia. However, spinal anesthesia is an option for mild to moderate fetal distress. The author recommends administering oxygen to the mother and continu-

TABLE 11–4
Local Anesthetic Agents Commonly Used for Spinal and Epidural Anesthesia

Spinal

Agent	*%*	*T10 Sensory Level (Outlet Forceps) (mg)*	*T4 Sensory Level (Mid Forceps) (mg)*
Lidocaine	5	30–50	60–100
Bupivacaine	0.75	5–7.5	12.5–15
Tetracaine	1	5–6	8–12

Epidural

Agent	*Outlet Forceps (%)*	*Mid Forceps (%)*	*Recommended Initial Dose* (ml)*	*Maximal Initial Dose (mg/kg)†*
Lidocaine	1–2	2	10–15	7.0
Chloroprocaine	2	3	10–15	15
Bupivacaine	0.25–0.5	0.5	10–15	2.5

*Dosing must be tailored to individual patient requirements.

†Recommended maximal dose applies only to the initial dose. Individual adjustments must be made for repeat doses and continuous infusions.

ing to monitor the fetal heart rate during placement of the spinal anesthesia. A preplanned time limit for successful spinal placement is necessary during fetal stress. Alternative forms of anesthesia should be pursued if the spinal cannot be placed in a timely manner. Continued communication with the obstetrician is vital.

Any attempted mid forceps delivery can result in emergency cesarean section. At the author's institution, differentiation is made between routine mid forceps deliveries (as defined by ACOG) and mid forceps deliveries that have a reasonable likelihood of leading to abdominal delivery (mid forceps trial). The author distinguishes between the two by direct communication with the obstetrician and does not rely on "second-hand" information. For routine mid forceps deliveries, if the patient has an existing, functioning epidural catheter, an attempt is made to achieve T8–S4 sensory and motor blockade and the delivery occurs in the labor and delivery room. In contrast, for mid forceps trials, the author's group optimally establishes a T4–S4 sensory and motor blockade that should provide adequate anesthesia for cesarean section. Mid forceps trials should occur in the operating room previously prepared for possible cesarean delivery (double setup). As discussed previously, the author's group administers spinal anesthesia only in the operating room. Maternal and neonatal resuscitation equipment, as well as qualified personnel, should be readily available to perform appropriate resuscitation (see "Obstetric Anesthesia Guidelines," in Chapter 3) regardless of where the delivery occurs.

The importance of communication between the anesthesia team and the obstetric team must be emphasized. Optimal patient care can occur only when effective communication exists. Anesthetic management varies with the anticipated procedure, and only by knowing the obstetrician's plans can management be optimized. For example, outlet forceps deliveries can be performed in a delivery room with one set of anesthetic requirements, but a mid forceps trial should be performed in an operating room with entirely different anesthetic requirements.

Regional anesthesia can be performed only when no contraindications to regional anesthesia exist (Table 11–5).[19, 22] If regional anesthesia is contraindicated, general anesthesia will be required for most mid forceps deliveries.

TABLE 11–5
Contraindications to Spinal or Epidural Anesthesia

Absolute	Relative
Patient refusal	Sepsis
Severe uncorrected hypovolemia	Neurologic disorder (preexisting)
Infection at the placement site	Heparinization
Coagulopathy	Spinal deformity
	Metastatic disease to lumbar spine
	Fetal distress

GENERAL ANESTHESIA

General anesthesia should be administered only when regional anesthesia is contraindicated or inadequate; the anesthetic technique resembles that for cesarean section anesthesia. Pregnancy increases maternal risk during general anesthesia and is discussed in detail in Chapter 7.

VACUUM EXTRACTION

Risks associated with vacuum extraction closely resemble the risks associated with forceps deliveries. Therefore, anesthetic considerations for forceps deliveries also apply to vacuum extraction deliveries. Once again, regional anesthesia is recommended over general anesthesia whenever possible.

In conclusion, as with any procedure, risks are associated with forceps deliveries. Anesthesiologists caring for obstetric patients must be aware of these risks and must be prepared to treat all complications. Effective communication between the anesthesia team and the obstetric team, along with diligent preoperative assessment and intraoperative management, may lessen the likelihood of a poor outcome to both mother and newborn.

TEN PRACTICAL POINTS

1. Difficult forceps deliveries increase maternal and fetal risk and can lead to cesarean delivery.

2. Adequate stage 1 labor epidural analgesia does not guarantee adequate sacral analgesia for forceps delivery.

3. Nevertheless, demonstrating a bilateral T10–L2 sensory blockade during stage 1 labor minimizes the risk of inadequate sacral analgesia for forceps delivery.

4. Mid forceps deliveries require perineal and pelvic muscle relaxation that is best provided by major regional anesthesia.

5. Augmentation of a preexisting epidural may be more expeditious than induction of spinal anesthesia.

6. Administer maternal oxygen and monitor fetal heart rate during mid forceps trials or spinal placement, especially in patients with preexisting fetal distress.

7. Quick spinals are retrospective; therefore, have a preplanned time limit for spinal placement in urgent circumstances.

8. The author recommends performing mid forceps trials in a fully equipped operating room.

9. Have maternal and neonatal resuscitation equipment readily available.

10. Effective communication between the anesthesia team and the obstetric team improves patient care.

REFERENCES

1. Pearse WH: Electronic recording of forceps delivery. Am J Obstet Gynecol 86:43, 1963.
2. Ullery JC, Teteris NJ, Botschner AW, McDaniels B: Traction and compressive forces exerted by obstetric forceps and their effect on fetal heart rate. Am J Obstet Gynecol 85:1066, 1963.
3. Nyirjesy I, Pierce WE: Perinatal mortality and maternal morbidity in spontaneous and forceps vaginal deliveries. Am J Obstet Gynecol 89:568, 1964.
4. Healy LD, Laufe LE: Survey of obstetric forceps training in North America in 1981. Am J Obstet Gynecol 151:54, 1985.
5. Cesarean childbirth: Report of a Consensus Development Conference. Washington, DC, U.S. Department of Health and Human Services, Public Health Services, National Institutes of Health, 1981.
6. Goodlin RC: On protection of the maternal perineum during birth. Obstet Gynecol 62:393, 1983.
7. American College of Obstetricians and Gynecologists: Obstetric Forceps. ACOG Committee Opinion 71. Washington, DC, American College of Obstetricians and Gynecologists, 1989.
8. Forceps and vacuum extractor. *In* Pauerstein CJ (ed): Clinical Obstetrics. New York, Wiley Medical, 1987, p 849.
9. O'Brien WF, Cefalo RC: Labor and delivery. *In* Gabbe SG, Niebyl JR, Simpson JL (eds): Obstetrics: Normal and Problem Pregnancies. New York, Churchill Livingstone, 1986, p 364.
10. Laufe LE, Leslie DC: The timing of the episiotomy. Am J Obstet Gynecol 114:773, 1972.
11. Bowes WA, Bowes C: Current role of the midforceps operation. Clin Obstet Gynecol 23:549, 1980.
12. Chez RA: Midforceps delivery: Is it an anachronism? Contemp Obstet Gynecol 15:82, 1980.
13. Hughey MJ, McElin TW, Lussky R: Midforceps operations in perspective. I. Midforceps rotation complications. J Reprod Med 20:253, 1978.
14. Dierker LJ, Rosen MG, Thompson K, Lynn P: Midforceps deliveries: Long-term outcome of infants. Am J Obstet Gynecol 154:764, 1986.
15. Gilstrap LC III, Hauth JC, Sciano S, Connor KD: Neonatal acidosis and method of delivery. Obstet Gynecol 63:681, 1984.
16. Bonica JJ: The nature of pain of parturition. Clin Obstet Gynecol 2:511, 1975.
17. Gutsche BB: Obstetric anesthesia and perinatology. *In* Dripps RD, Eckenhoff JE, Vandam LD (eds): Introduction to Anesthesia: The Principles of Safe Practice, 7th ed. Philadelphia, WB Saunders, 1988, p 293.
18. Vandam LD: Complications of spinal and epidural anesthesia. *In* Orkin FK, Cooperman LH (eds): Complications in Anesthesiology. Philadelphia, JB Lippincott, 1983, p 75.
19. Covino BG, Lambert DH: Epidural and spinal anesthesia. *In* Barash PG, Cullen BF, Stoelting RK (eds): Clinical Anesthesia. Philadelphia, JB Lippincott, 1989, p 755.
20. Albright GA: Local anesthetics. *In* Albright GA, Ferguson JE II, Joyce TH III, Stevenson DK (eds): Anesthesia in Obstetrics: Maternal, Fetal, and Neonatal Aspects. Boston, Butterworths, 1986, p 115.
21. Bromage PR: Choice of local anesthetics in obstetrics. *In* Shnider SM, Levinson G (eds): Anesthesia for Obstetrics, 2nd ed. Baltimore, Williams & Wilkins, 1987, p 59.
22. Covino BG, Scott DB (eds): Handbook of Epidural Anesthesia and Analgesia. Clinical Considerations. New York, Grune & Stratton, 1985, p 109.

TWELVE

Embolic Disease in Pregnancy

Marc A. Huntoon, M.D.

INCIDENCE

In 1985, Kaunitz and coworkers[1] reported mortality in the United States during the years 1974 through 1978. Excluding aborted pregnancies, the leading cause for maternal mortality was embolism, accounting for nearly 20% of all deaths. Of a total 491 of embolic causes, 271 were thrombotic emboli, 189 were amniotic fluid emboli, and 25 were air emboli. Recent awareness of the magnitude of this problem has generated a great deal of research, particularly with respect to air embolism.

AIR EMBOLISM

Massive air emboli, frequently diagnosed at postmortem examination, have been the subject of case reports during cesarean section. Younker and associates[2] describe a massive air embolism occurring during cesarean section in a patient with placenta previa. The patient, who fortunately survived, developed brisk hemorrhage after operative delivery. During hysterectomy to obtain hemostasis, idioventricular rhythm, profound hypotension, and loss of end-tidal carbon dioxide waveform occurred. At this time, air bubbles were noted in the surgical field, and air embolism therapy was initiated, including 100% fractional inspired oxygen ($F_{I_{O_2}}$), advanced cardiac life support protocols, and placement of a central venous line to aspirate frothy air from the right side of the heart.

Pulmonary emboli, whether air or particulate (thrombus, fat, amniotic fluid), increase dead space ventilation by producing areas that are ventilated but not perfused. As a result, less carbon dioxide from mixed venous return will be measured by the capnograph; likewise, end-tidal nitrogen (from the inspired gas) may increase. Thus, patients with air emboli may present with sudden hypotension, dyspnea, hypoxemia, arrhythmias, and decreased end-tidal carbon dioxide partial pressure (P_{CO_2}) (Table 12–1). Although the patient previously described survived, emboli can cause significant morbidity and mortality in parturients, emphasizing the need for vigilance and prompt treatment (Table 12–2).

Asymptomatic air emboli also occur and can be detected in 11 to 65% of patients undergoing cesarean sections.[3–6] Although "asymptomatic," Doppler-detected air emboli during cesarean section have been implicated as causing spontaneous complaints of dyspnea, desaturation,[3] and chest pain,[4, 5] the significance of these emboli remains unclear. Questions of paramount importance are (1) Which patients are at risk? (2) When are emboli most likely to occur? (3) Do air emboli cause maternal complaints of dyspnea and chest pain? (4) Can one effectively

TABLE 12–1
Signs and Symptoms of Air Emboli

Hypotension	Chest pain
Dyspnea	Arrhythmia
Hypoxemia	Cardiovascular collapse

TABLE 12–2
Treatment of Air Embolus

Manage airway (including intubation, 100% oxygen, discontinuation of nitrous oxide)
Support circulation, including vasoactive drugs if necessary
Correct positioning (right atrium at highest point, surgical site below level of heart)
Alert the surgeon, flood the surgical field
Insert a multiorifice central venous catheter, positioned at the junction of the superior vena cava and the right atrium
If available, and if intracerebral or intracoronary air occurs, institute cardiopulmonary bypass/ hyperbaric medicine for effective therapy

monitor for air emboli? and (5) If one can monitor for air emboli, when and to what extent should one intervene?

A pressure gradient may exist between the atmosphere and the patient's vasculature. For example, a gradient may occur whenever the operative site is higher than the level of the heart and allow entrainment of air into the circulation. With large collections of air in the right ventricle, an airlock may form that may greatly increase pressure in the right ventricle and decrease cardiac output. Increased right-sided pressure may also cause air to paradoxically move through atrial-ventricular communications to the left side of the heart, leading to potentially fatal intracerebral or intracoronary air. Theoretically, uterine exteriorization that places the uterine incision above the level of the heart and profound hypotension associated with severe hypovolemia or hemorrhage may allow air entrainment into the vasculature and may return the air to the right side of the heart, causing obstruction. Patients particularly susceptible to vascular air embolism include those with placenta previa, abruptio placentae, and hypovolemia.

No consensus exists in the literature regarding the timing of venous air emboli during cesarean section. Most air emboli occur at hysterotomy, hysterotomy repair, or placental separation,[3–5] but they may occur at any time from skin incision to closure. Theoretically, hypotension from regional anesthesia may create a more favorable situation for air emboli owing to venous dilatation and decreased blood pressure. However, Fong and colleagues[6] identified no statistical association in venous air emboli incidences with anesthetic technique.

The precordial Doppler apparently effectively detects intraoperative air emboli. The authors know the detected emboli consist of air because simultaneous echocardiography, by differentiating echo density, confirms the presence of air. Noninvasive Doppler ultrasound is readily available in most operative suites and, when placed in the left parasternal area at the fourth intercostal space, will detect air emboli. Indeed, Robinson and Albin[7] advocate routine precordial Doppler monitoring in all cesarean section patients. However, although significant morbidity from air embolism occurs, injury is rare relative to the frequency of Doppler-detected air emboli.[1, 2] Unfortunately, routine monitoring does not differentiate between "asymptomatic" emboli and catastrophic emboli, producing frequent false-positive results. Clinically significant symptoms suggestive of air emboli indicate the need for treatment, *not* the presence or absence of detectable air embolism.

The best approach is selective monitoring of patients with known right to left shunts, or when symptoms suggestive of air embolus mandate intervention. If a patient is suspected of having a clinically significant air embolus—that is, is experiencing dyspnea, chest pain, hypotension, and hypoxemia—then initiate the previously described resuscitation sequence (see Table 12–2).

AMNIOTIC FLUID EMBOLISM

Catastrophic amniotic fluid embolism (AFE) occurs in approximately 1 in 20,000 deliveries.[8] AFE predisposition relates to abruptio placentae in 50% of patients and commonly associates with hypertonic labors as well as tumultuous, rapidly progressing labors. However, AFE has also occurred postpartum, preterm, and during spontaneous or induced abortion. Classically, large amounts of amniotic fluid enter the maternal circulation, causing cardiovascular collapse, hypoxia, hypotension, and coagulopathy. Reported mortality rates are uniformly dismal, with rates as high as 80%. Although this disorder is speculated to be a major cause of maternal death, its true incidence is uncertain, since postmortem studies demonstrating amniotic and fetal tissue emboli are often lacking or inconclusive, and the differential diagnoses are numerous (Table 12–3).

Lee and coworkers[9] examined pulmonary artery aspirates of patients with pulmonary artery catheters placed for reasons other than suspected AFE. They identified fetal squamous and trophoblastic cells in 3 of 14 aspirates from patients without clinical signs of AFE. This implies that additional factors in or associated with amniotic fluid are required to produce the AFE syndrome, and amniotic fluid alone may not produce symptoms. Azagami and Mori identified a leukotriene that may be that factor.[10]

Although AFE pathophysiology is difficult to study, work by Clark and associates[11, 12] has been enlightening. The pathophysiology probably involves a biphasic reaction, beginning with pulmonary vasospasm and leading to pulmonary hypertension, and symptoms of acute cor pulmonale. Presenting symptoms include sudden dyspnea and hypotension, usually without chest pain. Following the initial phase, for unknown reasons, primary left ventricular failure appears (Fig. 12–1) with depressed left ventricular stroke work and elevated pulmonary wedge pressures. Forty percent of patients ultimately develop consumptive coagulopathy.[11]

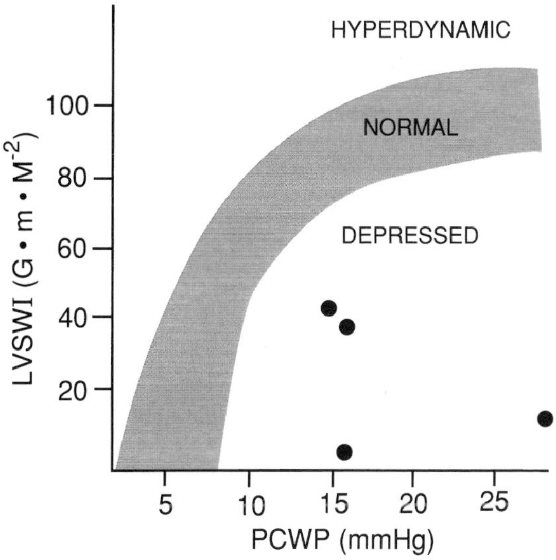

Figure 12–1. Ventricular function in amniotic fluid embolism. (*Abbreviations:* LVSWI = left ventricular stroke work index; PCWP = pulmonary capillary wedge pressure.) (From Clark SL, Cotton DB, Gonik B, et al: Central hemodynamic alterations in amniotic fluid embolism. Am J Obstet Gynecol 158:1124–1126, 1988.)

Differential Diagnosis

The sudden and catastrophic cardiorespiratory collapse of AFE has many imitators. Differentiation of AFE from other conditions such as aspiration, seizure, eclampsia, anaphylaxis, sepsis, and cardiogenic shock is aided by quickly evaluating the surgical field for evidence of profuse hemorrhage or frothy air; the temporal relations of symptoms, for example, recent emesis (possible aspiration syndrome); interventions by the surgeon or anesthesiologist (e.g., antibiotic infusion [drug reaction]); and preexisting medical problems, for example, questionable seizure activity (eclampsia) in the patient with pregnancy-induced hypertension. Historical clues and presentation may allow one to quickly rule out many conditions in the differential diagnosis (see Table 12–3).

TABLE 12–3
Differential Diagnosis of Amniotic Fluid Embolus

Hemorrhage/hypovolemia
Abruptio placentae (possibly concurrent with amniotic fluid embolus)
Placenta previa
Uterine atony
Retained placental fragment
Uterine inversion (eversion)
Severe supine hypotension
Preeclampsia/eclampsia
Seizure
Intracerebral event, bleeding
Mendelson syndrome (pulmonary aspiration of gastric contents)
Drug reaction/overdose
Gram-negative sepsis (septic shock)
Other emboli (e.g., air, thrombus)

TREATMENT

Treatment of massive air embolism begins with standard cardiopulmonary resuscitation (i.e., airway, breathing, and circulation) (Table 12–4). If advanced cardiac life support measures are not quickly successful, expeditious delivery of the fetus may be lifesaving. Case reports of "postmortem" delivery have been associated with sudden and dramatic maternal cardiovascular improvement.[13] Delivery may improve ve-

TABLE 12–4
Treatment of Amniotic Fluid Embolus

Treat airway, breathing, circulation
Intubate and ventilate with 100% oxygen
Support circulation with basic cardiopulmonary resuscitation and vasoactive drugs
Consider early delivery of fetus
Continue fetal monitoring
Improve cardiac preload and contractility
Initiate fluid challenge with crystalloid
Consider dopamine, digitalization
Install pulmonary artery catheter
Obtain distal heparinized sample for buffy coat examination
Examine ventricular function curves to optimize preload, prevent overzealous fluid administration (pulmonary edema)
Treat disseminated intravascular coagulation with fresh frozen plasma and packed red blood cells and monitor coagulation parameters until underlying cause is reversed

Data from Clark SL: Amniotic fluid embolism. Clin Perinatol 13:801–811, 1986.

nous return and vital organ circulation. If delivery is not appropriate, the patient should be moved to an intensive care setting, where better physician-nursing assets and monitoring capabilities exist when hemodynamic stability is achieved. Past treatments emphasizing vasodilators such as aminophylline, tolazoline, papaverine, or isoproterenol are not selective for the pulmonary vasculature. Pulmonary vasoconstriction occurs early, and rational treatment should focus on improving left ventricular function and careful central pressure monitoring. Pulmonary artery pressure monitoring can be very helpful, both for obtaining a pulmonary arterial blood sample for buffy coat examination and for more precise control of fluid administration, diuretics, and vasoactive drugs. Buffy coat examinations involve special staining procedures (Giemsa, Attwood) that may demonstrate fetal squames, lanugo hair, mucin, and other amniotic debris over the white blood cell smear layer.[14]

Disseminated intravascular coagulation may occur and requires regular checks of coagulation parameters. Amniotic fluid initially causes hypercoagulability that may rapidly consume Factors I, II, V, VIII, and XIII and platelets and increase fibrin degradation products. In acute disseminated intravascular coagulation, laboratory studies demonstrate prolongation of the partial thromboplastin time (PTT), variable platelet counts, decreased fibrinogen, and increased fibrin degradation products. Heparin therapy is relatively ineffective and may worsen clinical bleeding if clotting factors have been consumed. Fresh frozen plasma and red cell transfusion treat severe bleeding.[11] Platelet therapy is often not required. Treatment and resolution of the underlying problem, AFE, is achieved over time with supportive therapy, as no specific leukotriene or other factor in the amniotic fluid can yet be implicated (and blocked) with certainty.

VENOUS THROMBOEMBOLISM

Venous thromboembolism accounts for more than half of embolic mortality during pregnancy, making it a major focus of clinical prevention strategies. Pregnancy is a hypercoagulable state and is associated with increased Factors V, VII, VIII, IX, X, XII, and fibrinogen. Concomitantly, fibrinolytic activity decreases and venous stasis increases. The incidence of deep vein thrombosis (DVT) is estimated at up to 3 per 1000 cases, and pulmonary embolus (PE) occurs in 15 to 24% of pregnant patients with untreated DVT.[15] Approximately three fourths of all patients who die from PE, die within 2 hours of symptoms.[16] Sadly, since the mid-1980s, the case-fatality ratio has not changed for PE,[17] and this lack of improvement may relate directly to slow implementation of thrombolytic therapy. Although the U.S. Food and Drug Administration approved human tissue type plasminogen activator as of June 1990, pregnancy is a major contraindication to this form of therapy,[18] owing to the risk of maternal hemorrhage and unknown fetal effects. Thus, the clinician caring for the parturient with PE is limited to standard anticoagulation regimens utilizing heparin, hemodynamic support, and surgery. The following discussion concentrates on management of perioperative PE and anesthesia for the parturient receiving prophylactic therapy for DVT/PE.

Diagnosis of DVT

The clinical signs of DVT encompass pain, erythema, inflammation, increased temperature over the thrombotic site, positive Homan sign (calf pain with passive dorsiflexion), positive

Lowenberg test (pain occurring below a thigh cuff rapidly inflated to 180 mmHg), and a palpable venous cord. However, DVT can be clinically silent. Noninvasive testing, in the parturient, includes impedance plethysmography and B-mode Doppler ultrasound with color Doppler imaging. Impedance plethysmography has sensitivity of 90% for proximal venous obstruction.[19] Likewise, the sensitivity-specificity for Doppler ultrasound with color Doppler imaging exceeds 90% for "proximal" thrombosis, that is, common femoral, superficial femoral, or popliteal vein.[20] Venography may be performed if ultrasound is equivocal in the face of high clinical suspicion.

PULMONARY EMBOLUS

Signs of PE are acute dyspnea, cyanosis, tachycardia, and possibly hypotension. Progression to acute cor pulmonale or pulmonary infarction is catastrophic. Hemoptysis, pleuritic pain, and pleural friction rub should alert the clinician to possible PE.

The pathophysiology of PE is increased right ventricular outflow obstruction, causing increased pressure loading of the ventricle (Fig. 12–2). The right ventricle, thinly muscled and compliant compared with the left ventricle, compensates for increased afterload with coronary vasodilatation, decreased coronary resistance, and overall increased coronary flow. Unlike the left ventricle, which receives coronary perfusion primarily during diastole, the right ventricle is perfused during both systole and diastole. Hypotension (decreased aortic pressure) compromises coronary perfusion pressure during both parts of the cardiac cycle. Thus, maintenance of aortic pressure is vital to the right ventricle's continued compensation for heightened afterload stress. Enhanced preload (fluid infusion) also aids in compensating for increased afterload, but this mechanism is useful only so long as extreme right ventricular dilatation does not occur. At the extreme of right ventricular fluid overload, increased wall tension (increased oxygen demand), tricuspid regurgitation, and decreased *left* ventricular compliance can occur, all of which are deleterious. Thus, fluid infusion, maintenance of aortic pressure, and oxygenation are appropriate therapies when PEs occur.[21]

In patients without previous heart disease, the earliest signs of pulmonary vascular obstruction are systemic arterial hypoxemia and pulmonary hypertension. Interestingly, mean pulmonary artery pressures do not acutely exceed 40 mmHg, implying that the previously healthy right ventricle cannot acutely develop pressures above this level.[22] This differs from the response of the right ventricle to chronic obstruction where mean pressures and cor pulmonale may reach 60 to 90 mmHg or greater. Unlike in AFE, the cardiac index is usually elevated in PE except in massive cases with heart failure.

Testing

Ventilation-perfusion (V/Q) lung scanning, although noninvasive, poorly diagnoses PE. The Prospective Investigation of Pulmonary Embolism Diagnosis (PIOPED) investigators[23] found

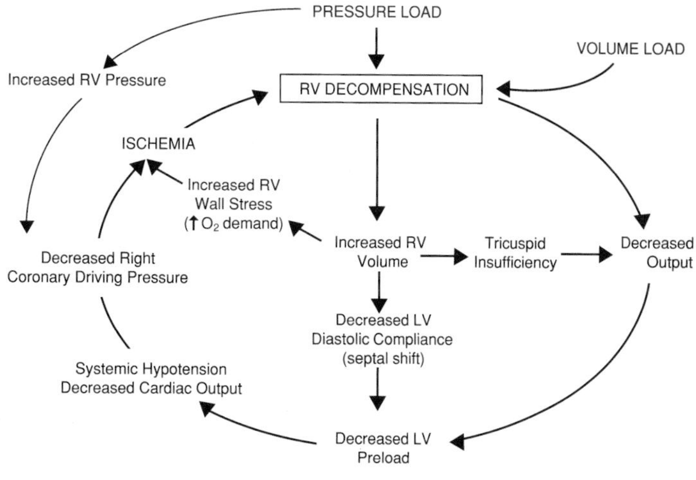

Figure 12–2. The pathophysiology of acute right ventricular failure (the "vicious circle") is depicted schematically. (*Abbreviations:* RV = right ventricular; LV = left ventricular.) (From Wiedemann HP, Matthay RA: Acute right heart failure. Crit Care Clin 1:631–661, 1985.)

only 41% of patients with angiographically proven PE had high-probability V/Q scans. This may not be true, however, in parturients. V/Q scanning remains useful to many clinicians. Since mortality rates with pulmonary arteriograms should not exceed 0.3%,[24] utilize this procedure when low or moderate probability V/Q scans occur in patients with clinically suspected PE and the clinical condition warrants.

Treatment

In the pregnant patient, full anticoagulation with heparin, along with hemodynamic support, remains the treatment of choice for acute PE. Warfarin crosses the placenta and has adverse fetal effects. Heparin does not cross the placenta and is not secreted in breast milk. Initial doses of 10,000 to 15,000 units, followed by infusions of 1000 units/hour should be used with regular checks of PTT or activated clotting time. A goal of 2 to 2.5 times prolongation of PTT for acute PE is reasonable. Heparin should help prevent further thrombus formation, but may not aid dissolution of existing thrombi.

Hypotension, although not common, may be best treated by increasing right ventricular filling pressures (high normal central venous pressure).[25] However, inotropes should be used prior to delivery only if the practitioner considers uterine blood flow, as the patient's condition will have to be weighed against the concern for fetal well-being. Choice of inotrope should be tailored to that patient's particular hemodynamics; for example, if the patient has a low cardiac index with adequate systemic vascular resistance then dobutamine may be indicated. α-agonists reduce uterine blood flow. Inotropes such as norepinephrine[25, 26] or dopamine[27] may be better than isoproterenol following delivery because they produce less tachycardia and maintain systemic pressures better. Vasodilators such as hydralazine may be helpful,[27] providing systolic blood pressure is maintained. Administration of a pulmonary vasodilator prostaglandin E_1 via pulmonary artery catheter in conjunction with norepinephrine systemically may be theoretically sound, but data in this population are lacking. Surgical options for treatment of acute massive PE include open pulmonary thrombectomy,[28] vena caval ligation, and caval filter placement.[29] Sasahara and colleagues' guidelines for surgery[30] include obstruction of greater than 50% of the pulmonary vasculature, $P_{A_{O_2}}$ less than 60, systolic blood pressure less than 90 mmHg, and urine output less 20 ml/hour despite maximal medical therapy for more than 1 hour.

HEPARIN PROPHYLAXIS

Although controversy exists regarding who should receive prophylaxis,[31] thromboembolism recurs in up to 12% of those women who experienced thromboembolism during a prior pregnancy.[32] Thus, given the morbidity of thromboembolism, some clinicians advocate prophylaxis. Patients with antithrombin III deficiencies and protein C or S deficiencies are among those with the strongest indications for prophylaxis. Long-term heparin therapy is well tolerated in most patients, in doses ranging from 5000 to 10,000 units twice a day subcutaneously. Osteoporosis may be seen more frequently with doses above 15,000 units per day for periods greater than 6 months.[33] Bone demineralization may occur in most patients on sustained heparin for long periods and may present as back pain.[34]

Fully anticoagulated patients are probably not candidates for regional anesthesia.[35] However, Odoom and Sih[36] report 1000 patients who received epidural anesthesia while receiving oral anticoagulants or intravenous heparin, or both. None of the patients developed epidural hematoma. The prudent clinician obtains coagulation parameters, platelet counts, and bleeding times in patients receiving heparin. If regional anesthesia is strongly indicated, and coagulation parameters are normal or near-normal (i.e., bleeding time within 2 minutes of upper limit), then the clinician might choose to proceed with regional anesthesia despite the fear of spinal hematoma. For example, an obese parturient with a difficult airway and a bleeding time of 12 minutes (normal, 10 minutes) may risk less morbidity from epidural anesthesia than from aspiration or loss of airway during a general anesthetic. If regional anesthesia is elected, it may be wise to use intermittent dosing schedules, with neurologic assessment between doses.[35] In this way, early detection of neurologic deficits may allow surgical decompression within 4 to 6 hours and may lessen chances for permanent damage.

TEN PRACTICAL POINTS

1. Massive air emboli can cause severe morbidity and mortality.

2. Precordial Doppler monitoring effectively detects air emboli but does not differentiate between "asymptomatic" air emboli and clinically significant emboli.

3. Routine precordial Doppler monitoring for air emboli is not indicated for all cesarean sections.

4. Amniotic fluid emboli, although difficult to diagnose, associate with high mortality rates and are major contributors to embolic maternal mortality.

5. Treatment of amniotic fluid embolism is primarily supportive and often requires invasive monitoring, inotropic agents, and blood products.

6. When selecting inotropic agents, consider both the mother and the fetus.

7. Pulmonary emboli increase right ventricular afterload, and treatment includes providing optimal preload and ensuring oxygenation and may require inotropic agents.

8. Thrombolytic agents are contraindicated during pregnancy, and treatment for pulmonary embolism requires full heparinization.

9. Epidural anesthesia in patients on minidose heparin is probably safe.

10. When considering regional anesthesia for patients receiving minidose heparin, evaluate the laboratory values and carefully consider the risks of both general and regional anesthesia.

REFERENCES

1. Kaunitz AM, Hughes JM, Grimes DA, et al: Causes of maternal mortality in the United States. Obstet Gynecol 65:605–612, 1985.
2. Younker D, Rodriguez V, Kavanagh J: Massive air embolism during cesarean section. Anesthesiology 65:77–79, 1986.
3. Vartikar JV, Johnson MD, Datta S: Precordial Doppler monitoring and pulse oximetry during cesarean delivery: Detection of venous air embolism. Reg Anesth 14:145–148, 1989.
4. Malinow AM, Naulty JS, Hunt CO, et al: Precordial ultrasonic monitoring during cesarean delivery. Anesthesiology 66:816–819, 1987.
5. Karuparthy VR, Downing JW, Husain EJ, et al: Incidence of venous air embolus during cesarean section is unchanged by the use of a 5 to 10 degree head up tilt. Anesth Analg 69:620–623, 1989.
6. Fong J, Gadalla F, Pierri MK, Druzin M: Are Doppler detected venous emboli during cesarean section air emboli? Anesth Analg 71:254–257, 1990.
7. Robinson DA, Albin MS: Venous air embolus and cesarean sections. Anesthesiology 66:93–94, 1987.
8. Chatelain SM, Quirk JG: Amniotic and thromboembolism. Clin Obstet Gynecol 33:473–481, 1990.
9. Lee W, Ginsburg KA, Cotton DB, Kaufman RH: Squamous and trophoblastic cells in the maternal pulmonary circulation identified by invasive hemodynamic monitoring during the peripartum period. Am J Obstet Gynecol 155:999–1001, 1986.
10. Azagami M, Mori N: Amniotic fluid embolism and leukotrienes. Am J Obstet Gynecol 155: 1119–1124, 1986.
11. Clark SL: Amniotic fluid embolism. Clin Perinatol 13:801–811, 1986.
12. Clark SL, Cotton DB, Gonik B, et al: Central hemodynamic alterations in amniotic fluid embolism. Am J Obstet Gynecol 158:1124–1126, 1988.
13. Marx GF: Cardiopulmonary resuscitation of late pregnant women. Anesthesiology 56:156, 1982.
14. Resnik R, Swartz WH, Plumer MH, et al: Amniotic fluid embolism with survival. Obstet Gynecol 47:295–298, 1976.
15. Rutherford SE, Phelan JP: Thromboembolic disease in pregnancy. Clin Perinatol 13:719–738, 1986.
16. Bell WR, Simon TL: Current status of pulmonary thrombolytic disease: Pathophysiology, diagnosis, and treatment. Am Heart J 103:239–262, 1982.
17. Goldhaber SZ: Pulmonary embolism death rates. Am Heart J 115:1342–1343, 1988.
18. Thrombolytic therapy in thrombosis: A National Institutes of Health Consensus Development Conference. Ann Intern Med 93:141–144, 1980.
19. Weiner CP: Diagnosis and management of thromboembolic disease during pregnancy. Clin Obstet Gynecol 28:107–118, 1985.
20. Lewis BD, James EM, Welch TJ: Current applications of duplex and color Doppler ultrasound imaging: Carotid and peripheral vascular system. Mayo Clin Proc 64:1147–1157, 1989.
21. Wiedemann HP, Mathay RA: Acute right heart failure. Crit Care Clin 1:631–661, 1985.
22. McIntyre KM, Sasahara AA: The hemodynamic response to PE in patients without prior cardiopulmonary disease. Am J Cardiol 28:288–294, 1971.
23. PIOPED Investigators: Value of the ventilation perfusion scan in acute pulmonary embolism. Results of the Prospective Investigation of Pulmo-

nary Embolism Diagnosis (PIOPED). JAMA 263:2753–2759, 1990.
24. Goldhaber SZ: Recent advances in the diagnosis and lytic therapy of pulmonary embolism. Chest 99:S173–S179, 1991.
25. Mathru M, Venus B, Smith RA, et al: Treatment of low cardiac output complicating acute pulmonary hypertension in normovolemic goats. Crit Care Med 14:120–124, 1986.
26. Molloy WD, Lee KY, Girling L, et al: Treatment of shock in a canine model of pulmonary embolism. Am Rev Respir Dis 130:870–874, 1984.
27. Dehring DJ, Arens JF: Pulmonary thromboembolism: Disease recognition and patient management. Anesthesiology 73:146–164, 1990.
28. Esposito RA, Grossi EA, Cappa G, et al: Successful treatment of postpartum shock caused by amniotic fluid embolism with cardiopulmonary bypass and pulmonary artery thromboembolectomy. Am J Obstet Gynecol 163:572–574, 1990.
29. Hux CH, Wapner RJ, Chayen B, et al: Use of the Greenfield filter for thromboembolic disease in pregnancy. Am J Obstet Gynecol 155:734–737, 1986.
30. Sasahara AA, Sharma GVRK, Barsamian EM, et al: Pulmonary thromboembolism: Diagnosis and treatment. JAMA 249:2945–2950, 1983.
31. Tengborn L, Bergqvist D, Mätzsch T, et al: Recurrent thromboembolism in pregnancy and puerperium. Is there a need for thromboprophylaxis? Am J Obstet Gynecol 160:90–94, 1989.
32. Badaracco MA, Vessey M: Recurrence of venous thromboembolism disease and use of oral contraceptives. Br Med J 1:215–217, 1974.
33. Bonnar J: Venous thromboembolism in pregnancy. Clin Obstet Gynecol 8:455–473, 1981.
34. De Swiet M, Ward PD, Fidler J, et al: Prolonged heparin therapy in pregnancy causes bone demineralization. Br J Obstet Gynecol 90:1129–1134, 1983.
35. Owens EL, Kasten GW, Hessel EA II: Spinal subarachnoid hematoma after lumbar puncture and heparinization: A case report, review of the literature and discussion of anesthetic implications. Anesth Analg 65:1201–1207, 1986.
36. Odoom JA, Sih IL: Epidural analgesia and anticoagulant therapy. Anaesthesia 38:254–259, 1983.

THIRTEEN

Shoulder Dystocia

David M. Dewan, M.D.

Shoulder dystocia represents a true obstetric emergency and is the obstetrician's version of the anesthesiologist's "can't intubate and can't ventilate." Shoulder dystocia associates with significant maternal and fetal morbidity, and good outcomes require swift, skilled problem resolution. Although shoulder dystocia is an obstetric complication, the anesthesia care provider must be prepared to provide appropriate conditions for safe, rapid problem solving. The prepared anesthesia care team has sufficient knowledge and understanding of the complication to anticipate its occurrence and understand the maneuvers necessary to achieve delivery and is able to participate in and supply appropriate delivery conditions.

Shoulder dystocia occurs in 0.15 to 1.7% of deliveries, and the frequency may be increasing.[1] Shoulder dystocia occurs when, following delivery of the head, the shoulders impact against the bony pelvis, preventing delivery of the body. During normal vaginal delivery, the fetal head traverses the maternal pelvis in the oblique lie, which offers the greatest space for passage (Fig. 13–1). Importantly, despite maneuvering of the fetal head to the anteroposterior position following delivery, the fetal shoulders usually follow the same oblique course through the maternal pelvis. However, during shoulder dystocia, the shoulders attempt entrance into the pelvis in the more constricted anteroposterior lie (Fig. 13–2). Thus, shoulder dystocia is a result of maternal-fetal disproportion and is a *bony* obstruction to delivery, which

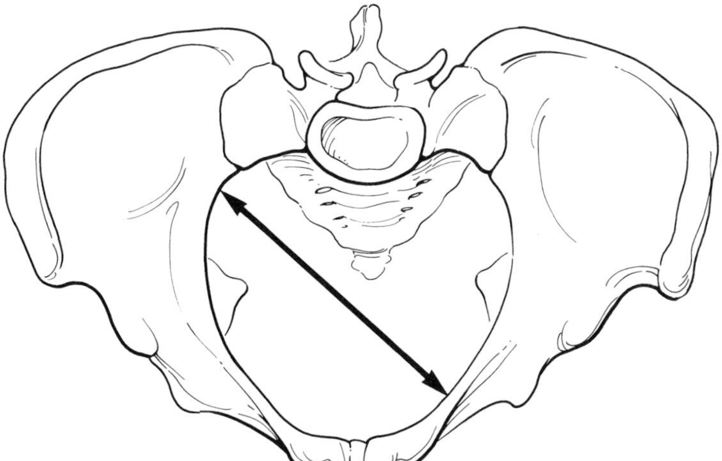

Figure 13–1. The pelvis has a greater diameter in the oblique lie.

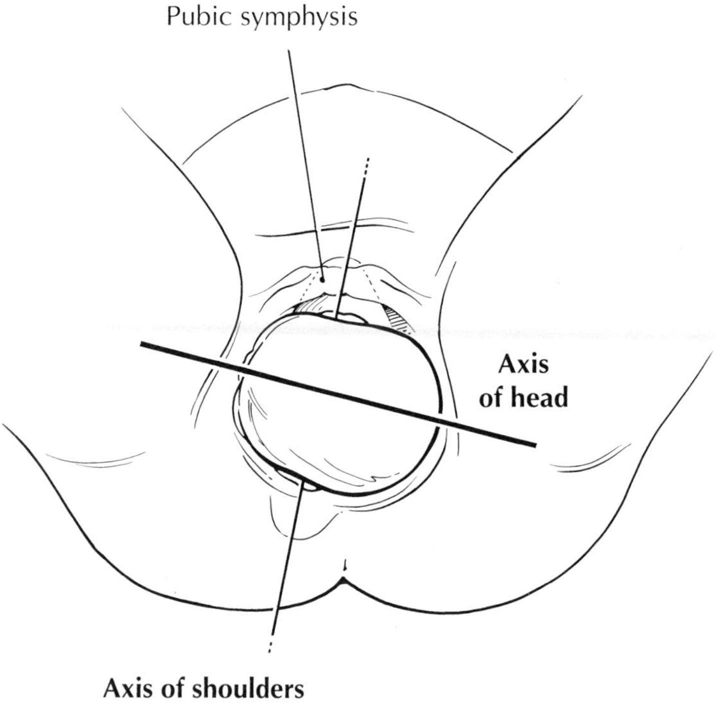

Figure 13–2. The pubic symphysis impedes the descent of the fetal shoulders.

occurs independent of the uterus or maternal soft tissue. Further maternal expulsive efforts, use of forceps, or *fundal* pressure are futile maneuvers and may worsen the degree of impaction and the complication rate, since they result in abduction of the shoulders, which increases shoulder dimensions (Fig. 13–3).[2] These efforts may evoke the turtle sign, a hallmark

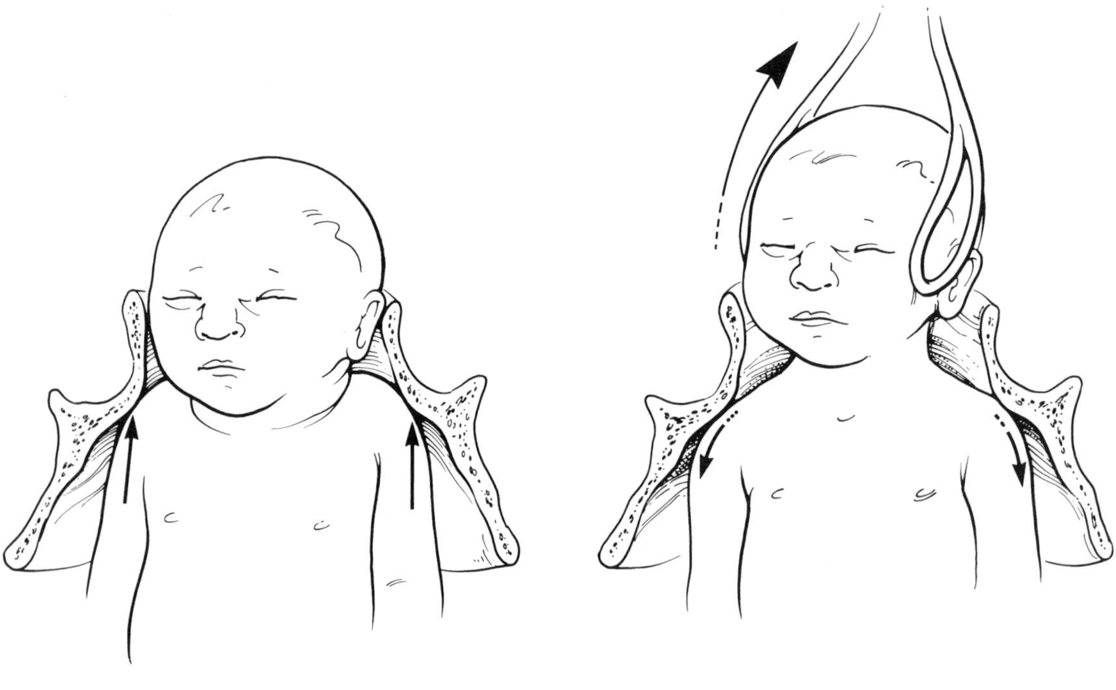

Figure 13–3. Shoulder dystocia is worsened with forceps, maternal expulsion efforts, or uterine fundal pressure. Note the increased shoulder dimensions with shoulder abduction.

TABLE 13–1
Risk Factors for Shoulder Dystocia

Unusually large mother's birth weight
Obesity
Diabetes
Known fetal macrosomia > 4000 gm
Prolonged gestation
Previous macrosomic infant
Previous difficult delivery
Mid forceps delivery
Epidural analgesia
Prolonged delivery phase
Prolonged second stage
Greater parity
Older maternal age

of shoulder dystocia, whereby the fetal head, following delivery, retracts into the maternal vagina. Without expeditious delivery, fetal death may follow secondary to interruption of effective fetal perfusion.

RISK FACTORS

Recognizing the risk factors associated with shoulder dystocia is essential and allows anticipation and advance preparations for this complication (Table 13–1). Two obvious factors that contribute to maternal-fetal disproportion are a contracted maternal pelvis and fetal macrosomia. Maternal pelvic abnormalities are usually discovered antepartum and documented in the obstetric records. Fetal macrosomia, a more common cause of dystocia, associates with multiple factors. Maternal age, parity, pregnancy weight gain, diabetes (both insulin-dependent and gestational), and obesity are antepartum factors increasing the likelihood of fetal macrosomia. Maternal obesity increases risk markedly. When maternal weight exceeds 250 pounds, the incidence of shoulder dystocia may increase eightfold compared with women who weigh less than 200 pounds.[3] Diabetes is particularly worrisome and increases the risk for any given newborn weight. According to Acker, when infants weigh more than 4000 gm, the incidence of shoulder dystocia is 23% in diabetic mothers and 10% in nondiabetic mothers.[4] The greater disparity between head and shoulder girth among infants with diabetic mothers may account for the difference.[5] Surprising, the *mother's* birth weight also associates with fetal macrosomia.[6] Finally, a history of a previous difficult delivery and a previous delivery of a macrosomic infant are significant risk factors. The alert anesthesia care provider may note a history of any of the preceding factors during anesthetic evaluation by questioning the patient and reviewing the obstetric record.

Other clues may appear at the time of admission or during the course of labor. For example, gestations greater than 41 weeks may associate with up to 40% of shoulder dystocia occurrences in nondiabetic patients,[1] and nearly one third of diabetic patients experience shoulder dystocia when ultrasonic examination reveals a fetal weight of greater than 4000 gm.[4] O'Leary and Leonetti believe that whenever estimated fetal weight exceeds 4500 gm, delivery should occur by elective cesarean section.[7] Clues may also present during labor. Prolongation of the deceleration phase of labor provides one clue. When unusual slowing of labor progress occurs between cervical dilatations of 8 and 10 cm, this may herald future problems. Similarly, prolongation of the second stage of labor may be a sign of an impending delivery problem. When these clues exist, communication between the anesthesia care team and the obstetrician is important. Whereas low forceps and outlet forceps deliveries may offer little fetal threat, mid forceps delivery, when associated with the factors previously discussed, should alert the anesthesia care team to potential shoulder dystocia problems. Be especially wary of "trial of forceps." When you hear this phrase, there should be direct communication between the obstetrician and the anesthesia provider. Nevertheless, 70% of patients who develop shoulder dystocia have normal labor patterns and 85% have spontaneous deliveries.[4] Not surprisingly, epidural anesthesia also associates with shoulder dystocia, albeit perhaps not in a causal relationship. In the author's institution, epidural anesthesia is more likely to be requested during long and painful labors and when abdominal delivery is likely.

Importantly, although the preceding risk factors associate with shoulder dystocia, they fall far short of predicting the majority of shoulder dystocias and may, in fact, identify only a minority of dystocias. For example, birth weight, prolonged deceleration phase, and duration of the second stage of labor predicted only 16% of dystocias causing trauma.[8] Alertness must be an

TABLE 13–2
Treatment

Complete episiotomy
McRoberts procedure to increase pelvic outlet size
Suprapubic pressure
Manual rotation of anterior shoulder
Extraction of posterior arm
Replacement of head in vagina and downward pressure on anterior shoulder
Tocolysis, cephalic replacement, and cesarean section
Abdominal rescue to allow vaginal delivery

integral characteristic of all caregivers at all deliveries, and close scrutiny of the delivery process and the obstetrician's demeanor by the anesthesia team may also provide early clues of an impending problem. When possible, observe the delivery, noting the amount of forceps traction and the ease of fetal descent, and watch for successful delivery of the anterior shoulder, which usually suggests successful vaginal delivery. Do not relax until the anterior shoulder is delivered!

TREATMENT

When shoulder dystocia presents, treatment begins with a proctoepisiotomy to relieve any soft tissue obstruction (Table 13–2). At the author's institution, the McRoberts procedure is the usual second step.[9] The McRoberts procedure involves removing the maternal legs from the stirrups and abducting them toward the chest (Fig. 13–4). This procedure rotates the pubic symphysis cephalad and straightens the sacrum, thereby increasing the size of the pelvic inlet. If this maneuver is not successful, suprapubic pressure, without fundal pressure, allows the anterior shoulder to slide underneath the pubic symphysis (Fig. 13–5). At this point, the obstetrician may attempt manual rotation of the anterior shoulder to an oblique lie, allowing further descent of the shoulder with gentle downward cephalic traction. Extraction of the posterior arm allows for more room and frequently permits successful manual rotation of the anterior shoulder. At this point, if all attempts to deliver the shoulders fail, the obstetrician may flex the head and replace it in the vagina, as described by Zavanelli.[10] This procedure may improve fetal perfusion while the obstetrician prepares for cesarean section. During cephalic replacement, the obstetrician may also administer tocolytics to relax the uterus, to allow easier return of the fetus into the uterus prior to performing a cesarean section. Finally, there is one report of abdominal rescue in which the surgeon performed an abdominal hysterotomy, gained access to the fetal shoulder, and rotated the shoulder under the pubic symphysis, which allowed vaginal delivery.[11]

As always, keys to success for these procedures are communication between the anesthesia and the obstetric care providers and having calm, cooperative patients with sufficient analgesia and skeletal muscle relaxation to allow performance of these maneuvers. For example, a rigid abdominal wall, frequently accompanying abdominal pain, may impair downward displacement of the anterior shoulder during suprapubic pressure. Inadequate vaginal anesthesia also

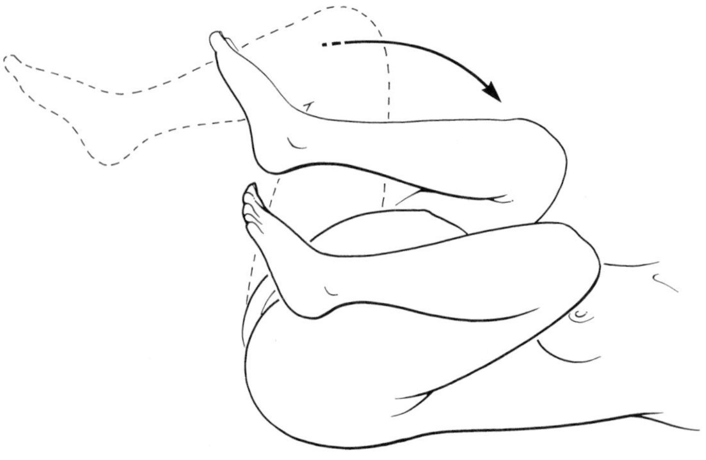

Figure 13–4. The McRoberts procedure: Abducting the legs toward the chest, straightening the sacrum, rotating the pubic symphysis cephalad, thus increasing the size of the pelvic inlet.

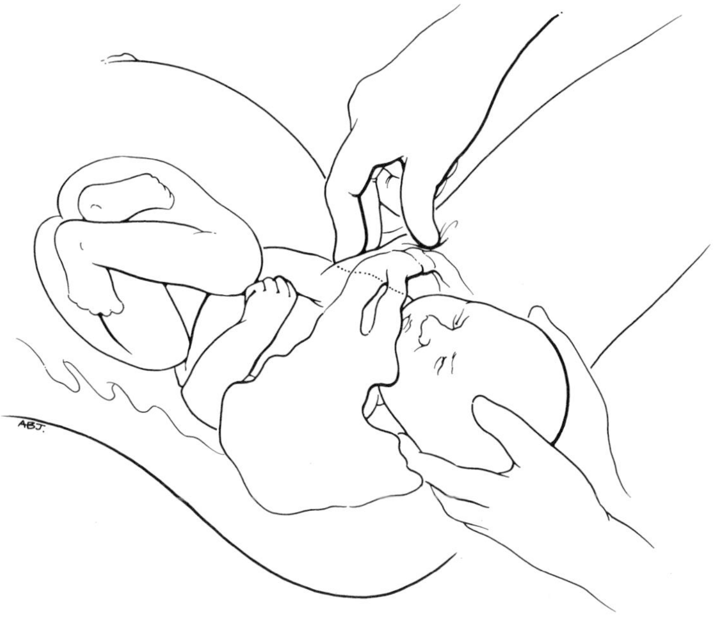

Figure 13–5. Suprapubic pressure assists anterior shoulder passage under the pubic symphysis.

impedes fetal manipulation. Communication between the obstetrician and the anesthesiologist is of the utmost importance for a successful outcome following shoulder dystocia. Mental, and perhaps actual, preparations for cesarean section anesthesia should accompany initiation of any of these maneuvers, as should anesthesiologist-obstetrician communication.

COMPLICATIONS

Maternal complications following shoulder dystocia include hemorrhage, uterine atony, uterine rupture, cervical and vaginal lacerations, and unintentional fourth-degree lacerations. Blood loss may be large and rapid. The anesthesia care team must prepare for volume resuscitation and maternal drug administration to control hemorrhage. Preparations for abdominal exploration or extensive vaginal surgery, despite apparent successful vaginal delivery, should also occur when hemorrhage persists.

Neonatal morbidity ranges from minor injury to death. As many as 2.9% of infants die,[12] and 20 to 42% of infants experience complications during true shoulder dystocia.[13, 14] Consistent with the earlier discussion, fundal pressure, unless accompanied by other maneuvers, may be harmful and produce a 77% newborn complication rate.[14] Plexus injury, either Erb, Duchenne, or Lumpke palsy, fracture of the clavicle or humerus, and neonatal asphyxia are significant dystocia-related morbidities. Not surprisingly, the degree of fetal asphyxia correlates directly with the delay in delivery, emphasizing the urgency of this complication. Umbilical artery pH declines at a rate of 0.4 pH units/min, documenting the urgency of this complication.[5]

Prior to considering anesthetic management, Hopwood's analysis of a typical dystocic event is worth noting. "Shoulder dystocia develops cataclysmically. What began as a difficult delivery now assumes catastrophic proportions. Frequently, consultation is not readily available, and one is left with untrained help, possibly inadequate anesthesia, an anxious husband, and a personal sense of doom and foreboding. An organized plan of attack is essential and involves a step-like progression of action."[1] This characterization aptly describes the ramifications of this harrowing experience.

ANESTHETIC MANAGEMENT

Anesthetic management begins prior to delivery. Ideally, both the obstetrician and the anesthesia care provider are aware of this potential "high-risk" delivery. At the author's institution, subarachnoid or general anesthesia is not administered in the labor, delivery, and recovery rooms. The high-risk nature of these deliveries, combined with the possible requirement for either subarachnoid or general anesthesia, mandates delivery in the operating room.

The author's group believes that labor epidural analgesia and the capability to provide profound surgical anesthesia are the best management for patients at risk for shoulder dystocia. Existing epidural anesthesia affords maximal flexibility to provide appropriate delivery conditions, whether for abdominal or difficult vaginal delivery. Epidural narcotics may mask inadequate epidural anesthesia. For this reason, the author's group avoids epidural narcotics until convinced that the epidural can provide surgical anesthesia in emergent circumstances. Alternatively, spinal anesthesia at the time of delivery may be appropriate. In this setting, after communicating with the obstetrician regarding prognosis for successful vaginal delivery, the author would suggest achieving cesarean section levels of either epidural or spinal anesthesia for these high-risk patients in the event that vaginal delivery is impossible. If there is no existing epidural anesthetic, and successful vaginal delivery is questionable, combined spinal-epidural anesthesia is also a reasonable choice. Higher levels of blockade should not impede delivery, since maternal expulsive efforts will probably not be necessary and may be detrimental. Select agents with an appropriate duration of action. Pudendal and local anesthesia, although alternatives, may provide inadequate anesthesia and ultimately require the administration of general anesthesia. Irrespective of the selected anesthetic technique, the obstetrician and anesthesiologist must decide the appropriate place for attempted delivery, and preparations should be made for complicated delivery, including the potential requirement for general endotracheal anesthesia.

The team must also prepare for potential management of the depressed newborn. The anesthesia care provider's primary responsibility is to the mother, and thus, alternative team members must be available to provide immediate expeditious and skillful newborn resuscitation. The patient should receive continuous oxygen during the delivery process. Continuous maternal oxygen administration elevates fetal arterial oxygen tension (Pa_{O_2}) and may provide reserve if effective fetal perfusion diminishes. Additionally, maternal oxygenation serves as denitrogenation in the event general endotracheal anesthesia is necessary.

Remember, the primary obstruction to delivery is bone. Therefore, uterine relaxation is not a prerequisite for successful vaginal delivery. Nevertheless, the patient must be calm, cooperative, and ideally, pain-free. The obstetrician must have sufficient maternal skeletal muscle relaxation to perform the required maneuvers. However, if cephalad replacement of the fetus becomes necessary and tocolysis for fetal reinsertion fails, uterine relaxation with general anesthetic agents may be required for successful fetal replacement into the uterine cavity.

General endotracheal anesthesia may be necessary to provide appropriate vaginal conditions for successful delivery when major regional blockade is not present. In this instance, the anesthetic technique should resemble that discussed in Chapter 7. In theory, tocolytic administration preceding the induction of general anesthesia might elevate the risk of maternal dysrhythmias. However, in the author's group's experience, tocolytic administration for other indications has not been a problem. The author would not withhold general anesthesia because of these theoretical concerns. Finally, ample support personnel should be available to execute the plan. Remain observant and, when appropriate, be available to assist. The author's group has occasionally assisted in performance of the McRoberts maneuver and the application of suprapubic pressure. Do not, however, abandon the mother—your primary responsibility. Maternal blood loss may be profound. Be observant and be prepared!

SUMMARY

Shoulder dystocia is a life-threatening complication with potential severe maternal and fetal complications. As with failed intubations, no assessment reliably predicts all instances. Knowing the obstetrician's needs and the fetal and maternal hazards and having a plan that minimizes delay are major steps in improving outcome.

TEN PRACTICAL POINTS

1. Shoulder dystocia is an acute emergency requiring rapid resolution.
2. If shoulder dystocia is suspected, deliver in an operative setting.
3. A properly functioning epidural provides the best flexibility for problem management.

4. Although shoulder dystocia is the result of a bony obstruction, effective treatment requires a calm, cooperative patient.

5. General anesthesia is rarely indicated if the previous conditions are met.

6. Administer 100% oxygen during delivery.

7. Have a newborn-resuscitation team available.

8. Maternal complications can be severe.

9. Be alert for warning signs!

10. Communicate!

REFERENCES

1. Hopwood H: Shoulder dystocia: 15 years' experience in a community hospital. Am J Obstet Gynecol 144:162–164, 1982.
2. Carlan S, Angel J, Knuppel R: Shoulder dystocia. Am Fam Physician 43:1307–1311, 1991.
3. Johnson SR, Kolberg BH, Varner MW: Maternal obesity in pregnancy. Surg Gynecol Obstet 164:431–437, 1987.
4. Acker DB, Sachs BP, Friedman EA: Risk factors for shoulder dystocia. Obstet Gynecol 66:762–768, 1985.
5. Hernandez C, Wendel G: Shoulder dystocia. Clin Obstet Gynecol 33:526–534, 1990.
6. Hackman E, Emanuel I, van Belle G, Daling J: Maternal birth weight and subsequent pregnancy outcome. JAMA 250:2016–2019, 1983.
7. O'Leary J, Leonetti H: Shoulder dystocia: Prevention and treatment. Am J Obstet Gynecol 162:5–9, 1990.
8. Gross T, Sokol R, Williams T, Thompson K: Shoulder dystocia: A fetal-physician risk. Am J Obstet Gynecol 156:1408–1418, 1987.
9. Gonik B, Stringer C, Held B: An alternate maneuver for management of shoulder dystocia. Am J Obstet Gynecol 145:882–884, 1983.
10. Sandberg EC: The Zavanelli maneuver: A potentially revolutionary method for resolution of shoulder dystocia. Am J Obstet Gynecol 152:479–484, 1985.
11. O'Leary J: Abdominal rescue after failed cephalic replacement. Obstet Gynecol 80:514–516, 1992.
12. Sandmire HF, O'Halloin TJ: Shoulder dystocia: Its incidence and associated risk factors. Int J Gynaecol Obstet 26:65–73, 1988.
13. Benedetti T, Gabbe S: Shoulder dystocia: A complication of fetal macrosomia and prolonged second stage of labor with mid-pelvic delivery. Obstet Gynecol 52:526–529, 1978.
14. Gross S, Shime J, Vereen D: Shoulder dystocia: Predictors and outcome, a 5-year review. Am J Obstet Gynecol 156:334–336, 1987.

FOURTEEN

Anesthesia in the Febrile Parturient

Connie E. Taylor, M.D.

The febrile parturient presents the anesthesia provider with a therapeutic dilemma. In the presence of bacteremia or viremia, the introduction of needles into the epidural or subarachnoid space risks allowing contaminated blood to enter the normally insulated central nervous system. Additionally, tissue trauma may derange regional host defenses, creating an area of diminished resistance vulnerable to infection. Given the morbidity associated with neuroaxial infection, many practitioners view the presence of fever as a contraindication to the administration of regional anesthesia.

Denying the option of regional anesthesia to the parturient is not, however, medically benign. The most compelling consideration is the risk associated with the induction of general anesthesia in the pregnant patient. Despite the technologic advances in monitoring and the capability for fiberoptic intubation, the primary cause of anesthetic-related obstetric morbidity and mortality remains airway management complications. In contrast, regional analgesia provides excellent pain relief, amelioration of the physiologic stress of labor, controlled conditions for vaginal or abdominal delivery, and hopefully an alternative to general anesthesia.

DIFFERENTIAL DIAGNOSIS

The parturient presenting with fever requires a thorough medical history and physical examination as well as appropriate laboratory tests and cultures. These initial data should guide the practitioner in distinguishing chronic from acute processes and surgical from nonsurgical infectious entities.

Spurious elevations in temperature may occur with dehydration when the body's ability to dissipate heat is diminished by the contracted intravascular volume. This frequently occurs in obstetric patients who receive nothing by mouth (NPO) from the onset of labor and are denied the benefit of intravenous fluids. Hydration with a balanced salt solution should result in normalization of body temperature and is a first step in evaluating fevers of uncertain cause.

The differential diagnosis must also include drug-induced fever. The most common drug-related fever occurring in obstetric patients results from prostaglandin E_2 (Prostin E_2), administered by vaginal suppository to induce uterine contractions. In addition to fever, prostaglandin E_2 administration is associated with nausea, vomiting, and respiratory symptoms. Frequently, the temporal association of symptoms with the initiation of drug therapy establishes the diagnosis and should permit regional anesthesia. However, when serial doses of prostaglandin are given on successive days to "ripen the cervix," the possibility of another cause for the fever must be considered because the relationship between drug and fever is less clear.

Viral infections, either gastrointestinal or upper respiratory, may present with fever. Virus-associated symptoms are often mild, and the presumptive diagnosis can be made on the basis of epidemiologic findings—either a community outbreak of viral illness or illness among the patient's family members or social contacts. At Wake Forest University, the author's group permits regional anesthesia when viral infection is present, unless the patient demonstrates significant compromise suggesting possible hemodynamic instability.

Bacterial infections may be a greater concern. Rarely, obstetric patients present with documented bacterial infections of known cause and source. Patients with known diagnoses usually present either already receiving or preparing to receive appropriate therapy. In this setting, anesthetic choice is dictated by the organ system involved and by the extent of involvement. For example, a treated pneumonia process may indicate regional anesthesia to avoid the deleterious effects of general anesthesia on the pulmonary system. In contrast, pulmonary infection with coexistent severe hypoxemia may warrant general anesthesia to ensure adequate oxygenation during surgical procedures.

More commonly, the source of infection is initially uncertain. Acute chorioamnionitis, the most common bacterial infection during pregnancy, complicates between 0.5 and 1.3% of all pregnancies.[1] When purulent amniotic fluid is observed, the diagnosis is straightforward. More often, however, chorioamnionitis is a diagnosis of exclusion made when a maternal fever of 38° C or greater accompanies prolonged ruptured membranes.[2] Indeed, chorioamnionitis, secondary to prolonged rupture of membranes, may account for up to one third of cases of idiopathic preterm labor or rupture of the membranes, and the diagnosis must be considered whenever premature labor exists.[3] Although chorioamnionitis precludes tocolysis, it is not an indication for cesarean section. Thus, some parturients face several hours of labor, and denying regional anesthesia to these patients has obvious major implications.

Once the diagnosis of chorioamnionitis is established, many obstetricians initiate intrapartum antibiotic therapy to reduce neonatal sepsis.[1, 4–6] The implications of antibiotic therapy are discussed later.

DIAGNOSIS

Management of nonamniotic bacterial infection will be dictated by the source of infection. Ideally, anesthesia providers would like concrete parameters defining safe conditions for administering regional anesthesia in the presence of fever without risking neuroaxial infection. These do not exist.

"Fever" may be the first presenting sign of bacterial infection. Nineteenth-century investigators identified 37° C as normal body temperature, with a diurnal variation between 36.2° and 37.5° C. Temperatures exceeding 38° C were considered abnormal. Although the precision of these measurements and the precise values obtained have recently been challenged,[7, 8] this definition of normal body temperature persists. Although originally described to define puerperal sepsis occurring postpartum, temperatures exceeding 38° C are still considered by many to define obstetric fever and significant clinical infection, and anesthesiologists frequently use the same criteria for dictating therapy.

When the nonpregnant patient's temperature rises, the white blood cell count assists diagnosis of clinically significant infections associated with viremia or bacteremia. However, pregnancy and labor influence the leukocyte count. The white count rises during pregnancy, with normal counts ranging from 5000 to 12,000 per μl. During stress, the leukocyte count may increase dramatically, producing counts as high as 25,000 per μl,[9] making this parameter an unreliable diagnostic tool. A recent retrospective study of women with chorioamnionitis who received regional anesthesia could not identify differences in either mean body temperature or mean leukocyte count between bacteremic and nonbacteremic patients.[10] Therefore, anesthesiologists cannot rely on body temperature or leukocyte count for identification of patients at risk for iatrogenic neuroaxial infection.[10] At Wake Forest University, whenever possible, the author's group attempts to delineate between bacteremic and nonbacteremic infections based on both clinical and laboratory findings. When the infection is not considered bacterial in origin, regional anesthesia is believed safe, unless systemic toxicity exists. But what about bacteremic infections?

Bacteremic Infections

A 1992 study by Carp and Bailey,[11] published in *Anesthesiology*, rekindled the practitioners' concerns regarding the appropriateness of potential dural puncture in the presence of bacteremia. The authors developed a model of chronic bacteremia in rats. Twelve of 40 rats who had blood culture–proven bacteremia at the time of percutaneous cisternal dural puncture developed meningitis. "Bacteremic animals not undergoing percutaneous cisternal dural punctures always had sterile spinal fluid, and dural puncture in the absence of bacteremia did not result in infection." They also identified a positive correlation between the extent of bacteremia (colony-forming units per milliliter) and the development of meningitis. These findings question the wisdom of performing dural puncture in the presence of bacteremic infection.[12, 13]

Other information conflicts, as seen in two early retrospective studies. In 1919, Wegeforth and Latham[14] presented clinical observations made during an epidemic of meningococcemia and concluded that lumbar puncture was a causative factor in the cases of meningitis they treated. In 1941, Pray[15] reported 207 cases of meningitis in children from 1912 to 1938, 80% of which occurred in patients under 2 years of age, the population in which meningitis is most prevalent. One of the earliest to examine the relationship between bacteremia and dural puncture, Pray concluded from his data that ". . . in general lumbar puncture is not hazardous for the patient with bacteremia." More recently, Eng and Seligman,[16] in a retrospective clinical study in 1981 examining lumbar puncture meningitis, reported that the incidence of cases of meningitis that had clinical features consistent with lumbar puncture–induced meningitis did not differ from the expected incidence of spontaneous meningitis.

Are there reliable human studies supporting a causal relationship between the administration of spinal or epidural anesthesia, the presence of bacteremia, and the development of neuroaxial infection? Regional anesthesia is often employed for compromised patients undergoing urologic or intestinal surgeries associated with fever, leukocytosis, and bacteremia. Although there are case reports of neuroaxial infection following regional anesthesia,[17–20] large series of spinal and epidural anesthetic administration have been reviewed and fail to identify an association. In a classic survey, Dripps and Vandam[21] prospectively evaluated 8460 patients who received 10,098 spinal anesthetics between 1948 and 1951. Spinal anesthesia was utilized for any procedure below the diaphragm, including in patients with cardiac or pulmonary disease, advanced age, obesity, or intestinal obstruction or in those considered at risk for general anesthesia. The authors identified no "evidence of a septic process in the meninges or epidural region."

Similarly, Phillips and associates[22] prospectively examined 10,440 patients receiving spinal anesthesia between 1964 and 1966. Ninety-three percent of these blocks were placed for obstetric delivery, either vaginal or abdominal. No infectious complications were reported.

Scott and Hubbard[23] retrospectively reviewed 505,000 extradural blocks performed between 1982 and 1986. Eighty-five percent were performed for labor analgesia and 16% were for cesarean section. Epidural abscesses occurred in 2 patients; 1, which developed in a diabetic patient 11 months postpartum, was not considered to be associated with the anesthetic.

Finally, Crawford[24] reported 27,000 consecutive epidural anesthetics performed in obstetric patients between 1968 and 1985. One patient developed an epidural abscess requiring laminectomy.

Although the inclusion-exclusion criteria for these studies did not address the presence of fever, almost certainly the cohorts included febrile patients with possible bacteremia in temporal proximity to block placement. Nevertheless, the infectious complication rate is astoundingly low. The large number of regional anesthetics administered and the very few cases of neuroaxial infections reported in which the anesthetic technique may have played a role argue for the benefits of regional anesthesia in the presence of fever.

Further, several previously mentioned studies speak to the benefit of antibiotic treatment prior to regional anesthesia for prevention of neuroaxial infection. Wegeforth and Latham[14] suggested a role for antibiotics: "With the exception of the fulminating case, those who had received intravenous serum therapy before lumbar puncture was done showed subsequently no evidence of meningeal infection." Eng and Seligman[16] observed: "None of the five patients in the current study with possible lumbar puncture–induced meningitis was receiving antibiotics when the lumbar punctures were performed." Carp and Bailey[11] found evidence for the value of antibiotic therapy in their study of rats. Their investigation included a group of 30 animals, all of which had documented bacteremias of a sufficient degree to cause meningitis and who received a dose of appropriate antibiotic prior to dural puncture. None developed meningitis.

At Wake Forest University, when the author's group's group was requested to do an epidural anesthetic or spinal anesthetic on a febrile patient, an obstetrician was consulted regarding her or his planned usage of antibiotic therapy. If the obstetrician intended antibiotic therapy and there was no urgency, the regional anesthesia was frequently withheld until the patient had received initial therapy and then the regional anesthesia was instituted.

However, when the obstetrician does not intend antibiotic usage, the decision is less clear. In such a case, if one is asked to perform epidural or spinal anesthesia on a febrile patient whose pregnancy has been uneventful, whose vaginal delivery is imminent, and whose airway anatomy is reassuring, the author's group sometimes chose not to expose her to the associated risks, however small. On the other hand, in an obese patient with a difficult airway, the risk of possible airway complications is of far greater concern than her risk of neuroaxial infection.

Central Nervous System Infection

The anesthesia practitioner often elicits complaints of backache and headache on postoperative rounds, symptoms that may be caused by prolonged NPO status, caffeine withdrawal, back strain, bruising at the site of regional block administration, or postdural puncture headache. Puerperal infection with fever may complicate the clinical picture.

These common complaints need to be distinguished from clinical presentations that may be consistent with meningitis or spinal epidural abscess. Although the incidence of neuroaxial infection is very low, the associated morbidity and mortality warrant a high index of suspicion and aggressive intervention.

Spinal epidural abscess presents with a progression of symptoms from backache to nerve root pain followed by weakness and paralysis. Symptoms in catheter-related cases have presented from as little as 72 hours to as long as 5 months after block placement. Associated findings include fever, leukocytosis, and signs of meningeal irritation, stiff neck and headache. Myelography is the definitive diagnostic test.

Therapy comprises surgical exploration and drainage and antibiotics. Outcome is directly related to duration of symptoms at the time treatment is initiated, since delay can cause injury. If there is any suspicion that spinal epidural abscess could be the diagnosis, emergency neurosurgical consultation is mandatory.[20, 25]

The diagnosis of meningitis is suggested by the presence of fever, headache, photophobia, stiff neck and back, positive Kernig and Brudzinski signs, seizures, vomiting, and a change in sensorium.[26] When these findings exist, obtain neurologic consultation along with cerebrospinal fluid chemistry and hematologic and microbiologic studies, followed by institution of antibiotic therapy if appropriate.

SUMMARY

Among the many causes of fever in the parturient, bacteremia presents perhaps the greatest dilemma. In the presence of bacteremia, the clinician must weigh the usual advantages of regional anesthesia against its small potential to cause neuroaxial infection. Following parenteral antibiotic therapy, the author's group usually administered regional anesthesia for labor and delivery or cesarean section if the benefits were judged to outweigh the minimal risks. However, regional anesthesia is considered contraindicated when there is local infection at the site of intended needle placement or serious system infection (primarily herpes simplex II infection). When regional anesthesia is performed in the bacteremic patient, extra care must be taken postpartum in evaluating for infection.

TEN PRACTICAL POINTS

1. The presence of fever does not necessarily indicate an infectious process; there are other causes for elevated body temperatures.
2. Try hydration as the initial therapy if no clear source of infection is readily identified.
3. The febrile parturient needs a thorough evaluation to identify the cause of her fever and to guide appropriate treatment.
4. There are reports of neuroaxial infections associated with regional anesthesia in patients who may have been bacteremic, but these are the exceptions, especially when compared with the number of regional anesthetics administered.

5. Neither the leukocyte count nor the degree of fever has been correlated with the parturient who has positive blood cultures.

6. The major cause of anesthetic-related morbidity and mortality in parturients remains airway complications associated with the induction of general anesthesia.

7. The decision to administer regional anesthesia to a febrile patient must reflect a careful consideration of the benefits and risks.

8. There is good experimental evidence that administration of antibiotics prior to dural puncture is protective, even in the setting of documented bacteremia.

9. Antibiotics administered intrapartum in the patient presumed to have chorioamnionitis have been shown to decrease the incidence of neonatal sepsis.

10. Once parenteral antibiotics have been administered, epidural or spinal anesthesia may be given unless serious systemic infection is present.

REFERENCES

1. Gilstrap LC, Leveno KJ, Cox SM, et al: Intrapartum treatment of acute chorioamnionitis: Impact on neonatal sepsis. Am J Obstet Gynecol 159:579–583, 1988.
2. Cunningham FG, MacDonald PC, Gant NF (eds): Williams Obstetrics, 18th ed. Norwalk, CT, Appleton & Lange, 1989, p 751.
3. Cunningham FG, MacDonald PC, Gant NF (eds): Williams Obstetrics, 18th ed. Norwalk, CT, Appleton & Lange, 1989, p 748.
4. Sperling RS, Ramamurthy RS, Gibbs RS: A comparison of intrapartum versus immediate postpartum treatment of intra-amniotic infection. Obstet Gynecol 70:861–865, 1987.
5. Mead PB: When to treat intra-amniotic infection. Obstet Gynecol 72:935–936, 1988.
6. Gibbs RS, Dinsmoor MJ, Newton ER, Ramamurthy RS: A randomized trial of intrapartum versus immediate postpartum treatment of women with intra-amniotic infection. Obstet Gynecol 72:823–828, 1988.
7. Mackowiak PA, Wasserman SS, Levine MM: A critical appraisal of 98.6° F, the upper limit of the normal body temperature, and other legacies of Carl Reinhold August Wunderlich. JAMA 268:1578–1580, 1992.
8. Weiger WA: 98.6° F [Letter]. JAMA 268:1249, 1992.
9. Cunningham FG, MacDonald PC, Gant NF (eds): Williams Obstetrics, 18th ed. Norwalk, CT, Appleton & Lange, 1989, p 143.
10. Bader AM, Gilbertson L, Kirz L, Datta S: Regional anesthesia in women with chorioamnionitis. Reg Anesth 17:84–86, 1992.
11. Carp H, Bailey S: The association between meningitis and dural puncture in bacteremic rats. Anesthesiology 76:739–742, 1992.
12. Weed LH, Wegeforth P, Ayer JB, Felton LD: The production of meningitis by release of cerebrospinal fluid during an experimental septicemia: Preliminary note. JAMA 72:190–193, 1919.
13. Petersdorf RG, Swarner DR, Garcia M: Studies of the pathogenesis of meningitis. II. Development of meningitis during pneumococcal bacteremia. J Clin Invest 41:320–328, 1962.
14. Wegeforth P, Latham JR: Lumbar puncture as a factor in the causation of meningitis. Am J Med Sci 158:183–201, 1919.
15. Pray LG: Lumbar puncture as a factor in the pathogenesis of meningitis. Am J Dis Child 62:295–308, 1941.
16. Eng RHK, Seligman SJ: Lumbar puncture–induced meningitis. JAMA 245:1456–1459, 1981.
17. Roberts SP, Petts HV: Meningitis after obstetric spinal anaesthesia. Anaesthesia 45:376–377, 1990.
18. Berman RS, Eisele JH: Bacteremia, spinal anesthesia, and development of meningitis. Anesthesiology 48:376–377, 1978.
19. Loarie DJ, Fairley HB: Epidural abscess following spinal anesthesia. Anesth Analg 57:351–353, 1978.
20. Ngan Kee WD, Jones MR, Thomas P, Worth RJ: Extradural abscess complicating extradural anaesthesia for caesarean section. Br J Anaesth 69:647–652, 1992.
21. Dripps RD, Vandam LD: Long-term follow-up of patients who received 10,098 spinal anesthetics: Failure to discover major neurological sequelae. JAMA 156:1486–1491, 1954.
22. Phillips OC, Ebner H, Nelson AT, Black MH: Neurologic complications following spinal anesthesia with lidocaine: A prospective review of 10,440 cases. Anesthesiology 30:284–289, 1969.
23. Scott DB, Hubbard BM: Serious non-fatal complications associated with extradural block in obstetric practice. Br J Anaesth 64:537–541, 1990.
24. Crawford JS: Some maternal complications of epidural analgesia for labour. Anaesthesia 40:1219–1225, 1985.
25. Baker AS, Ojemann RG, Swartz MN, Richardson EP: Spinal epidural abscess. N Engl J Med 293:463–468, 1975.
26. Wilson JD, Braunwald E, Isselbacher KJ, et al (eds): Harrison's Principles of Internal Medicine, 12th ed. New York, McGraw-Hill, 1991, p 2024.

FIFTEEN

Preeclampsia

David D. Hood, M.D.

Pregnancy-induced hypertension (PIH) is a serious complication of pregnancy, capable of producing significant morbidity and mortality in otherwise healthy women. Despite research efforts, there is an incomplete understanding of the disease. Although some causative factors are understood, the disease is not preventable and the most effective treatment remains delivery of the fetus. At present, treatment is essentially restricted to addressing the manifestations and side effects of the disease.

This chapter discusses the management of PIH from a practical approach—emphasizing treatments that are considered efficacious—and, with respect to anesthesia, illustrates approaches to care that are practical and safe.

DEFINITION

The American College of Obstetricians and Gynecologists separates the hypertensive disorders of pregnancy into three general categories: chronic hypertension that precedes pregnancy, chronic hypertension with superimposed preeclampsia/eclampsia, and PIH. By definition, women who become hypertensive during pregnancy have PIH and those who also develop proteinuria or pathologic edema after the 20th week of gestation in addition to hypertension have preeclampsia. Table 15–1 illustrates the criteria for applying the diagnosis of preeclampsia. Note that the diagnosis of severe preeclampsia requires only the diagnosis of preeclampsia and one or more additional complicating conditions. Preeclampsia or severe preeclampsia rarely develops before the 20th week of gestation, usually in the presence of hydatidiform mole or triploidy. Eclampsia is simply seizure or coma that occurs during preeclampsia and that is not caused by concurrent neurologic disease such as epilepsy.

EPIDEMIOLOGY AND OUTCOME

Preeclampsia complicates approximately 6% of all pregnancies. Several predisposing factors associate with preeclampsia: (1) primiparous women (85% of cases), (2) chronic hypertension, (3) renal disease, (4) insulin-dependent diabetes, (5) obesity, (6) history of previous pregnancy complicated by preeclampsia, (7) history of close relatives developing the disease, and (8) conditions with associated rapid uterine growth (e.g., multifetal gestation and macrosomia).

Mortality Risk

Significant mortality risk associates with hypertensive disease during pregnancy (Table 15–2). Note that despite improvements in medical care during the 15-year period covered in Table 15–2, hypertensive disease still ranks number one among all direct causes of maternal death. In contrast, maternal death secondary to anesthesia declined from number three to number eight, and the absolute percentage of maternal anesthetic deaths declined fivefold.

TABLE 15–1
Diagnosis of Preeclampsia and Severe Preeclampsia

Preeclampsia	Severe Preeclampsia
Hypertension	*Preeclampsia* + Any of These Complications
Diastolic blood pressure ≥ 90 mmHg [or] Systolic blood pressure ≥ 140 mmHg [or] Rise of ≥ 15 mmHg diastolic or 30 mmHg systolic on two occasions at least 6 hr apart	***Blood pressure*** Immediate diagnosis if diastolic blood pressure > 110 mmHg. Blood pressure ≥ 160 mmHg systolic or 110 mmHg diastolic on two occasions, at least 6 hours apart
and	
Proteinuria ≥ 300 mg protein/24 hr [or] ≥ 1 gm/L in two random specimens, at least 6 hr apart	***Proteinuria*** 3–4+ on semiquantitative urine analysis [or] ≥ 5 gm in a 24-hr urine collection
and/or	***Pulmonary Edema*** Diagnosis of pulmonary edema or cyanosis
Edema Generalized edema (>1+) after 12 hr of bed rest [or] Weight gain > 5 pounds in 1 wk	***Abdominal Pain*** Epigastric or right upper quadrant pain (liver edema → Glisson capsule stretch/pain)
	Hepatic Rupture
	Impaired Liver Function
	Cerebral or Visual Disturbances Headache, blurred vision, loss of consciousness (including seizure—by definition, *eclampsia*)
	Thrombocytopenia <150,000 platelets/dl
	HELLP Syndrome *H*emolysis, *el*evated *l*iver enzymes, *l*ow *p*latelets

Data from the American College of Obstetricians and Gynecologists: Management of preeclampsia. ACOG Technical Bulletin No. 91, 1986.

Table 15–3 lists the causes of maternal death in the most recent maternal mortality study from the United Kingdom (1988–1990) that were judged to be related to hypertensive disease. Most maternal deaths were due to either cerebral hemorrhage or adult respiratory distress syndrome, and most importantly, care was considered substandard in 24 of 27 cases (89%). These lapses in care illustrate the pitfalls of managing the severely preeclamptic patient.

The most common factor leading to maternal death was delay in treating the patient's disease aggressively. Other lapses in clinical care include poorly controlled blood pressure, delaying delivery in the hopes of allowing the fetus to mature, ignoring worsening symptoms, and providing inadequate postpartum management. As can be appreciated from Table 15–3, inadequate control of blood pressure leading to cerebral hemorrhage is still a common cause of preventable maternal death. Inadequate prophylaxis and treatment of eclamptic seizure was also a common factor leading to maternal death. Finally, a common circumstance leading to fatal consequences was inappropriate follow-up and management in the postpartum period. In this report from the United Kingdom, 12 of 27 fatalities were judged to have occurred owing to inappropriate postpartum management—emphasizing the need for following patients closely after delivery. Failure to adequately monitor blood pressure, failure to note worsening symptoms, and failure to recognize ominous symptoms were common themes in the postpartum period.

Medical management failures account for most maternal deaths secondary to hypertensive disease, and appropriate medical management

TABLE 15-2
Causes of Direct Maternal Death (England and Wales)

Cause	1973–1975 Rank (%)	1988–1990 Rank (%)
Hypertensive disease	1 (15.0%)	1 (18.4%)
Pulmonary embolism	2 (14.5%)	2 (16.9%)
Anesthesia	3 (11.9%)	8 (2.2%)
Abortion	4 (11.9%)	6 (5.1%)
Hemorrhage	5 (9.3%)	3 (15.4%)
Sepsis	6 (8.4%)	7 (4.4%)
Ectopic pregnancy	7 (8.4%)	4 (11.0%)
Amniotic fluid embolism	8 (6.2%)	5 (7.4%)
Ruptured uterus	9 (4.8%)	9 (1.5%)
Other complications	(9.7%)	(17.6%)

*Rank = rank among direct causes of maternal death; % = percent of all direct causes of maternal death.
Data from Hibbard BM, Anderson MM, O'Drife JO, et al: Report on Confidential Enquiries Into Maternal Deaths in the United Kingdom, 1988–1990, 36th ed. London, Her Majesty's Stationery Office, 1994.

can contribute significantly to successful outcomes for both mother and baby. The anesthesiologist must, therefore, be aware of appropriate management principles and understand what was done, why it was done, and how to conduct the anesthetic to minimize the possibility of poor outcome.

PATHOPHYSIOLOGY AND TREATMENT

Etiology

Although the cause of preeclampsia is complex and incompletely understood, patients with preeclampsia clearly develop an imbalance between plasma thromboxane and prostacyclin, allowing thromboxane's effects to predominate. The practical effects of excessive thromboxane activity are increased vasoconstriction and venoconstriction, increased platelet aggregation, increased uterine activity, and decreased uteroplacental blood flow. In addition, increased thromboxane concentrations relate to placental abnormalities that perpetuate and encourage disease progression. Delivery of the placenta is the definitive treatment.

Aspirin (ASA), which inhibits thromboxane synthesis by platelets, has been studied as a possible prophylactic treatment of preeclampsia. Initial trials examined the effectiveness of low-dose prophylactic ASA administered to women considered at risk for developing preeclampsia in preventing the disease. Dekker and Sibai[1] reviewed the results of all randomized trials between 1985 and 1991 and concluded that prophylactic ASA reduced both the incidence and the severity of preeclampsia and reduced the incidence of intrauterine growth retardation (IUGR). Subsequently, Sibai and colleagues[2] reported the results of a multicenter trial involving over 3000 healthy pregnant women who were not preselected as having risk factors for developing preeclampsia. There was a 2% reduction in the incidence of preeclampsia in the ASA-treated group (6.3% in the placebo group versus 4.6% in the ASA-treated group). Importantly, ASA did *not* increase the incidence of either postpartum hemorrhage or neonatal hemorrhage. However, birth weights and the incidence of IUGR were similar in the two groups, and perinatal morbidity was not improved by ASA therapy. However, ASA did associate with a fivefold increased incidence of abruptio placentae (p = .01). Finally, many women in these studies of ASA therapy received epidural anesthesia without reported anesthetic complications attributed to ASA therapy. Fur-

TABLE 15-3
Causes of Maternal Death Related to Hypertensive Disease, United Kingdom 1988–1990

Cerebral	
Hemorrhage-intracerebral	10
Subarachnoid	2
Infarction	1
Edema	1
Total Cerebral Deaths	**14**
Pulmonary	
Adult respiratory distress syndrome	9
Edema	1
Total Pulmonary Deaths	**10**
Hepatic	
Necrosis	1
Other	2
Total Deaths	**27**

Data from Hibbard BM, Anderson MM, O'Drife JO, et al: Report on Confidential Enquiries Into Maternal Deaths in the United Kingdom, 1988–1990, 36th ed. London, Her Majesty's Stationery Office, 1994.

ther investigation of prophylactic ASA continues for "at-risk" women.

Intravascular Volume

Intravascular volume may be normal or decreased in preeclamptic women compared with the volume in normal pregnant women. In general, the severity of the disease correlates with the likelihood of reduced intravascular volume, and severely preeclamptic women may have plasma volumes that are 30 to 40% less than those of normal pregnant women. The implications of this finding for anesthesia is discussed later.

Colloid Osmotic Pressure

Reductions in colloid osmotic pressure (COP) correlate with the severity of preeclampsia. In normal pregnancy, COP is approximately 20 mmHg in early labor, and it falls to 16 mmHg in the postpartum period (Table 15–4).[3] In contrast, the severely preeclamptic patient's initial COP is approximately 16 mmHg, and it falls to 13 mmHg by the postpartum period. Reduced COP contributes to the reduction in intravascular volume and the peripheral edema, and most significantly, it increases the risk of developing pulmonary edema.

Colloid Osmotic Pressure and Pulmonary Edema

Reduced COP may make normally acceptable intravenous (IV) fluid volumes excessive for several reasons. First, cardiac filling pressures in a "normal range" can produce pulmonary edema because the COP is low in severely preeclamptic patients. Remember, that when the COP-PCWP (pulmonary capillary wedge pressure) gradient is less than 4, pulmonary edema usually results.[4, 5] For example, pulmonary edema might develop in a severely preeclamptic patient with a PCWP of 10 and a COP of 13. This is one reason arbitrary administration of fluids to increase PCWP to "normal" is dangerous. In addition, since pulmonary capillary membrane defects are common in patients with severe preeclampsia, these defects may also make pulmonary edema more likely, increasing the risk of administering an arbitrary fluid volume. Finally, venous distensibility is impaired in preeclampsia, particularly in severe preeclampsia, when compared with distensibility in normal pregnant or nonpregnant women.[6] This may be manifested clinically by a more rapid increase in cardiac filling pressures following IV fluid administration.

For these reasons, the author's group resists administering large volumes of fluids prior to initiating regional anesthesia (see "Regional Analgesia: Technical Considerations," later in this chapter) or administering excessive crystalloid as a carrier for oxytocin during cesarean section. All too often, IV fluids are administered in volumes that are either followed out of habit and without efficacy data or given without proper awareness of the potential for precipitating pulmonary edema.

TABLE 15–4
Plasma Colloid Oncotic Pressure in Normotensive and Severely Preeclamptic Women

Women*	Normotensive Women* (N = 9)	Preeclamptic Women (N = 9)
Early labor	19.9 ± 0.7	16.1 ± 0.6
At delivery	17.2 ± 0.6	14.1 ± 0.5
Postpartum (16–18 hr)	16.2 ± 0.8	13.8 ± 0.5
6 wk postpartum	22.7 ± 0.8	26.2 ± 1.1

*Mean ± SD (mmHg).

Data from Zinaman M, Rubin J, Lindheimer MD: Serial plasma oncotic pressure levels and echoencephalography during and after delivery in severe preeclampsia. Lancet 1:1245–1247, 1985.

Blood Pressure

Blood pressures are significantly increased by the second trimester in women who will develop preeclampsia (Fig. 15–1).[7] Increased sensitivity to catecholamines occurs in women who develop preeclampsia, and this increased sensitivity to direct-acting pressor amines may be present before baseline blood pressure elevations are recognized.[8] Although, theoretically, ephedrine in usual doses might produce hypertension, the author's group routinely uses 5- to 10-mg bolus dose ephedrine to reverse hypotension during regional anesthesia (see "Regional Analgesia: Technical Considerations," later in this chapter). Lower doses are generally ineffective and delay the reversal of hypotension. The lack of an excessive hypertensive response to ephed-

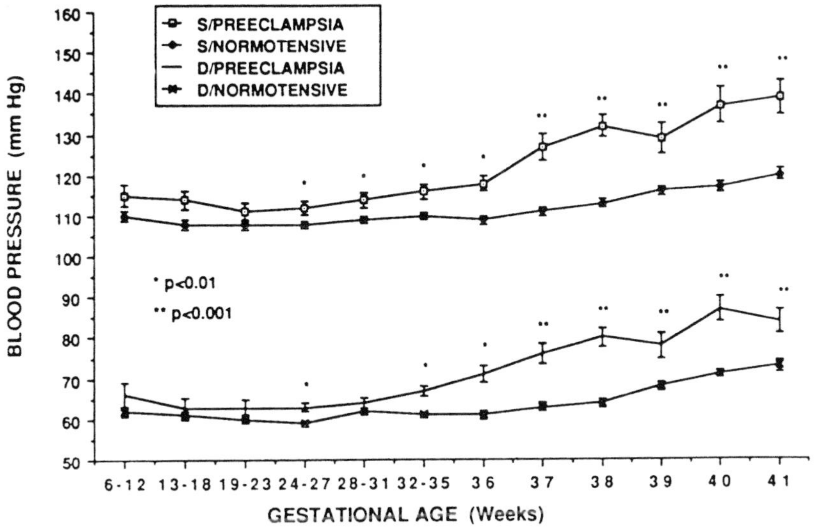

Figure 15–1. Systolic and diastolic blood pressures in normotensive pregnant women and in women destined to develop preeclampsia. (*Abbreviations:* S/preeclampsia = systolic blood pressure in the preeclamptic group; S/normotensive = systolic blood pressure in the normotensive group; D/preeclampsia = diastolic blood pressure in the preeclamptic group; D/normotensive = diastolic blood pressure in the normotensive group. Values are expressed as mean ± standard error of the mean [SEM]. $*p < .01$; $**p < .001$.) (From Villar MA, Sibai BM: Clinical significance of elevated mean arterial blood pressure in second trimester and threshold increase in systolic or diastolic blood pressure during third trimester. Am J Obstet Gynecol 160:419–423, 1989.)

rine probably relates to ephedrine's indirect pressor effects.

Hypertension Treatment

Treatment of hypertension is one of the primary interventions that clearly reduces maternal morbidity and mortality. In general, the goal of antihypertensive treatment is to reduce the diastolic blood pressure to 90 to 100 mmHg and the mean arterial blood pressure to less than 110 mmHg. Reductions in maternal blood pressure below these targets are generally not tolerated by the fetus and may produce signs of fetal stress. Diastolic blood pressures less than 100 mmHg are usually not treated. Table 15–5 lists the antihypertensive agents commonly used in severe preeclampsia.

Hydralazine

Hydralazine remains the most commonly used antihypertensive drug for treating PIH. Hydralazine dilates arterial smooth muscle while improving renal and uterine blood flow,[9] provided excessive blood pressure reductions do not occur.[10] Fortuitously, elevated systemic vascular resistance (SVR) is the most common element of severe preeclampsia pathophysiology, and hydralazine's afterload reduction is exactly the indicated treatment. Because hydralazine is relatively slow-acting, requiring 15 to 20 minutes for onset and up to 1 hour for peak effect, hydralazine infusions are difficult to titrate and may be prone to overdosage.[10] In general, most experts recommend 5- to 15-mg bolus increments of hydralazine, 20 to 30 minutes apart. Compensatory increases in heart rate are predictable. Hydralazine may produce hypotension and fetal stress in the presence of unrecognized severe hypovolemia. Despite these limitations, hydralazine has a long history of effective use by obstetricians and rarely fails to control hypertension. The author's group finds that small amounts (0.25–0.5 mg/kg) of the β blocker labetalol reduces hydralazine requirements, probably by blunting the compensatory tachycardia occurring with hydralazine.

Labetalol

Labetalol may be administered orally or intravenously and has both β-adrenergic-receptor antagonist and α_1-antagonist properties. (Rela-

TABLE 15–5
Acute Antihypertensive Drugs: Characteristics

Drug	Solution	Dose	Onset	Comments
Hydralazine	20 mg/ml	IV: 5–10 mg q 20 min up to 40 mg	15–20 min	Considerable variation in onset and effect; marked tachycardia common; peak effects up to 1 hr
Nifedipine	10-mg capsule	10 mg sublingual q 30 min	5–10 min	Tachycardia, headache, facial flushing; possible increased tocolysis and toxicity from $MgSO_4$
Labetalol	5 mg/ml	IV: 10–20 mg q 10 min up to 250–300 mg	5 min	Tachyphylaxis in 10% of patients; consider concurrent hydralazine use
Nitroglycerin	50 mg/500 ml	0.5 μg/kg/min, increase q 2 min, until effective	1 min	Ineffective after intravascular volume expansion; works well in combination with labetalol
Sodium nitroprusside	50 mg/500 ml	0.1 μg/kg/min, increase q 2 min, until effective or 8 μg/kg/min	1 min	May require intravascular volume expansion to prevent severe hypotension; works well in combination with labetalol
Trimethaphan	500 mg/500 ml	0.5 mg/min, increase q 2 min, until effective	1 min	Less cerebral vasodilatation than sodium nitroprusside or nitroglycerin; tachyphylaxis common; pupillary dilatation common; inhibits plasma cholinesterase

tive blockade ratio—α_1:β = 1:3–7). IV labetalol, compared with hydralazine, has a more rapid onset with peak effects within 10 to 15 minutes (see Table 15–5). Approximately 10% of severely preeclamptic patients are relatively resistant to labetalol's effects; these patients require the largest labetalol doses and experience the shortest duration of effect.[11] Unlike other β-adrenergic antagonists such as esmolol and propranolol, little labetalol crosses the placenta, avoiding the fetal/neonatal effects of β blockade.

Since the pathophysiology of most patients with severe preeclampsia is one of excessively increased SVR and left ventricular hyperdynamics, labetalol generally works well to reduce blood pressure. However, some severely preeclamptic patients have markedly elevated SVRs and depressed cardiac outputs. In this circumstance, labetalol may not be the first choice for blood pressure control. In these cases, afterload reduction should precede β blockade. For these reasons, when the author's group has no invasive hemodynamics to guide therapy and labetalol 0.5 mg/kg has not reduced blood pressure, we prefer to titrate additional hydralazine (5–20 mg) rather than continue with labetalol alone and risk cardiac depression.

Nifedipine

Nifedipine, an oral calcium channel blocking drug, is a second-line treatment for uncontrolled hypertension in severe preeclampsia. Calcium channel blocking drugs have several theoretical and practical complications that have limited investigations into their use. Infusion of nicardipine in pregnant monkeys produces progressive fetal acidosis and hypoxemia.[12] Furthermore, all calcium channel blocking drugs may interact with magnesium, producing exaggerated hypotension, tocolysis, and possible respiratory or cardiac toxicity. In isolated, perfused rat hearts, the combination of nifedipine and magnesium sulfate produces additive cardiac depression.[13] In one report, a patient receiving nifedipine for tocolysis developed acute respiratory insufficiency following IV magnesium administration.[14] Despite these limitations, oral nifedipine has successfully treated antepartum and postpartum hypertension.[15] Although nifedipine reduces blood pressure in women with severe preeclampsia, unique perinatal benefit has yet to be established.[15]

Methyldopa

Methyldopa is still the oral antihypertensive drug most commonly used for treatment of chronic hypertension during pregnancy (see Chapter 5 for details). In general, the drug is discontinued during labor, and other antihypertensive drugs are utilized as needed.

Potent Intravenous Antihypertensive Drugs

Sodium nitroprusside (SNP), nitroglycerin (NTG), and rarely, trimethaphan are used for acute blood pressure control in severely preeclamptic patients. Although these agents are occasionally used for blood pressure control or cardiac afterload reduction antepartum or postpartum, anesthesiologists primarily use them for blood pressure control during general anesthesia. Table 15–5 lists the properties of these drugs.

Sodium Nitroprusside. SNP has rapid onset and short duration (half-life <12 sec). SNP decreases SVR, and severe hypotension can occur. Direct arterial monitoring is advisable. Compensatory tachycardia is common, and uterine blood flow is usually preserved if hypotension is avoided.[16] SNP is a cerebral vasodilator; it will increase intracranial pressure (ICP) and may be contraindicated in patients with known or suspected increased ICP. SNP may not be the drug of choice in postsurgical patients unless a normal neurologic examination can be documented.

Naulty and coworkers[17] raised concerns about using SNP during pregnancy and reported cyanide toxicity and fetal death in sheep. However, the sheep that developed cyanide toxicity were resistant to the SNP's effects and received doses up to 25 μg/kg/min to reduce blood pressure. In contrast, the maximal acceptable dose of SNP in humans is approximately 8 μg/kg/min. Control of severe hypertension using SNP's normal dose ranges has been successful in parturients.[18–21] Wasserstrum reported that some patients with severe preeclampsia receiving SNP developed extreme hypotension and bradycardia.[18] He characterized these patients as responding like patients with severe, sudden hemorrhage who demonstrate cardiac and vasomotor depression. He recommended considering blood volume expansion before starting SNP. The author's group believes that some concurrent blood volume expansion will often be necessary in the subset of patients requiring SNP to treat refractory hypertension, since SNP will dramatically reduce the markedly elevated SVR, and without volume expansion, cardiac output falls precipitously. SNP is most useful when there has not been enough time to reduce the blood pressure with first-line drugs, and urgent cesarean section and general anesthesia are needed. Labetalol (10–20 mg) often reduces compensatory tachycardia, smooths the blood pressure reduction, and reduces the dose of SNP required to effect desired blood changes.

Nitroglycerin. NTG reduces both cardiac preload and afterload, but the predominant effect is on preload. Like SNP, NTG is rapid acting and has a duration of action measured in seconds. NTG partially restores uterine blood flow in hypertensive animals.[16, 22] Like SNP, NTG can increase ICP, and similar considerations apply to its use for women with known or suspected increased ICP. Since the antihypertensive effect of NTG in most severely preeclamptic patients is to reduce cardiac output secondary to preload reduction, the clinical effect of NTG depends on the parturient's intravascular volume. Patients who are severely volume contracted are very sensitive to NTG and may exhibit sudden, profound hypotension. As with patients receiving SNP, these patients require some volume expansion to tolerate the venodilatory effects of NTG. NTG will rapidly and smoothly reduce blood pressure in patients who receive moderate amounts of fluids and are not severely hypovolemic. If patients have received significant vol-

TABLE 15–6
Hemodynamic Parameters in Untreated Severely Preeclamptic Women

Authors	No. of Patients	CI	SVR	PCWP	CVP
Cotton et al[63]	14	4.8	1350	12	6
Groenendijk et al[64]	10	2.8	1943	3.3	—*
Belfort et al[65]	10	3.0	2392	5	2
Belfort et al[66]	9	3.2	1965	6	6
Wallenburg[67]	44	3.0	—	4	4

Abbreviations: CI = Cardiac index (L/min/m^2); SVR = systemic vascular resistance (dynes/sec/cm^{-5}); PCWP = pulmonary capillary wedge pressure (mmHg); CVP = central venous pressure (mmHg).

*— = Data not available.

Data from Sibai BM, Mabie WC: Hemodynamics of preeclampsia. Clin Perinatol 18:727–747, 1991.

ume expansion, NTG is often ineffective in reducing blood pressure.

NTG has been used in severely preeclamptic patients to treat pulmonary edema associated with elevated preload. Although NTG has also been used successfully to treat suspected renal artery vasospasm, its primary use is for short-term reductions in blood pressure in conjunction with general anesthesia.[23] Remember, if the patient has had significant intravascular volume expansion, NTG will be relatively ineffective.[24]

Trimethaphan. Trimethaphan's antihypertensive affect is secondary to sympathetic ganglionic blockade. Reduction in blood pressure often occurs without compensatory tachycardia; however, tachyphylaxis may develop during prolonged infusions. Unlike SNP and NTG, trimethaphan is not a direct cerebral vasodilator. However, animal investigation has shown that transient increases in ICP occur following rapid reductions in blood pressure when trimethaphan is used to induce hypotension. Remember, pupillary dilatation is a common side effect of this drug. As with NTG, with trimethaphan initial resistance or tachyphylaxis is more common in women receiving intravascular volume expansion.

Hemodynamics

The hemodynamics of preeclampsia are extremely variable, and no typical, predictable, hemodynamic profile exists. Studies of women who have not received medical treatment for their disease may have one pattern of hemodynamic profile, whereas women who have received treatment may have a different hemodynamic profile. Table 15–6 demonstrates that *women with untreated disease* have either low or normal cardiac outputs, high-normal to very elevated SVRs, and low to normal cardiac filling pressures. Severely preeclamptic *patients who have received treatment* of their disease (e.g., antihypertensive drugs, magnesium, and fluids), as a group, usually have elevated SVRs, normal to elevated cardiac outputs, and normal cardiac filling pressures (Table 15–7). Obviously, predicting the individual patient's hemodynamic values is difficult. Figure 15–2 illustrates the wide spectrum of hemodynamic values.[4]

Invasive Hemodynamic Monitoring

Although many clinical investigations involving invasive hemodynamic monitoring in the severely preeclamptic patient were conducted in the 1980s, today, invasive hemodynamic monitoring is reserved for women with specific complications of severe preeclampsia. As a result of the invasive hemodynamic studies of the 1980s, the pathophysiology of preeclampsia is better understood today, making Swan-Ganz catheter monitoring unnecessary in most instances, especially when the relative risks and benefits of Swan-Ganz catheter monitoring are considered.

Practically speaking, placement of the Swan-Ganz catheter or central venous pressure (CVP) catheter has well-documented complications. Furthermore, placing these catheters in a labor suite, providing the trained personnel to monitor for complications, and most importantly, appropriately using the catheter make the technique impractical in many hospitals, especially when personnel may be maximally tasked. Placing intensive care–level trained nurses in specialized obstetric intensive care areas is inefficient in all but the largest obstetric services. At Wake Forest, the author's group rarely elects

TABLE 15–7
Hemodynamic Parameters in Severely Preeclamptic-Eclamptic Women Who Have Received Medical Treatment

Parameter	Cotton et al[4] (n = 22*)	Wallenburg[67] (n = 45†)	Mabie et al[68] (n = 41‡)
Diastolic blood pressure (mmHg)	110	110±2	106±2
Pulmonary artery pressure (mmHg)	19	17±1	15±0.5
Cardiac index (L/min · m²)	3.8	4.1±0.1	4.4±0.1
SVRI (dynes · sec · cm⁻⁵ · M²)	2475	2726±120	2293±65
PCWP (mmHg)	8	10±1	8.3±0.3
CVP (mmHg)	2	4±1	4.8±0.4

Abbreviations: SVRI = systemic vascular resistance index; PCWP = pulmonary capillary wedge pressure; CVP = central venous pressure.
*Values expressed as median.
†Values expressed as mean ± SEM, includes 2 patients with pulmonary edema.
‡Values expressed as mean ± SEM, excludes 8 patients with pulmonary edema.
Data from Sibai BM, Mabie WC: Hemodynamics of preeclampsia. Clin Perinatol 18:727–747, 1991.

to place a Swan-Ganz catheter antepartum or intrapartum, even though the group has the luxury of dedicating senior resident/fellow physicians to monitor the patient—essentially performing nursing care in many respects. The alternative is to admit the patient to a medical or surgical intensive care unit where the nursing staff is familiar with invasive monitors but unfamiliar with the requirements for monitoring the fetus and the laboring parturient. Luckily, in most severely preeclamptic patients, appropriate care can be rendered without the use of invasive monitoring. The author's group reserves the use of Swan-Ganz catheter monitoring for patients with *malignant hypertension unresponsive to conventional antihypertensive treatment, pulmonary edema unresponsive to diuretics and morphine, hypotension and shock of unknown etiology,*

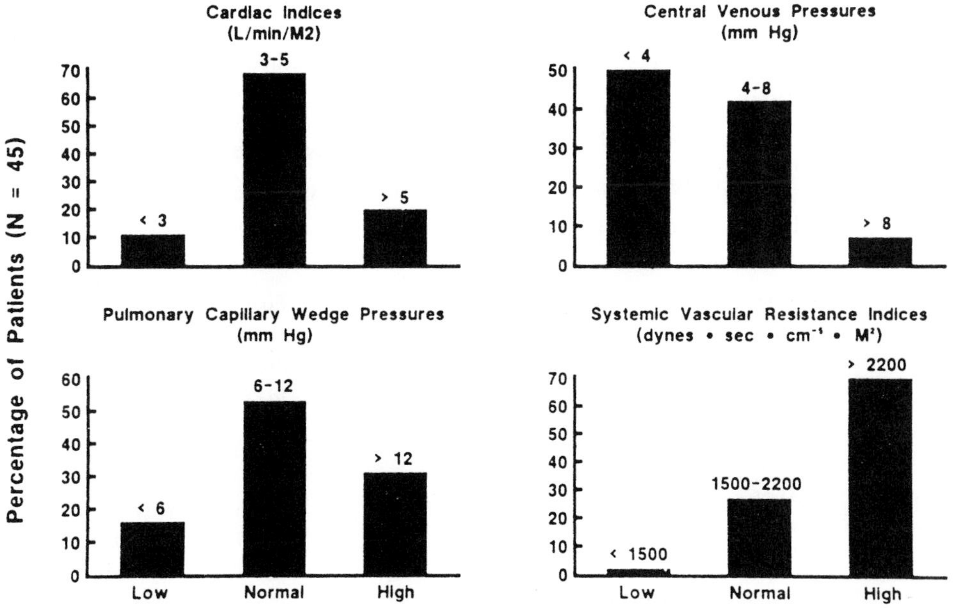

Figure 15–2. Hemodynamic subsets in 45 untreated subjects with severe preeclampsia. (From Cotton DB, Lee W, Huhta JC, Dorman KF: Hemodynamic profile of severe pregnancy-induced hypertension. Am J Obstet Gynecol 158:523–529, 1988.)

TABLE 15–8
Indications for Swan-Ganz Catheter Monitoring in Severe Preeclampsia

Malignant hypertension unresponsive to conventional antihypertensive therapy
Pulmonary edema unresponsive to diuretics, morphine, and oxygen
Persistent oliguria unresponsive to fluid challenge
Hypotension/shock of unknown cause

and persistent oliguria unresponsive to fluid challenge (Table 15–8).

Central Venous and Arterial Pressure Monitoring

CVP monitoring has risks, and the limitations of the technique should be understood when these risks are considered. In general, no predictable correlation exists between CVP and PCWP other than that PCWP is usually higher than CVP. Unfortunately, PCWP may be *much higher* than CVP (>10 mmHg), so that "normal" CVP values may be misleading and associated with PCWPs indicating borderline or frank pulmonary edema (Fig. 15–3).[25] Remember, the reduced COP associated with severe preeclampsia increases the risks for pulmonary edema at "normal" PCWP values.

However, as discussed previously, the difficulty of safely and reliably using a Swan-Ganz catheter in the labor suite may make a CVP catheter preferable in some circumstances. For example, when considering administering a fluid bolus, a CVP catheter provides useful information if the value is low (<6 mmHg), by indicating potential hypovolemia. In this circumstance, when conservative fluid boluses have not resolved oliguria (see "Renal Complications," later in this chapter) and the CVP is less than 6 mmHg, it is unlikely that the PCWP will be so high that pulmonary edema is imminent. Additional cautious fluid administration may be warranted. In contrast, a CVP of greater than 6 mmHg provides little information other than indicating that Swan-Ganz catheterization is necessary. Other factors such as renal artery spasm, low cardiac output, and excessively high SVRs, in addition to truly low cardiac filling pressures, can only be diagnosed with the use of a Swan-Ganz catheter.

TABLE 15–9
Indications for Intra-Arterial Pressure Monitoring

Sustained diastolic blood pressures > 105 mmHg, despite conservative antihypertensive therapy
Morbid obesity where accurate blood pressure measurement is impossible using noninvasive monitoring devices
Need for repeated, frequent blood sampling in patients with coagulopathy or those who present with very difficult venipuncture secondary to obesity or edema
Patients requiring continuous potent antihypertensive drug therapy that mandates beat-to-beat blood pressure monitoring

Potential indications for intra-arterial pressure monitoring are listed in Table 15–9.

Cardiopulmonary Complications

Pulmonary edema is one of the most common and significant complications of severe

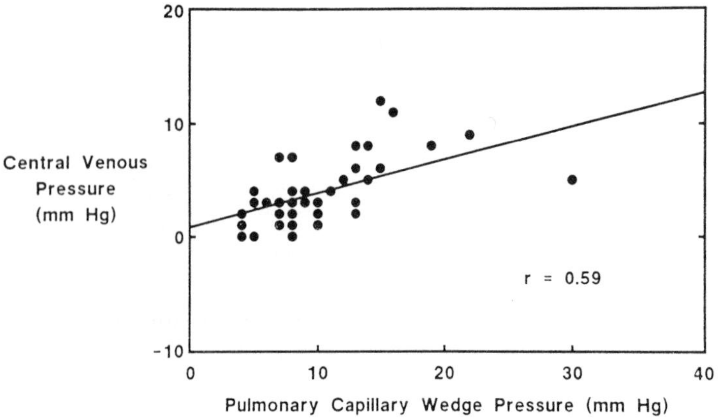

Figure 15–3. Relationship between central venous pressures and pulmonary capillary wedge pressures in women with severe pregnancy-induced hypertension. Multiple patients with the same data values are represented by a single point. (From Cotton DB, Lee W, Huhta JC, Dorman KF: Hemodynamic profile of severe pregnancy-induced hypertension. Am J Obstet Gynecol 158:523–529, 1988.)

preeclampsia, occurring in approximately 3% of patients.[26] Pulmonary edema presents most commonly in the postpartum period (70 to 80%) and is believed to be secondary to fluid mobilization from the periphery, further reducing COP and producing rapid increases in PCWP. Pulmonary edema may occur as late as 72 hours postpartum. As discussed previously, decreased COP makes pulmonary edema more likely when the PCWP rises.

Pulmonary edema is most commonly associated with multiple organ dysfunction and other complications of severe preeclampsia. Benedetti and associates[27] described the 3 pathophysiologic circumstances that cause pulmonary edema in severely preeclamptic patients (Fig. 15–4).

The most common cause of pulmonary edema is relative fluid overload; the left ventricular stroke work index is normal but intravascular hydrostatic pressure is too high (relative to the reduced COP). Remember, a COP-PCWP under 4 mmHg will usually lead to pulmonary edema. Women with relative fluid overload pulmonary edema often receive excessive IV fluids. In Sibai and coworkers'[26] series of 37 cases of pulmonary edema, fluids administered in conjunction with regional anesthesia did not contribute to pulmonary edema in any case. Other reports have, however, implicated pulmonary edema with excessive fluids associated with regional anesthesia.[27] Clearly, an awareness of the potential for relative fluid overload should help prevent iatrogenic pulmonary edema.

Treatment of fluid overload-induced pulmonary edema includes diuretics, morphine, and oxygen to reduce intravascular volume and hydrostatic pressure and improve oxygenation. IV NTG has successfully reduced PCWP in cases of hydrostatic-induced pulmonary edema; however, rapid improvements in oxygenation do not reliably occur.[28, 29]

The second most common cause of pulmonary edema is left ventricular failure. Excessive cardiac afterload and decreased cardiac indices are common in these patients. Afterload reduction with hydralazine, nifedipine, or SNP is the treatment of choice.

Finally, pulmonary capillary leak can develop in severe preeclampsia and lead to pulmonary edema. Importantly, the degree of peripheral edema does not correlate with risks for pulmonary capillary leak. In this setting, hemodynamic findings are variable with PCWPs that are low-normal while left ventricular stroke work indices are normal or elevated. The diagnosis can be made only with invasive hemodynamic monitoring. Significant pulmonary edema from this cause can occur in the presence of normal cardiac outputs and low PCWPs. Therapy is supportive and directed to minimizing PCWP consistent with reasonable cardiac output. Ultimately, delivery and resolution of the disease process is the only definitive treatment.

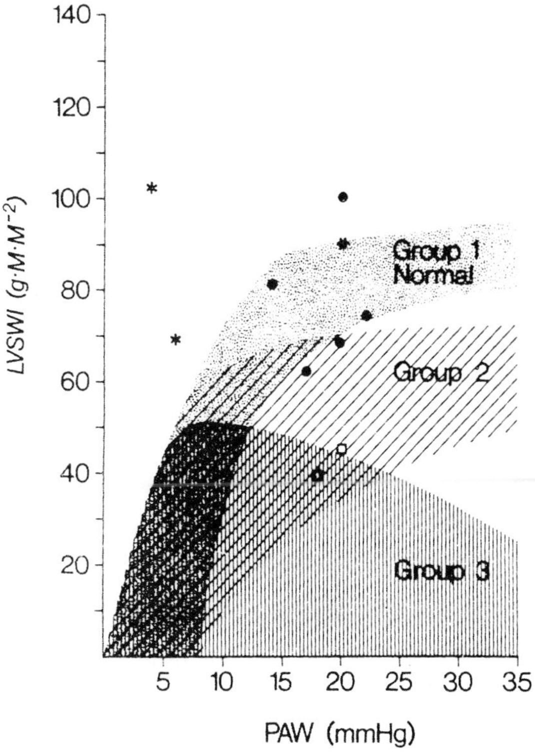

Figure 15–4. Ventricular function curve illustrating myocardial performance in severely preeclamptic patients with pulmonary edema. (*Abbreviations:* LVSWI = left ventricular stroke work index; PAW = pulmonary artery wedge pressure; *solid dots* = patients demonstrating alterations in hydrostatic/oncotic forces; *asterisks* = patients demonstrating capillary permeability pulmonary edema; *open squares* = patients demonstrating evidence of left ventricular failure.) (From Benedetti TJ, Kates R, Williams V: Hemodynamic observations in severe preeclampsia complicated by pulmonary edema. Am J Obstet Gynecol 152:330–334, 1985.)

Since the vast majority of cases of pulmonary edema develop in the postpartum period and are due to relative fluid overload, conservative therapy with diuretics such as furosemide, oxygen supplementation, and morphine will successfully treat many cases of pulmonary edema. A high index of suspicion is warranted when obstetric complications necessitate administering large amounts of fluids and colloids. Certainly, invasive hemodynamic monitoring with a Swan-Ganz catheter is indicated in fulminant pulmonary edema or milder cases where conservative therapy is unsuccessful.

Renal Complications

The glomerular filtration rate decreases as a result of a characteristic lesion, leading to glomerulopathy and proteinuria. The degree of proteinuria correlates with the severity of hypertension.[30] Urate clearance also decreases in severe preeclampsia, and elevated serum uric acid concentration correlates with the disease severity. Although normal nonpregnant serum creatinine levels are approximately 1 mg/dl, these levels indicate significant renal compromise in preeclamptic women. Reduced doses of drugs that are cleared by the kidney, such as magnesium, may be required to avoid excessive accumulation and toxic side effects.

Although oliguria (urine output <500 ml/24 hr) occurs commonly in severe preeclampsia, renal failure is rare in this previously healthy patient population unless hemorrhage and hypotension, complicated by bilateral renal cortical necroses, occur. In contrast, patients with chronic hypertension or concurrent renal disease are at much higher risk for developing renal failure in association with severe preeclampsia.

Most treatment regimens counsel active management when urine output falls to 25 to 30 ml/hr for 2 consecutive hours. Clark and colleagues[30] defined three subsets of hemodynamic pathophysiology presenting as oliguria. In their study, all patients whose oliguria persisted despite acute IV fluid crystalloid challenges of 500 ml over 20 minutes received pulmonary artery catheterization to delineate hemodynamics. Table 15–10 illustrates the three hemodynamic subsets in this study of oliguria. Five of nine patients had PCWPs below 8 mmHg, hyperdynamic left ventricular function, and mildly increased SVR, indicating mild intravascular hy-

TABLE 15–10
Common Hemodynamic Profiles of Severely Preeclamptic Women With Oliguria*

Category I	
Finding	Low PCWP, elevated SVR, low-normal CI
Interpretation	Intravascular volume depletion
Treatment	Additional IV fluid
Result	↑ PCWP, ↑ CI, ↓ SVR, urine output ↑
Category II	
Finding	High-normal to elevated PCWP, normal to slightly low SVR, low-normal CI
Interpretation	Renal artery vasospasm
Treatment	Cardiac afterload reduction with nifedipine, hydralazine, NTG, SNP, and cautious additional fluids
Result	Normal PCWP, normal CI, ↓ SVR, urine output ↑
Category III	
Finding	*Markedly elevated SVR,* depressed CI, elevated PCWP
Interpretation	Cardiac depression in response to markedly elevated cardiac afterload
Treatment	Cardiac afterload reduction with nefedipine, hydralazine, NTG, SNP, and cautious additional fluids
Result	Normal PCWP, normal CI, ↓ SVR, urine output ↑

Abbreviations: PCWP = pulmonary capillary wedge pressure; SVR = systemic vascular resistance; CI = cardiac index; NTG = nitroglyerine; SNP = sodium nitroprusside.

*Urine output unresponsive to 500 ml IV crystalloid bolus.

Data from Clark SL, Greenspoon JS, Aldahl D, Phelan JP: Severe preeclampsia with persistent oliguria: Management of hemodynamic subsets. Am J Obstet Gynecol 154:490–494, 1986.

povolemia. These patients' urine outputs increased following additional fluid administration.

The second group of patients had what Clark and colleagues[30] characterized as selective renal artery vasospasm, which responded to vasodilator therapy with hydralazine and additional fluids. These patients had normal-high PCWP and hyperdynamic left ventricular function, indicating that renal artery vasospasm was preventing adequate renal perfusion despite reasonable cardiac output and intravascular volume. In this circumstance, other authors have successfully used other vasodilator therapies including low-dose dopamine, NTG, and SNP combined with additional fluids as needed.

The third group of patients (one in nine) had depressed cardiac contractility and associated markedly elevated SVR. Following afterload reduction, cardiac output increased to normal, renal artery vasospasm probably diminished, and oliguria resolved.

Neither urine indices nor urine output reliably indicate intravascular volume or adequacy of renal perfusion. Lee and associates[31] correlated urinary diagnostic indices with hemodynamic parameters in severely preeclamptic patients with oliguria. No urinary diagnostic marker reliably predicted intravascular volume status. In fact, PCWPs were within normal range in five of seven patients. Pulmonary artery or CVP catheterization should be strongly considered when oliguria persists despite one or two IV fluid challenges of 500 ml (see "Hemodynamics," earlier in this chapter). Further "blind" fluid challenges risk inducing pulmonary edema.

Uteroplacental Complications

In normal pregnancies, the spiral arteries lose their smooth muscle, develop adrenergic denervation, and are thought to be maximally dilated. In contrast, the preeclamptic patient's placenta can be characterized by a persistence of spiral artery smooth musculature that retains adrenergic innervation and demonstrates greater than normal vasculature reactivity. Increased spiral artery resistance, blood hyperviscosity, and arterial intimal changes, including fibrin deposition and arterial occlusion, contribute to placental infarcts and placental insufficiency. These placental changes and systemic hypertension predispose preeclamptic patients to suffer placental abruption.

Abruptio placentae occurs in approximately 2% of all preeclamptic women, particularly those with preexisting chronic hypertension.[32] Disseminated intravascular coagulation (DIC) may occur in association with severe placental abruption and hemorrhage and is treated by immediate delivery, replacement of blood volume, and clotting factors as needed (see Chapter 9). Fetal death occurs in as many as 50% of patients with placental abruption.[33]

Fetal/Neonatal Outcome

Decreased uteroplacental blood flow and placental infarcts lead to chronic placental insufficiency and fetal IUGR. Uterine irritability predisposing to premature labor and preterm labor induction for worsening preeclampsia leads to a high incidence of premature delivery. Premature delivery accounts for most of the increased neonatal morbidity/mortality. However, other obstetric complications associated with PIH may also predispose the fetus to increased morbidity/mortality.

Hepatic Complications

Epigastric or right upper quadrant pain in the preeclamptic patient may indicate liver swelling from edema or subcapsular hemorrhage. This is a worrisome sign because, rarely, subcapsular hemorrhage produces liver capsule ruptures leading to life-threatening intraperitoneal hemorrhage, necessitating emergency surgery. Early indications of this complication in addition to pain include fetal distress and maternal hypotension. Maternal mortality following liver rupture approaches 75%. Diagnosis of liver swelling or subcapsular hemorrhage is usually made by sonography or computed tomography (CT) scan. As with many complications of preeclampsia, the only treatment is immediate delivery.

Elevation of serum transaminase is relatively common in mild preeclampsia. Significant elevation of other liver enzymes usually indicates hemolysis, elevated liver enzymes, and low platelets (HELLP syndrome), which may be confused with hepatitis, acute fatty liver of pregnancy, or gallbladder disease. Prolongation of prothrombin time (PT) is rare and indicates either significant liver involvement by the disease process, HELLP syndrome, or DIC.

HELLP Syndrome

HELLP syndrome is a subset of severe preeclampsia that is associated with high fetal mortality and significant maternal morbidity/mortality. The acronym represents the hallmarks of the disease: *h*emolysis, *e*levated *l*iver enzymes, and *l*ow *p*latelets. Although the exact laboratory criteria are somewhat controversial, the one most commonly used was advocated by Sibai in 1990.[34] The laboratory diagnosis requires (1) hemolysis, defined by abnormal peripheral smear, increased bilirubin (1.2 mg/dl), and increased lactic dehydrogenase (LDH) (>600 U/L); (2) elevated liver enzymes, defined as increased serum glutamic-oxaloacetic transaminase (SGOT) (70 U/L) and increased LDH; and (3) decreased platelet numbers, defined as platelet count <100,000/mm^3 (Table 15–11).

Maternal morbidity is significant, and in one large study of 442 pregnancies complicated by HELLP syndrome, maternal mortality was 1.1%.[35] Serious maternal morbidity included DIC (21%), abruptio placentae (16%), acute renal failure (7.7%), and pulmonary edema (5.9%). Fifty-five percent of patients required transfusion of blood products, and 2% required emergency laparotomy for intra-abdominal bleeding.

Perinatal mortality usually attributed to intrauterine asphyxia, abruptio placentae, and extreme prematurity ranges from 7.7% to 60%.[34] However, if the neonate survives the initial neonatal period, survival and morbidity are similar to those for gestational age–matched neonates.[36]

Of women who develop HELLP syndrome, 70% develop it antepartum, usually before 36 weeks' gestation, but 30% develop it postpartum.[34] Hypertension and proteinuria may be absent or mild. Patients complain of malaise (90%) and epigastric pain (90%) and may have nonspecific viral syndrome symptoms including nausea and vomiting (50%). These vague signs and symptoms, especially when hypertension is mild or absent, can lead to misdiagnosis. The rapid progress in symptoms is also important, and many patients develop clear laboratory evidence of HELLP syndrome within a 6- to 12-hour period. Therefore, all severely preeclamptic patients and patients exhibiting symptoms suspicious for possible HELLP syndrome should have laboratory screening tests repeated every 6 hours.

The treatment for the HELLP syndrome is immediate delivery. Delay often leads to deterioration of both the mother and the fetus.

TABLE 15–11
Diagnosis of HELLP Syndrome

***H*emolysis**
- Abnormal peripheral smear
- Serum bilirubin ≥ 1.2 mg/dl
- Lactic dehydrogenase > 600 units/L

***E*levated *L*iver Enzymes**
- SGOT ≥ 70 unit/L
- Increased lactate dehydrogenase

***L*ow *P*latelets**
- Platelet count < 100,000/mm^3

Data from Sibai BM: The HELLP syndrome (hemolysis, elevated liver enzymes, and low platelets: Much ado about nothing? [See comments]. Am J Obstet Gynecol 162:311–316, 1990.

Coagulation Abnormalities

Severe preeclampsia or HELLP syndrome may frequently produce abnormal coagulation indices. Abnormally low platelet counts are necessary for the diagnosis of HELLP but also occur among preeclamptic patients appearing in up to 20% of women with eclampsia.[37] Indeed, thrombocytopenia is the most common coagulation abnormality (platelet count <150,000/mm^3) in preeclampsia. Unfortunately, the severity of thrombocytopenia necessary to increase risk of bleeding is controversial. Some obstetricians will transfuse platelets when platelet counts are less than 50,000/mm^3, whereas others permit lower counts unless spontaneous bleeding occurs. Acceptable minimal platelet counts also vary with the anticipated mode of delivery, with higher platelet counts required for cesarean section. As discussed later in this chapter, the minimal platelet count necessary for performing safe regional anesthesia is also controversial. Clearly, most authorities regard obvious bleeding from needle punctures as abnormal and a contraindication to regional anesthesia.

The role of bleeding times, supposedly measuring platelet function, produced some confusion about the risk of bleeding in preeclamptic patients. Kelton and associates reported that 25% of preeclamptic patients with platelet counts above 150,000/mm^3 had prolonged bleeding times, suggesting that platelet counts alone were insufficient to predict bleeding.[36] However, a later report failed to find prolonged bleeding times when the platelet count was above 100,000/mm^3, but it suggested measuring bleeding times only when the platelet count was between 50,000 and 100,000/mm^3.[38] Subsequently, Rodgers and Levin[39] reviewed the world literature with respect to bleeding time and surgical blood loss. They concluded that bleeding time does not predict risk for bleeding, and most authorities do not utilize the bleeding time. The author's group's approach to thrombocytopenia is discussed later in this chapter.

Any parturient with significant thrombocytopenia also requires measurement of fibrinogen levels as well as fibrin degradation products, PT, and activated partial thromboplastin time (aPTT). Decreased fibrinogen and increased fibrin degradation products may indicate early or "compensated" DIC. When PT or aPTT, or both, is prolonged in association with increased fibrin degradation products and thrombocytopenia, frank or uncompensated DIC exists. Remember, although significant DIC is most commonly associated with abruptio placentae, it can also occur *without* placental abruption.

Thromboelastography (TEG), which measures the viscoelastic changes that occur when blood coagulates, has an undelineated role in preeclampsia and, at present, should be considered experimental.[40] TEG suffers the same predictive problems as the bleeding time. That is, investigators can define "abnormal values" for TEG whose efficacy in predicting bleeding is unknown.

Central Nervous System

Central nervous system (CNS) involvement is presumed for all preeclamptic patients. CNS involvement is most commonly manifested by hyperreflexia, visual disturbances, and headache, but it can also produce seizures (eclampsia, by definition), cerebral edema, increased ICP, and cortical blindness. The origin of CNS changes is unknown, but proposed causes include hypertensive encephalopathy, cerebral vasospasm, thrombosis, microinfarctions, and cerebral edema. Seizures during pregnancy are considered eclamptic seizures until proved otherwise. Prophylactic prevention of seizures and aggressive treatment of seizures, occurring despite prophylactic treatment, help minimize morbidity/mortality. Anesthetic implications of seizures are described subsequently.

Although most eclamptic seizures are considered "avoidable" and possibly anticipated, 27% of first eclamptic seizures occur in the *postpartum* period, and up to 31% of all convulsions may be "unavoidable."[41] Remember, the risk of convulsion is correlated poorly to the perceived disease severity. That is, seizure risk relates poorly to the severity of blood pressure elevation, the degree of proteinuria, or any other identifiable marker for preeclampsia. Therefore, all women identified as preeclamptic should be considered at risk for eclampsia antepartum, intrapartum, and for the first 24 to 72 hours postpartum and should be treated appropriately. Risk does not cease with delivery!

In North America, eclamptic seizure prophylaxis is usually accomplished with IV magnesium sulfate ($MgSO_4$). The antiepileptic mechanism of $MgSO_4$ is unknown; however, it is highly effective in preventing convulsions. In one large obstetric center, only 0.3% of patients receiving prophylactic $MgSO_4$ convulsed.[41]

The most common $MgSO_4$ regimen is to "load" the patient with 4 to 6 gm IV, over 20 minutes, followed by a continuous IV infusion of 1 to 2 gm/hr. "Breakthrough" or recurrent seizures are usually treated with an additional 2 to 4 gm of IV $MgSO_4$. When seizure occurs and $MgSO_4$ is not immediately available, drugs such as benzodiazepines will suppress the seizure. Remember, these drugs also depress the level of consciousness even after the seizure wanes. Thiopental 50 to 100 mg is a highly effective antiepileptic, and its effects on the level of consciousness are brief, permitting early postseizure neurologic assessment. Airway management skills are essential if considering using thiopental. Remember, the treatment should not have more risk than the seizure.

Magnesium is excreted by the kidneys, and blood levels should be checked frequently to verify therapeutic concentrations (see Chapter 5) and to avoid excessive levels in patients with deteriorating renal function. Loss of deep tendon reflexes may be an indicator of developing toxic magnesium blood levels (check upper extremity if epidural analgesia is in effect). Remember, a significant number of women will have their first seizure in the postpartum period, so $MgSO_4$ prophylaxis should continue postpartum until most of the signs of preeclampsia are resolving (hypertension, edema, and hyperreflexia).

Phenytoin and diazepam are the other relatively common antiepileptic drugs used outside the United States for prophylaxis and treatment of eclamptic seizures. A prospective Collaborative Eclampsia Trial reported the results of preventing recurrent seizures with these drugs compared with $MgSO_4$.[42] Women receiving $MgSO_4$ had a 52% lower risk of recurrent convulsions compared with those receiving diazepam and a 67% lower risk compared with women receiving phenytoin. At present, $MgSO_4$ is the most effective therapy to prevent eclamptic convulsions.

Convulsions rarely indicate immediate delivery. Women predictably become hypoxemic and acidotic during the seizure and in the immediate postictal period. The fetal heart rate will consistently demonstrate signs of stress. Administer oxygen, place the woman on her side, and wait for maternal and fetal hypoxemia/acidosis to resolve. Convulsions that occur despite therapeutic serum magnesium concentrations, particularly if they are focal seizures, might indicate intracerebral hemorrhage or other intracerebral lesions. Consider neurology consultation and possible CT or magnetic resonance imaging (MRI) scan when this occurs.

ANESTHETIC MANAGEMENT

All patients with preeclampsia are not identical. The anesthesiologist should evaluate each patient, assess which organ systems are most involved, and develop a management plan that reflects both the disease severity and the pattern of organ system involvement. For example one patient may have very severe hypertension with normal urine output. Another patient may have barely recognizable blood pressure elevations with significant renal compromise or seizures. The anesthetic considerations may differ markedly for these patients. As in all complicated obstetric cases, consultation with the attending obstetrician is mandatory prior to initiating the anesthetic plan. Only the attending obstetrician can convey his or her assessment, expectations, and plans for managing this particular patient. The author's group's approach is discussed in the following sections.

Screening Laboratory Tests

Initial laboratory screening evaluation should assess hemoglobin and hematocrit platelet numbers and include at least a semiquantitative urinary analysis for specific gravity, protein, and glucose. Severe preeclampsia indicates further screening laboratory studies including blood urea nitrogen, partial thromboplastin time, PT, fibrinogen, serum creatinine, and liver function tests. Severely preeclamptic patients require repeat screening every 6 hours during labor and within 6 hours before cesarean section because of potential rapid disease progression.

The hematocrit may identify intravascular volume contraction. Although, in normal pregnancies, the hematocrit seldom exceeds 36%, severe preeclampsia with significant vasospasm and intravascular volume contraction may significantly elevate hematocrits. Hematocrits between 40 and 45% usually indicate severe disease and intravascular volume contraction.

Assessing platelet numbers is essential. Platelet numbers under 150,000/mm^3, particularly in combination with hematocrits indicating hemoconcentration, strongly suggest severe preeclampsia, and additional laboratory screens are recommended.

Coagulation Abnormalities and Regional Anesthesia

Possible coagulation abnormalities are a primary concern when considering regional anesthesia. Thrombocytopenia occurs commonly and carries risks for spinal or epidural hematoma following regional anesthesia. Although a prudent concern, there are no reported cases of epidural hematoma in preeclamptic patients following epidural anesthesia. Whether this lack of documented morbidity is the result of conservative patient selection or exaggerated risks is unknown. Because of this uncertainty, absolute laboratory values that indicate risks contraindicating regional anesthesia are controversial.

Many anesthesiologists adopt arbitrary platelet counts below which they will not perform regional anesthesia, most commonly values under 100,000/mm^3. This number was initially selected based on studies of bleeding time, although the same number has traditionally been used in nonpreeclamptic patients as well. Unfortunately, bleeding time values do not predict bleeding in this patient population and have no validated ability to predict risks of epidural hematoma. The author's group does not order bleeding time tests, believing they provide no benefit.

In the absence of ecchymosis, petechiae, or bleeding from needle stick sites, the safe lower limit of platelets is unknown. Some anesthesiologists have decreased the lowest platelet count contraindicating regional anesthesia to 50,000/mm^3. Since women with other platelet deficiency diseases, such as autoimmune thrombocytopenic purpura, tolerate cesarean section without excessive blood loss, and women with unrecognized thrombocytopenia have received epidural anesthesia without incident, utilizing the arbitrary platelet count limit of 100,000/mm^3 needs further examination.[43–45] Unfortunately, at present, each anesthesiologist must use her or his clinical judgment to decide relative risks of alternative anesthetic techniques when considering what platelet counts contraindicate regional anesthesia in the thrombocytopenic preeclamptic patient.

The author's group encourages serial platelet counts (every 6 hours) on all severely preeclamptic patients and, if serial platelet counts decline significantly, try to place the epidural before the count declines below 100,000/mm^3. This sometimes necessitates placing the epidural catheter and testing placement with a small amount of local anesthetic prior to active labor. In these cases, the author's group must have a commitment from the obstetrician that delivery is planned within 24 hours. This approach often avoids the dilemma of trying to decide whether to place an epidural later in the face of low platelet counts.

The author's group is much more likely to perform regional anesthesia for women with platelet counts above 90,000/mm^3 than for those with platelet counts in the 50,000 to 90,000/mm^3 range. When considering low platelet counts, the author's group then tries to weigh any special considerations unique to the patient. For example, the author's group is more likely to perform regional anesthesia for a morbidly obese parturient or one with significant and obvious facial/oral edema, despite thrombocytopenia, than for a patient with a normal airway. If the author's group believes general anesthesia has excessive risk and the low platelet count precludes regional anesthesia, the obstetrician is consulted and possible platelet transfusion prior to regional anesthesia is considered.

A "single-shot" spinal anesthetic with a small needle may pose less risk than a 17-gauge epidural needle in the face of thrombocytopenia, especially considering possible vessel trauma by the relatively large epidural needle/catheter. However, these are theoretical considerations, without published evidence that morbidity is reduced by using a small spinal needle instead of an epidural needle and catheter. Clearly, one could argue that multiple attempts with a spinal needle might be more traumatic than a single attempt with an epidural needle. In the end, clinical judgment that considers relative risks dictates the choice of anesthesia, and the same concerns regarding spinal anesthesia in this population remain.

Finally, the last consideration is when to remove the epidural catheter when significant thrombocytopenia exists. No outcome studies justify a particular course of action. Waiting until the platelet count recovers above 100,000/mm^3 may require keeping the epidural catheter in place for 5 to 6 days postpartum and risking infection and unrecognized catheter dislodgment and vessel trauma.[46] Alternatively, unless DIC or significant bleeding exists the catheter may be removed and the patient monitored closely for 6 to 12 hours and questioned about increasing back or leg pain or changes in leg sensation. In the presence of significant bleeding diathesis or DIC, wait for laboratory resolution of DIC before removing the epidural catheter.

ANALGESIA FOR LABOR AND DELIVERY

Most anesthesiologists consider epidural analgesia techniques to be relatively indicated for preeclamptic, particularly severely preeclamptic, patients. Several theoretical and practical reasons exist for this preference: (1) epidural analgesia reduces circulating catecholamines, potentially improving uteroplacental blood flow, reducing exacerbations in maternal blood pressure and fluctuations in cardiac output,[47–50] (2) epidural analgesia provides the superior labor pain relief, (3) a functioning labor epidural can provide emergent anesthesia for forceps or cesarean delivery, avoiding the risks of general anesthesia. Although the theoretical benefits of improving placental blood flow are appealing, there is no clinical evidence of improved neonatal outcome when using epidural labor analgesia. The author's group believes the most important reasons for using epidural analgesia for labor are maternal comfort, a stable cardiovascular response to labor, and most importantly, a decreased requirement for general anesthesia.

Regional Analgesia: Technical Considerations

"How much fluid" is controversial in normal parturients and even more so for the preeclamptic patient. Traditional anesthesia teaching advocates prophylactic IV fluids prior to labor epidural anesthesia to "decrease the incidence of hypotension" and is believed more important prior to cesarean section anesthesia because of the greater extent of blockade. However, the effectiveness of this practice has been questioned for normal parturients,[51] and the effectiveness of prophylactic fluid administration in the preeclamptic patient has never been examined. The author's group uses the following approach.

The author's group first tries to clinically assess the possible degree of intravascular hypovolemia, utilizing the hematocrit and urine output. As discussed earlier, if the hematocrit does not indicate severe hemoconcentration and the urine output is reasonable (>0.5–1.0 ml/kg/hr), less than 500 ml of crystalloid is administered before initiating epidural labor analgesia, and less than 1000 ml is administered prior to cesarean section anesthesia. If the patient has urine output above 1 ml/kg/hr or has evidence of possible excess fluids (input>>urine output), the author's group frequently avoids or reduces arbitrary fluid "preloads." The epidural local anesthetic is administered in 5-ml increments, with frequent blood pressure measurements. If hypotension develops (blood pressure falls below 30%) or signs of fetal stress develop, additional fluids and ephedrine will be administered. Despite texts warning of excessive hypertensive response to usual doses of ephedrine, the author's group believes that ephedrine 5 to 10 mg is generally needed to reverse hypotension and that smaller doses are relatively ineffective. Severity and rapidity of onset of hypotension dictate whether 5- or 10-mg boluses of IV ephedrine are used. If hypotension does not promptly respond to therapy (less than 2 min), a second larger dose of ephedrine is often administered. In the author's group's experience, additional fluids and ephedrine are not usually needed when establishing epidural labor analgesia and are frequently not required when initiating cesarean section anesthesia. Nevertheless, severe maternal hypotension can occur, and vigilance is required to promptly initiate appropriate treatment. Remember, maintain uterine displacement or position the patient in the lateral decubitus position. Supplemental oxygen may be prudent.

The author's group does not believe regional anesthesia requires invasive hemodynamic monitoring for severely preeclamptic patients unless there are other indications. If invasive monitors are in place, treat other hemodynamic derangements before initiating epidural anesthesia, and when a patient already has an existing CVP or Swan-Ganz catheter, administer fluids and raise the CVP into positive values (if it is negative to start with) or increase the PCWP into the 5- to 10-mmHg range before inducing epidural anesthesia. Invasive monitors guide additional intrapartum hemodynamic treatments.

Epinephrine and Epidural Anesthesia

Testing the epidural catheter to rule out intrathecal and intravascular placement is a controversial topic for normal parturients and is more so for the preeclamptic patient. The primary concern regarding using epinephrine in preeclamptic patients is the potentially severe response to IV epinephrine that could accompany a "positive" IV test. Sudden, severe, systemic hypertension may follow. In addition, since the uterine and placental vasculature "hyperrespond" to catecholamines, IV epinephrine may compromise the fetus by severely reducing uterine blood flow. Furthermore, appropriately placed epidural catheters can migrate intravenously, or epinephrine-containing local anesthetic may be accidentally administered IV when multiport catheters have ports residing simultaneously in the epidural and the intravascular spaces. Absorption from the epidural space also has the potential to cause hypertension. Hadzic and coworkers[52] reported a case of malignant hypertension requiring treatment with SNP that developed in a preeclamptic parturient after administering 2% epidural lidocaine with 1:200,000 epinephrine. Hypertension developed despite a normal epidural block that provided sensory levels sufficient to produce cesarean section anesthesia. For these reasons, the author's group avoids epinephrine-containing local anesthetics for testing the epidural catheter placement and avoids epidural infusions containing epinephrine during labor. The author's group believes that the safest course is to test for the location of catheter placement with either lidocaine or 2-chloroprocaine to rule out subarachnoid and IV placement. Bupivacaine and 2-chloroprocaine are satisfactory alternatives for both labor analgesia and cesarean section anesthesia and do not require epinephrine use.

Labor Analgesia

All analgesic options discussed in Chapter 6 are available to preeclamptic patients, and the techniques are essentially identical. As discussed previously, epidural analgesia offers significant benefits and is the author's group's preferred technique. The newest technique of combined spinal/epidural using intrathecal narcotics followed by epidural local anesthetics, if required, is also equally indicated.

Lidocaine clearance is reduced in preeclamptic patients.[53] Therefore, the author's group avoids lidocaine infusions in preeclamptic patients. We prefer to test the catheter with 2% lidocaine (2 + 5 ml), and, following block establishment with additional 2% lidocaine or 0.25% bupivacaine, maintain analgesia with either a continuous infusion or a patient-controlled epidural analgesia (PCEA) infusion of bupivacaine, 0.0625 to 0.125% with or without fentanyl 1 to 2 μg/ml.

Cesarean Section Anesthesia

The author's group tries to avoid general anesthesia for cesarean section if possible. Similar to labor analgesia, there are theoretical and practical reasons to avoid general anesthesia.

Hemodynamic Response

In a classic study, Hodgkinson and colleagues[54] demonstrated the dramatic hemodynamic responses accompanying both tracheal intubation and tracheal suction/extubation (Fig. 15–5). Note the transient pulmonary wedge pressures of 25 to 30 mmHg and mean arterial blood pressures exceeding 155 mmHg in the group receiving general anesthesia. These severe hemodynamic changes could potentially produce a cerebrovascular accident, pulmonary edema, or cardiac failure. Contrast the stable hemodynamics associated with epidural anesthesia. Anticipating and controlling these blood pressure changes when general anesthesia is selected requires very potent vasodilators for blood pressure control.

Stress Response

Epidural anesthesia suppresses the significant increases in stress response hormones that accompany general anesthesia. When compared with levels in women receiving epidural anesthesia, plasma catecholamines, adrenocorticotropic hormone, and β-endorphin, immunoactivity markedly increases when women with severe preeclampsia receive general anesthesia.[55] Preventing this stress response using epidural anesthesia is potentially beneficial compared with general anesthesia. Newborn 1-minute Apgar scores improve when patients receive epidural.

As discussed under "Labor Analgesia," earlier in this chapter, epidural anesthesia may improve uteroplacental perfusion, and epidural anesthesia avoids the sudden surges of catecholamines associated with general anesthesia. Although it could be extrapolated that uteroplacental perfusion improves when regional anesthesia is used for cesarean section and improves neonatal outcome, there is no convincing evidence demonstrating this. The improved 1-minute Apgar scores noted earlier following regional anesthesia could be due to the transient sedative effects of general anesthesia on the neonate. Nonetheless, these theoretical benefits of regional anesthesia are appealing.

The practical and compelling indications for preferentially using epidural anesthesia have to

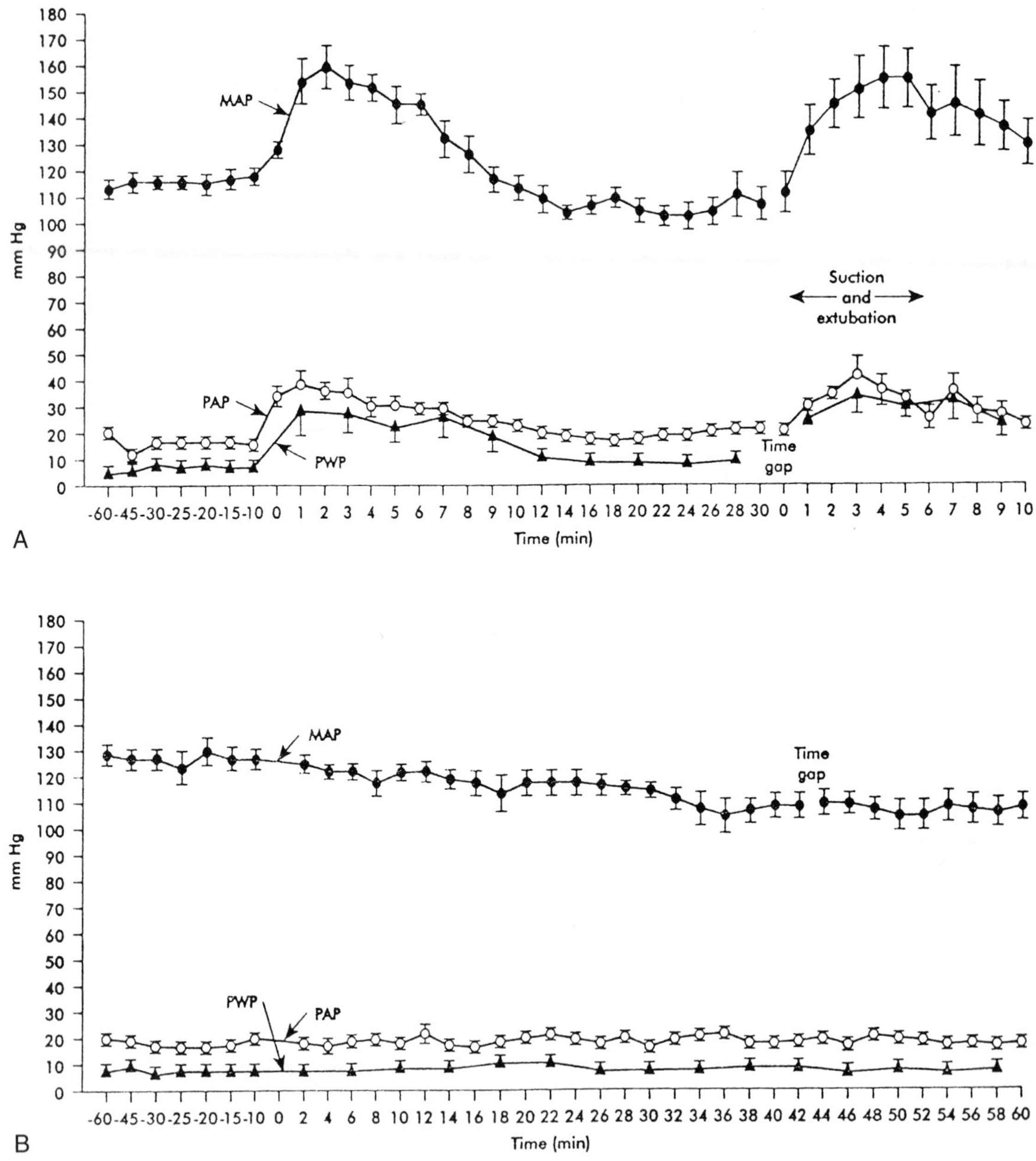

Figure 15–5. *A*, Mean ± SEM of mean arterial pressure (MAP), pulmonary artery pressure (PAP), and pulmonary wedge pressure (PWP) in 10 preeclamptic patients who underwent cesarean section under thiopental, nitrous oxide (40%), and halothane (0.5%) anesthesia. Measurements before induction of anesthesia are indicated at -60 to -10 min. The start of induction is indicated by the first 0. The second 0 refers to the start of suction and extubation. *Time gap* refers to the time elapsed between the completion of the first 30 min of anesthesia and the start of suction and extubation. *B*, Mean ± SEM of MAP, PAP, and PWP in 10 preeclamptic patients who underwent cesarean section under epidural bupivacaine anesthesia. Measurements before epidural injection of bupivacaine (at 0 min) are indicated at −60 to −10 min, and measurements during epidural anesthesia are indicated at 2 to 60 min. (*A* and *B*, From Hodgkinson R, Husain FJ, Hayashi RH: Systemic and pulmonary blood pressure during caesarean section in parturients with gestational hypertension. Can Anaesth Soc J 27:389–394, 1980.)

do with risks for difficult tracheal intubation, potential hypoventilation and hypoxemia, and the risk of pulmonary aspiration.

Airway Edema

Generalized edema, particularly facial and mucosal edema, are hallmarks of severe preeclampsia. Edema can make visualization of the glottic opening impossible. Potential mucosal bleeding associated with instrumentation, further complicating tracheal intubation, is also more likely in these patients. Respiratory distress or stridor can be a presenting symptom in severe preeclampsia.[56] Glottic edema can be more severe than anticipated from the degree of facial edema.[57]

Hypoxemia during induction of general anesthesia is also more likely in the severely preeclamptic patient. Subacute or overt pulmonary edema can lessen the pulmonary reserve necessary to tolerate the apnea accompanying induction of general anesthesia. If tracheal intubation is at all difficult, these women will often demonstrate arterial desaturation. In contrast to normal pregnancy, which is associated with a right shift in the oxyhemoglobin dissociation curve, preeclampsia has an associated left shift in the oxyhemoglobin dissociation curve, inhibiting oxygen release to the tissues (and fetus), further contributing to the potential adverse effects of hypoxemia.[58]

General anesthesia, particularly emergency general anesthesia, increases the maternal death risk when compared with regional anesthesia. The most common causes of anesthesia-related death in normal parturients—that is, tracheal intubation/ventilation difficulties and pulmonary aspiration—are a greater concern for the severely preeclamptic patient. When considering these risks and the malignant hemodynamic responses to tracheal intubation, the author's group prefers to avoid general anesthesia whenever possible in the severely preeclamptic patient.

Epidural Anesthesia for Cesarean Section

Women with a functioning labor epidural catheter should have their block extended with either 3% 2-chloroprocaine or 0.5% bupivacaine. Either epidural local anesthetic provides excellent anesthesia, and the choice is primarily dictated by the anticipated duration and urgency of surgery. As mentioned previously, the author's group avoids epinephrine-containing solutions. Since the author's group believes that epidural lidocaine without epinephrine produces poor cesarean section anesthesia, lidocaine is avoided.

If time permits, the epidural block should be slowly extended to at least the T4 dermatomal level. The author's group administers local anesthetic in 5-ml aliquots and closely monitors the blood pressure. When a preexisting epidural block is extended, the author's group does not administer more than 500 ml of IV fluid. The author's group administers additional crystalloid only when the blood pressure decreases more than 20%. If the blood pressure declines approximately 30% or the fetal heart rate indicates stress, the author's group will administer IV ephedrine in 5- to 10-mg increments, every 1 to 2 minutes until the blood pressure stabilizes. If the epidural block has been extended with 2-chloroprocaine, the author's group will reinforce the block with approximately 8 to 12 ml of the drug every 30 minutes and maintain the block.

In the author's group's experience, it is often not necessary to administer additional fluids or ephedrine when extending labor blocks. On occasion, the group has administered additional labetalol and hydralazine to treat severe hypertension during regional anesthesia, despite excellent epidural or spinal anesthesia and apparent block heights above T4.

Severe obstetric emergencies, even in the presence of a functioning labor epidural, complicate decision making. If there is significant hemorrhage such as accompanies placentae abruptio, general anesthesia is used. If there is *severe, sustained, fetal bradycardia,* general anesthesia will often be selected. However, for most circumstances, including fetal stress, the author's group rapidly extends the epidural block using 3% 2-chloroprocaine. In this situation, the catheter is tested for subarachnoid migration with 2 ml of the local anesthetic, and motor block is reassessed 2 to 3 minutes later. If there is no dramatic increase in the density of motor block following testing, the author's group will administer a total of 15 to 20 ml of 3% 2-chloroprocaine in 5-ml aliquots every 1 to 2 minutes, querying the patient about possible IV CNS symptoms. In these *urgent* circumstances, the author's group also infuses the crystalloid rapidly, monitors the blood pressure every 1 to 2 minutes, and treats any reduction in blood pressure greater than 15 to 20% with ephedrine until the blood pressure stabilizes. Again, in the author's group's experience, these women do not require unusually large amounts of either ephedrine or IV fluid.

Spinal Versus Epidural Anesthesia

For many years, spinal anesthesia, with its more rapid onset, was believed to have a greater likelihood of producing severe hypotension when compared with epidural anesthesia in preeclamptic patients. Although the frequency of hypotension is greater following spinal anesthesia than epidural anesthesia in normal parturients, no recent studies have tested this hypothesis in severely preeclamptic patients.

At the author's institution, spinal anesthesia is frequently used for uncomplicated preeclamptic patients and has been performed with increasing frequency in *severely* preeclamptic patients. The author's group conducted a retrospective record review of all epidural and spinal anesthetics performed in severely preeclamptic women for cesarean section during the years 1989 to 1994. Only women with the most severe hypertension were included and the lowest recorded blood pressures corresponding to preinduction, induction to delivery, and after delivery were compared. Fifty-nine patients received spinal anesthesia and 69 received epidural anesthesia. Blood pressure changes associated with spinal and epidural anesthesia were similar (Fig. 15–6). Apgar scores were similar, as was antihypertensive therapy and ephedrine use. Patients having spinal anesthesia did receive significantly more IV fluid (approximately 2100 ml of IV fluid in the spinal group and 1500 ml in the epidural group). Whether this increased fluid administration was needed or was a result of "prophylactic preloading" is unknown. Maternal and neonatal outcomes were also similar in the spinal and epidural groups.

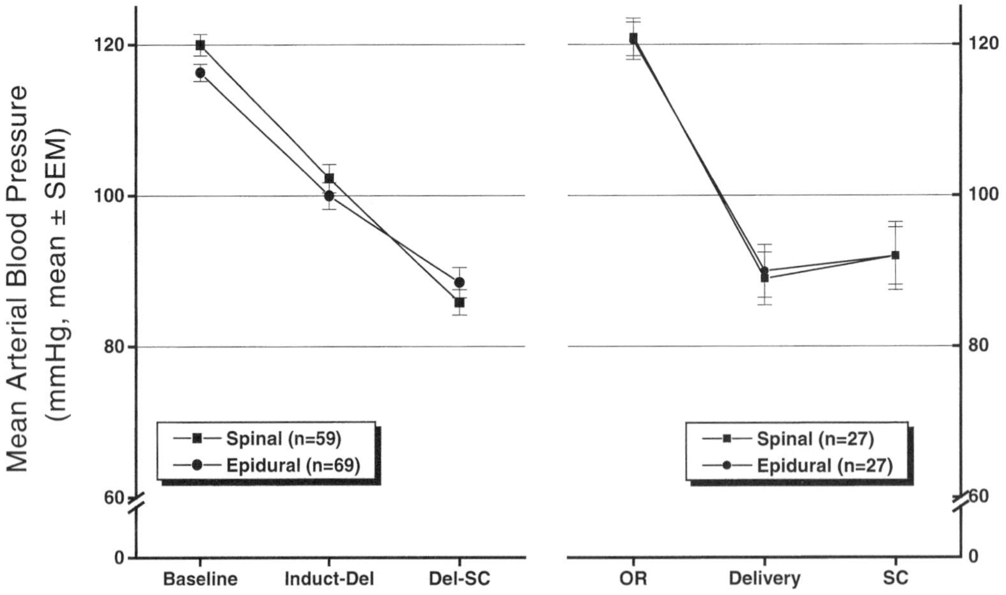

Figure 15–6. Spinal versus epidural anesthesia for cesarean section in severely preeclamptic parturients. *Left,* Retrospective review of Wake Forest University patients. Blood pressures are the lowest recorded in each time period. (*Time periods:* Baseline = 15-min period before induction of regional anesthesia; Induct-Del = period from regional anesthesia induction until delivery; Del-SC = period from delivery until skin closure.) *Right,* Prospective study. Spinal = combined spinal-epidural technique; however, the dose of spinal local anesthetic was bupivacaine, 0.75% with dextrose, 11.25 mg. Blood pressures are the mean pressure recorded at the time point. (*Time periods:* OR = operating room; Delivery = delivery; SC = skin closure.) (Data from Wallace DH, Leveno KJ, Cunningham FG, et al: Randomized comparison of general and regional anesthesia for cesarean delivery in pregnancies complicated by severe preeclampsia. Obstet Gynecol 86:193–199, 1995.)

A study by Wallace and associates[59] also supports the contention that blood pressure response to spinal anesthesia of severely preeclamptic patients may be clinically similar to that seen with epidural anesthesia. In this small prospective study, severely preeclamptic patients requiring cesarean section were randomized to receive spinal anesthesia using a combined spinal/epidural technique, epidural anesthesia, or general anesthesia. The combined spinal/epidural group received 1.5 ml of 0.75% bupivacaine in 7.5% dextrose, followed by additional epidural lidocaine if needed. This dose of spinal bupivacaine would probably produce a total sympathectomy and sensory blockade sufficient to perform cesarean section on most patients, although some patients in the combined spinal/epidural group received additional epidural bupivacaine. Patients in the epidural group received lidocaine or bupivacaine. Reductions in blood pressure were similar following either anesthetic technique (see Fig. 15–6). The author's group believes that this small study, along with our larger retrospective experience, supports prospective study of spinal versus epidural anesthesia for cesarean section in severely preeclamptic patients.

When considering epidural versus spinal anesthesia for cesarean section for severe preeclampsia, the author's group prefers epidural anesthesia. The primary reason is the slower onset and the ability to slowly titrate the level of the block. Slow block titration facilitates administering only the minimal amount of fluid indicated by the patient's response to the block. The rapid onset of spinal anesthesia and the occasional rapid decline in blood pressure make overinfusion of IV fluids more likely. When using spinal anesthesia, the author's group also feels compelled to administer more "prophylactic preload," trying to prevent the circumstance of needing to infuse large amounts of fluids rapidly to treat developing hypotension. The author's group does not alter the dose of spinal anesthetic and usually administers 1000 ml of fluid immediately before spinal injection. Despite the group's successful use of spinal anesthesia, until definitive, prospective studies are completed in the severely preeclamptic patient, we *do not recommend* performing spinal anesthesia in severe preeclampsia unless the urgent need for cesarean section precludes the additional time needed for epidural anesthesia and patient safety militates against general anesthesia.

General Anesthesia for Cesarean Section

Management of the airway and blunting the blood pressure response to laryngoscopy and tracheal intubation are the primary challenges associated with general anesthesia for cesarean section. Thorough evaluation of the airway is required before initiating general anesthesia. If there is any stridor, dysphonia, hoarseness, difficulty swallowing, or respiratory distress, consider glottic edema, regardless of the apparent severity of facial edema. Awake intubation is indicated for suspected difficult airway management.

Because some glottic edema is often present, the author's group now routinely uses a 6.0- to 6.5-mm endotracheal tube as the first choice for endotracheal intubation, since, on occasion, it is impossible to pass a 7.0-mm endotracheal tube through the glottic opening in patients with severe preeclampsia. Have smaller cuffed endotracheal tubes available! One patient at the author's institution required a 5.5-mm endotracheal tube. It is much easier to start with a smaller than average endotracheal tube than to repeat airway instrumentation.

Blood Pressure Control

Severely preeclamptic patients with diastolic blood pressures greater than 105 mmHg require additional preinduction blood pressure control, anticipating the 20 to 30% increase in blood pressure that is associated with airway instrumentation. If time permits, the author's group prefers to have a "base" of hydralazine and labetalol. Most often, these antihypertensives lower the baseline blood pressure sufficiently, so that the transient increase in blood pressure that accompanies tracheal intubation is not dangerous. If there is inadequate time for hydralazine to affect blood pressure reduction, the author's group administers up to 0.25 mg/kg of labetalol IV combined with a potent vasodilator. The labetalol blunts compensatory tachycardia that accompanies the vasodilator, making blood pressure control easier. NTG is the first choice. Although it is less potent than SNP, the author's group believes it is easier to titrate. Remember, patients who have received intravascular volume expansion, particularly with colloids, may be resistant to NTG's antihypertensive effects. When patients are resistant to NTG, the author's group switches to SNP. We do not require intra-arterial blood pressure monitoring when using NTG; however, safe use of SNP requires beat-to-beat blood pressure monitoring. Regardless of the potent vasodilator used, the author's group tries to reduce the baseline blood pressure by 20 to 30%, then induces general anesthesia with thiopental, 4 to 6 mg/kg. This regimen does *not* prevent an increase in blood pressure; it only lowers the starting point and secondarily the peak pressure. Often, the vasodilator is not needed intraoperatively; however, anticipate that significant pressor responses with oral suctioning and tracheal extubation at the end of the operation may temporarily require increasing or reinstituting the vasodilator infusion (see Fig. 15–5).

Other ancillary techniques may also blunt the pressor response to airway instrumentation. These include IV lidocaine 1.5 mg/kg if given 2 minutes in advance of instrumentation[60] and IV alfentanil 10 μg/kg[61] given immediately prior to general anesthesia induction. If opioids are administered, the pediatrician must be notified of the possibility of associated neonatal depression, particularly for premature neonates.

Magnesium Sulfate

All severely preeclamptic patients should be receiving $MgSO_4$ for eclampsia prophylaxis. $MgSO_4$ prolongs nondepolarizing *and* depolarizing muscle relaxants in vitro. However, only the interaction with nondepolarizing relaxants is clinically significant. For example, note the marked prolongation of vecuronium effect in a patient receiving $MgSO_4$ 2 gm/hr IV (Fig. 15–7).[62] Careful titration of neuromuscular blocking drugs mandates monitoring with a peripheral nerve stimulator. Also, be aware that there is a potential for "recurarization" in the postanesthesia care unit in patients receiving continuous $MgSO_4$ therapy. This complication is more likely when longer-acting nondepolarizing blockers such a pancuronium are used.

The issue of whether to continue the $MgSO_4$ intraoperatively is unclear regardless of the anesthetic technique. Some authors discontinue the drug intraoperatively, fearing accidental infusion and overdose. Others continue the infusion, believing that the $MgSO_4$ smooths blood pressure control. Continuation of $MgSO_4$ may make sustained uterine contraction following delivery less likely (tocolytic effect) and produce increased blood loss. Oxytocin infusion immediately after delivery is needed to counteract this tocolytic effect; however, decrease the oxytocin infusion rate after sustained uterine contractions are evident. It is all too easy to administer excessive fluids during oxytocin infusion postdelivery. The author's group usually discontinues $MgSO_4$ infusion intraoperatively and continues the infusion immediately after completing the operation. However, the infusion is continued for eclamptic patients, believing that they have demonstrated a propensity for convulsions.

CONCLUSION

Medical and anesthetic management of severely preeclamptic patients is challenging. A large part of the challenge associates with a lack of knowledge. The cause of the disease is not understood. Effective treatments other than delivery do not exist. And there are few anesthetic outcome studies to guide anesthetic choices. Successful care of these high-risk patients depends on close collaboration and cooperation with the obstetrician and appropriate application of the limited understanding of options and possible outcomes. Dogma must be challenged so that treatment is guided by science rather than by extrapolation.

TEN PRACTICAL POINTS

1. Treat hypertension aggressively—cerebral hemorrhage is the most common cause of death.
2. The risk of seizure does not correlate with the severity of hypertension.
3. Women needing invasive hemodynamic monitoring intrapartum require continued monitoring in the postoperative period (24 to 72 hours).
4. When possible, place and test epidural catheters before developing thrombocytopenia becomes frank thrombocytopenia.
5. Avoid using bleeding time tests—they do not indicate risks of bleeding.
6. Platelet counts less than 100,000/mm^3 do

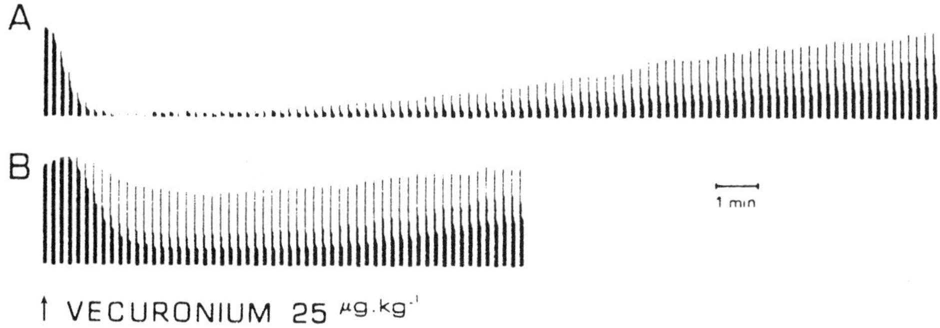

Figure 15–7. Electromyographic tracing comparing the neuromuscular blockade achieved by vecuronium, 25 μg·kg^{-1}, in an eclamptic patient *(A)* receiving intravenous magnesium sulfate at 2 gm/hr to that achieved in a control parturient *(B)*. *(A* and *B,* From Baraka A, Yazigi A: Neuromuscular interaction of magnesium with succinylcholine vecuronium sequence in the eclamptic parturient. Anesthesiology 67:806–808, 1987.)

not always contraindicate regional anesthesia. Use clinical judgment.

7. Severely preeclamptic patients require repeat laboratory screening every 6 hours—significant abnormalities can develop during the 6-hour period.

8. Severely preeclamptic patients may require less IV crystalloid than normal pregnant women during regional anesthesia.

9. Preferentially use regional anesthesia for cesarean section.

10. Suspect glottic edema in the presence of dysphonia, stridor, or respiratory distress.

REFERENCES

1. Dekker GA, Sibai BM: Low-dose aspirin in the prevention of preeclampsia and fetal growth retardation: Rationale, mechanisms, and clinical trials. Am J Obstet Gynecol 168:214–227, 1993.
2. Sibai BM, Caritis SN, Thom E, et al: Prevention of preeclampsia with low-dose aspirin in healthy, nulliparous pregnant women. The National Institute of Child Health and Human Development Network of Maternal-Fetal Medicine Units. N Engl J Med 329:1213–1218, 1993.
3. Zinaman M, Rubin J, Lindheimer MD: Serial plasma oncotic pressure levels and echoencephalography during and after delivery in severe preeclampsia. Lancet 1:1245–1247, 1985.
4. Cotton DB, Lee W, Huhta JC, Dorman KF: Hemodynamic profile of severe pregnancy-induced hypertension. Am J Obstet Gynecol 158:523–529, 1988.
5. Benedetti TJ, Carlson RW: Studies of colloid osmotic pressure in pregnancy-induced hypertension. Am J Obstet Gynecol 135:308–311, 1979.
6. Sakai K, Imaizumi T, Maeda H, et al: Venous distensibility during pregnancy. Comparisons between normal pregnancy and preeclampsia. Hypertension 24:461–466, 1994.
7. Villar MA, Sibai BM: Clinical significance of elevated mean arterial blood pressure in second trimester and threshold increase in systolic or diastolic blood pressure during third trimester [see Comments]. Am J Obstet Gynecol 160:419–423, 1989.
8. Gant NF, Daley GL, Chand S, et al: A study of angiotensin II pressor response throughout primigravid pregnancy. J Clin Invest 52:2682–2689, 1973.
9. Ring G, Krames E, Shnider SM, et al: Comparison of nitroprusside and hydralazine in hypertensive pregnant ewes. Obstet Gynecol 50:598–602, 1977.
10. Kirshon B, Wasserstrum N, Cotton DB: Should continuous hydralazine infusions be utilized in severe pregnancy-induced hypertension? Am J Perinatol 8:206–208, 1991.
11. Mabie WC, Gonzalez AR, Sibai BM, Amon E: A comparative trial of labetalol and hydralazine in the acute management of severe hypertension complicating pregnancy. Obstet Gynecol 70:328–333, 1987.
12. Ducsay CA, Thompson JS, Wu AT, Novy MJ: Effects of calcium entry blocker (nicardipine) tocolysis in rhesus macaques: Fetal plasma concentrations and cardiorespiratory changes. Am J Obstet Gynecol 157:1482–1486, 1987.
13. Thorp JM Jr, Spielman FJ, Valea FA, et al: Nifedipine enhances the cardiac toxicity of magnesium sulfate in the isolated perfused Sprague-Dawley rat heart. Am J Obstet Gynecol 163:655–656, 1990.
14. Snyder SW, Cardwell MS: Neuromuscular blockade with magnesium sulfate and nifedipine. Am J Obstet Gynecol 161:35–36, 1989.

15. Levin AC, Doering PL, Hatton RC: Use of nifedipine in the hypertensive diseases of pregnancy. Ann Pharmacother 28:1371–1378, 1994.
16. Wheeler AS, James FMI, Meis PJ, et al: Effects of nitroglycerin and nitroprusside on the uterine vasculature of gravid ewes. Anesthesiology 52:390–394, 1980.
17. Naulty J, Cefalo RC, Lewis PE: Fetal toxicity of nitroprusside in the pregnant ewe. Am J Obstet Gynecol 6:708–711, 1981.
18. Wasserstrum N: Nitroprusside in preeclampsia: Circulatory distress and paradoxical bradycardia. Hypertension 18:79–84, 1991.
19. Shoemaker CT, Meyers M: Sodium nitroprusside for control of severe hypertensive disease of pregnancy: A case report and discussion of potential toxicity. Am J Obstet Gynecol 149:171–173, 1984.
20. Baker AB: Management of severe pregnancy-induced hypertension, or gestosis, with sodium nitroprusside. Anaesth Intensive Care 18:361–365, 1990.
21. Stempel JE, O'Grady JP, Morton MJ, Johnson KA: Use of sodium nitroprusside in complications of gestational hypertension. Obstet Gynecol 60:533–538, 1982.
22. Craft JBJ, Co EG, Yonekura ML, Gilman RM: Nitroglycerin therapy for phenylephrine-induced hypertension in pregnant ewes. Anesth Analg 59:494–499, 1980.
23. Hood DD, Dewan DM, James FM III, et al: The use of nitroglycerin in preventing the hypertensive response to tracheal intubation in severe preeclampsia. Anesthesiology 63:329–332, 1985.
24. Longmire S, Leduc L, Jones MM, et al: The hemodynamic effects of intubation during nitroglycerin infusion in severe preeclampsia. Am J Obstet Gynecol 164:551–556, 1991.
25. Cotton DB, Gonik B, Dorman K, Harrist R: Cardiovascular alterations in severe pregnancy-induced hypertension: Relationship of central venous pressure to pulmonary capillary wedge pressure. Am J Obstet Gynecol 151:762–764, 1985.
26. Sibai BM, Mabie BC, Harvey CJ, Gonzalez AR: Pulmonary edema in severe preeclampsia-eclampsia: Analysis of thirty-seven consecutive cases. Am J Obstet Gynecol 156:1174–1179, 1987.
27. Benedetti TJ, Kates R, Williams V: Hemodynamic observations in severe preeclampsia complicated by pulmonary edema. Am J Obstet Gynecol 152:330–334, 1985.
28. Cotton DB, Longmire S, Jones MM, et al: Cardiovascular alterations in severe pregnancy-induced hypertension: Effects of intravenous nitroglycerin coupled with blood volume expansion. Am J Obstet Gynecol 154:1053–1059, 1986.
29. Cotton DB, Jones MM, Longmire S, et al: Role of intravenous nitroglycerin in the treatment of severe pregnancy-induced hypertension complicated by pulmonary edema. Am J Obstet Gynecol 154:91–93, 1986.
30. Clark SL, Greenspoon JS, Aldahl D, Phelan JP: Severe preeclampsia with persistent oliguria: Management of hemodynamic subsets. Am J Obstet Gynecol 154:490–494, 1986.
31. Lee W, Gonik B, Cotton DB: Urinary diagnostic indices in preeclampsia-associated oliguria: Correlation with invasive hemodynamic monitoring. Am J Obstet Gynecol 156:100–103, 1987.
32. Dildy GA, Cotton DB: Management of severe preeclampsia and eclampsia. Crit Care Clin 7:829–850, 1991.
33. Pritchard JA, Mason R, Corley M, Pritchard S: Genesis of severe placental abruption. Am J Obstet Gynecol 108:22–27, 1970.
34. Sibai BM: The HELLP syndrome (hemolysis, elevated liver enzymes, and low platelets): Much ado about nothing? [see Comments]. Am J Obstet Gynecol 162:311–316, 1990.
35. Sibai BM, Ramadan MK, Usta I, et al: Maternal morbidity and mortality in 442 pregnancies with hemolysis, elevated liver enzymes, and low platelets (HELLP syndrome). Am J Obstet Gynecol 169:1000–1006, 1993.
36. Kelton JG, Hunter DJ, Neame PB: A platelet function defect in preeclampsia. Obstet Gynecol 65:107–109, 1985.
37. Sibai BM, Abdella TH, Taylor HA: Eclampsia in the first half of pregnancy. A report of three cases and review of the literature. J Reprod Med 27:706–708, 1982.
38. Ramanathan J, Sibai BM, Vu T, Chauhan D: Correlation between bleeding times and platelet counts in women with preeclampsia undergoing cesarean section. Anesthesiology 71:188–191, 1989.
39. Rodgers RPC, Levin J: A critical reappraisal of the bleeding time. Semin Thromb Hemost 16:1–20, 1990.
40. Orlikowski CE, Payne AJ, Moodley J, Rocke DA: Thrombelastography after aspirin ingestion in pregnant and non-pregnant subjects. Br J Anaesth 69:159–161, 1992.
41. Sibai BM, Abdella TN, Spinnato JA, Anderson GD: Eclampsia. V. The incidence of nonpreventable eclampsia. Am J Obstet Gynecol 154:581–586, 1986.
42. Anonymous: Which anticonvulsant for women with eclampsia? Evidence from the Collaborative Eclampsia Trial. Lancet 345:1455–1463, 1995.
43. Rolbin SH, Abbott D, Musclow E, et al: Epidural anesthesia in pregnant patients with low platelet counts. Obstet Gynecol 71:918–920, 1988.
44. Rasmus KT, Rottman RL, Kotelko DM, et al: Unrecognized thrombocytopenia and regional anes-

thesia in parturients: A retrospective review. Obstet Gynecol 73:943–946, 1989.
45. Hew-Wing P, Rolbin SH, Hew E, Amato D: Epidural anaesthesia and thrombocytopenia. Anaesthesia 44:775–777, 1989.
46. Martin JN Jr, Blake PG, Lowry SL, et al: Pregnancy complicated by preeclampsia-eclampsia with the syndrome of hemolysis, elevated liver enzymes, and low platelet count: How rapid is postpartum recovery? Obstet Gynecol 76:737–741, 1990.
47. Abboud T, Artal R, Sarkis F, et al: Sympathoadrenal activity, maternal, fetal, and neonatal responses after epidural anesthesia in the preeclamptic patient. Am J Obstet Gynecol 144:915–918, 1982.
48. Jouppila P, Jouppila R, Hollmen A, Koivula A: Lumbar epidural analgesia to improve intervillous blood flow during labor in severe preeclampsia. Obstet Gynecol 59:158–161, 1982.
49. James FM III, Davies P: Maternal and fetal effects of lumbar epidural analgesia for labor and delivery in patients with gestational hypertension. Am J Obstet Gynecol 126:195–201, 1976.
50. Ramos-Santos E, Devoe LD, Wakefield ML, et al: The effects of epidural anesthesia on the Doppler velocimetry of umbilical and uterine arteries in normal and hypertensive patients during active term labor. Obstet Gynecol 77:20–26, 1991.
51. Rout CC, Rocke DA, Levin J, et al: A reevaluation of the role of crystalloid preload in the prevention of hypotension associated with spinal anesthesia for elective cesarean section. Anesthesiology 79:262–269, 1993.
52. Hadzic A, Vloka J, Patel N, Birnbach D: Hypertensive crisis after a successful placement of an epidural anesthetic in a hypertensive parturient. Case report. Reg Anesth 20:156–158, 1995.
53. Ramanathan J, Bottorff M, Jeter JN, et al: The pharmacokinetics and maternal and neonatal effects of epidural lidocaine in preeclampsia. Anesth Analg 65:120–126, 1986.
54. Hodgkinson R, Husain FJ, Hayashi RH: Systemic and pulmonary blood pressure during caesarean section in parturients with gestational hypertension. Can Anaesth Soc J 27:389–394, 1980.
55. Ramanathan J, Coleman P, Sibai B: Anesthetic modification of hemodynamic and neuroendocrine stress responses to cesarean delivery in women with severe preeclampsia. Anesth Analg 73:772–779, 1991.
56. Heller PJ, Scheider EP, Marx GF: Pharyngolaryngeal edema as a presenting symptom in preeclampsia. Obstet Gynecol 62:523–524, 1983.
57. Jouppila R, Jouppila P, Hollmen A: Laryngeal oedema as an obstetric anaesthesia complication. Acta Anaesthesiol Scand 24:97–98, 1980.
58. Kambam JR, Handte RE, Brown WU, Smith BE: Effect of normal and preeclamptic pregnancies on the oxyhemoglobin dissociation curve. Anesthesiology 65:426–427, 1986.
59. Wallace DH, Leveno KJ, Cunningham FG, et al: Randomized comparison of general and regional anesthesia for cesarean delivery in pregnancies complicated by severe preeclampsia. Obstet Gynecol 86:193–199, 1995.
60. Wilson IG, Meiklejohn BH, Smith G: Intravenous lignocaine and sympathoadrenal responses to laryngoscopy and intubation. The effect of varying time of injection. Anaesthesia 46:177–180, 1991.
61. Allen RW, James MF, Uys PC: Attenuation of the pressor response to tracheal intubation in hypertensive proteinuric pregnant patients by lignocaine, alfentanil and magnesium sulphate. Br J Anaesth 66:216–223, 1991.
62. Baraka A, Yazigi A: Neuromuscular interaction of magnesium with succinylcholine-vecuronium sequence in the eclamptic parturient. Anesthesiology 67:806–808, 1987.
63. Cotton DB, Gonik B, Dorman KF: Cardiovascular alterations in severe pregnancy-induced hypertension: Acute effects of intravenous magnesium sulfate. Am J Obstet Gynecol 148:162–165, 1984.
64. Groenendijk R, Trimbos JB, Wallenburg HC: Hemodynamic measurements in preeclampsia: Preliminary observations. Am J Obstet Gynecol 150:232–236, 1984.
65. Belfort MA, Anthony J, Buccimazza A, Davey DA: Hemodynamic changes associated with intravenous infusion of the calcium antagonist verapamil in the treatment of severe gestational proteinuric hypertension. Obstet Gynecol 75:970–974, 1990.
66. Belfort M, Uys P, Dommisse J, Davey DA: Haemodynamic changes in gestational proteinuric hypertension: The effects of rapid volume expansion and vasodilator therapy. Br J Obstet Gynaecol 96:634–641, 1989.
67. Wallenburg HCS: Hemodynamics in hypertensive pregnancy. *In* Rubin PC (ed): Hypertension in Pregnancy. Amsterdam, Elsevier, 1988, pp 66–101.
68. Mabie WC, Ratts TE, Sibai BM: The central hemodynamics of severe preeclampsia. Am J Obstet Gynecol 161:1443–1448, 1989.

SIXTEEN

Anesthesia for the Morbidly Obese Pregnant Patient

David M. Dewan, M.D.

The morbidly obese pregnant patient presents the anesthesia care provider with major challenges. Morbid obesity alters normal physiology, complicates the antepartum and intrapartum course, influences anesthetic management, and worsens postpartum outcome. Unfortunately, consistent with the increased prevalence of obesity in the general population, morbid obesity is also occurring with greater frequency among the obstetric population. At Wake Forest, the author's group's incidence of patients exceeding 300 pounds at the time of delivery increased from 0.18% to 0.35% between 1978 and 1989. Unless the anesthesia care provider understands the obstetric and anesthetic implications of morbid obesity, disasters may follow.

PATHOPHYSIOLOGY

Although obese patients have a normal basic metabolic rate, the increased body mass increases total body metabolism markedly. Obese pregnant patients consume more oxygen and produce more carbon dioxide in supporting their excess weight. These changes in turn increase ventilatory requirements, and in the absence of the pickwickian syndrome, alveolar ventilation increases and meets demands. However, ventilatory reserve diminishes. These ventilation requirements, superimposed on the metabolic demands of pregnancy, challenge the patient's ability to meet the metabolic demands of labor and delivery.

Obesity decreases functional residual capacity (FRC), inspiratory reserve volume, expiratory reserve volume, and total lung capacity. Reduced FRC may allow closing volume to occur within normal tidal ventilation and lead to hypoxemia, especially in the supine position. Although FRC, expiratory reserve volume, and residual volume usually decline during pregnancy, the decline in FRC among obese pregnant patients is less than in obese nonpregnant patients, perhaps offering some protection from hypoxemia, which might occur if the conditions were additive.[1] Furthermore, the greater chest wall weight and the pressure of the protuberant abdomen on the diaphragm compress alveoli in the dependent portion of the lungs. These less compliant alveoli promote preferential ventilation to the nondependent, more compliant portions of the lungs while pulmonary blood flow continues preferentially to the dependent portion of the lungs, producing ventilation-perfusion mismatch and hypoxemia. Thus, the morbidly obese pregnant patient may demonstrate hypoxemia. Eng and coworkers[1] and Blass[2] reported a maternal Pa_{O_2} of approximately 85 mmHg in morbidly obese pregnant patients, which is significantly lower than that observed in normal pregnant patients. However, these values do exceed those obtained in morbidly obese nonpregnant patients presenting for gastric bypass. Nevertheless, these values are abnormal and must be considered in light of the demands of labor and delivery and potential abdominal delivery.

Both pregnancy and obesity increase cardiac output and blood volume. Obesity increases blood volume proportionate to total body mass and this increase is superimposed on the 30 to 45% increase accompanying pregnancy. Cardiac output and cardiac work obviously increase concomitantly. Although systemic blood pressure usually decreases during pregnancy, hypertension occurs with greater frequency among obese patients. However, pulmonary artery pressure usually remains normal during pregnancy and in most obese patients, except when hypoxemia and compression of the pulmonary vessels produce pulmonary hypertension. Circulatory shifts may occur with position changes and airway obstruction. For example, changing from the sitting to supine position elevates wedge pressure by as much as 30%,[3] and airway obstruction may increase pulmonary wedge pressure approximately 30 mmHg.[4] Indeed, cardiac arrest has occurred when morbidly obese nonpregnant patients were placed supine for surgical procedures.[5] Thus, the morbidly obese pregnant patient's cardiovascular system may be unstable at the time of anesthetic intervention.

Both pregnancy and obesity increase the likelihood of large acidic gastric volumes. Eighty-eight percent of obese patients have a pH less than 2.5, and 86% have gastric volumes exceeding 25 ml.[6] These gastric volumes, combined with an increased likelihood of hiatal hernia, place the morbidly obese pregnant patient at great risk for pulmonary aspiration.

OBSTETRIC CONSIDERATIONS

Morbid obesity detrimentally influences the antepartum and intrapartum course. Chronic hypertension, pregnancy-induced hypertension, and diabetes all occur with greater frequency among obese patients. At Wake Forest, chronic hypertension occurred in 28% of patients whose weight exceeded 300 pounds at the time of delivery. This contrasted with a 2% incidence among control patients. These findings are comparable to those of Garbaciak and associates,[7] who noted an eightfold to ninefold increase of chronic hypertension among patients whose prepregnant weight exceeded 150% of ideal. Similarly, gestational and insulin-dependent diabetes occur with significantly greater frequency. At Wake Forest, diabetes, not delineated as either gestational or nongestational, increased fourfold; this was consistent with the increased incidences in gestational and insulin-dependent diabetes among morbidly obese patients reported by others.[8] Although pregnancy-induced hypertension occurs with greater frequency, the increases are not nearly as marked as those observed with chronic hypertension and diabetes. The author's group observed incidences of preeclampsia that increased from 10 to 16%, whereas Garbaciak and associates[7] noted an increase from 4.4 to 6.9%.

Nevertheless, the message is clear. Morbidly obese patients are frequently ill before labor commences. The author's group's overall observed incidence of antepartum medical disease was 47%, clearly demonstrating that the morbidly obese pregnant patient requires close scrutiny regarding systemic disease prior to the onset of labor. Indeed, complicating medical disease may categorize the obese patients as "high risk" *independent of obesity*. The validity of this high-risk category is apparent in the markedly increased death rate of morbidly obese pregnant patients. Representative findings are the disproportionate increases in maternal deaths among morbidly obese pregnant patients reported by Maeder and colleagues[9] in Minnesota and the identification of obesity as a significant risk factor contributing to maternal anesthetic deaths in Michigan covered in the excellent review by Endler and coworkers.[10] The anesthesia care provider *must* understand that morbid obesity increases the risks of maternal death!

Effect on Obstetric Course

The historical obstetric concerns regarding the high frequency of complicated vaginal delivery and cesarean sections among morbidly obese patients are valid. What remains unclear are the explanations. Although it would be tempting to speculate that the high incidence of complicating medical disease and the associated increase in oxytocic inductions could account for the increased frequency of cesarean sections among obese pregnant patients, this explanation does not hold true for morbidly obese patients. Both the author's group and Garbaciak and associates[7] noted that morbidly obese pregnant patients undergo more cesarean sections compared with normal-weight controls, even after complicating medical disease is accounted for. Speculation also exists regarding labor quality among morbidly obese pregnant patients. However, no controlled series substantiates the clinical impression that uterine activity is suboptimal in this patient population.

Intrapartum complications could also contribute to increased frequency of abdominal delivery. Although Garbaciak and associates[7] noted more fetal distress among obese patients, the present author's group failed to substantiate this finding. Certainly, fetal macrosomia complicates the intrapartum course. Obesity and diabetes may act independently and increase the likelihood of large-for-gestational-age infants.[11] Fetal macrosomia increases both the likelihood of shoulder dystocia during attempted vaginal delivery and the likelihood of failure to progress or cephalopelvic disproportion among laboring patients. However, fetal macrosomia does not fully explain the large cesarean section rate in this patient population. There is speculation that "fatty dystocia" exists in obese pregnant patients, whereby fat deposits along the pelvic side walls impair fetal descent, resulting in failure to progress.[12] Fetal macrosomia does account for the greater likelihood of shoulder dystocia, a true obstetric emergency! Indeed, at the author's institution, the indications for cesarean section among morbidly obese pregnant patients resemble those for normal-weight controls, except for the diagnosis of failure to progress, which increased more than fourfold and accounted for 49% of cesarean sections. Even more astounding was the overall cesarean section rate of 63%, including 50% of laboring patients.

The implications for the anesthesiologist are clear. Morbid obesity increases the requirement for anesthetic intervention, and considering the high anesthetic risk status of morbidly obese patients, early awareness and intervention by the anesthesia team may improve outcome and avoid disasters.

Neonatal Outcome

Whether or not obesity influences neonatal outcome is unclear. Morbidly obese patients are less likely to delivery prematurely; thus, accurate analysis of fetal outcome directly related to obesity is complicated by decreased death rate secondary to prematurity.[13] The wise anesthesia care provider, however, anticipates neonatal resuscitation requirements and has ample, trained personnel available for resuscitation of the newborn.

ANESTHETIC CONCERNS

Obese patients, especially those with concurrent diabetes mellitus, may present significant challenges for the anesthesia care provider. After a thorough preoperative examination early in the course of labor and appropriate laboratory evaluations to investigate concurrent disease, addressing technical concerns is the next step in management of the morbidly obese patient. In light of the high likelihood of abdominal delivery and difficult IV placement, early IV cannulation is imperative. Although the progesterone-related venodilatation accompanying pregnancy offers some protection, central venous access, with its own problems in the obese patient, may be the only accessible route. The greater depth of the epidural and subarachnoid space among this patient population suggests that longer needles must be available for regional anesthesia. Indeed, Blass performed a series of cesarean sections with the patient under spinal anesthesia when epidural needles were of insufficient length to identify the epidural space.[2] However, in the author's group's experience, the standard 3½-inch needles present on our spinal and epidural trays suffice for the overwhelming majority of patients weighing up to 500 pounds. The varied fat distribution among obese patients, which may spare the lumbar area, suggests that early attempts should utilize standard equipment. Inability to identify the epidural or subarachnoid space is more likely misdirection than inadequate needle length. Nevertheless, in rare cases, longer spinal and epidural needles may be required and are commercially available.

Although, in theory, some patients may require larger than normal operating tables, the experience at the author's institution does not support this. However, in one instance, the foot of an operating table collapsed while the patient was being shifted to the lithotomy position. More important than the width of the operating table is the immediate availability of additional personnel to aid in transport. Transporting anesthetized patients from the labor area to the operating room for cesarean section requires moving an immobile patient who is unable to assist in transport and dictates available support personnel. Furthermore, catheter dislodgement is always a threat during transport. A hand placed at the insertion site during movement may prevent this undesirable outcome. When transport help is unavailable, consider dosing the epidural in the operating room.

Anesthesia for Vaginal Delivery

The same options exist for vaginal delivery in the morbidly obese patient as for the normal-weight pregnant patient, including parenteral medications, inhalation analgesia, local infiltration, pudendal block, epidural analgesia, and spinal anesthesia. Parenteral analgesics supplemented at delivery with pudendal and local anesthesia, and occasionally inhalation analgesia, offer the advantages of simplicity. However, the pain relief provided by parenteral narcotics and local infiltration or pudendal block, even when supplemented with inhalation analgesia, is insufficient in a significant number of patients, especially in light of the increased likelihood of complicated vaginal delivery that may require profound anesthesia. This selection of a "simple" anesthetic may increase the probability of having to provide a "stat" major anesthetic and lessens the desirability of these "simple" techniques.

Spinal anesthesia obviates the disadvantage of inadequate anesthesia at vaginal delivery, but it may require placement under urgent circumstances in patients in whom placement is technically difficult. Subarachnoid lidocaine 30 to 40 mg or bupivacaine 6 to 7 mg administered with the patient sitting should provide adequate low spinal anesthesia. However, should abdominal delivery become necessary after unsuccessful attempted vaginal delivery, the distribution of analgesia following this dose regimen may be insufficient to provide cesarean section anesthesia. Because of its flexibility, epidural anesthesia is the technique of choice at the author's group's institution.

Epidural anesthesia offers the advantages of potentially easier placement, titratability, less motor block than spinal anesthesia, and most importantly, the ability for rapid augmentation to provide anesthesia for cesarean section, thus avoiding general anesthesia and its attendant airway hazards. Theoretical advantages also include the associated decreased oxygen consumption and attenuated fluctuations in cardiac output associated with epidural anesthesia in laboring pregnant patients. These could theoretically be important in the morbidly obese pregnant patient whose respiratory and cardiovascular systems are stressed because of her weight and the superimposed demands of pregnancy.

Epidural anesthesia is clearly feasible among morbidly obese pregnant patients. The author's group's 94% success rate of epidural anesthesia, documented by adequate pain relief or the presence of demonstrable dermatomal changes, provides sufficient evidence. This success rate did not differ from the group's success rate among control patients. We believe early placement offers significant advantages. First, a calm, cooperative patient able to position herself adequately for epidural placement eases the challenge of less than ideal anatomy. Furthermore, and most importantly, early epidural catheter placement provides an available anesthetic when urgent abdominal delivery becomes necessary early in the labor course. At the author's institution, catheters are sometimes placed and tested for adequacy of anesthesia before the onset of active labor. Further injections are then avoided until active labor develops. This plan eases placement and provides the patient with rapid pain relief when requested. However, even under ideal conditions, placements can be difficult. Although a 94% success rate was achieved for epidural anesthesia among obese pregnant patients, obese patients required significantly more catheter placements to achieve adequate analgesia than normal-weight patients. Some patients required as many as five epidural catheters prior to achieving satisfactory anesthesia. The author's group believes the effort was worth it. An honest preoperative discussion with the patient regarding potentially difficult catheter placement frequently results in a patient who accepts multiple punctures and catheter placements and understands the importance of utilizing epidural anesthesia.

The author's group also believes it is imperative to accept nothing less than a perfect block because of the predisposition to use the catheter for surgical anesthesia. Remember the 63% cesarean section rate! Any epidural catheter that does not provide *complete* labor pain relief with bupivacaine 0.25% or less without the addition of narcotics may not provide adequate surgical anesthesia. Therefore, the author's group meticulously tests epidural catheters and closely scrutinizes the analgesic effects. When any doubt exists as to the quality of block, the catheter is replaced. For the same reasons, the author's group avoids the combined spinal-epidural technique in this patient population. Indeed, following this practice in the author's group's series of morbidly obese pregnant patients undergoing cesarean section, only one patient required intraoperative conversion to general anesthesia because of inadequate surgical anesthesia. The intraoperative conversion to general anesthesia can be far worse than the preoperative induction!

Although the author's faculty varies on desired patient position during placement, the sitting position offers the advantage of easier midline identification. However, also noted is a greater likelihood of unintentionally cephalad placement of epidural catheters when obese patients are anesthetized in the sitting position. The greater amount of fat on the iliac crest probably accounts for the misinterpretation of interspace (Fig. 16–1). Cephalad catheters frequently express themselves by inadequate sacral analgesia despite large volumes of local anesthetic. Unusual cephalad spread of anesthesia aids in confirming the diagnosis. If one observes a high block without sacral anesthesia, check the level of epidural insertion. Occasionally, withdrawing the catheter 1 to 2 cm corrects the problem. Otherwise, rely on re-placement. During placement, search for the spinous process—this is the driveway to one's home. When the spinous processes are identified, the needle is walked either caudad or cephalad to identify the appropriate interspace. The patient is the best source to determine if placement is lateral. Most patients can tell, if asked, whether the approach is to the left or the right of the midline.

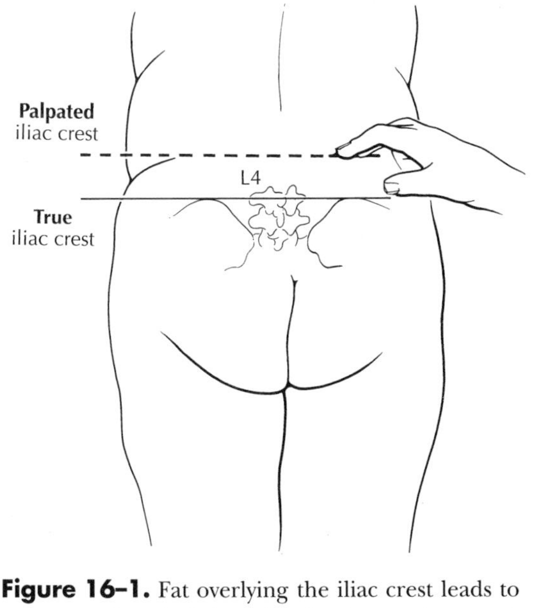

Figure 16–1. Fat overlying the iliac crest leads to unexpected cephalad epidural catheter placement.

Should unintentional dural puncture occur, continuous spinal anesthesia offers an alternative, but it is not the author's group's anesthetic of choice. On the group's busy labor service, confusion between a continuous spinal catheter and an epidural catheter is possible, and considering the consequences of confusion and possible total spinal anesthesia, we usually repeat placement at another interspace. In this setting, the catheter is carefully tested with *each* reinjection, looking carefully for excess spread. One of the author's group's normal-weight patients experienced total spinal anesthesia after two normal reinjections. Once the space is identified, we thread the catheter more than the customary 3 to 4 cm because the greater amount of adipose tissue predisposes to catheter displacement. Therefore, catheters are threaded 5, 6, or more cm into the epidural space, recognizing that this may increase the likelihood of asymmetric blocks. However, in the author's group's experience, the preponderance of epidural blocks are symmetric, regardless of catheter insertion length. When asymmetry exists, the catheter is simply pulled back until adequate symmetric anesthesia is provided. If minimal amounts (2–3 cm) of catheter remain in the epidural space, the author's group frequently removes the epidural catheter and replaces it, unless the patient is late in the course of labor. Short catheter distances and long labors lead to catheter dislodgement! Remember to caution nursing staff and the patient about appropriate movement to minimize catheter tension and risks for dislodgement.

Drug selection for analgesic maintenance during labor is relatively unimportant, provided the adequacy of the block has been demonstrated *without* supplemental narcotics. Bupivacaine should provide for complete comfort (10–15 ml 0.25% bupivacaine). Once the adequacy of the block has been proved, supplemental epidural narcotics are appropriate. The author's group's usual maintenance infusion is 0.125% bupivacaine at approximately 12 to 14 ml/hr. For perineal anesthetizing doses, the author's group predominantly utilizes 2% 2-chloroprocaine, 15 ml in divided doses, because of its rapid onset. A suitable alternative would be 2% lidocaine. Although obesity may influence both the drug requirement and the distribution of epidural anesthesia, fractionation of local anesthetic injections to 5 ml per aliquot renders these minimal changes clinically insignificant. The author's group is not convinced that obesity alters the drug requirement for labor analgesia.

TABLE 16–1
Preparation for Difficult Intubation

Assorted face masks
Oral and nasal airways
Short-handled laryngoscope handle
Assorted laryngoscope blades
Pulse oximeter and capnograph
Cricothyroidotomy kit and jet ventilator
Fiberoptic intubating bronchoscope
Additional experienced hands

Anesthesia for Cesarean Section

General Anesthesia

General anesthesia for cesarean section in this patient population poses significant threats and risks. General anesthesia presents major challenges for the anesthetic team, with airway difficulties predominating as a leading cause of maternal mortality. Early preparations begin with a thorough examination of the airway. Importantly, no assessment guarantees that intubation or mask ventilation may be possible. Furthermore, a history of uneventful intubation does not predict future success. The author's group had a patient who had a previous cesarean section, utilizing general anesthesia, and whose weight was greater than 300 pounds at the time of that anesthetic. Chart review revealed a previous uneventful rapid-sequence induction. When the patient refused regional anesthesia for this subsequent anesthetic and demanded general anesthesia, she required seven intubation attempts and difficult mask ventilation prior to securing the airway.

Obviously, when general anesthesia becomes necessary, or circumstances dictate or mandate general anesthesia, all preparations must be made in advance (Table 16–1). Minimal preparations should include: antacid therapy; equipment for difficult intubation (including assorted laryngoscope blades); various endotracheal tube sizes; a short-handled laryngoscope; and most importantly, additional experienced hands to assist during difficult establishment of the airway. Limited neck extension, increased chest wall size, and large pendulous breasts impede laryngoscopy utilizing standard laryngoscope handles (Fig. 16–2). A short-handled laryngoscope is preferable, and a fiberoptic laryngoscope should be immediately available. Additional experienced hands are vital because the primary anesthetist fatigues rapidly during re-

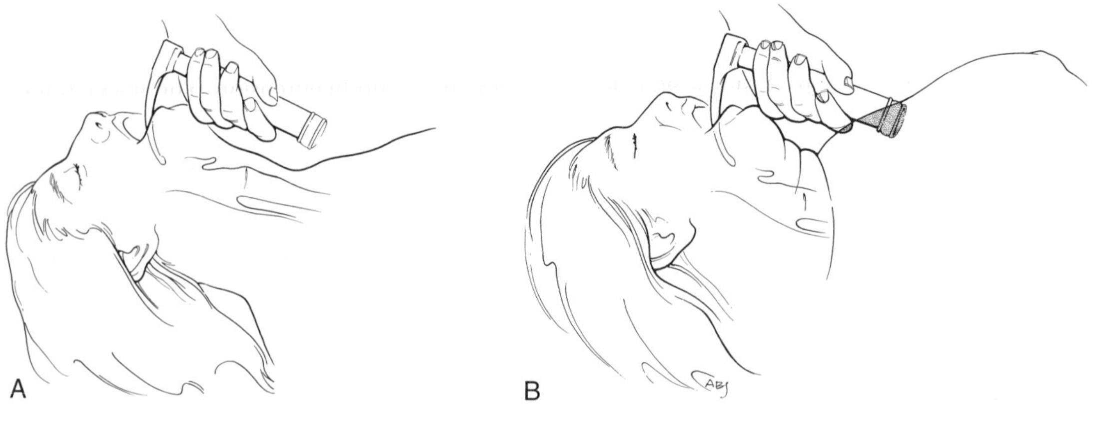

Figure 16–2. *A*, Normal laryngoscope/anatomic relationship. *B*, Obstructed laryngoscope placement in obese patients.

peated attempts at tracheal intubation, and mask ventilation may require two experienced individuals.

Unfortunately, in this patient population, fat tissue in the neck makes cricothyroid membrane identification difficult, compromising the anesthesia care provider's ability to establish emergency ventilation. Palpate the neck prior to selecting rapid-sequence induction and *do not* assume that cricothyroidotomy is a reliable backup for securing the airway. Adequate denitrogenation is essential, and although four deep breaths within 30 seconds is reported as sufficient in the nonobese population, and one preliminary report suggests its suitability in morbidly obese nonpregnant patients,[14] 3 minutes of ventilation of 100% oxygen is a preferable course because of the additional protection offered during prolonged periods of apnea.[15] During the 3 minutes of tidal ventilation, occasional deep breaths are advisable because airway closure may occur during normal tidal ventilation.

Thiopental is a suitable induction agent in most circumstances, and although the obese patient has a larger volume of distribution, 4 mg/kg, up to a maximum of 500 mg, has been the routine at the author's institution in this patient population. Similarly, succinylcholine is the agent of choice for a rapid-sequence induction. Pseudocholinesterase activity increases among morbidly obese patients and may offer reduced paralysis duration in the event intubation fails.[16] The author's group's usual dose of succinylcholine is 1.5 to 2 mg/kg, up to a maximum of 200 mg, for patients weighing up to 500 pounds. Pulse oximetry and capnography are, obviously, essential components of a rapid-sequence induction. Following securing of the airway, maintaining adequate oxygenation is imperative. Obese patients may require higher oxygen concentrations to maintain a Pa_{O_2} above 80,[17] limiting nitrous oxide administration. Pulse oximetry aids in determining the adequate oxygen concentration. Supplementation of nitrous oxide with a potent inhalation agent or narcotics, or both, is suitable for provision of maintenance anesthesia. However, as with nonobese pregnant patients, concentrations of the potent agents exceeding 1 minimal alveoler concentration (MAC) may produce unwanted uterine relaxation and fetal depression.

Although minor differences may exist regarding morbidly obese patients' handling of nondepolarizing muscle relaxants, all are suitable choices, providing the degree of neuromuscular blockade is monitored. Do not handicap the surgeon with poor relaxation! Following conclusion of the surgical procedure, adequate reversal is essential. However, even a fully conscious patient and adequate neuromuscular reversal do not guarantee maintenance of adequate oxygenation. At the author's institution, one patient required reintubation within 1 minute of extubation despite full consciousness and clearly adequate reversal and return of muscle function. Therefore, be prepared at the end of the case, too!

Finally, awake fiberoptic intubation is a reasonable alternative for elective securing of the airway, if time permits; otherwise, direct laryngoscopy may be the only choice. The author's group prefers oral intubation because the nasal passages of pregnant patients have extremely friable mucosa, making nasal intubation a less desirable alternative. Remember, stress accompanying unsedated fiberoptic intubation may produce stress-related reductions in uterine blood flow, whereas excessive sedation may depress the fetus. The author's group usually selects narcotic sedation because of its reversibility and advises the neonatal resuscitation team of this drug selection.

Regional Anesthesia

Regional anesthesia for cesarean section requires the same careful preparation as general anesthesia, including preparations for emergency airway securement (Table 16–2). Successful regional anesthesia also includes sufficient time for block placement, documentation of adequacy, and preparedness for treating complications, including a total blockade, inadequate ventilation, and hypotension. The selected technique must provide *both* the quality *and* the

TABLE 16–2
Requirements for Successful Regional Anesthesia

Preparations for emergency airway securement
Adequate time for block placement
Adequate anesthetic duration
Aggressive treatment of hypotension
Judgment

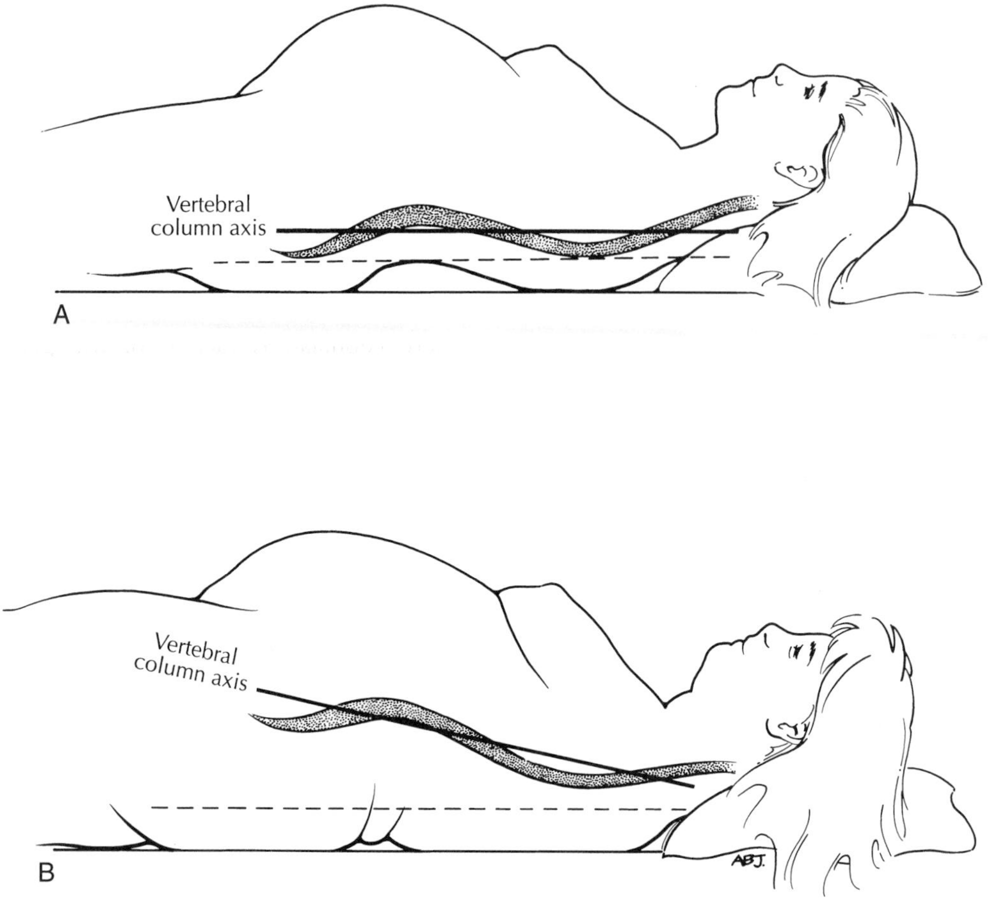

Figure 16–3. *A,* Vertebral column axis in horizontal, normal-weight patients. *B,* Altered vertebral column axis in horizontal, obese patients.

duration of blockade for the proposed procedure. Administer supplemental oxygen throughout the procedure. Judgment exercised preoperatively is the key to success.

Spinal Anesthesia

Spinal anesthesia offers an alternative to general anesthesia but is not the technique of choice at the author's institution. The disadvantages of spinal anesthesia include unpredictable spread, profound motor blockade, and limited duration of action. Although some evidence suggests that the role obesity plays in determining the distribution of spinal anesthesia may be small,[18] many anesthesiologists agree that there is unpredictable spread in this patient population. Greene believes the "exaggerated spread" of local anesthetic in this patient population, if it occurs, may be secondary to the enlarged buttocks, which place the patient in the Trendelenburg position, despite a level operating room table (Fig. 16–3).[19] A horizontal patient axis may require reverse Trendelenburg positioning of the operating table.

In contrast to epidural anesthesia, spinal anesthesia produces a greater degree of motor blockade for a given sensory level. Higher levels of motor blockade could impair ventilation if the patient depends on the accessory muscles of respiration to maintain ventilation. However, in the author's group's limited experience with spinal anesthesia, this has not posed a problem. All morbidly obese patients should receive supplemental oxygen, irrespective of anesthetic technique. Oxygen supplementation protects the fetus and serves as preoxygenation if conversion to general anesthesia becomes necessary. Therefore, maintain supplemental oxygen until the infant is delivered *and* the quality of block ensured. Continuously monitor oxygen saturation with pulse oximetry and continue supplementing oxygen as needed.

Finally, the author's group's most important reason for not selecting spinal anesthesia is that cesarean section in obese patients takes longer. The operating times at the author's institution, for patients weighing greater than 300 pounds, ranged from 13 to 190 minutes, the latter time being clearly beyond the range of the author's group's usual and customary spinal anesthetic duration. Continuous spinal anesthesia offers a potential alternative to single-shot spinal. Most authorities recommend limiting subarachnoid catheter length to 2 to 4 cm to minimize risks for spinal cord damage. Since skin and fat movement in these patients can easily dislodge a spinal catheter, reliable spinal redosing is questionable. One of the author's group's regional anesthetic failures occurred secondary to spinal catheter dislodgement. Spinal microcatheters are currently unavailable, making epidural catheters the only viable spinal catheter, potentially increasing the risk of spinal headache requiring epidural blood patch. There are no studies in this patient population delineating risks and benefits of spinal versus epidural catheters. However, the risks of continuous spinal, even with an epidural catheter, may be less than a single-shot spinal with inadequate anesthetic duration.

Epidural Anesthesia

Epidural anesthesia is the technique of choice for cesarean section at the author's institution. The same technical difficulties exist for providing for cesarean section anesthesia with epidural anesthesia as for providing labor analgesia. Morbidly obese pregnant patients may require less drug to obtain surgical anesthesia, as documented by Hodgkinson and Husain.[20] However, fractionation of local anesthetics makes this finding clinically insignificant. Following catheter testing, titrate the local anesthetic drug in 5-ml aliquots until the desired dermatomal distribution is demonstrated. Large bolus administration could produce extensive spread, and even titration may produce unwanted cephalad spread. However, in Hodgkinson and Husain's study, patients ventilated adequately despite high sensory levels (including cervical levels), and there was a surprisingly low incidence of hypotension. The author's group's experience is consistent with these findings, and when patients experience dyspnea, we found that elevating the head of the operating table approximately 10 to 30 degrees lessens patients' complaints without impeding the surgical field. Remember, use supplemental oxygen! Cephalad retraction of the panniculus during regional anesthesia can be catastrophic. Hodgkinson and Husain reported profound hypotension associated with fetal loss during cesarean section where cephalad retraction of the panniculus occurred.[21] This has not been the author's group's experience, but the anesthesia team must be cognizant of the potential role of panniculus retraction in producing unexpected severe systemic hypotension, even in the presence of adequate left uterine displacement.

Suitable choices for epidural analgesia for cesarean section are 3% chloroprocaine, 2% lidocaine with bicarbonate and epinephrine, and 0.5% bupivacaine. Circumstances should dictate the drug of choice. Chloroprocaine provides rapid onset but produces risk of inadequate duration of anesthesia, should the epidural catheter become dislodged, preventing redosing of the catheter. Bupivacaine provides a prolonged duration of anesthesia but has slow onset. The author's group may choose 0.5% bupivacaine when catheters are tenuous. Lidocaine with bicarbonate and epinephrine provides a third alternative and may be a reasonable choice, especially when the anesthesia team elects to use postoperative epidural narcotics. In the author's group's experience, required drug volumes are similar with all these drugs. Again, the author's group is not impressed with a dramatically reduced drug requirement among morbidly obese pregnant patients utilizing epidural anesthesia, but the consequences of excessively high block emphasize the importance of fractionation of local anesthetic injections. If time permits, dosing the patient in the operating room lessens the risk of catheter dislodgement, enabling the patient to assist in preoperative transport and providing immediately available equipment for airway securement.

POSTOPERATIVE CARE

Adequate pain relief is important in this patient population and may be provided with parenteral narcotics, epidural narcotics, and patient-controlled analgesia. Parenteral narcotics exhibit the same disadvantages and advantages in this patient population as in the normal-weight population. Ease of administration and variable quality are the major advantage and disadvantage of this choice. Although epidural narcotics provide excellent pain relief, especially following bupivacaine or lidocaine anesthetics, the rare risk of respiratory depression exists. The anesthesia team must weigh the potential catastrophic outcome of respiratory depression in this patient population versus the benefits of pain relief. At the author's institution, the author's group utilizes patient-controlled analgesia in this patient population, as is used in the group's normal-weight population. Adequate postoperative monitoring of respiratory function is essential in this population.

TEN PRACTICAL POINTS

1. Morbidly obese patients experience a high incidence of antenatal medical disease, increasing maternal and fetal risk.
2. Intrapartum complications, potential shoulder dystocia, and a remarkably high incidence of failure to progress increase the likelihood of abdominal delivery in this patient population.
3. Nearly 50% of laboring morbidly obese patients undergo cesarean section.
4. General anesthesia is a major contributor to maternal anesthetic mortality in this patient population. Avoid general anesthesia if possible.
5. Early anesthesia team involvement and adequate preoperative assessment of these patients are vital.
6. Early epidural placement during labor decreases the likelihood of requiring general anesthesia for cesarean section.
7. Accept nothing less than a perfect block and complete pain relief during labor, since the epidural may be utilized for cesarean section.
8. Have ample experienced hands available when general anesthesia is required.
9. Administer 100% oxygen during regional anesthesia until the newborn is delivered and the quality of block is ensured.
10. Obese patients die!

REFERENCES

1. Eng M, Butler J, Bonica JJ: Respiratory function in pregnant obese women. Am J Obstet Gynecol 123:241–245, 1975.
2. Blass NH: Regional anesthesia in the morbidly obese patient. Reg Anesth 4:20–22, 1979.
3. Paul B, Hoyt J, Boutrou A: Cardiovascular and respiratory changes in response to change of position in the very obese. Anesthesiology 45:73–78, 1976.
4. Teeple E, Ghia JN: An elevated pulmonary wedge pressure resulting from an upper respiratory obstruction in an obese patient. Anesthesiology 59:66–68, 1983.
5. Tseuda K, Debrand M, Zeok S, et al: Obesity supine sudden death syndrome: Report of two morbidly obese patients. Anesth Analg 58:345–347, 1979.
6. Vaughan RW, Bauer S, Wise L: Volume and pH of gastric juice in obese patients. Anesthesiology 43:686–689, 1975.
7. Garbaciak JA, Richter M, Miller S, Barton JJ: Maternal weight in pregnancy complications. Obstet Gynecol 152:238–245, 1985.
8. Gross T, Sokol RJ, King KC: Obesity and pregnancy: Risk and outcome. Obstet Gynecol 56:446–450, 1980.
9. Maeder EC, Barno A, Mecklenburg F. Obesity: A maternal high-risk factor. Obstet Gynecol 45:669–671, 1975.
10. Endler GC, Mariona FG, Solol RJ, Stevenson LB: Anesthesia-related mortality in Michigan 1972–1984. Am J Obstet Gynecol 159:187–193, 1988.
11. Gould SF, Makowski EL: Obesity in pregnancy. Perinatol Neonatol May-June 1981, pp 49–59.
12. Prough SG, Askel S: Overweight, endocrine function, and infertility. Obesity endocrinology. Contemp Obstet Gynecol October 1987, pp 63–78.
13. Kliegman RM, Gross TL: Perinatal problems of the obese mother and her infant. Obstet Gynecol 66:299–306, 1985.
14. Goldberg ME, Norris MC, Ghassem EL, et al: Preoxygenation in the morbidly obese: A comparison of two techniques. Anesth Analg 68:520–522, 1989.
15. Gambee M, Hetzka R, Fisher D: Preoxygenation techniques: Comparison of three minutes and four breaths. Anesth Analg 66:468–479, 1987.
16. Bentley JB, Borel JD, Vaughn RW, Gandolfi AJ: Weight, pseudocholinesterase activity, and succinylcholine requirement. Anesthesiology 57:48–49, 1982.
17. Vaughan RW, Wise L: Intraoperative arterial oxygenation of obese patients. Ann Surg 84:35–42, 1976.
18. Norris MC: Height, weight and spread of subarachnoid hyperbaric bupivacaine in the term pregnant patient. Anesth Analg 67:555–558, 1988.
19. Greene NM: Distribution of local anesthetics within the subarachnoid space. Anesth Analg 64:715–730, 1985.

20. Hodgkinson R, Husain FJ: Obesity and the cephalad spread of analgesia following epidural administration of bupivacaine for cesarean section. Anesth Analg 59:89–92, 1980.

21. Hodgkinson R, Husain FJ: Caesarean section associated with gross obesity. Br J Anaesth 52:919–923, 1980.

SEVENTEEN

Diabetes in Pregnancy

Desmond Writer, M.B., F.R.C.A., F.R.C.P.(C.)

Diabetes mellitus is the most common medical problem affecting pregnant women. The disorder challenges the mother's glucose control, increases her potential complication rate, and may also affect the fetus or neonate. Infrequently, diabetes antedates the pregnancy and becomes exacerbated by it (pregestational diabetes: Type I or II).[1, 2] However, 90% of the diabetic cases that complicate pregnancy are gestational diabetes mellitus (GDM), which has its onset or first recognition during pregnancy.

Women with Type I diabetes (insulin-dependent diabetes mellitus [IDDM]) secrete insufficient insulin because of damage to their pancreatic β cells by an autoimmune process or viral injury.[3] Typically nonobese, they have no family history of diabetes. The disease generally begins in their juvenile years, although onset may be postponed up to the age of 40 years. Type I subjects are prone to develop ketosis and require daily insulin when nonpregnant. Their insulin requirements characteristically increase during pregnancy. Type I diabetes presents the greatest potential for pregnancy-related complications, and risk increases with duration and severity of the disease.

Type II diabetes typically begins after the age of 40 years and is uncommon in women of childbearing age. Many of these individuals are obese. They demonstrate insulin resistance and have a relative impairment of insulin secretion. Frequently, there is a strong family history of diabetes. Although this type is usually referred to as *non–insulin-dependent diabetes mellitus* (NIDDM), patients with Type II diabetes may require treatment with exogenous insulin, or oral hypoglycemic agents, to supplement the inadequate endogenous secretion. Pregnancy contraindicates oral hypoglycemic drugs, all of which cross the placenta. Type II diabetes occurring in pregnancy must therefore be controlled with insulin.[4]

GDM increases in probability with advancing maternal age. Catalano and coworkers[5] found GDM in 7 of 1000 (0.7%) gravid women under 20 years of age, and 38 of 1000 (3.8%) in those aged 30 to 34 years. Overall, GDM affects approximately 3 to 5% of pregnancies in the United States.[6] Similarity exists between the pathogenesis of Type II diabetes and that of GDM, and up to 50% of women with GDM develop Type II diabetes in the 15 years following the affected pregnancy.[1] Gestational diabetes may be subclassified as Class A_1 (diet-controlled), and Class A_2 (requiring insulin).[7]

Regardless of the type of diabetes, improved understanding of the pathophysiology, coupled with treatment that achieves and maintains normoglycemia throughout pregnancy, has greatly reduced the fetal and neonatal mortality rates formerly associated with the condition. When pregnant diabetic patients receive appropriate care, whether with diet alone or with insulin, they can now expect a perinatal outcome comparable with that of healthy women (except for pregnancies complicated by IDDM, which result in a higher incidence of congenital malformations).[1] However, the incidence and severity of diabetic-related complications tends to increase with duration of the disease. In her "traditional" classification of diabetes, White noted that duration of the disease, and the presence of vascular complications, adversely influenced perinatal outcome (Table 17–1).[8] Although some obstetricians now consider White's classification obsolete because of the improved outcomes, many still consider it helpful because it precisely defines the severity and *potential* risks of the disorder. *From a practical viewpoint, anesthesiologists also should anticipate increased maternal, fetal, and neonatal complications in women who require insulin, especially those with long-standing disease and those who are insulin-dependent.*

GLUCOSE CONTROL DURING NORMAL PREGNANCY

Carbohydrate metabolism changes during normal pregnancy to provide for the needs of mother and fetus. The first half of pregnancy can be considered an anabolic phase. Increased levels of estrogen and progesterone lead to β

TABLE 17–1
White's Classification of Diabetes

Class	Characteristics	Implications
Gestational diabetes	Glucose intolerance diagnosed during pregnancy	Diagnosis before 30 wks' gestation important in prevention of macrosomia; treatment goal is fasting plasma glucose level ≤ 105 mg/dl (5.8 mmol/L) and 2-hr postprandial plasma glucose level <120 mg/dl (6.7 mmol/L); if insulin becomes necessary, manage as in classes B, C, and D
A	Chemical diabetes diagnosed before pregnancy; managed by diet alone, any age or onset (NIDDM)	Management as for gestational diabetes
B	Overt diabetes; insulin-dependent before pregnancy; onset ≥ age 20 years; duration <10 years	Some endogenous insulin secretion may persist; insulin resistance at the cellular level in obese women; management, and fetal and neonatal risk, equivalent to classes C and D
C	Overt diabetes; insulin-dependent; onset age 10–20 years, or duration 10–20 years	Insulin-dependent diabetes of juvenile onset (Type I IDDM)
D	Overt diabetes; insulin-dependent; onset < age 10 years, or duration > 20 years; or chronic hypertension (not preeclampsia); or benign retinopathy (tiny hemorrhages)	Severe Type I IDDM; IUGR possible; retinal "microaneurysms" may progress during pregnancy, then regress after delivery
F	Diabetic nephropathy with proteinuria	Anemia and hypertension common; proteinuria increases in third trimester, declines after pregnancy; IUGR common; perinatal survival ~85% under optimal conditions; bed rest necessary; Class T—postrenal transplant—outlook good
R	Malignant proliferative retinopathy	Neovascularization; risk of vitreous hemorrhage or retinal detachment; laser photocoagulation useful; delivery route controversial
H	Coronary artery disease	Grave maternal risk

Abbreviations: NIDDM = non–insulin-dependent diabetes mellitus; IDDM = insulin-dependent diabetes mellitus; IUGR = intrauterine growth retardation.

From Datta S, Kitzmiller JL, Naulty JS, et al: Acid-base status of diabetic mothers and their infants following spinal anesthesia for cesarean section. Anesth Analg 61(8):662–665, 1982.

cell hyperplasia and an increase in insulin secretion.[1, 9] The result is increased glycogen deposition in the peripheral maternal tissues and a concomitant decrease in hepatic glucose production. Maternal blood glucose levels fall to 55 to 65 mg/dl in the fasting state, a decrease of 15 to 20 mg/dl below those of the nonpregnant female. After an overnight fast, plasma ketone levels increase significantly, providing an alternative maternal energy source while sparing glucose for the fetus. Glucose is transported across the placenta to the fetus by a process of facilitated diffusion.

The second half of pregnancy represents a catabolic phase. As the placental size increases, insulin production must increase in an effort to overcome the insulin resistance promoted by "diabetogenic" placental hormones, including human placental lactogen, the strongest insulin antagonist, and pituitary prolactin. Because these hormones antagonize insulin at a postreceptor site, the maternal cells lack sufficient glucose, and the mother experiences "accelerated starvation," in which more rapid and profound diversion to fat metabolism occurs in the fasting state than in the first half of pregnancy. This results in ketonemia and increased plasma levels of free fatty acids. However, glucose transfer to the fetus increases as a result of these changes. *In short, the mother foregoes her main energy substrate, glucose, and uses fats, preserving glucose to satisfy the needs of an increasingly "demanding" fetus.*

GLUCOSE CONTROL IN THE DIABETIC PREGNANCY

Women with GDM usually first demonstrate decreased insulin reserve in the second half of pregnancy, when the production of contrainsulin hormones increases. Ten to 15% of these women require insulin. Obstetricians use varying criteria for starting insulin; some consider a fasting blood glucose above 95 mg/dl (5.3 mmol/L) to be the criterion, whereas others start insulin only when the level exceeds 105 mg/dl.

For insulin-dependent diabetics (Type I IDDM), pregnancy constitutes a metabolic challenge. In the first half of pregnancy, the transfer of maternal glucose and amino acids to the fetus significantly affects the mother's carbohydrate homeostasis, predisposing her to hypoglycemia. Diminished food intake, associated with morning sickness, can exacerbate this tendency. In women with good prepregnancy diabetic control, the insulin requirement in the early weeks of pregnancy characteristically remains unchanged and may even decrease, owing to the lowered plasma glucose levels. In contrast, from midpregnancy onward, the parturient's daily insulin needs increase to avoid the occurrence of ketosis, which adversely affects the fetus. Ultimately, the augmented insulin dose may be as much as 50 to 100% above the mother's nonpregnant requirements and insulin requirements usually persist at this level until the last few weeks of pregnancy.

The mother's insulin requirement usually decreases in the last weeks of pregnancy, and she becomes particularly susceptible to hypoglycemia, especially overnight and in the early morning, if her augmented insulin dose is not reduced. Formerly thought to indicate fetoplacental insufficiency, this decreased insulin requirement probably results from the continuous consumption of maternal fuels by the fetus at a stage when fetal growth increases considerably. *In summary, in late pregnancy, the fetus consumes a greater share of the mother's carbohydrate intake, necessitating a reduction in her daily insulin dosage.*

The Risk of Postpartum Hypoglycemia

During labor and delivery, insulin requirements in diabetic parturients fall significantly. Some women require no insulin for several hours during labor, whereas in others, doses approximating 1 to 2 units/hr suffice. In the immediate postpartum period, diabetic mothers demonstrate profound insulin sensitivity, and the augmented dose of the third trimester declines dramatically, even below the pre-pregnancy level. *Beware of giving a substantial dose of insulin before delivery—for example, before cesarean section—because of the significant danger of postpartum hypoglycemia!*

Over the days and weeks following delivery, as the mother's carbohydrate intake increases, and in the absence of the glucose-consuming fetus, the daily insulin requirement of women with Type I IDDM again rises.

DIABETES AND PREGNANCY

The Mother

As recently as the 1970s, diabetic women were counseled to avoid pregnancy because all major pregnancy complications occurred with increased frequency in diabetic gravidae.[10] Important developments since the mid-1980s, notably improved fetal surveillance, and more precise estimation of fetal lung maturity, along with treatment directed toward strict blood glucose control, led to better maternal and fetal outcomes. Maternal complications may still occur, however, especially in late pregnancy (Table 17–2). The incidence of preeclampsia is approximately 10%, slightly more than double that of nondiabetic mothers, and its severity increases with increasing severity of the diabetes. Diabetic parturients with vascular disease (e.g., hypertension, nephropathy, and chronic hypertension) present particular challenges. Type I diabetes may present during pregnancy (and usually presents as ketoacidosis) and also carries a poor pregnancy prognosis.[10]

The Fetus

Glucose crosses the placenta freely, and a close correlation exists between fetal glucose uptake and maternal blood levels.[1] In diabetic parturients, maternal hyperglycemia leads to fetal hyperglycemia that, in turn, increases fetal insulin secretion and promotes macrosomia. Fetal hyperinsulinism also contributes to an increased risk of intrauterine fetal death, respiratory distress syndrome, neonatal hypoglycemia, and other neonatal morbidity (Table 17–3). When preeclampsia complicates diabetes, the perinatal mortality rate increases sharply, from 9 per 1000 live births for all diabetic pregnancies to 60 per 1000.[11]

TABLE 17–2
Maternal Complications of the Diabetic Pregnancy

- Pregnancy-induced hypertension (approximately twofold increase, even in the absence of vascular or renal disease)
- Increased maternal susceptibility to infection
- Diabetes-induced fetal macrosomia, with increased incidence of difficult deliveries, e.g., shoulder dystocia, and consequent maternal/fetal injury
- Polyhydramnios (when associated with fetal macrosomia, this may increase maternal cardiorespiratory embarrassment)
- Increased incidence of cesarean delivery
- Postpartum hemorrhage

TABLE 17–3
Fetal and Neonatal Consequences of Diabetes

Complication	Possible Causes
Intrauterine fetal death (stillbirth)	Reduced uteroplacental blood flow Maternal hyperinsulinemia Maternal ketosis (Preeclampsia)
Congenital anomalies	Type I IDDM Maternal hyperglycemia Maternal ketosis Maternal hypoglycemia
Neonatal respiratory distress syndrome	Impaired surfactant production Fetal hyperglycemia Fetal hyperinsulinemia
Neonatal electrolyte disturbances	
Hypocalcemia	Impaired neonatal synthesis of parathyroid hormone
Hypomagnesemia	?

Abbreviation: IDDM = insulin-dependent diabetes mellitus.

Data from Landon MB, Gabbe SG: Diabetes mellitus and pregnancy. Obstet Gynecol Clin North Am 19:633–654, 1992.

Other factors adversely affecting the fetus include maternal hypoglycemia and high maternal plasma ketone levels. Even relatively mild hypoglycemia can impair fetal cardiac function,[9] and some studies implicate ketosis in the cause of intrauterine growth retardation (IUGR) and possibly fetal anomalies.

Major congenital anomalies occur in 7.5 to 13% of pregnancies in women with pregestational diabetes who register for care after conception. This represents a sevenfold increase over that of infants of nondiabetic women.[12] Fetal malformations now account for 30 to 50% of diabetes-related perinatal deaths.[1]

The greatest risk for development of structural fetal defects appears to be before the seventh week following conception. Women with pregestational diabetes must register *in advance of conception* and be closely observed in the critical 1 to 2 months following conception for the risk of major anomalies to fall significantly. Improved blood glucose control appears to be a key factor in reducing the incidence of congenital malformations. Methods to assess glucose control include daily self-monitoring of blood glucose levels (SMBG) and laboratory measurement of plasma glycosylated hemoglobin (mainly hemoglobin A_{1C}). The latter gives an index of control (unfortunately retrospective) over the previous 1 to 2 months. Normal values range from 4 to 6%. (Many laboratories now use total glycohemoglobin level, i.e., A_1 [normal 5–7%], which includes the a, b, and c fractions.)

The Neonate

Neonates of diabetic mothers experience an increased incidence of respiratory distress syndrome (RDS), hypoglycemia, hypocalcemia, and hyperbilirubinemia. Before the detection of pulmonary surfactant became routine, most infants of diabetic mothers (IDMs), especially those delivered at or around 36 weeks' gestation, demonstrated RDS to a greater or lesser degree. Strict metabolic control of diabetes near to term, intensive antepartum surveillance, and measurement of the phosphatidylglycerol (PG) level in amniotic fluid have since appreciably reduced this incidence.[1, 9] The appearance of PG in the amniotic fluid, especially in amounts greater than 0.5%, reliably indicates maturity of fetal/neonatal pulmonary surfactant. Its measurement has replaced the formerly used lecithin-syringomyelin ratio.

OBSTETRIC MANAGEMENT OF THE DIABETIC PREGNANCY

General Principles

Evidence now clearly supports enrollment of women with pregestational diabetes, and those who developed GDM in a previous pregnancy, in preconception programs. Such programs try to ensure (1) patient education; (2) instruction in daily, multiple SMBG; (3) periconceptional and first trimester measurement of glycosylated hemoglobin levels; (4) adjustment of the insulin dose to achieve near-normal glycemia; and (5) regular clinic visits.[12] In this way, obstetricians have the best possibility of diminishing the incidence of diabetes-related fetal anomalies.

Since 90% of the women with diabetes that complicates pregnancy have GDM, universal screening, undertaken at 24 to 28 weeks' gestation, now represents the standard of obstetric care. The screening test involves ingestion of an oral 50-gm glucose load (Trutol), followed 1 hour later by estimation of the plasma glucose. Mothers with an abnormal test require a full glucose tolerance test to exclude diabetes.

The careful monitoring of maternal blood glucose levels throughout the third trimester (when the risk of sudden intrauterine death increases) represents the single most important therapeutic intervention in the management of pregnancies complicated by diabetes.[13] The preferred methods of glucose surveillance differ greatly among obstetricians. Some determine fasting glucose levels on a weekly basis, whereas others instruct patients to perform daily SMBG. Self-monitoring significantly reduces the need for hospitalization. The blood glucose thresholds at which to commence insulin therapy also vary among specialists. Most perinatologists recommend insulin when the average fasting glucose level reaches 105 ± 7.0 mg/dl and the 2-hour postprandial level reaches 140 ± 15 mg/dl.

With respect to fetal surveillance, most obstetricians favor nonstress tests (NST) in women with GDM, on a weekly or twice-weekly basis, beginning at 28 to 32 weeks' gestation. A nonreactive NST requires further fetal assessment, for example, a full biophysical profile. Many obstetricians also recommend fetal movement counting.

Ultrasound plays a major role in the antepartum surveillance of diabetic gravidae. A detailed study, at 18 to 20 weeks' gestation, should exclude neural tube defects and other congenital anomalies. Repeat examinations, at 4- to 6-week intervals, enable assessment of fetal growth and exclude macrosomia or IUGR.[1]

The majority of obstetricians favor elective delivery, by either induction of labor or cesarean section, when amniocentesis confirms fetal lung maturity. The cesarean section rate in pregnancies complicated by diabetes approaches 50% in many institutions.[13]

INSULIN MANAGEMENT

Although many types of insulin exist, most parturients now receive human insulin. All forms of human insulin are highly purified and contain 100 units/ml (U-100).[4] Three principal

TABLE 17–4
Commonly Used Insulins

Type	Peak and Duration (hr)		Species
Short-acting (regular)	2–4	6–8	Human and animal
Intermediate-acting	4–10	18–22	Human
NPH/Lente	6–12	20–24	Animal
Long-acting	8–16	24–26	Human
Ultralente	12–24	30–34	Animal

TABLE 17–6
Peripartum Insulin/Dextrose Regimes

Blood Sugar	Insulin	IV Fluid
<100 mg/dl (<5.5 mmol/L)	0.5 U/hr	D5/LR 150 ml/hr
100–145 mg/dl (5.5–8 mmol/L)	1 U/hr	D5/LR 125 ml/hr
145–180 mg/dl (8–10 mmol/L)	1.5 U/hr	D5/LR 100 ml/hr

Abbreviations: IV = intravenous; D5/LR = 5% dextrose in water/lactated Ringer's solution.

groups exist—short-acting (regular), intermediate, and long-acting (Table 17–4).

Four common insulin regimes exist (Table 17–5), and in a small number of women, treatment comprises either multiple-dose regimes or (rarely) continuous insulin infusion via subcutaneous pump (CSII).

The maintenance of a normal blood sugar level (80–100 mg/dl) largely determines healthy outcome. Patients who achieve good control in early pregnancy can usually be managed as outpatients, with frequent SMBG. Less-motivated gravidae, and those with poor control, need hospitalization in early pregnancy to establish good control. All patients with IDDM (and their family members) should receive instruction in the use of glucagon for treatment of severe hypoglycemia.

Peripartum Insulin Therapy

Insulin requirements in labor may fall dramatically, and some women require no insulin for several hours. Nonetheless, strict maternal glucose control during labor, or before cesarean section, remains crucial to avoid rebound neonatal hypoglycemia. An intravenous (IV) dextrose infusion, at a rate of 5 to 10 gm/hr, and a continuous insulin infusion at 1 to 2 units/hr (or less), are adjusted appropriately (Table 17–6). Blood glucose levels should be monitored hourly using Chemstrip estimation, as well as serial blood glucose monitoring via a heparin lock. The goal should be to maintain the glucose level at 60 to 100 mg/dl. In the author's institution, the insulin is stopped at the time of delivery, but an infusion of 5% dextrose in wa-

TABLE 17–5
Common Insulin Regimes in Diabetic Pregnancies

A.M.	P.M.	Comments
1. Single injection: intermediate insulin		Peak effect in afternoon; A.M. fasting glucose (prebreakfast) reflects effectiveness of control
2. Single injection: short-acting, plus intermediate insulin		Short-acting controls A.M. glucose level, until intermediate reaches peak
3. Regular, plus intermediate prebreakfast	Intermediate insulin before evening meal, or at bedtime	Benefits women who develop afternoon hypoglycemia on regime #1, but have poor prebreakfast control
4. Regular, plus intermediate	Regular plus intermediate	Presupper regular insulin controls postsupper and bedtime glucose levels; intermediate P.M. component may cause nocturnal hypoglycemia

ter (D5/W), or 5% dextrose in lactated Ringer's solution (D5/W/RL), is maintained at a rate of 100 to 125 ml/hr, while blood glucose levels are monitored, every 1 to 2 hours in the first instance.

Patients with GDM, not receiving insulin, also require a glucose infusion in labor, along the lines previously described.

If a woman goes into spontaneous labor after taking her normal morning or evening dose of insulin, particular attention must be paid to the maintenance of euglycemia during labor, adjusting the dextrose infusion appropriately to ensure effective control.

Avoiding Hypoglycemia

Many diabetic mothers undergo elective cesarean delivery. The procedure should be scheduled early, to avoid a protracted fast. Although maintenance of a normal predelivery blood glucose level is a key requirement, anesthesiologists must remember that insulin requirements fall immediately postpartum following the delivery of the placenta, most likely the result of decreased production of contrainsulin hormones. Women then become *very sensitive* to insulin. Any preoperative insulin doses must be small, and sufficiently short-acting, to avoid the possibility of postdelivery hypoglycemia. *If in doubt, omit the dose!*

During the postpartum period, in women with IDDM, insulin requirements rarely exceed 50% of the dose required in the last weeks of pregnancy.

Diabetic Ketoacidosis in Pregnancy: A Major Emergency

Among all patients with diabetes, diabetic ketoacidosis (DKA) remains one of the most serious complications, which if misdiagnosed, untreated, or undertreated, carries a high mortality.[9, 14–16] Earlier reviews suggested an incidence of DKA approximating 10% in pregnancy, and perinatal mortality rates were estimated to vary from 30 to more than 50%. More recent publications report lower perinatal mortality rates, but DKA still occurs, almost always in Type I IDDM, and represents a major obstetric emergency.[15] Precipitating events include infection (especially pyelonephritis), the use of β agonists in the management of preterm labor, missed insulin doses, and insulin pump failure.

Two major metabolic derangements characterize DKA:

1. Alteration in the production and utilization of glucose, which leads to hyperglycemia, with resultant osmotic diuresis, volume depletion, and dehydration.
2. Accelerated ketogenesis and increased fat breakdown, which results in metabolic acidosis.

In pregnancy, it is particularly important to differentiate starvation ketosis ("accelerated starvation") from DKA.[16] Remember that blood ketone levels two to three times the nonpregnant value can occur normally. If low or normal blood glucose levels accompany the ketosis, this suggests starvation ketosis. However, to further confuse the issue, DKA in pregnancy may occur at plasma glucose levels lower than in the nonpregnant state. Thus, it becomes essential to obtain a careful history and to determine whether infection, cessation of insulin therapy, or severe metabolic stress precipitated the patient's deterioration.

Anesthesiologists may be called on to institute supportive measures (e.g., IV lines and arterial lines) or to provide airway control in unconscious diabetic parturients and must have a clear understanding of the pathogenesis and immediate treatment of DKA if the patient is to receive the best possible care.

Clinical Presentation of Diabetic Ketoacidosis

Classically, subjects with DKA present with vomiting, thirst, polyuria, dehydration, disturbed consciousness, and air hunger (Kussmaul respirations). On physical examination, they may demonstrate tachycardia, and up to 20% of them later show frank hypotension. Laboratory findings reveal elevated plasma glucose levels, which may range from nearly normal to very extreme. Plasma osmolality normally exceeds 340 mOsm/L in subjects with coma. Blood pH is less than 7.3, and even lower in comatose individuals. Serum sodium may be low, normal, or high, although total body sodium is always low because of the diuresis. Plasma potassium concentrations may be low, normal, or elevated but usually increase initially as a result of the metabolic acidosis, which dis-

TABLE 17–7
Management of Diabetic Ketoacidosis

Treatment	Monitoring
Insulin	
Administer 10 U/hr regular insulin, IV; decrease only when ketoacidosis reversed or blood glucose level decreases to 200–250 mg/dl (11–14 mmol/L)	Blood glucose Arterial blood gases Serum and urinary ketones Serum electrolytes
Administer "supportive" glucose infusion to avoid hypoglycemia, if insulin still required; switch to intermediate-acting insulin (e.g., NPH) after 24–36 hr	
Fluids	
Administer 0.9% NaCl, 1 L/hr (severely hypovolemic parturients may need 2–3 L initially); substitute 0.45% NaCl in hypernatremia and when vital signs return to normal	Urine output Serum Na^+, K^+, Cl^-, HCO_3^-, PO_4^{2-}, q 1–2 hr initially Blood urea nitrogen, creatinine
Use lactated Ringer's in hyperchloremia	Central line, if no improvement within 1–2 hr
Electrolytes	
Potassium: 20–40 mmol/h; start after 2–4 hr	Serum K^+, electrocardiogram
Sodium: See NaCl regimen above	
Phosphate: Adminster 40–60 mmol potassium phosphate, only if serum phosphate level is low	Serum Na^+, plasma osmolality Serum PO_4^{2-}

places potassium from within the cells. Subsequently, a significant fall in total body potassium occurs, owing to potassium loss through the urine and gastrointestinal tract. Potassium administration should be commenced only after insulin is started (Table 17–7). Plasma bicarbonate levels fall below 15 mEq/L in DKA, and serum ketones exceed 7 mmol/L.[14]

Treatment of Diabetic Ketoacidosis
(see Table 17–7)

The major cause of death in DKA is failure to treat the hyperosmolar state, which accompanies diabetic coma, and fluid administration represents a priority in the immediate management. The fluid deficit may range from 4 to 10 L, and adequate fluid replacement requires that approximately 50% of this deficit be replaced in the first 5 hours.[14] In the first 2 hours, 0.9% sodium chloride (NaCl) should be given at a rate of 1 L/hr, while urine output and clinical response are carefully monitored. More severely hypovolemic parturients may need 2 to 3 L of 0.9% NaCl, in the first hour. When the patient has a normal blood pressure, or if plasma sodium exceeds 145 mmol/L, normal saline should be replaced with 0.45% NaCl.

Fluid administration enhances glucose excretion, by causing a diuresis, and decreases the levels of counterregulatory hormones that stimulate hyperglycemia.

Potassium Replacement

The total body potassium deficit in DKA approximates 3 to 5 mmol/kg body weight, but it may reach 10 mmol/kg. After the initially high plasma levels decline, patients require potassium, but replacement should not be commenced until after insulin is started, to avoid producing hyperkalemia. Some physicians prefer to delay potassium administration until 2 to 4 hours after starting insulin therapy. The initial administration rate should not exceed 20 to 40 mmol/hr, with monitoring of serum potassium levels, every 1–2 hr, and continuous electrocardiogram (ECG) monitoring.

Phosphate and Bicarbonate Replacement

Although phosphate depletion in DKA can be severe, with an average deficit of 0.5 to 1.5 mmol/kg, there is little evidence that phosphate administration improves clinical outcome. Replacement is normally considered only if the serum phosphate is very low.[14] Controlled studies have demonstrated that bicarbonate administration does not influence ultimate outcome in DKA and may prove harmful. Because of its hyperosmolality, it should not be administered to comatose subjects. Small doses (e.g., 44 mmol) may be given to noncomatose individuals, if the serum pH is less than 7.

Insulin Therapy

Although insulin therapy is less critical than the initial fluid replacement in hyperosmolar subjects, insulin nonetheless remains key to the successful management of DKA. Insulin lowers the plasma glucagon level, counteracts glucagon's effects on the liver, and inhibits the flow of fatty and amino acids from the periphery. It also enhances glucose uptake and usage by the cells. Traditionally, patients with DKA received large insulin doses (up to 50–100 units every 1–2 hr), but since the 1980s, physicians have favored low-dose regimens. However, there is some concern about development of insulin resistance with low-dose schedules, and some authorities still commence with an initial bolus of approximately 30 units of regular insulin, followed by a continuous drip at a rate of 2 to 5 units/hr. Others recommend schedules with more cautious initial doses (e.g., 10 units, followed by an infusion rate of 5–10 units/hr). Regardless of schedule, if ketone levels do not fall, or pH does not increase within 3 to 4 hours of starting therapy, the patient requires larger insulin doses without delay.

When the plasma glucose level declines to 200 to 250 mg/dl, the insulin dose should be reduced and a "supportive" glucose infusion instituted to avoid hypoglycemia. The insulin infusion is normally reduced to 1 to 2 units/hr, to maintain blood glucose in the range of 80 to 120 mg/dl, until the patient reverts to her normal therapy.

Complications of Diabetic Ketoacidosis

Shock

Vascular collapse in DKA usually responds to the initial treatment with fluids and electrolytes, but in the absence of a prompt response, the possibility of gram-negative septicemia, or even silent myocardial infarction, should be considered.

Infection

Pyelonephritis, pneumonia, septicemia, and chorioamnionitis constitute the most common causes of infection, and these should be excluded as possibilities in every pregnant woman with DKA.

Vascular Thrombosis

Features such as dehydration, hypovolemia, low cardiac output, and increased blood viscosity predispose DKA subjects to vascular thrombosis. In addition, certain hemostatic changes favoring thrombosis, such as increased Factor VIII activity and Factor VIIIRAg, also occur. The well-documented hypercoagulability that accompanies pregnancy may worsen this situation.

Fetal Consequences of DKA

In all cases of DKA, continuous fetal monitoring should be undertaken during the mother's treatment. Fetal heart rate patterns consistent with fetal distress have been reported. They may be expected to resolve with effective management of the DKA, and cesarean section for fetal distress should not prove necessary.

ANESTHETIC CONSIDERATIONS IN DIABETIC PARTURIENTS

Predelivery Assessment of the Diabetic: A Multisystem Review

Although the improved management of diabetes has led to a significant decline in perinatal mortality, the likelihood of maternal complications increases with increasing severity of the disease. In Class C, and those with end-organ damage, obstetricians anticipate an increased complication rate, for example, premature labor, pregnancy-induced hypertension, and fetal macrosomia, all of which predict a higher cesarean section rate.

Ideally, anesthesiologists should assess the severity of diabetes, review the parturient's insulin dose and degree of glucose control, identify diabetes-related complications (e.g., nephropathy and peripheral neuropathy), and determine fetal status, *when the patient is admitted to the labor floor.* In women with more severe diabetes, anesthesiologists also should anticipate an increased incidence of complications, such as poor intrapartum glucose control, maternal hypotension following regional block, and fetal distress.

During preoperative assessment, the anesthesiologist must determine the degree of end-organ damage, which generally relates to the duration of the diabetes, and its severity. The well-known complications of diabetes result from involvement of large and small vessels, mainly in the following organ systems:

1. *Cardiovascular*—for example, hypertension, ischemic heart disease, peripheral vascular disease, and (rarely) cardiomyopathy.
2. *Renal*—for example, diabetic nephropathy, ultimately leading to renal failure.
3. *Nervous*—for example, peripheral and autonomic neuropathies.
4. *Eyes*—for example, diabetic retinopathy and cataract.

In the cardiovascular system, first exclude preexistent hypertension. If present, is this well controlled? Is the parturient taking antihypertensive medications? (If yes, when was her last dose?) What are the implications of her current therapy for regional or general anesthesia? Is the diabetes complicated by pregnancy-induced hypertension? (If so, assess its severity. Does the patient require magnesium sulfate [$MgSO_4$], or other perioperative steps to control hypertension, especially if the obstetricians plan cesarean section?)

Class H diabetes occurs in only a small number of women, although those with long-standing IDDM, of juvenile onset, may have evidence of coronary artery disease, even at the age of 25 to 30 years. When present, ischemic heart disease places the patient at greatly increased risk of morbidity/mortality during pregnancy. This applies particularly to the few women with a history of previous myocardial infarction, in whom mortality rates are estimated to exceed 50%.[1] If clinical assessment during pregnancy suggests any myocardial involvement, the parturient should have a full cardiovascular work-up before her anticipated delivery.

Diabetic nephropathy constitutes a well-recognized complication of severe diabetes, and anesthesiologists must pay particular attention to assessment of renal function in patients with Class F disease. Factors that predict poor perinatal outcome include proteinuria at or above 3 gm/24 hr, serum creatinine at or above 1.5 mg/dl, anemia (hematocrit $< 25\%$), and hypertension (mean arterial pressure > 107 mmHg).[1] These women have an increased risk of perioperative renal failure and require careful fluid management during labor and vigilant postpartum assessment. They should receive appropriate antibiotic prophylaxis because urinary stasis and the resultant sepsis increase the perioperative risk of acute renal failure.

The anesthesiologist must also assess all diabetic parturients for the possibility of cardiac autonomic neuropathy (CAN). (Symptoms such as orthostatic hypotension may suggest the diagnosis.) CAN is a well-recognized and serious complication, which does not correlate with maternal age, severity, or duration of the diabetes, that affects 20 to 40% of diabetics and causes degeneration of the afferent and efferent components of sympathetic/parasympathetic innervation to the heart and peripheral vessels. Nonpregnant diabetic patients with CAN have been noted to experience a greater decline in heart rate and arterial pressure following induction of general anesthesia compared with control subjects.[17] A smaller increase in these parameters occurred after tracheal intubation. Obstetric anesthesiologists should therefore be on the lookout for hypotension in these individuals, especially during regional anesthesia. Monitor blood pressure more frequently than usual, and remember that these patients are more likely to require intraoperative vasopressor therapy.

The existence of any peripheral neuropathy mandates particularly careful preoperative evaluation. The anesthesiologist must fully document its extent on the preoperative record, especially when planning regional anesthesia. Bromage[18] found variable increases in epidural segmental spread (ranging from 0 to 42% greater than that in nondiabetic patients) and related the increased spread to possible microangiopathy. Anesthesiologists should, therefore, anticipate unexpectedly extensive spread of epidural anesthesia in parturients with more severe IDDM, although careful fractionation of local anesthetic doses should avoid unnecessarily high block levels.

Because of autonomic dysfunction, diabetic

parturients may experience poor gastric emptying (diabetes-induced gastroparesis). The delayed gastric emptying of pregnancy, coupled with this complication, may place diabetic parturients at even greater risk of regurgitation and subsequent pulmonary aspiration.

From the anesthesiologist's viewpoint, the presence of retinopathy has little bearing on the choice of anesthetic technique. It should, however, be viewed as a marker of severe disease, and anesthesiologists should not overlook the possibility of severe visual impairment in these women.

"Stiff joint" syndrome, which occurs in approximately one of four adolescents with IDDM, represents an interesting complication of diabetes, of particular interest to anesthesiologists. Other features that may suggest this condition include rapidly progressive microangiopathy, short stature, tight waxy skin, and finger joint contractures, which lead to an inability to approximate the palmar surfaces of the phalangeal joints ("prayer sign") (Fig. 17–1).[19] Importantly, these women may have fixation of the atlanto-occipital joint, with limitation of head extension, and tracheal intubation may prove difficult or impossible.

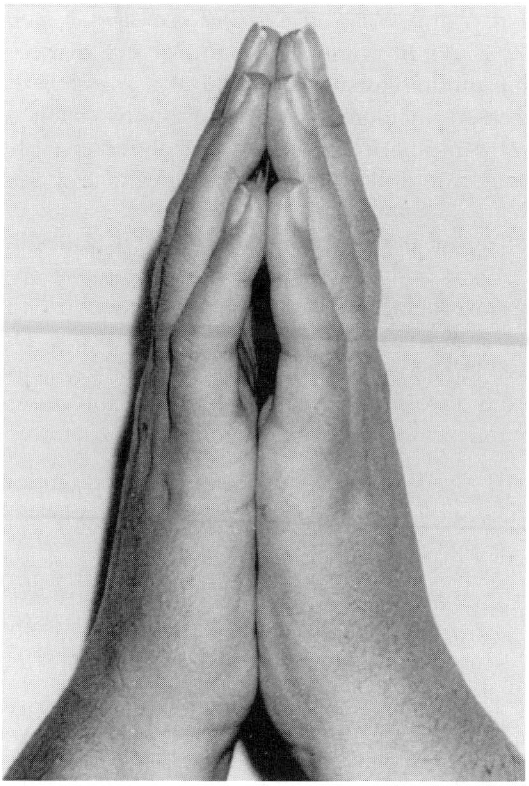

Figure 17–1. The "prayer" sign. (From Reissell E, Orko R, Maunuksela E-L, et al: Predictability of difficult laryngoscopy in patients with long-term diabetes mellitus. Anaesthesia 45:1024–1027, 1990.)

In nondiabetic subjects, the physiologic response to hypoglycemia involves enhanced secretion of glucagon, epinephrine, and cortisol. In IDDM, this response is frequently defective. Almost all Type I diabetics have deficient glucagon secretion in response to hypoglycemia after 5 years of disease, and approximately 40% of IDDM patients also have deficient epinephrine secretion because of adrenergic neuropathy. As a result, *some diabetics, when they experience hypoglycemia—for example, after the overnight fast before cesarean section—may have no symptoms.* The prolonged fasting of Type I IDDM patients must therefore be avoided by establishing a "background" infusion of D5W (e.g., 125 ml/hr), ensuring regular Chemstrip measurements, and placing severe diabetics in the first operating slot on the morning list. The administration of β blockers (e.g., propranolol) must particularly be avoided, as they can lead to further impairment of epinephrine secretion.

ANESTHETIC MANAGEMENT OF THE PREGNANT DIABETIC PATIENT

Five principles underlie the anesthesiologist's management of the diabetic parturient: (1) careful preoperative assessment of the patient's diabetic status and any associated complications; (2) rigid control of the *intrapartum* blood glucose level; (3) administration of a crystalloid (non–dextrose-containing) preload before regional anesthesia; (4) prevention and prompt treatment of hypotension; and (5) minimizing maternal stress.

Three further points deserve consideration for all diabetic parturients.[20] First, placental abnormalities may exist in the diabetic pregnancy and can significantly impair uteroplacental blood flow. Second, oxygen release at tissue level, and the placental interface, may be adversely affected. Third, IDMs have a reduced ability to handle an acid load and demonstrate an increased affinity of hemoglobin for oxygen. In consequence, they are more susceptible to intrapartum asphyxia.

Anesthesiologists must therefore be less tolerant of hypotension in diabetic patients than in normal subjects. These considerations also accent the hazards of impaired oxygen delivery at the placental interface in diabetic women. If oxygen delivery becomes compromised, for example, by hypotension or during a difficult attempted tracheal intubation, the diabetic mother, and especially her infant, may suffer severe hypoxemia. Anesthesiologists must be cognizant of these risks and be especially alert to changes that might affect maternal and fetal oxygen delivery.

Intrapartum Glucose Control: Aim for Euglycemia, Avoid Hypoglycemia

In the author's institution, patients with IDDM have team care throughout the intrapartum and postpartum periods. In general, the responsibility for monitoring insulin and glucose infusions rests with the obstetrician or diabetologist. Whenever anesthesiologists become involved in the care of diabetic parturients, they accept a responsibility to undertake regular Chemstrip estimation of blood glucose levels to avoid serious maternal hyperglycemia or hypoglycemia.

Ramanathan and colleagues[21] studied maternal and neonatal acid-base status and glucose metabolism in 20 women with IDDM who underwent elective cesarean section utilizing epidural anesthesia and compared them with non-diabetic patients also utilizing epidural anesthesia. All diabetics received their usual insulin therapy until the night before surgery. On the day of surgery, they received a glucose/insulin infusion, beginning at 6 A.M. (glucose 70 mg/kg body weight/hr; insulin 1 unit/hr). A nurse measured maternal blood glucose every 30 minutes (Chemstrip plus a reflectance glucometer) and adjusted the maternal insulin infusion to maintain capillary blood glucose between 70 and 120 mg/dl. In the control arm of the study, 30 healthy women received either 800 ml lactated Ringer's solution, plus 400 ml D5W over the 1 hour before induction of anesthesia (nondiabetic hyperglycemic controls) or 1200 ml lactated Ringer's solution (euglycemic controls). The authors found no significant difference among the three groups with respect to maternal and neonatal acid-base status or Apgar scores. However, neonatal umbilical vein glucose was significantly elevated in the diabetics and in the hyperglycemic controls, confirming the relationship between neonatal and maternal glucose levels. Seven of the 20 IDMs, but none of the control babies, subsequently developed neonatal hypoglycemia (<30 mg/dl). Thus, although the authors' insulin regime, plus epidural anesthesia for cesarean section, did not adversely affect neonatal status, it did not prevent the neonatal hypoglycemia that characterizes IDMs. The *practical* consequences of this study, with respect to insulin therapy, may seem puzzling to occasional obstetric anesthesiologists. These diabetic mothers received glucose/insulin therapy, and bolus injections, carefully adjusted to maintain near-normal capillary glucose levels. Despite this closely monitored regime, some infants developed neonatal hypoglycemia. These findings imply that anesthesiologists must accept, as inevitable, the occurrence of neonatal hypoglycemia in some IDMs. All IDMs therefore need careful observation and monitoring in the first 2 to 4 hours of life to exclude hypoglycemia. An attempt should be made to maintain near-normal maternal glucose levels (the type of regime advocated by Ramanathan and colleagues[21] represents one example), but *vigorous attempts to maintain maternal euglycemia must be avoided* because of the enhanced sensitivity to insulin that occurs immediately postpartum. Whether epidural or spinal anesthesia is given is probably of no consequence with respect to neonatal status.

The Preload: Omit Dextrose!

In the late 1970s, Datta and Brown[22] undertook comparative studies of the effects of general or spinal anesthesia for cesarean section in normal and diabetic women. They demonstrated that IDMs who received spinal anesthesia became more acidotic than IDMs whose mothers were undergoing general anesthesia. The extent of acidosis varied with the severity of the diabetes, the most acidotic infants being born to the severe diabetics. The lowest pH and base excess values occurred in infants whose mothers became hypotensive before delivery. Although the incidence of spinal hypotension in the normal controls (53%) actually exceeded that in the diabetic mothers (40%), neonatal depression occurred with much greater frequency in the diabetic group (53% vs. 0% in the healthy group). In short, in this study, hypotension, resulting from spinal anesthesia, had a significant adverse effect on the neonatal status of IDMs.

Datta and Brown[22] explained their findings by hypothesizing that spinal hypotension decreased uteroplacental blood flow and led to fetal compromise, probably as a result of the aforementioned placental abnormalities that occur in diabetes.

In a later study of diabetic women undergoing *epidural* anesthesia for cesarean section, Datta and associates[23] categorized neonates into two groups, based on the umbilical artery pH at birth. The acidotic infants, with a pH less than or equal to 7.2, were delivered from mothers with more severe diabetes, 50% of whom experienced significant predelivery hypotension after the induction of anesthesia.[23]

As a result of this work, many anesthesiologists preferred general anesthesia to spinal anesthesia for cesarean section for diabetic women, even though 40% of IDMs whose mothers received general anesthesia demonstrated neonatal depression (Apgar score <7 at 1 min) compared with 13% of neonates from healthy mothers.

In both of these studies, all mothers received a preload of D5/LR before anesthesia. The authors could not exclude the possibility that the dextrose-containing preload influenced neonatal status. In a third and definitive study, they therefore reevaluated acid-base data in 10 IDDM mothers and 10 healthy controls having spinal anesthesia for elective cesarean section at term, all of whom received dextrose-free solutions for volume expansion before induction of anesthesia.[24] The women received IV ephedrine boluses, 5 to 10 mg immediately, if they developed hypotension. The investigators found no significant difference in acid-base values between the diabetic group infants and the control group infants, and Apgar scores were similar in both groups. *They concluded that strict control of maternal diabetes (preoperative fasting glucose levels were 86 ± 4 mg/dl), prompt treatment of any maternal hypotension, and a crystalloid preload would maintain neonatal acid-base status.* (The author continues to follow these recommendations, but substitutes an ephedrine infusion, 50 mg/L, for intermittent bolus administration.)

Interestingly, Ammon[25] considers lactated Ringer's solution an inappropriate fluid and volume replacement in diabetics because it contains 28 mmol/L of lactate, a gluconeogenic substrate. He instead suggests 0.9% NaCl or Isolyte for maintenance therapy and third space replacement. To date, no prospective studies have compared NaCl with lactated Ringer's in diabetic parturients undergoing cesarean section, and obstetric anesthesiologists should consider the potentially adverse effects of an excessive sodium load, especially in women with pregnancy-induced hypertension. In the author's view, lactated Ringer's remains the standard in obstetric anesthesia until alternative evidence becomes available.

Maternal Stress

Diabetes increases maternal stress during pregnancy, and measures of psychological stress correlate highly with increased levels of blood glucose.[26] In addition to psychological stress, diabetic parturients may have the superimposed physical stresses of labor or cesarean section, which precipitate neuroendocrine responses, including excess production of growth hormone, adrenocorticotropic hormone, and glucocorticoids. Evidence from nondiabetic parturients with pregnancy-induced hypertension demonstrates that regional anesthesia, in contrast to general anesthesia, attenuates neuroendocrine stress responses, thus reinforcing the benefits of regional anesthesia.[27]

ANESTHESIA/ANALGESIA FOR THE DIABETIC PARTURIENT

Anesthesiologists may expect to care for pregnant diabetic women in a variety of situations, including premature labor; uncomplicated labor at term; complicating obstetric disorders (e.g., pregnancy-induced hypertension); and emergency or elective anesthesia for cesarean section. Less frequently, diabetics may require anesthesia for intercurrent surgery during pregnancy.

Analgesia for Labor and Delivery

Labor

Systemic narcotics (e.g., meperidine 25–50 mg IV; 100–125 mg IM) are an acceptable first-line pain therapy for women with GDM, who do not require insulin and have no apparent fetal compromise or other complicating features.

The advantages of narcotics include simplicity of administration and minimal requirements for patient monitoring. The main disadvantages include inadequate pain relief, frequent clouding of the mother's sensorium, and possible newborn depression. In addition, when administered intravenously, drugs such as meperidine increase the incidence of nausea and vomiting.

For all women with Type I IDDM, and those with more severe (insulin-dependent) GDM, the author recommends early epidural analgesia, in preference to systemic medication. The technique best achieves the aim of a stress-free labor in diabetic parturients. The mother gains improved pain relief and stable circulatory parameters (if the block is appropriately titrated) and will have lower plasma levels of maternal catecholamines and stress-related hormones. The extent of sensory blockade can readily be extended should cesarean section be required. From the fetal viewpoint, the advantages of regional analgesia include a lower incidence of drug depression and improved Apgar scores at delivery.

Before initiating regional block, carefully assess the parturient for the presence of any predelivery complications. In particular, determine the adequacy of blood glucose control, carefully assess the airway (to exclude the possibility of stiff joint syndrome), confirm the adequacy of renal function, and document or exclude peripheral neuropathy. After the baseline vital signs have been recorded, the author infuses lactated Ringer's, approximately 10 ml/kg, before instituting analgesia, to reduce the likelihood of maternal hypotension.

The author prefers to use 10 ml bupivacaine 0.125% containing 100 μg of fentanyl to establish the labor block. In more severe diabetics, great emphasis is placed on careful titration of the block with fractionated boluses of local anesthetics as the block develops. The fetal heart rate should be monitored continuously as the block develops during its establishment. Any decrease in systolic pressure should be treated immediately with an additional bolus of lactated Ringer's. Ephedrine rarely proves necessary during labor analgesia. The author's group prefers to maintain analgesia with a continuous bupivacaine infusion (0.0625–0.125%, plus fentanyl 2 μg/ml), commencing at 10 ml/hr. Patient-controlled epidural analgesia (PCEA) may be preferred by motivated parturients. We use 0.08-0.1% bupivacaine, plus fentanyl 2 mg/ml, with a bolus dose of 5 ml, and a lockout interval of 10 minutes.

Delivery

Because diabetic mothers belong to a high-risk category, obstetricians generally avoid a prolonged second stage of labor, since fetal pH deteriorates progressively with increased duration of second stage labor and maternal pushing. (Vigorous maternal efforts must especially be avoided in those few women with proliferative retinopathy, to reduce the risk of vitreous hemorrhage.)

Most obstetricians recommend continuous fetal heart rate monitoring to detect possible fetal distress. Inadequate fetal descent during the second stage of labor, fetal distress, and fetal acidosis may necessitate instrumental or cesarean delivery.

Before a mid forceps or trial of forceps procedure, we usually prefer to augment preexistent epidural blockade with pH-adjusted bupivacaine 0.5% or lidocaine 2% (plus epinephrine 1:200,000). The patient receives an additional preload of lactated Ringer's 8 to 10 ml/kg, depending on the state of her fluid balance and the volume infused during labor. Some anesthesiologists empirically avoid epinephrine-containing local anesthetics, especially in patients with severe IDDM, fearing these agents may promote hyperglycemia. No evidence exists to support the view, and diabetes does not represent an absolute contraindication to epinephrine-containing agents.

Continuous-infusion techniques usually provide adequate anesthesia for low forceps or spontaneous delivery, although it may occasionally be necessary to augment the block with bupivacaine 0.25% or 2-chloroprocaine 2 to 3%.

Occasionally, the anesthesiologist may be asked to initiate a block for mid forceps delivery or trial of forceps procedure in a diabetic parturient who has no preexisting anesthesia. If blood glucose is rigidly controlled, crystalloid solutions infused for volume preload, and maternal hypotension treated aggressively to avoid pressures below 100 mmHg, the author favors spinal anesthesia because of its rapid onset and superior pain relief compared with epidural anesthesia. In addition to a crystalloid preload approximating 1 L, the author uses an ephedrine infusion (50 mg/L) or intermittent bolus administration (5–10 mg) to minimize hypotension. Epidural anesthesia, with 2% pH-adjusted lidocaine plus epinephrine or 2-chloroprocaine 3% represents an acceptable alternative to subarachnoid block, if time permits.

Because fetal macrosomia may complicate pregnancy, especially in Type I IDDM parturients, shoulder dystocia may occur during vaginal delivery. A profound sensory and motor block is desirable for forceps delivery in an effort to provide good relaxation of the pelvic floor and lower birth canal.

Even in the presence of moderate to severe fetal distress, the author favors subarachnoid block over general anesthesia. (General anesthesia presents a significant hazard in pregnancy, and the possibility of diabetic gastroparesis compounds this hazard in women with severe IDDM.) After institution of the block, the blood pressure is measured at frequent intervals, for example, 3 to 5 minutes, ideally on the arm opposite to that which holds the IV line. Again, the author employs a prophylactic ephedrine infusion to reduce the likelihood of hypotension and does not hesitate to use additional ephedrine boluses, 5 to 10 mg, if necessary.

Regarding insulin therapy, laboring parturients have an IV dextrose infusion in situ (e.g., D5W at 100–125 ml/hr) in addition to their crystalloid maintenance line. The obstetrician or diabetologist will normally ensure the patient has a continuous insulin infusion, adjusted to a rate sufficient to maintain blood glucose at 60 to 100 mg/dl. A recent Chemstrip estimation should be available to the anesthesiologist before anesthesia. In the event blood glucose is less than 60 mg/dl, stop the insulin immediately and adjust the dextrose infusion as necessary.

Anesthesia for Cesarean Section

Elective

Despite improvements in fetal monitoring and the metabolic management of diabetes, many obstetricians still prefer to deliver IDDM parturients by elective cesarean section, which has the following advantages:

1. Delivery can be planned early in the day, avoiding the need for preoperative insulin therapy.

2. An elective procedure avoids the risks inherent in labor and vaginal delivery, notably fetal distress and shoulder dystocia owing to fetal macrosomia.

3. Planned delivery generally ensures the availability of a staff neonatologist. Since the infant requires admission to a special neonatal care unit, initial care can then be undertaken in daytime hours.

4. In those women at increased risk (e.g., having had a previous third trimester stillbirth, fetal macrosomia greater than 4000 gm, and poor diabetic control), elective cesarean section at 37 to 38 weeks' gestation (with prior confirmation of fetal lung maturity) reduces the likelihood of perinatal loss.

5. The anesthesiologist has the opportunity to make a careful preoperative assessment, review the management and severity of the maternal diabetes, and determine any possible fetal effects.

The Benefits of Regional Anesthesia

After the careful preoperative review, the author notes the complications and documents the extent of any peripheral neuropathy. (If present, it does not contraindicate regional anesthesia, but it does call for careful preoperative evaluation and postoperative review to demonstrate that no progression has occurred. As well, the presence of peripheral neuropathy may point to involvement of autonomic nerves, especially in the cardiovascular system.) After reviewing the choice of anesthetic techniques with the patient, we emphasize the advantages of regional anesthesia, either epidural or subarachnoid block. The former technique is considered preferable in severe diabetics with significant end-organ disease because of the greater incidence of hypotension that usually characterizes spinal anesthesia.

Since the patient usually has nothing by mouth from midnight on the evening before surgery, she requires some modification of her insulin regime. One common practice involves administration of the normal NPH evening dose on the preoperative day, plus a small morning dose (one quarter to one half the normal *prepregnancy* dose) on the operative day. (The author's group dislikes this regime because of the hypoglycemia risk; in the author's institution no preoperative insulin is given.) The goal of preparation should be to ensure preoperative glucose control, while avoiding the occurrence of postdelivery hypoglycemia. An IV line (D5W, approximately 100–150 ml/hr) should be established on the evening before to avoid the possibility of early morning hypoglycemia. (In some institutions, physicians allow diabetics to eat until 4 A.M. on the operative day to avoid hypoglycemia.)[21] On the operative day, diabetic parturients should be scheduled at the beginning of the day.

Because of the possibility of diabetic gastroparesis and the impaired gastric emptying of pregnancy, patients should receive ranitidine 150 mg by mouth on the evening before surgery (10 P.M.) and 150 mg by mouth 2 hours preoperatively. These doses can be doubled in women with marked reflux. When parturients insist on a general anesthetic (despite vigorous persuasion to the contrary), 0.3 M sodium citrate, 30 ml, is given in the operating room immediately before induction of anesthesia. A gastric prokinetic (e.g., metoclopramide 10 mg IV 30–60 min preoperatively) is also prescribed.

The D5W infusion must be in place when the mother arrives in the operating room, whether it is established 2 hours preoperatively or the evening before. The anesthesiologist should take blood for immediate laboratory estimation of blood glucose. (The author normally performs a Chemstrip estimation, in addition.) A second IV line should be inserted to administer the crystalloid preload (approximately 15 ml/kg).

After establishing the appropriate monitors—electrocardiogram, automatic blood pressure, pulse oximeter—for those patients having epidural anesthesia the author performs the block with the patient in the left lateral position, unless technical difficulties, such as obesity, are anticipated. We prefer to use pH-adjusted bupivacaine 0.5% and titrate the block slowly to minimize hypotension, while infusing additional lactated Ringer's, as necessary.

As the block progresses, the patient assumes the supine position, with the table tilted appropriately into a 15-degree right or left lateral tilt. To ensure stable circulatory parameters, the patient receives an ephedrine infusion 50 mg/L, as previously described, and oxygen, 6 to 8 L/min, via a facemask throughout the procedure and until completion of uterine closure.

When performing spinal anesthesia for cesarean section, the author administers a similar preload immediately before induction of anesthesia and establishes an IV ephedrine infusion. The block is again performed with the patient in the left lateral position, using a pencil-point needle (e.g., Sprotte 24-gauge, Whitacre 25- to 27-gauge), and hyperbaric bupivacaine 0.75% 1.6 to 1.8 ml is administered. (Additionally, patients receive intrathecal fentanyl 12.5–25 μg and preservative-free morphine 0.25–0.3 mg for postoperative analgesia.) As the block level rises, one needs to ensure the maximal rate of ephedrine infusion, or give frequent boluses, to avoid hypotension. Datta and coworkers[24] monitor blood pressure at 30-second intervals for the first 15 minutes, then every 3 minutes thereafter. The author's group considers this an overly intensive regime but agrees that measurement intervals should not exceed 3 minutes for the first 10 to 15 minutes of block. Usually, blood pressure readings stabilize at this point, although any persistent instability may suggest autonomic neuropathy.

General Anesthesia

In the unlikely event that diabetic parturients request general anesthesia (or when emergency situations contraindicate a regional technique), the author's group meticulously assesses the airway, especially in Type I IDDM. The author follows his normal practice of rapid sequence induction with thiopental 4 mg/kg and succinylcholine 1.5 mg/kg. Preoxygenation may be undertaken by the rapid three to four deep breaths technique or for the preoperative 3 to 5 minutes. An assistant maintains cricoid pressure until the endotracheal tube has been inserted and the airway secured. The fractional inspired oxygen approximates 50% through delivery to ensure fetal oxygenation. No single volatile agent has obvious advantages over the others; in these parturients, the author's group gives enflurane 1 to 1.5% or isoflurane 1%.

Following delivery, intraoperative analgesia should be maintained with IV narcotic (e.g., morphine 10 mg or fentanyl 100 μg), and the patient must be extubated only when fully awake and positioned on her left side in the operating room.

Other Measures

The author's group monitors glucose control by immediate preoperative blood sugar estimation and Chemstrip estimation *immediately following delivery*. Beware of maternal hypoglycemia, as insulin requirements fall rapidly!

In view of the increased infection risk in diabetics, IV antibiotics should also be administered immediately following delivery, according to the obstetrician's wishes.

Parturients with severe IDDM, and those with significant end-organ disease, require close observation in a high-dependency nursing care area or a high-risk perinatal unit for the 24 hours immediately following cesarean section. This allows careful monitoring and management of their glucose control. Diabetics with NIDDM can return to the regular postpartum floor following the appropriate period of observation in the recovery room.

Emergency

The principles discussed previously apply equally to diabetics requiring emergency cesarean section. However, factors such as full stomach, bleeding, and cord prolapse influence the choice of anaesthetic technique. In addition, the patient may recently have received a large insulin dose (e.g., A.M. regular, plus lente, or ultralente). In the presence of infection, such as chorioamnionitis, there may be hyperglycemia and other evidence of poor glucose control (e.g., ketosis and dehydration).

These situations call for expeditious preoperative assessment. Normoglycemia should be the goal, but it must not be secured at the expense of an increased hypoglycemia risk. If in doubt, err on the high side to maintain a glucose level approximating 100 to 140 mg/dl. Although this level increases the likelihood of neonatal hypoglycemia, it lessens the possibility of postpartum maternal hypoglycemia.

Following surgery, diabetic women who underwent emergency cesarean section require careful observation in a high-dependency environment until the blood glucose level stabilizes.

Postoperative Analgesia

In the IWK-Grace Health Centre, Halifax, Nova Scotia, the author's group believes that epidural or intrathecal opiates ensure the best postoperative pain relief. Following epidural block, patients receive epidural morphine 3.5 to 4 mg; women having spinal anesthesia receive intrathecal morphine 0.25 to 0.3 mg, on institution of the block. These agents are supplemented with oral/intramuscular (IM) analgesics (e.g., acetaminophen, acetaminophen-codeine; nonsteroidal anti-inflammatory drugs, such as ketoralac (IM), and diclofenac or naproxen, by mouth.) The author's group treats side effects, such as pruritus, nausea, and vomiting, with IM nalbuphine, and metoclopramide. Other institutions prefer IV patient-controlled analgesic opioids to neuraxial administration. These regimes offer less effective analgesia, with less pruritus, but a comparable incidence of nausea and vomiting.

Neonatal Care: The Neonatologist's Responsibility

Except in emergency situations, anesthesiologists cannot provide immediate neonatal care for IDMs. The neonatal team must be alerted preoperatively and, ideally, should meet the mother on the evening before elective cesarean section. All neonates require immediate admission to the special care neonatal unit, usually for 24 hours, and immediate investigations include umbilical cord blood gases, blood glucose, and serum electrolytes to exclude neonatal acidosis, hyperglycemia or hypoglycemia, and hypocalcemia. In view of the risk of fetal hyperinsulinemia and resultant neonatal hypoglycemia, at 1 to 2 hours of age, the neonatologists repeat these investigations at 30-minute intervals for 2 hours to monitor the neonate's progress. In the case of severe diabetics and macrosomic infants, the neonate may need to remain in the intensive care unit for 48 to 72 hours.

Although the incidence of neonatal RDS has decreased rapidly because of improvements in the estimation of fetal lung maturity, transient tachypnea of the newborn and RDS still occur in a small percentage of IDMs. These neonates therefore need careful observation for evidence of grunting, rib retractions, and tachypnea. Some IDMs show evidence of hemoconcentration, which, in its severest form, may lead to renal vein thrombosis.

TEN PRACTICAL POINTS

1. Maintaining euglycemia, from the prepregnancy period onward, improves maternal and neonatal outcome.
2. Anticipate maternal, fetal, and neonatal complications in insulin-dependent diabetic parturients.

3. Maternal insulin requirements decrease markedly in the postpartum period—beware of insulin!

4. No insulin is better than too much insulin prior to elective cesarean section.

5. Observe newborns closely for hypoglycemia.

6. Volume replacement is the cornerstone of management of diabetic ketoacidosis.

7. Aggressively treat maternal hypertension, which can severely threaten the fetus.

8. If selecting general anesthesia, beware of the "stiff joint" syndrome.

9. Do not preload with dextrose-containing solutions.

10. Beware of fetal macrosomia causing complicated vaginal delivery.

REFERENCES

1. Landon MB, Gabbe SG: Diabetes mellitus and pregnancy. Obstet Gynecol Clin North Am 19:633–654, 1992.
2. American Diabetes Association: Position statement on gestational diabetes mellitus. Am J Obstet Gynecol 156:488–489, 1987.
3. Milaskiewicz RM, Hall GM: Diabetes and anaesthesia: The past decade. Br J Anaesth 68:198–206, 1992.
4. Hare JW: Insulin management of Type I and Type II diabetes in pregnancy. Clin Obstet Gynecol 34:494–504, 1991.
5. Catalano PM, Bernstein IM, Wolfe RR, et al: Subclinical abnormalities of glucose metabolism in subjects with previous gestational diabetes. Am J Obstet Gynecol 155:1255–1262, 1986.
6. Mulford MI, Jovanovic-Peterson L, Peterson CM: Alternative therapies for the management of gestational diabetes. Clin Perinatol 20:619–634, 1993.
7. Coustan DR: Management of gestational diabetes. Clin Obstet Gynecol 34:558–564, 1991.
8. White P: Diabetes mellitus in pregnancy. Clin Perinatol 1:331–347, 1974.
9. Writer WD: The pregnant diabetic. Probl Anesth 3:69–89, 1989.
10. Jovanovic-Peterson L, Peterson CM: Pregnancy in the diabetic woman. Guidelines for a successful outcome. Endocrinol Metab Clin North Am 121:433–456, 1992.
11. Garner PR, D'Alton ME, Dudley DK, et al: Preeclampsia in diabetic pregnancies. Am J Obstet Gynecol 163:505–508, 1990.
12. Cousins L: Etiology and prevention of congenital anomalies among infants of overt diabetic women. Clin Obstet Gynecol 34:481–493, 1991.
13. Landon MB, Gabbe SG, Sachs L: Management of diabetes mellitus and pregnancy: A survey of obstetricians and maternal-fetal specialists. Obstet Gynecol 75:635–640, 1990.
14. Siperstein MD: Diabetic ketoacidosis and hyperosmolar coma. Endocrinol Metab Clin North Am 21:415–431, 1992.
15. Prihoda JS, Davis LE: Metabolic emergencies in obstetrics. Obstet Gynecol Clin North Am 18: 301–318, 1991.
16. Coustan DR, Felig P: Diabetes mellitus. *In* Burrow GN, Ferris TF (eds): Medical Complications During Pregnancy, 3rd ed. Philadelphia, WB Saunders, 1988, pp 34–64.
17. Burgos LG, Ebert TJ, Assiddao C, et al: Increased intraoperative cardiovascular morbidity in diabetics with autonomic neuropathy. Anesthesiology 70:591–597, 1989.
18. Bromage PR: Epidural Analgesia. Philadelphia, WB Saunders, 1978.
19. Reissel E, Orko R, Maunuksela E-L, et al: Predictability of difficult laryngoscopy in patients with long-term diabetes mellitus. Anaesthesia 45:1024–1027, 1990.
20. Datta S: Anesthetic management of the obstetric or pregnant patient with diabetes. Clin Anaesthesiol 4:275–289, 1986.
21. Ramanathan S, Khoo P, Arismendy J: Perioperative maternal and neonatal acid-base status and glucose metabolism in patients with insulin-dependent diabetes mellitus. Anesth Analg 73:105–111, 1991.
22. Datta S, Brown WU: Acid-base status in diabetic mothers and their infants following general or spinal anesthesia for cesarean section. Anesthesiology 47:272–276, 1977.
23. Datta S, Brown WU, Ostheimer GW, et al: Epidural anesthesia for cesarean section in diabetic parturients: Maternal and neonatal acid-base status and bupivacaine concentration. Anesth Analg 60:574–578, 1981.
24. Datta S, Kitzmiller JL, Naulty JS, et al: Acid-base status of diabetic mothers and their infants following spinal anesthesia for cesarean section. Anesth Analg 61:662–665, 1982.
25. Ammon JR: Perioperative management of the diabetic patient. 38th Annual Refresher Course Lectures, Atlanta, October 10–14, 1987. Park Ridge, IL, American Society of Anesthesiologists, 1987, p 272.
26. York R, Brown LP, Swank A, et al: Diabetes mellitus in pregnancy: Clinical review. J Perinatol 10:285–293, 1990.
27. Ramanathan J, Coleman P, Sibai B: Anesthetic modification of hemodynamic and neuroendocrine stress responses to cesarean delivery in women with severe preeclampsia. Anesth Analg 73:772–779, 1991.

EIGHTEEN

Cardiovascular Disease

Mary Louise Steward, B.Sc., M.Sc., M.D., F.R.C.P.(C.)

Cardiac disease complicates 1 to 2% of pregnancies.[1] Although rheumatic heart disease remains the most common cause of heart disorders presenting during pregnancy, recent advances in medical and surgical care allow more women with congenital heart disease (CHD) to reach the childbearing years. Whereas some cardiac lesions are associated with a very low risk of maternal mortality, others may result in death risks approaching 50% (Table 18–1).[2] The anesthesia provider must clearly understand the interaction of the underlying cardiac disease pathophysiology with the physiologic changes accompanying pregnancy, labor, and delivery. Optimal maternal and fetal outcome depends on rational anesthesia management. This chapter presents a practical approach to anesthetic management of cardiac patients.

TABLE 18–1
Risk of Mortality Associated With Specific Cardiac Lesions[2]

Low Risk of Maternal Mortality (<1%)
Uncomplicated atrial and ventricular septal defects
Patent ductus arteriosus
Pulmonary or tricuspid valve disease
Corrected tetralogy of Fallot
Porcine valve prosthesis
Mitral stenosis (New York Heart Association [NYHA] classes I and II)
Moderate Risk of Maternal Mortality (5–15%)
Mitral stenosis with atrial fibrillation
Mitral stenosis (NYHA classes III and IV)
Prosthetic valve
Aortic stenosis
Coarctation of the aorta—uncomplicated
Uncorrected tetralogy of Fallot
Previous myocardial infarction
Marfan syndrome without evidence of aortic disease
Symptomatic hypertrophic cardiomyopathy
High Risk of Maternal Mortality (25–50%)
Pulmonary hypertension
Coarctation of the aorta—complicated
Marfan syndrome with aortic involvement
Eisenmenger syndrome

Data from Clark SL: Labor and delivery in the patient with structural cardiac disease. Clin Perinatol 13:695–703, 1986.

CARDIOVASCULAR CHANGES DURING PREGNANCY AND DELIVERY

From 12 weeks' gestation, maternal cardiac output (CO) progressively increases, reaching 150% of normal at 28 to 32 weeks. At 20 weeks' gestation, there is a 40% increase in both stroke volume and CO (Table 18–2). After 20 weeks' gestation, heart rate increases, reaching 120% of normal at term. During labor and delivery, CO increases an additional 50 to 60%, but regional analgesia attenuates these additional cardiac demands, an advantage in many patients. Maximal CO occurs after delivery, secondary to the autotransfusion that follows placenta extrusion and subsequent uterine contraction. The anesthesia provider must be aware that risks do *not* end with delivery of the fetus and placenta.

TABLE 18–2
Cardiovascular Changes During Pregnancy

Parameter	% Change	Normal (Nonpregnant)
Heart rate	+10–20	71 + 10 bpm
Stroke volume	+20–30	73.3 + 9 ml
Cardiac output	+30–50	4.3 + 0.9 L/min
Blood volume	+20–100	5 L
Plasma	+70–80	
Red cells	+20–30 = relative anemia	
Oxygen consumption	+20	250 ml/min

These acute changes in cardiovascular dynamics may place an intolerable load on the compromised heart.

PRINCIPLES OF ANESTHETIC MANAGEMENT

The pregnant cardiac patient is best managed by utilizing a team approach involving early consultation among the anesthesiologist, the cardiologist, and the obstetrician. Maternal outcome correlates best with the New York Heart Association Functional Classification (Table 18–3).[3] Early evaluation, including a careful history and physical examination as well as appropriate laboratory and diagnostic tests, should determine the nature and severity of cardiac disease and subsequent management (Table 18–4). Anesthetic choices vary with the type and severity of the heart disease, the planned obstetric management, and the skills of the available personnel. Obstetric management is usually a planned vaginal delivery, reserving cesarean section for obstetric indications. Patients who may not tolerate a Valsalva maneuver usually undergo elective vacuum extraction or forceps delivery to decrease the length of second stage labor and minimize maternal pushing efforts. Importantly, patients with structural heart lesions must receive appropriate prophylactic antibiotics to prevent subacute bacterial endocarditis (Table 18–5).

TABLE 18–3
New York Heart Association Functional Classification of Cardiovascular Disease

Class I	No limitation of physical activity. Ordinary physical activity does not precipitate cardiovascular symptoms such as dyspnea, angina, fatigue, or palpitations.
Class II	Slight limitation of physical activity. Ordinary physical activity will precipitate cardiovascular symptoms, although patients are comfortable at rest.
Class III	Less than ordinary physical activity precipitates symptoms that markedly limit activity. Patients are comfortable at rest.
Class IV	Patients are unable to carry on any physical activity without discomfort. Cardiovascular symptoms may be present at rest.

Monitoring

Asymptomatic patients or those with only mild symptoms may be managed routinely. However, delivery in a hospital capable of managing cardiac decompensation is prudent. The fact that such patients have reached term with only mild symptoms is a testimony to their cardiac reserve. Standard practice, as for all patients, includes left uterine displacement and fetal monitoring. Continuous pulse oximetry should be used for all symptomatic cardiac patients. Patients with moderate or severe symptoms may benefit from invasive monitoring, including an arterial line and pulmonary artery (PA) catheterization to determine pulmonary wedge pressure and thermodilution CO, recognizing that invasive monitoring is often difficult to institute in awake laboring patients. Patients requiring invasive monitoring during labor and delivery will also need to be transferred to an intensive care unit following delivery, since CO increases maximally following delivery, and it may take a few days for the patient's cardiac and fluid status to stabilize. Obviously, patients requiring intensive monitoring should deliver in a tertiary care facility with an appropriate intensive care unit.

Postoperative Pain

The cardiac patient also benefits from good postoperative analgesia minimizing cardiac stress and encouraging early mobilization. Dis-

TABLE 18–4
Management of the Cardiac Patient

Symptoms	Recommended Laboratory Tests	Monitoring	Location
None—mild	Complete blood count Electrolytes, ECG Chest x-ray	ECG, BP Oximetry Urine output	Primary hospital
Moderate	Complete blood count Electrolytes, ECG, CXR Urinalysis, blood gas Echocardiogram Vital capacity	ECG, BP, pulse oximetry, arterial, CVP, ± PA pressure Urinary output	Tertiary hospital with ICU
Severe	As above	As above with Swan-Ganz catheter	As above

Abbreviations: ECG = electrocardiogram; BP = blood pressure; ICU = intensive care unit; CXR = chest x-ray; CVP = central venous pressure; PA = pulmonary artery.

cuss the analgesic plan in advance with the patient. There is now good evidence to suggest that regional analgesia or epidural opiates administered before surgery (preemptive analgesia) reduce postoperative pain. Consider using intrathecal or epidural narcotics, which may be combined with intravenous (IV) patient-controlled analgesia (PCA). Patients receiving a regional anesthetic for cesarean section may be given 0.1 to 0.2 mg morphine intrathecally or 3 to 5 mg of epidural morphine with good results. IV PCA narcotic infusion also provides adequate postoperative analgesia for patients receiving general anesthesia for cesarean section. Patients receiving intrathecal or epidural morphine must have appropriate nursing supervision and hourly monitoring of vital signs for 18 to 24 hours after their last neuraxial narcotic drug dose.

TABLE 18–5
Recommendations for Antibiotic Prophylaxis for Subacute Bacterial Endocarditis

1. Ampicillin—2 gm IV or IM 30 min preoperatively; 1 gm IV or IM 6 hr after the initial dose.
2. For patients allergic to penicillin—clindamycin—300 mg IV 30 min preoperatively; 150 mg IV 6 hr after the initial dose.
3. For patients considered to be at extreme risk and not candidates for the standard regimen—Ampicillin 2 gm IV, plus gentamicin 1.5 mg/kg (not to exceed 80 mg total) 30 min preoperatively, followed by amoxicillin 1.5 gm orally 6 hr after the initial dose. (Alternatively, the parenteral regimen may be repeated 8 hr after the initial dose.)
4. For patients considered to be at extreme risk and not candidates for the standard regimen and who are allergic to penicillin: vancomycin—1 gm IV administered slowly over 1 hr beginning 1 hr preoperatively. No follow-up dosage is necessary.

ANESTHETIC MANAGEMENT

General Principles

Aortocaval compression must be avoided at all times in high-risk cardiac patients. Reductions in venous return and CO secondary to aortocaval compression may be catastrophic for these women. The author's group recommends exaggerating uterine displacement and encouraging the patient to labor in a lateral decubitus position when practical. Ensure that *all* medical personnel involved with the care of these women are aware of the importance of avoiding aortocaval compression. For example, in the author's experience the most common time for a lapse in vigilance is during vaginal examination or placement of a Foley catheter.

Administering supplemental oxygen may be highly desirable for some high-risk women with cardiovascular disease. The author's group recommends supplemental oxygen using a nonrebreathing mask with reservoir for all parturients with moderate to severe cardiovascular disease, and as discussed earlier, continuous monitoring of oxygen saturation via pulse oximetry should be employed if possible.

The method of providing labor analgesia or cesarean section anesthesia must minimize risks of adversely affecting the pathophysiology of the parturient with severe cardiac disease while protecting the fetus. Table 18–6 summarizes the desirable hemodynamic parameters for specific cardiac lesions and the general advisability of employing epidural analgesia/anesthesia.

Analgesia for Labor and Vaginal Delivery

Several techniques are available for parturients for whom regional analgesia is contraindicated or refused. Systemic narcotic analgesia may be provided with intermittent IV meperidine or butorphanol. Alternatively, IV PCA with fentanyl (maximal dose 150 μg/hr) can provide systemic narcotic analgesia. Delivery analgesia can be supplemented with local infiltration or pudendal block. Inhalational analgesia supplementation with nitrous oxide or inhalational agents is an option if necessary and feasible. If more intralabor analgesia is required, intrathecal morphine 0.25 to 0.5 mg with fentanyl 12.5 to 25 μg provides long-lasting analgesia that is superior to systemic narcotics and minimizes the risk of hypotension.[4] Unfortunately, nausea and vomiting are relatively common, and if these potential side effects would compromise the patient, avoid this technique. Intrathecal sufentanil 5 to 10 μg provides rapid, reliable first stage labor analgesia that lasts 90 to 120 minutes.[5] However, second stage analgesia is usually less than satisfactory with intrathecal sufentanil. Importantly, some investigators, but not all, report that normal laboring patients can develop transient, mild hypotension within 5 to 15 minutes following sufentanil injection. Resolution usually occurs within 5 to 10 minutes and responds to additional fluids or vasopressors, or both. The cause of this transient hypotension, if real, is unknown at this time. However, even mild, transient hypotension is a significant risk factor for cardiac decompensation in some cardiac patients. Carefully consider the risk/benefit of intrathecal sufentanil for labor pain relief. Remember, the limited duration of analgesia accompanying intrathecal sufentanil requires repeated "single-shot" intrathecal injections or a continuous spinal technique. Either option has associated increased risks for postdural puncture headache. Headaches, however, are not life-threatening and, in most patients, can be relatively easily treated. Patients should not be denied the benefits of intrathecal narcotics out of fear of their developing a postdural puncture headache if these agents are the "best" option.

Epidural Analgesia

The author's group utilizes the following technique for "high-risk" patients. Patients with known or suspected intracardiac shunts should not be exposed to intravascular air and potential paradoxical air emboli. Be careful to avoid air bubbles in IV lines and use saline solution for the "loss of resistance" test when identifying the epidural space. Carefully test the epidural

TABLE 18–6
Summary of Desired Hemodynamics for Specific Cardiac Lesions

Lesion	Heart Rate	Preload	Contractility	SVR	Invasive Monitor	Epidural
Mitral stenosis	<110	↑	N ↑	N	if Sx	Yes
Mitral insufficiency	80–100	↑	N ↑	↓	if Sx	Yes
Aortic stenosis	80–120	↑	N ↑	↑	if Sx	No
Aortic insufficiency	80–100	↑	N ↑	↓	if Sx	Yes
Tetralogy of Fallot	<110	↑	↑ ↓	↑	if Sx	No
HOC	<100 (↓)	↑	↓	N ↑	if Sx	No
Eisenmenger	<100	↑	N	N ↑	Yes	No
Pulmonary HTN	<100	↑	N	↑	if Sx	No
Coronary artery	<100	N	N ↓	N ↓	if Sx	Yes

Abbreviations: SVR = systemic vascular resistance; Sx = symptoms; HOC = hypertrophic obstetric cardiomyopathy; HTN = hypertension.

catheter for accidental subarachnoid placement by administering a small dose of local anesthetic sufficient to produce a recognizable block while avoiding extensive spread. Typically, the author's group uses 30 to 45 mg of lidocaine. Closely observe for possible signs of subarachnoid block for 5 minutes following the spinal test dose.

Next, exclude IV catheter placement. Cardiac conditions in which tachycardia and increases in systemic vascular resistance (SVR) are dangerous preclude utilizing epinephrine for testing. In these circumstances, 100 mg of lidocaine or 2-chloroprocaine usually produces characteristic signs of mild transient systemic local anesthetic toxicity. Remember, if epidural narcotic supplementation is planned, avoid testing the epidural catheter with 2-chloroprocaine; use lidocaine 100 mg for IV testing. The editor's group has found that 2-chloroprocaine dramatically interferes with the efficacy of epidural narcotics (fentanyl or morphine) for many hours following administration.[6] A "funny taste" is the most common symptom of intravascular local anesthetic injection, with a "ringing and/or roaring noise" in the ears also a frequent complaint. However, these complaints are not an absolutely reliable indication of IV catheter placement, and good practice dictates that all subsequent doses of local anesthetics be administered in 5-ml aliquots and the patient repeatedly questioned for symptoms. Others prefer epinephrine 15 μg administered between contractions, followed by close observation of the maternal heart rate for changes. For IV testing, the editor's group believe, that, for most high-risk cardiac patients, using epinephrine to test for IV epidural catheter placement often adds risk and is potentially unreliable in this patient population because of either the cardiac lesion or concomitant drug treatment. Epinephrine mixed with local anesthetics may be acceptable in some circumstances after IV catheterization is excluded. Remember, IV catheter migration can occur. Thus, epinephrine is probably best avoided in high-risk patients who could deteriorate if they received IV epinephrine.

Following epidural catheter testing for intrathecal and IV placement, the author's group most commonly utilizes bupivacaine 0.0625 to 0.125% containing fentanyl 1 to 2 μg/ml, titrating drug administration slowly to achieve analgesia and dermatomal levels of approximately T10. The author's group believes fentanyl allows a decrease in the concentration of local anesthetic and hence the degree of motor blockade. Continuous infusion or patient-controlled epidural infusion is then used to maintain analgesia. Epidural infusion rates are typically 10 to 15 ml/hr. Pain occurring despite the epidural infusion is most commonly supplemented with bupivacaine 0.125 to 0.25% in 5-ml aliquots. Drug is titrated prior to delivery to provide a comfortable patient during spontaneous or forceps delivery. The location of delivery (operating room vs. labor room) varies with the severity of disease.

Cesarean Section Anesthesia

If regional anesthesia is planned, the author's group avoids "single-shot" spinal anesthesia and the resulting rapid sympathectomy. Epidural anesthesia allows slow block establishment and early recognition of cardiovascular side effects, permitting early, aggressive treatment. If necessary, epidural anesthesia can also be abandoned if early symptoms prove more difficult to treat than anticipated. Obviously, this is not an option with spinal anesthesia. Most commonly following catheter testing, the author's group uses 5-ml aliquots of bupivacaine 0.5% or 2-chloroprocaine 3% to establish anesthesia. Block onset is slower with bupivacaine. Occasionally, the author's group administers lidocaine 2% mixed with 1:300,000 epinephrine and bicarbonate, 1 mEq/ml, cognizant of the earlier considerations regarding epinephrine. The author's group believes epinephrine limits plasma lidocaine concentrations and improves the quality of the block. The group does not use lidocaine 2% without epinephrine. As discussed, if epinephrine administration is a concern, the group does not generally utilize epidural lidocaine.

General anesthesia may be preferable to regional anesthesia in some cases. The author's group always administers orally 0.3 M sodium citrate 30 ml immediately prior to transporting the patient to the operating room. If a slow general anesthetic induction is planned, the group may also administer IV metoclopramide (10 mg, 1 hr before surgery) or ranitidine (50 mg IV), or both. Patients receive ranitidine 150 mg by mouth the night before surgery and the morning of surgery with a sip of water. In urgent circumstances, the author's group administers IV ranitidine 50 mg 1 to 2 hours before surgery. If the group plans to use moderate to high-dose IV narcotics during induction, we generally use fentanyl or alfentanil and alert the neonatology team. If general anesthesia is induced slowly with narcotics or potent inhalational agents, prudence would dictate that a pediatrician or neonatologist attend the delivery to support the neonate until the general anesthetic drug effects wane. For some patients, the author's group follows a standard general anesthesia technique for cesarean section (see Chapter 7) employing pentothal 4 to 6 mg/kg, succinylcholine chloride 1 to 2 mg/kg, $N_2O:O_2$ = 50:50, a potent inhalational agent (less than ½ minimal alveolar concentration [MAC]), and IV narcotics after delivery. The general anesthetic techniques recommended for several types of disease are discussed subsequently.

SPECIFIC CARDIAC CONDITIONS

Figure 18–1, a reference for this discussion, illustrates normal cardiac function and contrasts with the cardiac conditions depicted in subsequent figures.

Rheumatic Heart Disease

Mitral Stenosis (Fig. 18–2)

Mitral stenosis is the most common valvular lesion occurring in pregnant women.[7] Ninety percent of pregnant women with a history of rheumatic heart disease have mitral stenosis.[8]

Pathophysiology. Following a group A β-hemolytic streptococcal infection and rheumatic carditis, mitral valve narrowing occurs in 10 to 15% of patients. Decreased left ventricular diastolic filling is the primary hemodynamic consequence of mitral valve stenosis. Left ventricular stroke volume is reduced, and left atrial and PA wedge pressures increase. Eventually, pulmonary hypertension and right ventricular hypertrophy occur in response to increased fluid volume in the pulmonary vasculature. Pulmonary congestion and atrial fibrillation may also occur. Tachycardia, impairing left ventricular diastolic filling, is poorly tolerated in patients with mitral stenosis and must be considered when selecting an anesthetic technique. Antepartum β-adrenergic blockade is often initiated to blunt tachycardia (remember to avoid epinephrine) and may improve maternal outcome.[9] Ventricular filling is also impaired if atrial fibrillation occurs. The relief of aortocaval compression and

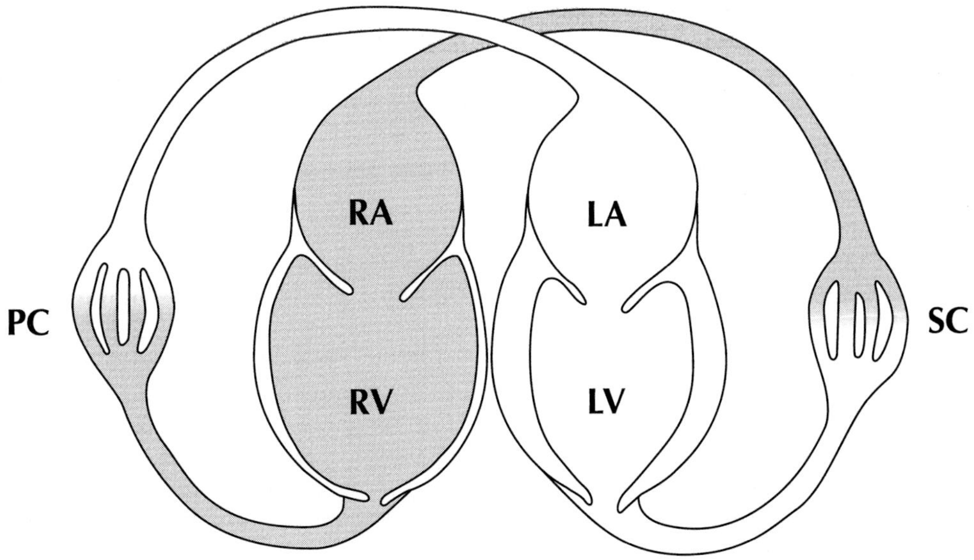

Figure 18–1. The normal heart. A diagram of normal cardiac anatomy to be compared with specific cardiac conditions illustrated in subsequent figures. Venous circulation is *shaded.* (*Abbreviations:* LA = left atrium; LV = left ventricle; RA = right atrium; RV = right ventricle; PC = pulmonary circulation; SC = systemic circulation.)

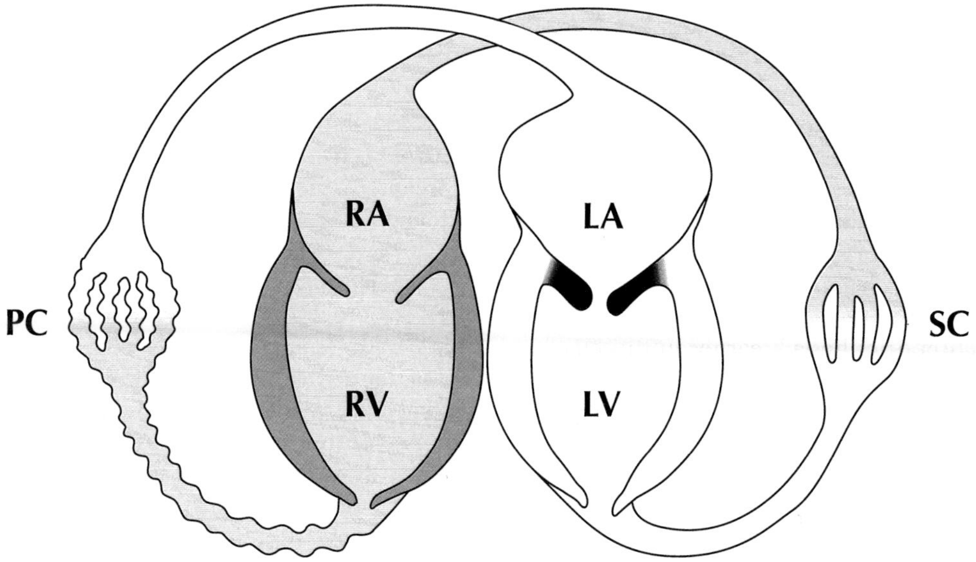

Figure 18–2. Mitral stenosis. Note the thickened, stenotic mitral valve, which eventually causes left atrial dilatation, pulmonary hypertension, and right ventricular hypertrophy. Venous circulation is *shaded.* (*Abbreviations:* LA = left atrium; LV = left ventricle; RA = right atrium; RV = right ventricle; PC = pulmonary circulation; SC = systemic circulation.) Refer to Figure 18–1 for normal cardiac anatomy.

the autotransfusion that occurs following placenta delivery rapidly increase venous return and may produce pulmonary edema secondary to increased pulmonary congestion.

Anesthetic Considerations. Patients with a history of pulmonary congestion require radial artery cannulation and PA pressure monitoring. Atrial fibrillation causing cardiac decompensation, with concurrent hypotension or pulmonary edema, should be treated with immediate cardioversion starting with 25 to 100 watt-sec of energy. If time permits (hours), and cardiac symptoms are benign, administer digoxin 0.5 mg IV over 10 minutes followed by 0.25 mg IV every 2 hours up to a total of 1.25 mg and maintain the ventricular rate below 110 beats per minute. Following full digitalization, procainamide or quinidine can usually restore a sinus rhythm. IV propranolol in 0.5-mg increments may be given, but this agent is associated with delays in neonatal initiation of sustained respiration. Always administer IV fluids judiciously in these patients and maintain uterine displacement. For labor analgesia, consider slowly titrating the epidural block and administering IV fluids as indicated. If preload is a concern, monitor central venous pressure (CVP) and, in the case of severe disease, pulmonary wedge pressures and cardiac outputs with a PA catheter. Arbitrary "preloads" are dangerous unless CVPs are monitored continuously. Avoid the Trendelenburg position since this markedly increases central blood volume and risks for pulmonary edema. Tachycardia is poorly tolerated, and if hypotension develops, treat with phenylephrine (50–100 μg) incrementally while administering additional fluid. Avoid decreasing SVR or precipitating hypercarbia, hypoxia, acidosis, and excessive ventilatory pressures during general anesthesia. All can lead to pulmonary hypertension and tachycardia.

Recommended Analgesic Technique for Vaginal Delivery. For labor and vaginal delivery, lumbar epidural analgesia provides good labor pain relief, helps block the tachycardia accompanying uterine contractions and pain, and provides a calm, cooperative patient at delivery. In general, the author's group recommends the epidural analgesia technique outlined in the section on "Analgesia for Labor and Vaginal Delivery" for the high-risk cardiac patient. IV narcotics and nitrous oxide with a pudendal block are poor alternatives because these analgesia techniques do not blunt the patient's response to pain as well as epidural analgesia does. Spinal anesthesia for vaginal delivery may cause a rapid reduction in SVR inducing compensatory tachycardia and hence should be used with extreme caution in cardiac patients with stenotic lesions. There are no cardiac advantages for caudal analgesia.

Cesarean Section. Lumbar epidural anesthesia may be used for cesarean section for patients with mitral stenosis. The author's group recommends using the technique outlined in "Cesarean Section Anesthesia," earlier in this chapter. Avoid epinephrine-containing local anesthetic solutions. If a vasopressor is required, administer phenylephrine (50–100 μg) incrementally. Epidural morphine (3–5 mg) may be given after delivery to provide postoperative analgesia. If the patient has received 2-chloroprocaine, the effectiveness may be less than desirable. Alternatively, IV PCA is acceptable.

General anesthesia is a reasonable option for cesarean section. Avoid tachycardia-inducing drugs such as ketamine, pancuronium, and possibly isoflurane. Moderate β-adrenergic-receptor blockade may be indicated. The author's group prefers propranolol to esmolol. Although esmolol is short-acting, it rapidly crosses the placenta, causing fetal bradycardia. Patients with symptomatic mitral stenosis may require a slow induction of anesthesia using IV narcotics and possible mask ventilation with continuous cricoid pressure prior to tracheal intubation.

Mitral Insufficiency (Fig. 18–3)

Patients with mitral regurgitation usually tolerate pregnancy well because the left ventricle accommodates the excess volume load. Indeed, such patients usually remain asymptomatic until after their childbearing years. They may, however, develop pulmonary edema, pulmonary emboli, or subacute endocarditis during pregnancy.

Pathophysiology. When the left ventricle contracts, a portion of the stroke volume regurgitates into the left atrium. The degree of regurgitation depends on the resistance to forward flow through the aortic valve compared with retrograde flow through the incompetent mitral valve. Similar to patients with mitral stenosis, these women are at increased risk for atrial fibrillation and poorly tolerate rapid ventricular responses. The extent of invasive monitoring required depends on the severity of the disease. Patients with a history of left ventricular failure require radial artery and PA catheterization. In

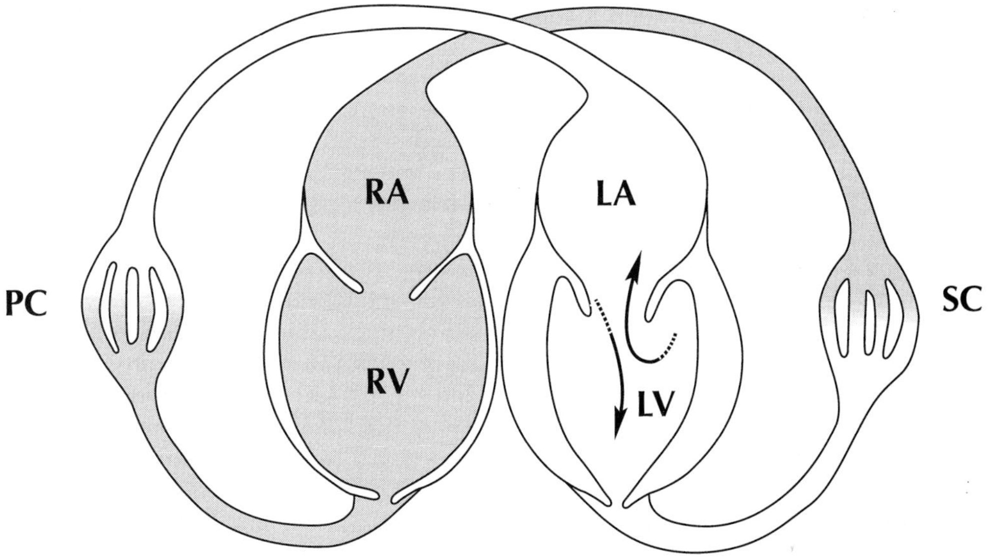

Figure 18–3. Mitral insufficiency. Note the retrograde blood flow through the incompetent mitral valve into the left atrium. Left ventricle dilatation eventually occurs in response to chronic volume overload and contractility becomes depressed. Venous circulation is *shaded. (Abbreviations:* LA = left atrium; LV = left ventricle; RA = right atrium; RV = right ventricle; PC = pulmonary circulation; SC = systemic circulation.) Refer to Figure 18–1 for normal cardiac anatomy.

contrast to mitral stenosis, bradycardia is not tolerated by patients with mitral insufficiency because slow heart rates increase regurgitation, and therefore, less of the left ventricular stroke volume enters the aorta during systole. Left ventricle dilatation occurs in response to chronic volume overload and diminishes myocardial contractility (Starling law). These patients may decompensate if myocardial depressants are given.

Recommended Analgesic Technique for Labor and Vaginal Delivery. For labor and delivery, it is important to be judicious with preload, particularly with patients who have signs of cardiac failure, since excess fluids may precipitate pulmonary edema. Avoid arbitrary "preloads." PA catheters are useful, but the left atrial compliance is very high and absolute pulmonary wedge numbers may be misleading. However, increases in pulmonary pressure V waveform indicate increased regurgitation. Lumbar epidural anesthesia (see "Epidural Analgesia" for modified anesthetic technique for labor and vaginal delivery in high-risk parturients) offers great benefit to these patients because sympathetic blockade decreases afterload and encourages forward flow. Furthermore, pain relief prevents catecholamine release, which would increase the SVR and produce tachycardia.

Cesarean Section. The author's group recommends lumbar epidural anesthesia for cesarean section. Treat hypotension with incremental ephedrine 5 to 10 mg IV. Fentanyl 50 to 100 μg may be added to the amide local anesthetic solution to provide additional analgesia. General anesthesia may be administered using thiopental, nitrous oxide, oxygen (50:50), relaxant, and narcotics after delivery. Utilize potent inhalation agents to diminish awareness and decrease the afterload; however, remember these agents are myocardial depressants and the concentration should be limited to less than ½ MAC. Labetalol or hydralazine in 5-mg increments IV may also be used to treat hypertension, but avoid bradycardia or excessive tachycardia. Avoid ketamine, which may produce hypertension and increase valvular regurgitation.

Mitral Valve Prolapse

Mitral valve prolapse occurs in 5 to 10% of the population and is the most common congenital valvular lesion. Although most patients are asymptomatic, those individuals with structurally abnormal valves that are prolapsing and regurgitant may suffer chest pains, arrhythmias, embolism, and transient ischemic attacks and may develop bacterial endocarditis.[10] Echocardiography confirms the diagnosis.

For symptomatic parturients, anesthetic management should ensure adequate preload (1–2 L) and early diagnosis and treatment of arrhythmias. Otherwise, anesthetic management is standard. If they have associated mitral regurgitation, the anesthetic considerations outlined previously for mitral regurgitation apply. Symptomatic patients should probably receive endocarditis prophylaxis, but this is controversial.

Aortic Stenosis (Fig. 18–4)

The decreased aortic valve orifice area reduces left ventricular stroke volume. Aortic valve stenosis increases left ventricular end-diastolic pressures and produces ventricular hypertrophy. Maintenance of stroke volume depends on adequate preload. The increased plasma volume of pregnancy helps to maintain preload and CO. Parturients with mild to moderate aortic stenosis usually tolerate pregnancy. However, with severe aortic stenosis, the mortality in pregnant patients with aortic gradients greater than 100 mmHg is 17%.[2]

Anesthetic Considerations. Symptoms of syncope, angina, or congestive heart failure suggest severe aortic stenosis, which warrants radial artery and PA catheterization. Since the left ventricle has a relatively fixed stroke volume, CO depends on heart rate, and bradycardia is poorly tolerated. Additionally, heart rates exceeding 130 beats per minute decrease diastolic filling time and time for perfusion of the hypertrophic left ventricle. Tachycardia decreases CO and increases myocardial oxygen demand. Therefore, decreases in diastolic perfusion, myocardial contractility, hemoglobin concentration, CO, or atrial oxygen saturation may lead to myocardial ischemia. Anesthetic goals include maintenance of a normal heart rate, sinus rhythm, adequate SVR, intravascular volume and venous return, and normal CO.

Recommended Analgesic Technique for Labor and Vaginal Delivery. If the woman has severe dis-

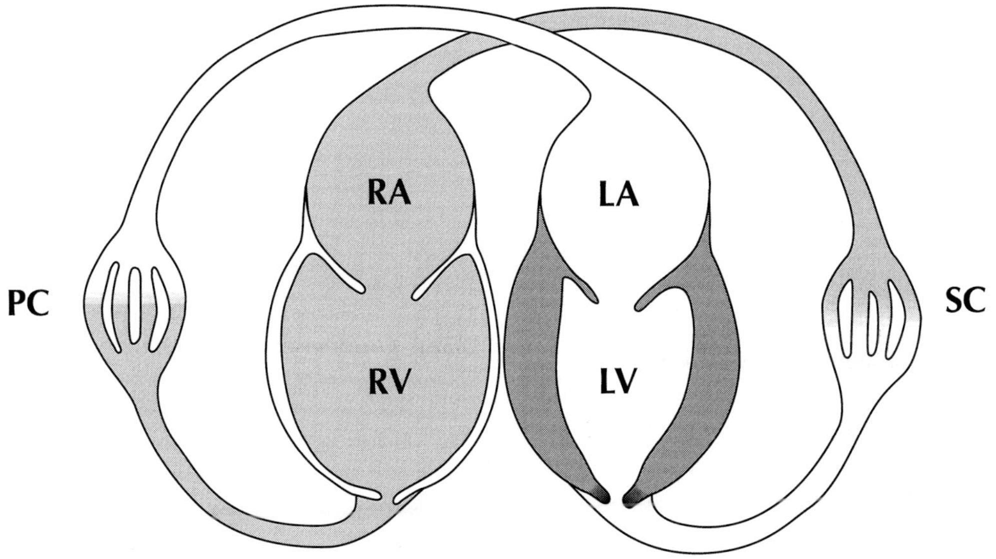

Figure 18–4. Aortic stenosis. Note the thickened, stenotic aortic valve, which reduces left ventricular stroke volume. Eventually, the left ventricle hypertrophies. Venous circulation is *shaded.* (*Abbreviations:* LA = left atrium; LV = left ventricle; RA = right atrium; RV = right ventricle; PC = pulmonary circulation; SC = systemic circulation.) Refer to Figure 18–1 for normal cardiac anatomy.

ease, sympathetic blockade is best avoided. The risks for decreases in SVR, venous return, and hypotension leading to myocardial ischemia are significant. Close attention must be paid to volume status, since an adequate preload is essential. Therefore, systemic narcotics, such as PCA fentanyl or Entonox (50:50 N_2O:O_2) provide desirable alternatives for labor management. Some authors recommend intrathecal narcotics, particularly intrathecal sufentanil, as a desirable first stage labor analgesia alternative. Remember, some patients may develop hypotension, and there are no reports documenting the relative safety of this technique in this patient population. Personal experience and judgment of the relative risk/benefit should dictate whether this technique is reasonable for a particular circumstance. A pudendal block or local anesthesia can be used to facilitate delivery. If regional anesthesia is selected for a patient with mild disease, the modified analgesic technique outlined under "Epidural Analgesia" is recommended.

Cesarean Section. For cesarean section, a "light" general anesthetic provided with a muscle relaxant, thiopental, N_2O:O_2 (50:50), and ½ MAC halogenated agent, is preferred over regional anesthesia. IV narcotics may be administered after delivery. Ketamine causes tachycardia and, therefore, should be avoided. Consider IV lidocaine or narcotics, or both, prior to intubation to help blunt the response to laryngoscopy. Etomidate combined with narcotics may represent an alternative induction agent for those women with severe disease. If narcotics are used prior to delivery, anticipate the need for neonatal resuscitation and possible reversal of narcotic-induced newborn respiratory depression.

Aortic Insufficiency (Fig. 18–5)

Severe aortic insufficiency usually develops after a woman completes her reproductive years. Therefore, most pregnant patients do not have severe disease and generally tolerate pregnancy well. Occasionally, aortic stenosis accompanies aortic insufficiency. In these women, the stenotic aspect is usually more significant, and patients with combined lesions should be treated primarily as having aortic stenosis.

Pathophysiology. During diastole, a portion of the previously ejected stroke volume regurgitates back into the left ventricle, elevating left ventricular end-diastolic volume and decreasing effective forward stroke volume. Increased left

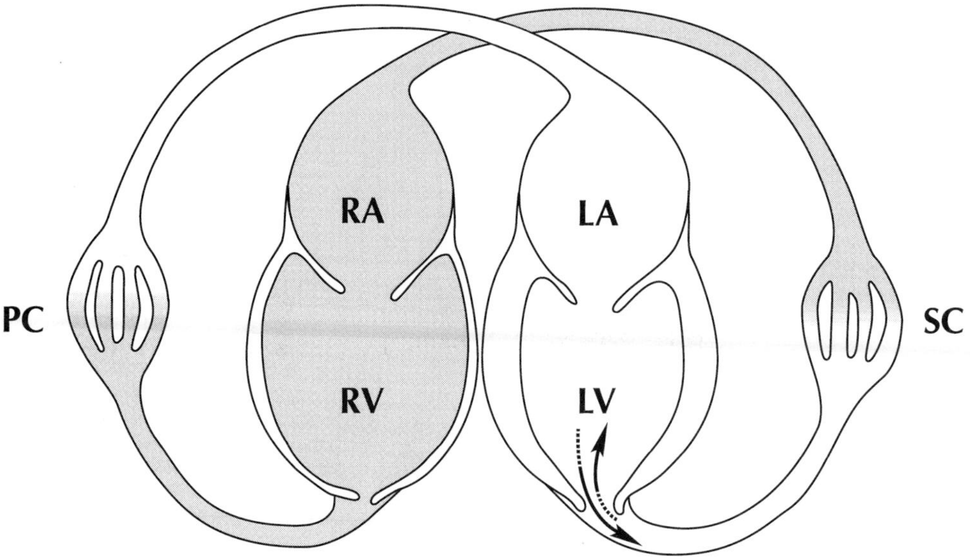

Figure 18–5. Aortic insufficiency. Note retrograde blood flow through the incompetent aortic valve into the left ventricle, elevating left ventricular end-diastolic volume. Eventually, the left ventricle dilates and fails. Venous circulation is *shaded*. (*Abbreviations:* LA = left atrium; LV = left ventricle; RA = right atrium; RV = right ventricle; PC = pulmonary circulation; SC = systemic circulation.) Refer to Figure 18–1 for normal cardiac anatomy.

ventricular volume produces left ventricular dilatation and failure. As with mitral insufficiency, bradycardia or increases in afterload exacerbate regurgitation into the ventricle and decrease cardiac output.

Recommended Analgesic Technique for Labor and Vaginal Delivery. Lumbar epidural analgesia, which prevents pain-induced increases in the SVR, is the preferred anesthetic technique for labor and delivery. The anesthetic principles are similar to those outlined under "Mitral Insufficiency," earlier in this chapter.

Cesarean Section. For cesarean section, lumbar epidural anesthesia is recommended for reasons similar to those given for mitral insufficiency. Hypotension should be treated with IV ephedrine. If general anesthesia is required, the author's group recommends a technique similar to the modified anesthetic technique outlined under "Cesarean Section Anesthesia."

Congenital Heart Disease

CHD is classified as producing either a left-to-right shunt, a right-to-left shunt, or an obstructive valvular or vascular lesion. In a report on maternal mortality in the United Kingdom for 1988 to 1990, 50% of the maternal deaths related to cardiac disease were associated with CHD.[11] The anesthesiologist must understand the basic pathophysiology of the disease, the implications of previously performed corrective surgical procedures, and the severity of existing hemodynamic derangements. For instance, consider patients with repaired ductus arteriosus or atrial septal defects (ASDs) cured.[12] In contrast with other lesions, some patients retain the original cardiac defect despite palliative procedures. Corrective surgery may produce new problems. For example, atrial incisions performed during repair may make the heart more prone to develop arrhythmias or conduction blocks. Similarly, ventriculotomy may result in residual scar tissue and lead to ventricular failure. The type and function of pacemakers also require consideration. Despite previous palliative/corrective surgery, current cardiac physiology must be known to properly plan anesthetic interventions.

Remember, there is an increased incidence of congenital heart lesions in babies of mothers with congenital heart lesions. The majority of CHD lesions follow a polygenic multifactorial mode of inheritance. Hypertrophic obstructive cardiomyopathy (HOC) and Marfan syndrome have an autosomal dominant mode of inheritance.

Left-to-Right Shunts

Ventricular Septal Defect (Fig. 18–6)

The majority of patients with ventricular septal defects (VSDs) require surgical correction during childhood and will not present significant problems during pregnancy. However, if the VSD is uncorrected, its size and any associated pulmonary hypertension determine risk.[13] Indicators of poor prognosis include hematocrits above 65%, Pa_{O_2} less than 70 mmHg, and syncopal episodes.

Pathophysiology. Left-sided cardiac pressures usually exceed right-sided pressures, and therefore, there is a left-to-right shunt through the VSD, leading to increased pulmonary blood flow and increased left ventricular work. Chronically increased pulmonary blood flow eventually causes pulmonary hypertension. Hence, right-sided heart failure, left-sided heart failure, and pulmonary edema may develop. If pulmonary resistance markedly increases or SVR decreases, the shunt may become a right-to-left shunt, producing hypoxemia if right-sided pressures exceed left ventricular pressure (see the discussion of "Eisenmenger Syndrome," later in this chapter).

Anesthetic Considerations. Overhydration or increased SVR (secondary to pain) may increase pulmonary blood flow and pulmonary congestion, producing pulmonary edema. Patients with pulmonary hypertension are at risk for developing right-to-left shunts. Avoid hypoxemia, hypercarbia, and excessive inspiratory ventilation pressures during general anesthesia because PA pressures may increase, producing a right-to-left shunt and hypoxemia. Similarly, in patients with PA hypertension, decreases in SVR can result in hypoxemia by lowering left-sided pressures below right-sided pressures, causing shunt reversal.

Recommended Analgesic Technique for Labor and Vaginal Delivery. Women with a history of VSD and heart failure or pulmonary hypertension require radial artery and CVP monitoring. During labor, lumbar epidural analgesia helps pre-

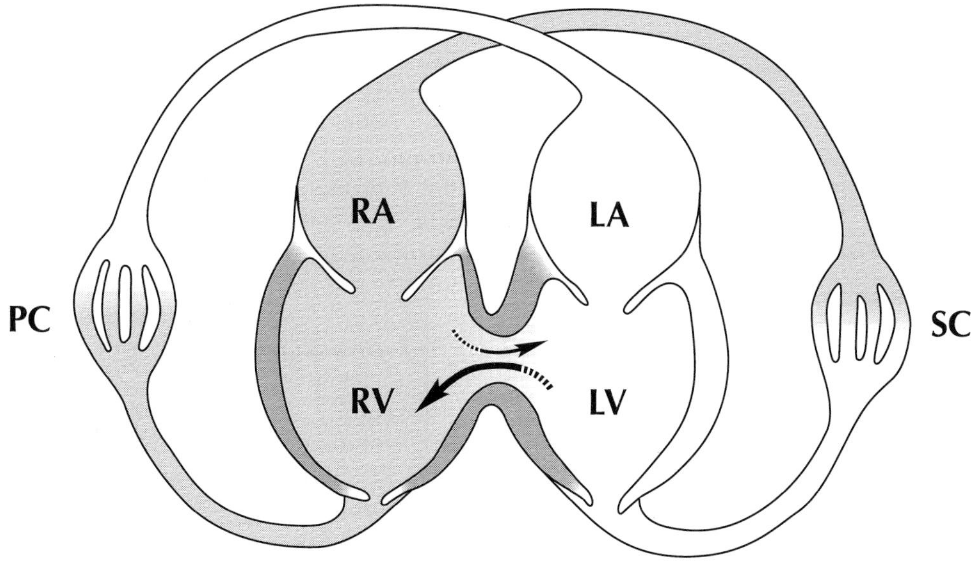

Figure 18–6. Ventricular septal defect. Note blood flow from the left ventricle through the ventricular septum into the right ventricle. Left ventricular pressure usually exceeds right ventricular pressure, leading to a left-to-right shunt. Eventually right ventricular failure will increase right ventricular pressure, equalizing or reversing the shunt. Shunt reversal, producing right-to-left shunt, will lead to peripheral cyanosis. Venous circulation is *shaded.* (*Abbreviations:* LA = left atrium; LV = left ventricle; RA = right atrium; RV = right ventricle; PC = pulmonary circulation; SC = systemic circulation.) Refer to Figure 18–1 for normal cardiac anatomy.

vent increases in SVR that potentially increase left-to-right shunt. However, avoid epidural anesthesia in patients with *severe* pulmonary hypertension or known right-to-left shunts, since they poorly tolerate SVR reductions (see "Eisenmenger Syndrome," later in this chapter).

Cesarean Section. For cesarean section, if epidural anesthesia is appropriate (no severe pulmonary hypertension, no right-to-left shunts), slowly titrate the epidural block sensory level to T4. Severe VSD symptoms mandate arterial and PA pressure monitoring to manage fluids and the patient's responses to anesthesia. For general anesthesia, use the modified anesthetic technique for cesarean section outlined previously. If significant pulmonary hypertension exists, apply the technique discussed under "Eisenmenger Syndrome," later in this chapter.

Atrial Septal Defect

Parturients with large uncorrected ASDs may develop supraventricular arrhythmias and tachycardia. If arrhythmias present acutely and produce cardiovascular instability, treat with direct current cardioversion (starting with 100 watt-sec). If the woman is relatively stable, administer propranolol in 0.5-mg increments in 5- to 10-minute intervals. These women may also develop right-sided heart failure and pulmonary hypertension if there is long-standing left-to-right shunt.

Recommended Analgesic Technique for Labor and Vaginal Delivery. Continuous lumbar analgesia, as previously described, prevents SVR increases and tachycardia while providing good analgesia.

Cesarean Section. Lumbar epidural anesthesia is preferred to general anesthesia. The same principles apply to ASD patients as to VSD patients.

Patent Ductus Arteriosus

Although this is a common congenital heart defect, patent ductus arteriosus (PDA) is usually corrected in childhood. If the shunt is small, patients tolerate the hemodynamic changes of pregnancy well. However, large shunts can lead to pulmonary hypertension and increased risk. Management should then include invasive monitoring by intra-arterial and PA catheters. Significant increases in pulmonary vascular resistance (PVR) or decreases in SVR are to be avoided, since these changes may lead to shunt reversal (right-to-left shunt) and produce hypoxemia. Epidural anesthesia is best avoided in women with severe pulmonary hypertension or known right-to-left shunts.

Recommended Analgesic Technique for Labor and Vaginal Delivery. As with the septal defects, *in the absence of pulmonary hypertension,* lumbar epidural analgesia moderates increases in SVR that may worsen left-to-right shunt.

Cesarean Section. Lumbar epidural anesthesia is preferred to general anesthesia. The same general principles apply to PDA patients as to VSD patients.

Right-to-Left Shunts

Tetralogy of Fallot (Fig. 18–7)

This is the most common cyanotic CHD among obstetric patients.[12] Significant maternal and fetal mortality occurs in women who have not had surgical correction. The lesion consists of four defects: (1) pulmonary valve or infundibular stenosis, (2) right ventricular hypertrophy, (3) an overriding aorta, and (4) VSD. Even with surgical correction, these patients may have right ventricular failure secondary to chronic right ventricular outflow tract obstruction. Indicators of poor prognosis include hematocrit greater than 65%, Pa_{O_2} less than 70 mmHg, increased right-sided heart pressures, and syncopal episodes.

Pathophysiology. Obstruction to the right outflow tract and elevated right ventricular pressures produce a right-to-left shunt through the VSD, resulting in systemic hypoxemia. If the right outflow tract obstruction is caused by dynamic infundibular hypertrophy rather than fixed valvular obstruction, increased myocardial contractility, as may occur with pain or hypotension, may worsen the obstruction. This pathophysiology is similar to HOC, which is discussed later.

Anesthetic Considerations. Women without surgical repair or those with residual right ventricu-

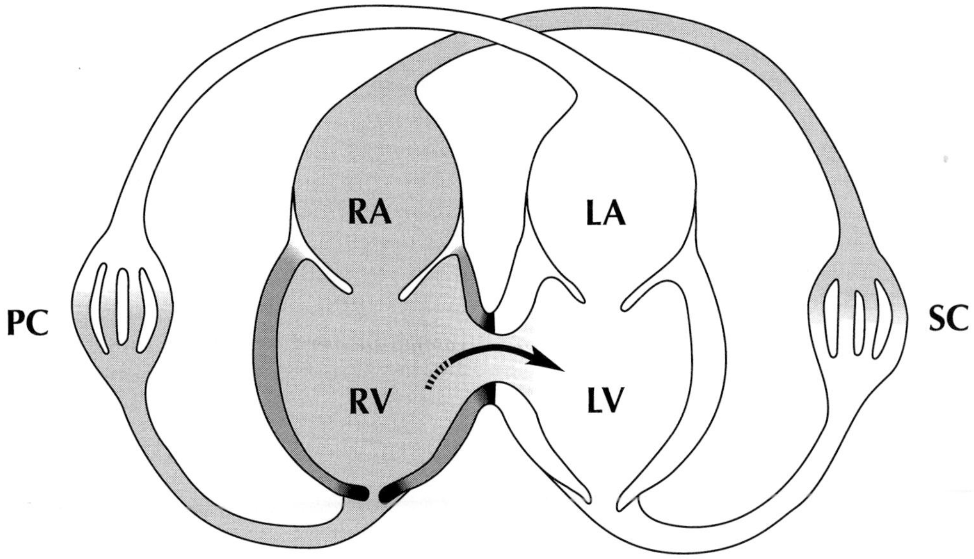

Figure 18–7. Tetralogy of Fallot. Note obstruction of the right ventricular outflow tract, elevating right ventricular pressure, producing a right-to-left shunt through the ventricular septal defect. Right ventricular outflow tract obstruction may be secondary to dynamic infundibular hypertrophy or valvular obstruction. Venous circulation is *shaded*. *(Abbreviations:* LA = left atrium; LV = left ventricle; RA = right atrium; RV = right ventricle; PC = pulmonary circulation; SC = systemic circulation.) Refer to Figure 18–1 for normal cardiac anatomy.

lar hypertension require CVP and radial artery pressure monitoring. Maintain central blood volume and venous return at baseline values by ensuring left uterine displacement, and monitor CVP pressures to guide fluid administration. In general, Swan-Ganz catheters are less useful in this patient population. They may be very difficult to float into correct position, and the calculated cardiac outputs may be meaningless. Decreases in SVR increase right-to-left shunt because PVR will be greater than SVR. Pulse oximetry monitoring will provide early noninvasive warning of worsening right-to-left shunt and hypoxemia. Administering oxygen during labor is benign and may moderate developing hypoxemia in these patients. If the pulmonary outflow obstruction is fixed, maintain contractility; if dynamic, it may be necessary to decrease right ventricular contractility with propranolol.

Recommended Analgesic Technique for Labor and Vaginal Delivery. Analgesia for labor/delivery and cesarean section is essentially similar to the techniques used for Eisenmenger syndrome (see later in this chapter for recommendations).

Eisenmenger Syndrome

Eisenmenger syndrome consists of pulmonary hypertension and right-to-left or bidirectional shunting through a long-standing ASD or VSD or PDA. Since PVR is fixed, surgical intervention offers no improvement. Maternal mortality approaches 70%, and chronic hypoxemia places the fetus at extreme risk.[12]

Anesthetic Considerations. Avoid hypoxemia, hypercarbia, and high inspiratory ventilation pressures during general anesthesia that increase PVR. Maintain central blood volume, venous return, and SVR to avoid worsening the shunt. Provide supplemental oxygenation and monitor with continuous-pulse oximetry.

Recommended Analgesic Technique for Labor and Vaginal Delivery. Regional anesthesia and the concomitant sympathetic blockade are best avoided in these patients. Intrathecal narcotics and intramuscular (IM)/IV meperidine 50 mg are options. The author's group has successfully used IV fentanyl via patient-controlled infusion (maximal dose 150 μg/hr). As discussed previously, mild, transient decreases in blood pressure may follow intrathecal sufentanil or fentanyl. This transient hypotension usually does not need treatment, but if treatment is needed (i.e., arterial saturation decreases), it responds to fluids and small boluses of dilute phenylephrine.

Cesarean Section. The author's group prefers a balanced general anesthetic for cesarean section. However, other institutions have successfully used epidural anesthesia.[14, 15] Those that use epidural anesthesia slowly induce anesthesia to allow compensatory vasoconstriction above the block and infuse dilute phenylephrine, IV as necessary to maintain preload, SVR, and oxygen saturation. When employing general anesthesia, it may be necessary to use greater than 50% O_2 if the Pa_{O_2} declines. When using oxygen concentrations greater than 50%, ensure amnesia with low-dose inhalational agents (<½ MAC). If the pulmonary outflow obstruction is dynamic, halogenated agents (½–1 MAC) may help to depress right ventricular contractility but also risk depressing uterine contractility and increasing bleeding. Treat hypotension aggressively with vasopressors. IV phenylephrine (Neo-Synephrine) may be needed to reverse hypotension. Use ephedrine cautiously, since it may increase PVR or worsen dynamic ventricular obstruction.

Other Congenital Heart Disease

Congenital Pulmonic Stenosis (Fig. 18–8)

Pulmonary valvular stenosis is a common congenital heart lesion. Right ventricular outflow obstruction may be either valvular or infundibular (subvalvular). Patients with significant stenosis usually undergo valvulotomy and tolerate pregnancy well.

Pathophysiology. Right ventricular outflow obstruction leads to right ventricular hypertrophy. Right ventricular failure eventually develops when the right ventricle cannot withstand high intraventricular pressures. If right ventricular output decreases, then left ventricular output decreases, producing syncope symptoms and fatigue.

Anesthetic Considerations. Patients with a history of right ventricular failure should be monitored with CVP and radial artery catheters. Systemic hypotension and an elevated CVP usually indicate increased right-sided heart failure. Avoid bradycardia and tachycardia, both of which may decrease CO. Maintain preload in the normal range; do not allow the patient to become dehydrated or administer excess IV fluids. Rapidly increasing intravascular volume may precipitate right ventricular failure, whereas rapid reductions in intravascular volume lead to decreased right ventricular stroke volume. Avoid potent inhalational anesthetic agents in concentrations known to be myocardial depres-

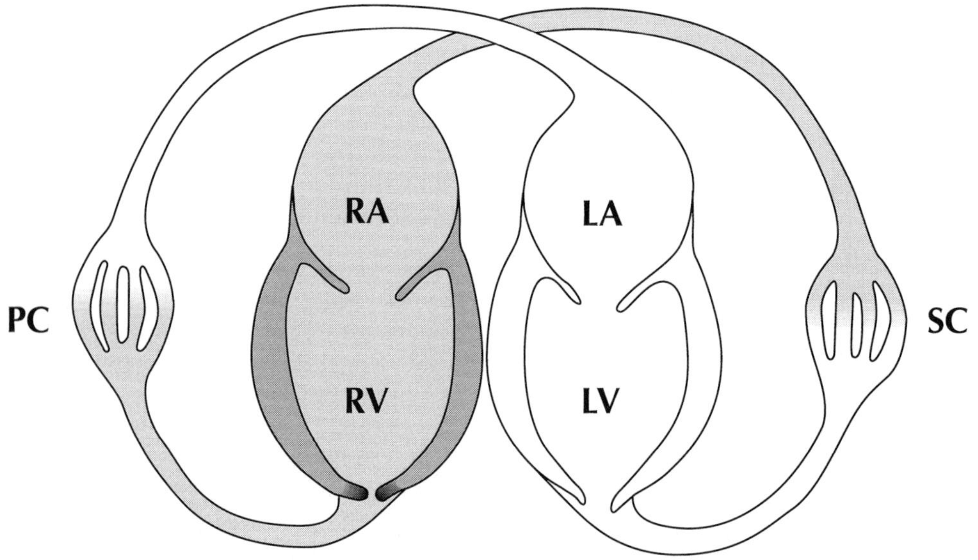

Figure 18–8. Congenital pulmonic stenosis. Note right ventricular outflow obstruction leading to right ventricular hypertrophy. Outflow obstruction may be valvular or infundibular (subvalvular). Elevated right ventricular pressures eventually lead to ventricular failure. Venous circulation is *shaded.* (*Abbreviations:* LA = left atrium; LV = left ventricle; RA = right atrium; RV = right ventricle; PC = pulmonary circulation; SC = systemic circulation.) Refer to Figure 18–1 for normal cardiac anatomy.

sants in patients with evidence of right-sided heart failure.

Recommended Analgesic Technique for Labor and Vaginal Delivery. The author's group prefers systemic narcotics for labor analgesia. Narcotics avoid the risks of decreased venous return and hypotension following epidural analgesia. Intrathecal narcotics may be an acceptable alternative. Administer a pudendal block for delivery. Occasionally, for women with poor pain control with the techniques previously described, the author's group uses epidural analgesia as outlined under "Epidural Analgesia."

Cesarean Section. General anesthesia is the preferred technique for cesarean section. To avoid possible pulmonary hypertension secondary to light anesthesia during intubation, some authors recommended using a slow inhalation induction with halothane. An inotropic infusion, such as dopamine, may be necessary to maintain blood pressure. Epinephrine, even in low doses, markedly decreases uterine blood flow. Thus, dopamine, in doses less than 10 μg/kg/min, may be a better choice, since it restores maternal blood pressure following spinal anesthesia hypotension in normal patients without compromising the neonate.[16]

Coarctation of the Aorta (Fig. 18–9)

Most patients with significant coarctation of the aorta will have undergone surgical repair prior to pregnancy and have an uneventful course. Stenosis may recur in later years. Patients with significant lesions risk aortic rupture or dissection and rupture of associated berry aneurysms of the circle of Willis. Endocarditis may also occur. The fetus is at risk if the coarctation is severe and inadequate collateral circulation impairs uterine blood flow. Some obstetricians advocate elective cesarean section to prevent the adverse effects of labor in patients with uncorrected coarctation of the aorta.

Pathophysiology. As in aortic stenosis, the left ventricle hypertrophies in response to the pressure load against a fixed obstruction and eventually fails. Avoid tachycardia and the resultant decreased diastolic time that produces inadequate ventricular filling and may lead to cardiac failure and hypotension. Avoid bradycardia or significant decreases in SVR, since stroke volume is fixed and compensation limited. Because stroke volume is fixed, anything leading to decreased ventricular filling should be avoided. Therefore, maintain venous return (hydration and uterine displacement). Blood pressure is

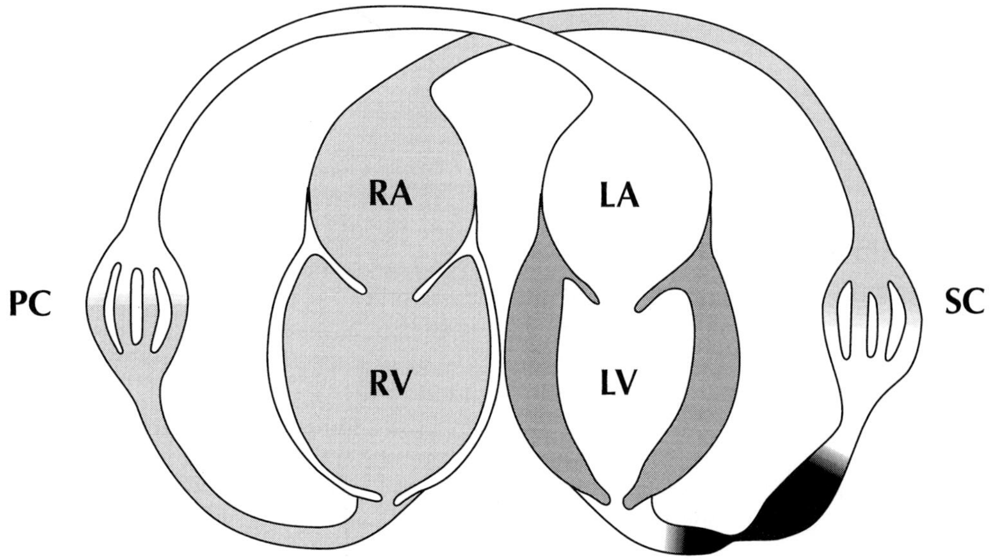

Figure 18–9. Coarctation of the aorta. Note aortic narrowing and poststenotic dilatation. Blood pressure proximal to the aortic lesion is markedly elevated; distal to the lesion, blood pressure is decreased. The left ventricle hypertrophies in response to increased back pressure and eventually fails. Venous circulation is *shaded. (Abbreviations:* LA = left atrium; LV = left ventricle; RA = right atrium; RV = right ventricle; PC = pulmonary circulation; SC = systemic circulation.) Refer to Figure 18–1 for normal cardiac anatomy.

increased proximal to the lesion, increasing risks for intracranial hemorrhage. Distal to the lesion, blood pressure decreases, potentially compromising uterine blood flow.

Recommended Analgesic Technique for Labor and Vaginal Delivery. Patients with a significant coarctation or symptoms of left ventricular failure should have radial artery and PA monitoring. Monitor blood pressure in both the upper (prestenotic) and the lower (poststenotic) extremities and guide therapy appropriately. Remember, lower limb blood pressure (poststenotic) correlates with uterine blood flow. Narcotics (IM, intrathecal, or IV) may be used for first stage of labor analgesia and a pudendal block administered for second stage analgesia. If lumbar epidural analgesia is selected, slowly and carefully titrate the block, remembering to monitor poststenotic blood pressure, which determines uterine blood flow.

Cesarean Section. One must weigh the possible risks of decreased SVR from an epidural anesthetic versus the hypertensive response to tracheal intubation. Both epidural[17] and general anesthesia for cesarean section have been successfully used. If general anesthesia is chosen, deeply anesthetize the patient with pentothal (4–6 mg/kg), and possibly fentanyl, prior to intubation. If narcotics are used, the neonatologist should be aware of risks for neonatal narcotic depression.

Other Cardiac Diseases

Hypertrophic Obstructive Cardiomyopathy (Fig. 18–10)

HOC is an autosomal dominant condition characterized by varying degrees of ventricular septal hypertrophy. During ventricular systole, the ventricular septum contracts and thickens, causing a dynamic obstruction to the left ventricular outflow tract. Symptoms of decreased left ventricular output such as exertional dyspnea, chest pain, or syncope are common, although many patients are asymptomatic and diagnosed by echocardiography. Patients with HOC are prone to atrial arrhythmias, which should be treated with propranolol or, if compromising, direct current conversion to preserve CO.

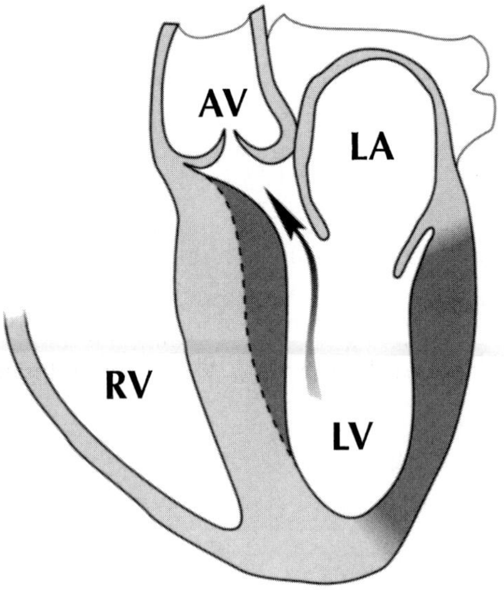

Figure 18–10. Hypertrophic obstructive cardiomyopathy. Note the hypertrophied interventricular septum causing left ventricular outflow obstruction. Increased myocardial contractility increases the outflow obstruction. Hypertrophic tissue is *shaded.* (*Abbreviations:* LA = left atrium; LV = left ventricle; RV = right ventricle; AV = aortic valve.) Refer to Figure 18–1 for normal cardiac anatomy.

Pathophysiology. With each left ventricular contraction, the hypertrophied septum contracts, increasing the obstruction to the left ventricular outflow tract. Factors that affect the obstruction are listed in Table 18–7 and must be considered when devising the anesthetic plan.

Recommended Analgesic Technique for Labor and Vaginal Delivery. Monitor significantly symptomatic patients with radial artery and PA catheters. Labor pain may increase the obstruction; therefore, good labor analgesia is desirable. The challenge is providing good analgesia without excessive sympathetic blockade. Many authors use narcotics (intrathecal, IM, or IV) to provide analgesia and utilize pudendal nerve blockade during the second stage of labor. Unfortunately, pain and tachycardia may still accompany these analgesia techniques, worsening cardiac outflow obstruction. The anesthesiologists at Wake Forest often use lumbar epidural analgesia to minimize the patient's response to pain. If epidural analgesia is used, give adequate preload (guided by PA catheter in severe cases) and consider epidural narcotics combined with weak bupiva-

TABLE 18-7
For Hypertrophic Cardiomyopathy—Factors Affecting Obstruction

Increased Obstruction	Decreased Obstruction
Increased contractility	Decreased contractility
Pain	β blockers
β-adrenergic drugs	Inhalational anesthesia
Digitalis	Ca^{2+} channel blockers
Decreased preload	Increased preload
↓ Intravascular volume	Intravenous infusion
Vasodilator drugs	Bradycardia
Valsalva maneuver	
Tachycardia	
Decreased afterload	Increased afterload
Vasodilator drugs	α-adrenergic drugs
Sympathetic blockade	Squatting
Hypovolemia	↑ Intravascular volume

caine solutions (discussed earlier). Hypotension should be treated with increased fluids and low-dose phenylephrine or metaraminol infusion. Avoid ephedrine because it may increase contractility and outflow obstruction.

Cesarean Section. A balanced general anesthetic technique supplemented with a potent inhalation agent may be used. The negative inotropic and chronotropic effects of halothane produce less tachycardia and reduction in SVR than isoflurane or enflurane. Avoid ketamine because tachycardia may decrease stroke volume and CO. Regional anesthesia for cesarean section and the accompanying total sympathectomy are best avoided.

Primary Pulmonary Hypertension

A mean PA pressure greater than 25 mmHg with no evidence of cardiorespiratory or thromboembolic disease defines primary pulmonary hypertension (PPH). Unlike the pulmonary hypertension of Eisenmenger syndrome, PPH may be responsive to vasodilator agents. Maternal mortality exceeds 50%, and therefore, these patients should deliver in a tertiary care setting.[18] PPH increases right ventricular afterload. Right ventricular hypertrophy and dilatation follow. Since CO is fixed, decreases in venous return reduce CO. Hypovolemia or decreased SVR commonly decrease CO in women with PPH.

Anesthetic Considerations. These patients should have PA and radial artery pressure monitoring. Avoid hypoxia, hypercarbia, acidosis, and mechanical hyperventilation of the lungs during general anesthesia. All can increase PVR, leading to cardiac failure. Administer oxygen during labor.

Recommended Analgesic Technique for Labor and Vaginal Delivery. Systemic or intrathecal narcotics with pudendal block for delivery are preferred to regional analgesia.

Cesarean Section. Utilize general anesthesia; however, avoid the conventional rapid-sequence induction with pentothal and succinylcholine, since this technique may precipitate increased pulmonary hypertension, myocardial depression, and cardiac failure. Since halothane or isoflurane may decrease PVR, provided SVR is maintained (see "Recommended Analgesic Technique for Labor and Vaginal Delivery," under "Eisenmenger Syndrome," earlier in this chapter), these may be desirable agents. Other authors suggest a high-dose opioid induction to minimize hemodynamic changes.[19]

Peripartum Cardiomyopathy

Peripartum cardiomyopathy is the onset of congestive heart failure in the last 4 weeks of pregnancy or the first 6 months postpartum in a patient with no previous history of cardiac disease. Parturients usually show signs and symptoms of left or right ventricular failure. The cause of the disease is unknown, and the diagnosis is made by excluding other causes of congestive heart failure.[20]

Anesthetic Considerations. Prenatal management for patients with congestive heart failure consists of fluid and sodium restriction, diuretics, and digitalis as their condition demands. Invasive monitoring by PA and radial artery catheters may be necessary during the intrapartum and immediate postpartum period. Avoid myocardial depression. In addition, painful uterine contractions may place excessive hemodynamic demands, precipitating further CO reduction. The vasodilatation that accompanies sympathetic blockade is usually beneficial, improving CO. Adequate preload must be maintained in the normal to slightly hypervolemic range and is best assessed by PA catheterization. Echocardiographic evidence of left ventricular failure 6 months' postpartum carries a poor prognosis.

Recommended Analgesic Technique for Labor and Vaginal Delivery. Epidural analgesia is the analgesic technique of choice. Labor pain that causes tachycardia, hypertension, and increased afterload worsens cardiac failure. Regional analgesia blocks these responses to pain and also may improve CO by reducing SVR. Maintain venous return with judicious IV fluids as needed and uterine displacement. Prophylactic ephedrine or arbitrary fluid preloads are not recommended.

Cesarean Section. Either general or regional anesthesia is acceptable. The author's group prefers epidural anesthesia because the block can be slowly titrated and significant changes in SVR or preload can be treated. Ephedrine is the vasopressor of choice; however, in cases of significant reductions in afterload that are unresponsive to ephedrine, phenylephrine infusion may be necessary. General anesthesia should be a nitrous/narcotic technique. Avoid inhalational agents in concentrations greater than ½ MAC, since these drugs are myocardial depressants. Remember, pentothal 4 to 6 mg/kg is a significant myocardial depressant. Induction supplementation with fentanyl 2 to 10 μg/kg and concurrent pentothal dose reductions (1–2 mg/kg) may be necessary, depending on the severity of cardiac failure. During general anesthesia, afterload reduction may be necessary. The author's group recommends sodium nitroprusside infusion guided by CO and SVR when needed during general anesthesia.

Coronary Artery Disease

The incidence of coronary artery disease in the pregnant population is 1 in 10,000.[21] Myocardial infarctions occurring during pregnancy carry a maternal mortality of up to 40%, especially if delivery occurs within 2 weeks of the infarction. Optimal anesthetic management should improve myocardial oxygen supply:demand ratio. Therefore, avoid tachycardia and elevated SVR and maintain optimal preloads. Consider invasive monitoring for patients with significant disease or unstable hemodynamics.

For labor and delivery, lumbar epidural analgesia decreases the hemodynamic stress of painful contraction, thus minimizing the risk of tachycardia and hypertension.

If cesarean section is required, lumbar epidural anesthesia combined with postdelivery epidural morphine to provide postoperative pain relief is preferable. Hemodynamically unstable patients may require high-dose narcotic general anesthesia.

Cardiac Surgery During Pregnancy

Patients with cardiac disease who deteriorate hemodynamically during pregnancy in spite of optimal medical treatment may require open heart surgery. Maternal mortality is low following surgery and cardiopulmonary bypass, but fetal mortality is high.[22] Perioperative monitoring of the fetal heart is essential, and drugs that decrease uterine blood flow should be avoided. If the parturient is near term, it may be advisable to perform a cesarean section at the beginning of the cardiac surgery.

Anesthetic Considerations. Monitor fetal heart rate in the perioperative period. An obstetric team should be available to perform an emergency cesarean section for fetal stress if indicated. Higher than normal pump flows with short bypass times are preferable.

Management of Patients With Prosthetic Valves

Several factors must be considered in the management of patients with prosthetic valves.[23] They may have residual ventricular dysfunction, arrhythmias, or pulmonary hypertension. In addition, women with mechanical valves require full anticoagulation in addition to bacterial endocarditis prophylaxis. Warfarin is relatively contraindicated, as it has associated fetal teratogenic effects. Heparin is, therefore, preferred because it does not cross the placental barrier.

Regional anesthesia is controversial in these patients. If heparin must be continued throughout labor and delivery, systemic narcotics should be used for labor and general anesthesia for cesarean section. An alternative approach is to discontinue heparin for 6 hours and administer lumbar epidural anesthesia if the prothrombin time and partial thromboplastin time values at that time are normal. Six hours after the removal of the epidural catheter heparin therapy may be restarted.

Marfan Syndrome

Marfan syndrome is a autosomal dominant collagen vascular disease. In addition to musculoskeletal abnormalities, patients may develop mitral valve prolapse, progressive dilatation of the aortic root, aortic incompetence, dissecting aortic aneurysm, and rupture of the aorta. In one review of 32 pregnant women with Marfan syndrome, one half died and 4 survived acute aortic dissection.[24] The incidence of aortic dissection increases during pregnancy, and parturients may develop aortic dissection during labor.[25, 26]

Signs and symptoms of aortic dissection include back or chest pain, shortness of breath, syncope, tachycardia, or extremity ischemia. Chest x-ray may reveal a widening mediastinum or hemothorax. Magnetic resonance imaging may be useful, but aortic dye radiography is the definitive diagnostic test.

Treatment of aortic dissection includes management of hypertension with vasodilators and β-adrenergic-blocking drugs and surgery. Small, nonprogressing dissections may be followed medically, and these women may tolerate a well-controlled labor and vaginal delivery.

Anesthetic Considerations. Women with Marfan syndrome should be managed according to their symptoms. Women without symptoms and demonstrating good exercise tolerance can be managed in a standard fashion. Patients with signs of aortic root enlargement are often placed on β-adrenergic-blocking drugs to decrease the ventricular ejection force and the aortic wall shear stress. However, all women with Marfan syndrome, regardless of the disease severity, should be observed for the possibility of developing aortic dissection during the stress of labor. Women with significant disease should avoid the additional hemodynamic stress of expulsive efforts. This is best accomplished by dense epidural anesthesia throughout the course of labor, with delivery accomplished by forceps or vacuum extraction. Remember, consider aortic dissection if the patient complains of persistent back pain during or after epidural anesthesia.

Cardiac Arrest

If cardiopulmonary resuscitation (CPR) is required, it is important to maintain left uterine displacement in the mother, and CPR should be performed on a hard surface. The primary concern should be survival of the mother. Standard advanced cardiac life support (ACLS) protocols should be utilized. Direct current cardioversion with energy settings as high as 100 watt/sec have been used with no adverse effects to the fetus.[27] No indicated resuscitation drugs or energy settings for direct current cardioversion should be withheld out of fear of harming the fetus. In general, CPR is relatively ineffective in near-term pregnancy. To resuscitate the mother, it may be necessary to deliver the baby by emergency cesarean section. Maternal and fetal survival are best when cesarean sections are performed within 10 minutes of maternal arrest.

SUMMARY

First, the anesthesiologist must understand the pathophysiology of the specific cardiac lesion. These patients are best managed by a team, consisting of anesthesiologist, cardiologist, and obstetrician. Patients with symptomatic or high-risk cardiac disease are best managed with invasive monitors. The information gained from invasive monitoring often outweighs the risks associated with insertion. If tachycardia or increased cardiac outputs are harmful, slowly establish a lumbar epidural anesthetic. If decreases in SVR will compromise the patient, avoid lumbar epidural anesthesia or slowly titrate the block. If fentanyl 2 μg/ml is added to the local anesthetic as a continuous infusion, 0.125% or 0.0625% bupivacaine can be used with minimal hemodynamic changes. As in all term parturients, left uterine displacement is essential. As an alternative, use narcotics (intrathecal, IM, or IV PCA); however, intrathecal sufentanil may have associated hypotensive risks. Epidural morphine, patient-controlled epidural analgesia, or IV narcotic infusions provide excellent postpartum analgesia and will minimize cardiovascular stress.

TEN PRACTICAL POINTS

1. Compulsively ensure uterine displacement; reductions in preload and cardiac output may be catastrophic in these patients.

2. Use saline solution to identify the epidural space by loss of resistance; intravascular air should be avoided in all women with possible right-to-left intracardiac shunts.

3. Labor analgesia using intravenous patient-controlled analgesia fentanyl is a reasonable alternative when regional anesthesia is contraindicated.

4. Remember that small risk of mild, transient hypotension may accompany the use of intrathecal fentanyl or sufentanil.

5. Supplemental oxygen via a nonrebreathing mask is always benign and often beneficial.

6. Avoid testing the epidural catheter for intravenous placement with epinephrine solutions; sudden tachycardia may be undesirable.

7. Avoid the use of epidural 2-chloroprocaine if epidural narcotics are desirable.

8. Avoid arbitrary prophylactic infusions.

9. Back pain during labor in women with Marfan syndrome may be an indication of aortic root dissection.

10. Remember, maternal and fetal survival are best when emergency cesarean section is performed within 10 minutes of cardiac arrest.

REFERENCES

1. Mason SJ: Cardiac failure and arrhythmias during pregnancy. *In* Berkowitz RL (ed): Critical Care of the Obstetric Patient. New York, Churchill Livingstone, 1983, pp 481–504.
2. Clark SL: Labor and delivery in the patient with structural cardiac disease. Clin Perinatol 13:695–703, 1986.
3. Hess DB, Hess LW: Management of cardiovascular disease in pregnancy. Obstet Gynecol Clin North Am 19:679–695, 1992.
4. Leighton BL, DeSimone CA, Norris MC, Ben-David B: Intrathecal narcotics for labor revisited: The combination of fentanyl and morphine intrathecally provides rapid onset of profound, prolonged analgesia. Anesth Analg 69:122–125, 1989.
5. D'Angelo R, Anderson MT, Philip J, Eisenach JC: Intrathecal sufentanil compared to epidural bupivacaine for labor analgesia. Anesthesiology 80:1209–1215, 1994.
6. Grice SC, Eisenach JC, Dewan DM: Labor analgesia with epidural bupivacaine plus fentanyl: Enhancement with epinephrine and inhibition with 2-chloroprocaine. Anesthesiology 72:623–628, 1990.
7. Ueland K: Rheumatic heart disease and pregnancy. *In* Elkayam U (ed): Diagnosis and Management of Maternal and Fetal Disease, 2nd ed. New York, Alan R Liss, 1990, pp 99–107.
8. Braunwald E: Valvular heart disease. *In* Braunwald E (ed): Heart Disease: A Textbook of Cardiovascular Medicine, 4th ed. Philadelphia, WB Saunders, 1992, pp 1007–1077.
9. al Kasab SM, Sabag T, al Zaibag M, et al: Beta-adrenergic receptor blockade in the management of pregnant women with mitral stenosis. Am J Obstet Gynecol 163:37–40, 1990.
10. Rayburn WF: Mitral valve prolapse and pregnancy. *In* Elkayam U (ed): Diagnosis and Management of Maternal and Fetal Disease, 2nd ed. New York, Alan R Liss, 1990, pp 181–188.
11. Report on Confidential Enquiries into Maternal Deaths in the United Kingdom 1988–1990. London, HMSO, 1994.
12. Ramin SM, Mayberry MC, Gilstrap LC III: Congenital heart disease. Clin Obstet Gynecol 32:41–47, 1989.
13. Patton DE, Lee W, Cotton DB, et al: Cyanotic maternal heart disease in pregnancy. Obstet Gynecol Surv 45:594–600, 1990.
14. Spinnato JA, Kraynack BJ, Cooper MW: Eisenmenger's syndrome in pregnancy: Epidural anesthesia for elective cesarean section. N Engl J Med 304:1215–1217, 1981.
15. Johnson MD, Saltzman D: Cardiac disease. *In* Datta S (ed): Anesthetic and Obstetric Management of High-Risk Pregnancy. St. Louis, CV Mosby, 1991, pp 245–248.
16. Clark RB, Brunner JA III: Dopamine for the treatment of spinal hypotension during cesarean section. Anesthesiology 53:514–517, 1980.
17. Mangano DT: Anesthesia for the pregnant cardiac patient. *In* Shnider SM, Levinson G (eds): Anaesthesia for Obstetrics, 2nd ed. Baltimore, Williams & Wilkins, 1987, pp 345–381.
18. Roberts NV, Keast PJ: Pulmonary hypertension and pregnancy—A lethal combination. Anaesth Intensive Care 18:366–374, 1990.
19. Ferguson JE II, Wyner J, Albright GA, Brodsky JB: Maternal health complications. *In* Albright GA, Ferguson JE II, Joyce TH III, Stevenson DK (eds): Anaesthesia in Obstetrics: Maternal, Fetal and Neonatal Aspects. Boston, Butterworths, 1986, pp 374–420.
20. Lee W, Cotton DB: Peripartum cardiomyopathy: Current concepts and clinical management. Clin Obstet Gynecol 32:54–67, 1989.
21. Nolan TE, Hankins GD: Myocardial infarction in pregnancy. Clin Obstet Gynecol 32:68–75, 1989.
22. Spielman FJ: Anaesthetic management of the ob-

stetric patient with cardiac disease. Clin Anesth 4:247–260, 1986.
23. McColgin SW, Martin JN Jr, Morrison JC: Pregnant women with prosthetic heart valves. Clin Obstet Gynecol 32:76–88, 1989.
24. Pyeritz RE: Maternal and fetal complications of pregnancy in the Marfan syndrome. Am J Med 71:784–90, 1981.
25. Schnitker MA, Bayer CA: Dissecting aneurysm of the aorta in young individuals, particularly in association with pregnancy. Ann Intern Med 20:486–511, 1944.
26. Ferguson JE II, Ueland K, Stinson EB, Maly RP: Marfan's syndrome: Acute aortic dissection during labor, resulting in fetal distress and cesarean section, followed by successful surgical repair. Am J Obstet Gynecol 147:759–762, 1983.
27. Vogel JHK, Pryor R, Blount SG Jr: Direct-current defibrillation during pregnancy. JAMA 193:970–971, 1965.

NINETEEN

Complex Medical Problems

M. Joanne Douglas, M.D., F.R.C.P.(C.)

Parturients with complex medical problems present a challenge to the anesthesiologist, since the choice of anesthesia may be limited owing to involvement of the airway and back as well as to changes in coagulation and neuromuscular function. This chapter outlines the anesthetic management of parturients with scoliosis (corrected and uncorrected), spinal cord injury, multiple sclerosis (MS), coagulation problems, connective tissue disorders (systemic lupus erythematosus [SLE], systemic sclerosis, rheumatoid arthritis [RA]), muscular dystrophy, myasthenia gravis, and acquired immunodeficiency syndrome (AIDS). As a first rule, consider referral to an anesthesiologist or institution with additional expertise and facilities managing more complex problems. In the following discussion, when specific problems are not identified, routine drug dosage and obstetric anesthetic management are implied.

ORTHOPEDIC AND NEUROLOGIC DISORDERS

Scoliosis

Scoliosis is a rotational deformity of the spine and ribs, which is either idiopathic or secondary to neuromuscular or connective tissue disorders. Depending on the severity of the curvature, impairment of respiratory and cardiac functions can occur.[1] Often the deformity increases with time, ultimately requiring surgical correction to prevent deterioration of cardiorespiratory function. Patients with corrected or stabilized defects usually tolerate pregnancy and delivery well.

Severe scoliosis (Cobb angle greater than 90 degrees) reduces lung volumes, produces ventilation-perfusion inequalities, decreases the response to carbon dioxide, and increases pulmonary vascular resistance. During pregnancy, in patients with uncorrected kyphoscoliosis, hypoxia risk increases with gestation owing to the progressive increases in oxygen consumption and alveolar ventilation requirements imposed by pregnancy and secondary to encroachment on the thorax by the enlarging uterus. Maternal dyspnea may necessitate early delivery. Despite delivery, cardiorespiratory failure can occur postpartum, and the anesthesia and obstetric care teams must remain alert throughout the peripartum period.

Labor Analgesia

The usual forms of analgesia are appropriate for parturients with corrected or mild scoliosis.[2, 3] In early labor, massage, heat, Lamaze techniques, and transcutaneous electrical nerve stimulation (TENS) are useful (Table 19–1). Inhalational analgesia (nitrous oxide and oxygen), if available, provides short-term analgesia and is particularly helpful for the multiparous patient. Parenteral narcotics (intramuscular, intravenous) are useful when regional analgesia is unsuccessful or contraindicated.[4] Indeed, regional techniques may prove technically difficult in these parturients, and some anesthesiolo-

TABLE 19–1
Alternatives to Epidural Analgesia

Alternative	Methods
Nonpharmacologic	Heat Massage Lamaze techniques TENS
Inhalational	Self-administered nitrous oxide and oxygen 50:50 mixture—inhaled during contractions
Narcotics	*Intramuscular* *Intravenous PCA fentanyl:* 1 μg/kg loading dose, 25 μg bolus, lockout 5–15 minutes *Intrathecal:* Morphine 250 μg and fentanyl 25 μg

Abbreviations: TENS = transcutaneous electrical nerve stimulation; PCA = patient-controlled analgesia.

Data from Coalson DW, Glosten B: Alternatives to epidural analgesia. Semin Perinatol 15:375, 1991.

gists only reluctantly attempt them. Persistent back pain frequently accompanies scoliosis, and considering the potentially difficult placement, it is important to explain the risks and benefits of regional analgesia to the patient prior to its initiation. When utilized, epidural analgesia requires usual incremental injections of local anesthetics, and management resembles that of normal parturients.

Potentially easier identification of the subarachnoid space makes spinal opioids a reasonable alternative to the usual epidural technique or when epidural analgesia fails. The recommended doses of spinal opioids are 250 to 300 μg of morphine with or without 25 μg of fentanyl. Remember, although intrathecal morphine and fentanyl produce analgesia for the first stage of labor,[5] delivery may require pudendal or saddle block anesthesia.

Anesthesia for Cesarean Section

Both general and regional anesthesia are suitable for cesarean section in parturients with mild or corrected scoliosis. However, when scoliosis is secondary to muscular disease, it is important to assess cardiorespiratory function prior to surgery to identify additional risk factors. Patients with muscle disorders, such as muscular dystrophy, may have poor pulmonary function and may experience an increased risk of cardiac abnormalities. In this setting, pulmonary function studies are useful to identify patients at risk for postoperative respiratory failure. Close monitoring in an intensive care unit setting may be required for 24 to 48 hours. Parturients with underlying valvular heart disorders require antibiotic prophylaxis.

The parturient with severe scoliosis is frequently underweight, so the doses of local anesthetics and intravenous agents (narcotics, anesthetic induction agents, sedatives) must be carefully titrated to avoid overdose. Slow incremental administration allows more precise drug titration.

Although the indications for blood transfusion are the same as for other parturients, small patients, such as those with severe scoliosis, require transfusion of blood products after a smaller absolute blood loss than normal-sized adults. However, difficulty in estimating fluid and blood requirements may lead to fluid overload and cardiac failure. A central venous pressure monitoring line is useful in managing fluid balance in the parturient with severe scoliosis.

Compared with regional anesthesia for cesarean section, spinal anesthesia may be technically easier to perform and provides a clearly defined end-point, namely identification of cerebrospinal fluid. Theoretically, scarring in the epidural space from previous surgery (fusion, Harrington rod insertion) may increase the risk of unintentional dural puncture while the anesthesiologist attempts an epidural or inadequate epidural block secondary to poor spread of local anesthetic following placement.[2, 6]

In the author's experience, there is an increased incidence of complications and an increased degree of difficulty in identifying the epidural space. However, once the epidural space is identified, it is generally possible to obtain a successful block. Success may depend on using increased volume or concentration of local anesthetic or adding an opiate, such as fentanyl, or epinephrine. Although it is wise to caution the parturient with a history of previous spinal surgery to expect a higher incidence of difficulty in initiating the block or complications, one can reassure her that the chances of a patchy or incomplete block are similar to those in patients without a history of spinal surgery.

Problems With General Anesthesia
(Table 19–2)

In parturients with severe, uncorrected scoliosis, ventilation problems may be encountered

TABLE 19–2
General Anesthesia: Problems and Their Management

Problem	Management
Oxygenation	Increase inspired oxygen concentration Monitor oxygen saturation
Muscle relaxation	Avoid succinylcholine if muscle wasting is present Use nondepolarizing agents Use awake intubation
Postoperative respiratory depression	Titrate induction agents and narcotics Ventilate postoperatively
Restricted pulmonary function	Ventilate postoperatively as required

secondary to the underlying disease process (e.g., spinal muscular atrophy, polio, osteogenesis imperfecta) and may require postpartum mechanical ventilation. Intraoperatively, higher inspired oxygen concentrations may be required, emphasizing the need for monitoring oxygen saturation. Succinylcholine is relatively contraindicated in parturients with severe muscle wasting, as there may be a massive release of potassium, resulting in cardiac arrhythmias and arrest. Precurarization with a nondepolarizing muscle relaxant to avoid fasciculations does not prevent potassium release. Awake intubation or nondepolarizing agents provide alternatives. Carefully titrated induction agents and narcotics avoid the risk of postoperative respiratory depression.

Problems With Regional Anesthesia (Table 19–3)

Difficulty is often encountered in performing regional anesthesia owing to problems in accurately identifying the midline. The sitting position tends to eliminate additional distortion from lateral flexion and may improve the chance of identifying the epidural-intrathecal space. Positioning the sterile drapes for an unobstructed view of the entire spine allows one to follow the curvature from the neck to the buttocks. Select the widest available intervertebral space. For example, if the patient has had surgery and the scar extends to L2–3, attempt L3–4.

Infiltrate the area well with local anesthetic. Adequate analgesia increases the patient's tolerance during difficult placement. If performed for an elective procedure, consider applying topical local anesthetic (lidocaine-prilocaine mixture [EMLA cream]) at least 1 hour prior to the procedure, followed by local infiltration. Bicarbonate increases local anesthetic pH and decreases the pain of local infiltration. Explain the procedure as it is performed and enlist the parturient's cooperation in identifying the middle of her neuraxis. Ask her to tell where she "feels the pressure of the needle." If the pressure is not in the midline she will say that it is to the right or the left. Direct the needle according to her instructions.

If unintentional dural puncture occurs, consider converting to a continuous spinal using the epidural catheter.[7] Use small doses of preservative-free local anesthetic (1 ml of 0.25% bupivacaine [2.5 mg] or 1 ml of 0.5 to 1% lidocaine [5 to 10 mg]) and monitor the level of the block frequently.

When a patchy or inadequate epidural block occurs, use a larger volume of bupivacaine (12 ml of 0.125%) combined with epinephrine (1:400,000 to 1:800,000). A bolus dose of epidural fentanyl 1 μg/kg in a volume of 10-ml saline solution is also helpful. Continuous infusions of 0.1 to 0.125% bupivacaine, with or with-

TABLE 19–3
Regional Anesthesia: Problems and Their Management

Problem	Management
Insertion of epidural	Place patient in sitting position Ask patient where she "feels the needle"
Patchy block	Use a large-volume, dilute local anesthetic in the epidural catheter Add epinephrine 2.5 μg/ml Add fentanyl 2 μg/ml
Accidental dural puncture	Convert to continuous spinal anesthesia with epidural catheter
Backache	Position carefully during labor

out 1 to 2 μg/ml of fentanyl, at a rate of 8 to 12 ml/hour, reduce the need for repeated bolus doses of local anesthetic. Remember, block failure is not always secondary to the disease process. Replacement may work.

Finally, emphasize to the patient and obstetrician the importance of good back care (frequent position changes and a pillow under or between the knees) during the duration of the epidural. This may decrease the incidence and severity of postpartum backache. Maintain left uterine displacement.

The awake parturient with severe scoliosis and respiratory compromise may not tolerate the supine and wedged position for surgery. Rarely, general anesthesia may be required to ensure adequate ventilation.

Spinal opiates for post–cesarean section analgesia allow early ambulation and improve the respiratory status. Close monitoring of respiratory function is necessary.

The Spinal Cord–Injured Parturient

An increasing number of women with spinal cord injury are becoming pregnant.[8, 9] Patients with spinal cord injury frequently experience repeated urinary tract infections, anemia, muscle atrophy, decubitus ulcers, and thromboembolic events. With spinal cord injuries above T5, postural hypotension, respiratory compromise, and autonomic hyperreflexia (AH) occur. AH, characterized by hypertension, headache, anxiety, sweating, piloerection, and bradycardia, arises in response to stimuli occurring below the level of the cord injury. In parturients, stimuli such as uterine contractions (labor), delivery, vaginal examinations, and bladder distention may trigger AH.

AH is common with lesions above T5, but it may also occur with lower lesions. As discussed, uterine contractions (labor) or delivery may trigger an episode of AH. Anxiolytics such as midazolam may decrease stress-induced catecholamine release. Arteriolar vasodilators (sodium nitroprusside, phentolamine) may control the hypertension but can also cause wide fluctuations in blood pressure (hypertension to hypotension). Hypertension is best controlled by decreasing afferent impulses to the spinal cord using regional analgesia. Evidence suggests that most spinal and epidural narcotics are ineffective in preventing AH. Epidural fentanyl does not prevent AH[10] but will improve the quality of a local anesthetic block. However, epidural meperidine alone has successfully prevented AH,[11] probably secondary to its local anesthetic properties.

Labor Analgesia (Table 19–4)

Determine the level of injury and the duration of the paralysis in order to estimate the risk of AH. When AH first appears is unpredictable, but AH does not occur during the period of spinal shock (areflexia at or below the level of injury) that may last up to a few months following injury. Question the patient regarding AH and its frequency. Remember, a negative history of AH does not eliminate its possible occurrence during labor.

The spinal cord–injured patient may not experience labor pain. Indeed, the obstetrician may plan elective induction of labor, since spinal cord–injury patients frequently have premature silent labor. Although the level of injury may be high enough to preclude pain during labor, epidural analgesia is, nevertheless, indicated to prevent AH. Place the epidural catheter early in labor. If the patient is not in labor, apply a topical local anesthetic (lidocaine-prilocaine mixture) 1 hour before epidural placement. Importantly, reflex spasm and AH may occur during positioning, local anesthetic infil-

TABLE 19–4
The Spinal Cord–Injured Parturient: Potential Problems During Labor and Their Management

Problem	Management
Hypothermia	Use warm intravenous fluids Provide warm room, blankets
Hypotension	Ensure adequate fluid preload
Autonomic hyperreflexia	Establish epidural analgesia, secure catheter (tincture benzoin) Use anxiolytics, antihypertensives
Hypoxia	Supplement oxygen
Bladder distention	Use Foley catheter
Decubitus ulcers	Change patient's position frequently Cushion pressure areas

tration, or epidural catheter insertion. Be prepared!

Closely monitor the blood pressure with an automatic, noninvasive blood pressure monitor. If cardiovascular instability occurs or the epidural is ineffective, it may be necessary to insert a central venous catheter and arterial catheter to allow accurate control of hypertension with potent vasoactive drugs. Pulse oximetry is useful to assess ventilation, and supplemental oxygen may be required with higher spinal cord lesions.

An intravenous preload (500 to 1000 ml of Ringer lactate or normal saline solution) is essential because these patients are prone to hypotension owing to impaired vasomotor autoregulation. Incremental injection (3 to 5 ml at a time) of local anesthetic (0.125% bupivacaine) to a total volume of 10 to 12 ml lessens the likelihood of maternal hypotension by slowing the onset of blockade. Assessment of the level of epidural block may be difficult if the level of the spinal cord lesion extends above T8. Control of the symptoms of AH may be the only guideline.

Secure the epidural catheter well. During AH, sweating increases and the tape may "peel off." Application of tincture of benzoin increases tape adherence.

These patients are prone to develop hypothermia. Use warm intravenous fluids and keep the environmental temperature warm. Position the patient carefully during labor to prevent decubitus ulcers. Remember, epidural analgesia may mask bladder distention, which can evoke AH, so these patients usually require a Foley catheter.

Monitor patients closely for at least 12 hours following delivery, since AH can occur postpartum, and do not remove the epidural catheter until the patient is transferred to the ward.

Anesthesia for Cesarean Section

The major anesthetic concerns during cesarean section resemble those for labor and include possible AH, respiratory embarrassment problems (including the need for ventilatory assistance), and hypotension. In parturients with spinal cord injury levels above T8, avoid general anesthesia, if possible, since fairly deep levels of general anesthesia are required to prevent AH. Deep general anesthesia increases the risk of uterine hypotonia and bleeding and newborn depression. It may be necessary to combine general anesthesia with regional anesthesia in order to assist ventilation and avoid the problems of AH in the parturient with respiratory compromise.

General anesthesia requires direct arterial and central venous monitoring. Succinylcholine is contraindicated in patients with recent spinal cord injury (1 week to 12 months) or severe muscle wasting, since severe hyperkalemia and cardiac arrest may occur (Table 19–5). Increased depths of anesthesia are essential to prevent AH; thus, the neonatologist should be alerted to the risk of a depressed newborn from the volatile anesthetic. Have drugs to treat hypertension (sodium nitroprusside) and hypotension readily available. If administered briefly, vasoactive drugs should not affect the newborn.

Regional anesthesia for cesarean section prevents AH. With higher spinal cord lesions, utilize a slow induction of epidural anesthesia with incremental boluses (3 to 5 ml) of local anesthetic (2% lidocaine with 5 μg/ml epinephrine). Monitor the blood pressure closely and treat hypotension with additional intravenous fluids and incremental boluses of ephedrine (5 to 10 mg). If an unintentional dural puncture occurs, a continuous spinal technique with incremental administration of lidocaine (5 to 10 mg) or bupivacaine (2.5 to 5.0 mg) is a useful alternative. Spinal anesthesia is suitable for parturients with lesions below T6. With lesions above this level, anesthesia is not required for surgery but is still required to prevent AH.

Invasive hemodynamic monitoring during cesarean section may be advantageous in quadriplegic parturients for accurate monitoring of blood pressure and titration of fluids. Noninvasive monitoring is suitable for parturients with levels of spinal cord injury below T8, without evidence of AH. Parturients with levels of injury above T2 may not tolerate lying supine. Supplemental oxygen and adjustment of the operating room table to provide a head-up position may overcome this problem. Prior discussion with

TABLE 19–5
Alternatives to Succinylcholine for Intubation

Awake intubation under topical anesthesia
Vecuronium 0.25 mg/kg or atracurium 1.5 mg/kg

the obstetrician should allow a suitable compromise between surgical exposure and patient comfort. Induction of general anesthesia with endotracheal intubation and positive-pressure ventilation may rarely be required. The combination of general anesthesia (to overcome respiratory embarrassment) and epidural anesthesia (to prevent AH) is a reasonable compromise for these parturients.

Multiple Sclerosis

Multiple sclerosis (MS) is a demyelinating disease of the brain and spinal cord, usually occurring in young adults and characterized by exacerbations and remissions over a period of years. The symptoms and signs of MS depend on the areas of demyelination. Vision, gait, bladder function, sensation, and motor power are commonly affected. Pregnancy does not appear to increase the risk of exacerbation.

Anesthetic Considerations

Anesthesiologists are often reluctant to administer spinal or epidural anesthesia to these patients, fearing the procedure might be blamed for an exacerbation of MS.[12] There is no evidence that epidural anesthesia causes exacerbation. Theoretically, spinal anesthesia might cause an exacerbation owing to the close proximity of the local anesthetic to demyelinated areas. Thus, epidural anesthesia is probably the preferable technique.

Labor Analgesia

TENS, inhalational analgesia, and narcotics (intramuscular, intravenous, and subarachnoid) are acceptable for labor analgesia in parturients with MS. Continuous spinal analgesia with local anesthetics is probably best avoided for the reasons noted previously. Do not deny patients epidural analgesia-anesthesia for labor and delivery, provided the risks and benefits are fully explained and alternatives offered (see Table 19–1). Management resembles that for normal patients.

Anesthesia for Cesarean Section

Epidural anesthesia is preferable to spinal anesthesia for the reasons listed earlier. Drug selection does not differ from normal. General anesthesia risks potential exaggerated response to nondepolarizing muscle relaxants such as atracurium or vecuronium. Use a peripheral nerve stimulator to titrate neuromuscular-blocking agents. When possible, avoid succinylcholine if severe muscle wasting exists because of potential excess potassium release and cardiac arrest. Precurarization may attenuate fasciculations but does not prevent potassium release.

HEMATOLOGIC DISORDERS

Pregnancy has been termed a "hypercoagulable" state, since several clotting factors increase and some anticoagulant factors decrease (Table 19–6). Normal parturients are prone to thrombosis, especially in light of the increased venous stasis accompanying pregnancy.

Parturients who have "hypocoagulable" disorders pose special anesthetic concerns.[13] Coagulation abnormalities increase the risk of life-threatening hemorrhage at delivery and postpartum and may also limit available anesthetic options. For example, regional anesthesia (epidural or spinal) is relatively contraindicated in parturients with coagulation abnormalities because of the risk of epidural hematoma. In approximately 10% of patients, an epidural vein is punctured during routine epidural needle placement.[14] Subsequent bleeding into the epidural space in patients with a coagulation abnormality may produce an epidural hematoma and possible neurologic deficit. The incidence of epidural hematoma related to epidural analgesia in parturients is rare, approximately 1 in 500,000 epidurals.[15] (The incidence of epidural hematoma in hypocoagulable patients is un-

TABLE 19–6
Changes in Coagulation Factors That Occur With Pregnancy

Coagulation Factor	Change
Factor VII	Increased
Factor VIII	Increased
Factor X	Increased
Fibrinogen	Increased
Antithrombin III	Normal or decreased
Protein S	Decreased

known.) The diagnosis of epidural hematoma centers on complaints of severe back pain and tenderness associated with neurologic signs (sensory and motor). Radiologic confirmation with myelography should be promptly followed by surgical exploration and evacuation of the clot. Importantly, recovery appears to be related to the duration of symptoms. Act quickly!

When considering regional anesthesia in patients at risk for hypocoagulability, select appropriate screening tests for coagulation abnormalities based on the history and physical examination. Although the bleeding time is useful to screen Von Willebrand disease, it is not useful as a screening test for platelet abnormalities. A history of clinical bleeding or bruising requires further investigation. Platelet count, prothrombin time, partial thromboplastin time (PTT), and fibrinogen level are useful initial screening tests. Insufficient information exists at present to determine the value of thromboelastography as a screening tool.

Platelet Disorders

Platelets are an integral part of the coagulation process, forming the initial plug when a vessel is cut or punctured. Bleeding may result from quantitative (not enough platelets) or qualitative (poor platelet function) disorders. Platelets decrease in parturients with gestational thrombocytopenia (low platelets without apparent cause); idiopathic thrombocytopenic purpura (ITP); hemolysis, elevated liver enzymes, low platelets (HELLP) syndrome; and disseminated intravascular coagulation. Although in the past the bleeding time was used to assess platelet function, recent reviews suggest that it is an unreliable test[16] for predicting clinical bleeding in this setting.

Gestational Thrombocytopenia

Women with gestational thrombocytopenia have lower than normal platelet counts ($<150 \times 10^9$/L) during pregnancy unrelated to a pathologic process. Platelet counts return to normal postpartum. Usually the platelet count exceeds 100×10^9/L, and these patients do not risk bleeding.[17]

Idiopathic Thrombocytopenic Purpura

ITP typically affects young adults, including parturients.[18] The platelets in this disorder are more susceptible to premature destruction, resulting in a lower platelet count. The remaining platelets are generally young platelets and more hemostatically competent. Bleeding tends to occur when the platelet count declines below 50×10^9/L. Importantly, the antibody that leads to the destruction of the platelets can cross the placenta, leading to newborn thrombocytopenia, increasing the risk of intracranial hemorrhage in the newborn during vaginal delivery. These patients often deliver by cesarean section.

Although 100×10^9/L has been considered the lowest acceptable platelet count for regional anesthesia, providing there is no evidence of clinical bleeding or bruising and the platelet count is above 75×10^9/L, the author believes regional anesthesia is not contraindicated in the parturient with ITP. When the platelet count is between 50 and 75×10^9/L, the author uses a regional technique, provided there is no evidence of clinical bleeding or bruising and that other alternatives, such as patient-controlled analgesia (PCA) narcotics for labor or general anesthesia for cesarean section, *are not suitable.* Spinal anesthesia with its smaller needle may pose less risk than epidural anesthesia.

Other Disorders of Coagulation

Von Willebrand Disease

This inherited disorder affects approximately 1 in 10,000 people and is clinically suspected when there is a history of prolonged bleeding, usually at surgery. A prolonged bleeding time confirms the diagnosis. During pregnancy, mild Von Willebrand disease may completely resolve, reducing the risk of hemorrhage.[19] In contrast, if the severe form is present, the parturient may require cryoprecipitate to prevent hemorrhage.

Severity of illness dictates anesthetic options. In the milder forms, which have a normal bleeding time, regional anesthesia may be safely given. If the severe form is present, regional anesthesia is contraindicated.

Iatrogenic: Aspirin and Heparin

In addition to the normal "hypercoagulable" state of pregnancy, certain disorders increase the pregnant patient's risk for thrombosis. Examples of these disorders are the inherited Protein C, Protein S, and anti–thrombin III deficiencies. Lupus anticoagulant and anticardiolipin antibodies also increase the tendency for thrombosis and may be responsible for recurrent pregnancy loss.[20]

Parturients with a history of deep venous thrombosis or pulmonary embolism or with lupus anticoagulant or anticardiolipin antibodies may receive prophylactic low-dose aspirin or heparin to prevent deep venous thrombosis. The dose of heparin is designed to maintain *normal* coagulation but prevent thrombosis. Parturients who develop a deep venous thrombosis during the current pregnancy receive *therapeutic* doses of heparin that prolong the PTT to 1.5 to 2 times normal.

Low-dose aspirin (80 mg) therapy attempts to prevent preeclampsia and treats intrauterine growth retardation.[21] Similarly, patients with lupus anticoagulant or anticardiolipin antibodies receive low-dose aspirin prophylactically to prolong pregnancy and prevent thrombosis.

Management of Parturients With Altered Coagulation

Take a complete history with respect to abnormal bleeding in the parturient or her family and ascertain the nature of the problem: bleeding from the gums, spontaneous nosebleeds, bleeding after surgery or delivery. Inquire about previous testing or hematologic consultation.

Examine the parturient for evidence of bleeding: petechiae (look at the blood pressure cuff site), bruising, overt bleeding from venipuncture sites, vaginal bleeding.

Order and check the appropriate blood work: hemoglobin, platelet count, prothrombin time, PTT, serum fibrinogen concentration. Remember, fibrinogen levels increase during pregnancy (Table 19–7).

TABLE 19–7
Coagulation Tests*

Test	Normal Value
Platelet count	150–440 × 10^9/L
Prothrombin time	8–12 seconds
Partial thromboplastin time	24–36 seconds
Serum fibrinogen	2.5–6.5 g/L

*Absolute values are dependent on the laboratory.

Labor Analgesia

If evidence of a coagulopathy exists, either drug-induced or secondary to disease, consider alternative methods of analgesia-anesthesia to regional anesthesia (see Table 19–1). These include TENS, nitrous oxide and oxygen in a 50% mixture, and narcotics (intravenous—infusion, PCA [see Table 19–1]).[22] Explain the risks and benefits of each technique to the patient and fully answer all questions. Document the risks and the discussion on the chart.

Regional analgesia is contraindicated in parturients receiving therapeutic heparin and those with evidence of a coagulopathy. Regional anesthesia in patients receiving aspirin or prophylactic heparin is controversial.[13] Although aspirin inhibits platelet function, the bleeding time is not a reliable method of assessing platelet function.[16] The author does not inquire about aspirin ingestion prior to regional block but does ask about a history of easy bleeding or bruising. Coagulation is usually not impaired with prophylactic, low-dose heparin, and if the PTT is normal, regional anesthesia is not contraindicated.[23] *Do* check the PTT 3 to 4 hours after the last dose of heparin to ensure that it is within the normal range, since there are reports of markedly prolonged PTTs following prophylactic low-dose heparin.

If performing a regional anesthetic in a parturient with a coagulation abnormality or receiving prophylactic heparin or aspirin, an experienced anesthesiologist should perform the block. Midline approaches decrease the risk of trauma to the epidural veins, which are located laterally in the epidural space. The author's group uses short-acting local anesthetics such as lidocaine or chloroprocaine that allow early block regression and permit earlier neurologic assessment. Following delivery, visit the patient frequently to rule out development of an epidural hematoma. Leave specific orders for anesthesia to be called in the event of severe backache, back tenderness, or motor or bowel or bladder dysfunction. If these develop, a myelogram or contrast computed tomography scan establishes the diagnosis. Remember, early clot evacuation provides the best prognosis.

The question is frequently asked about when to remove an epidural catheter in the parturient who develops a coagulopathy during parturition. The author would suggest removal once coagulation returns to normal, as removal may cause bleeding in the epidural space.

Anesthesia for Cesarean Section

Assess the risks and benefits of each technique. Examine the airway. If a difficult or impossible intubation is anticipated, an awake intubation may be necessary. Spinal anesthesia using a small needle, potentially decreasing the risk of venipuncture, may be a reasonable alternative in these parturients with bad airways. The author would use spinal anesthesia only for parturients who refuse general anesthesia or who have a potentially difficult airway. Completely inform the patient of the risks and benefits of the proposed treatment-management and fully document the discussion and consent on the chart. Follow the patient carefully to identify possible complications related to the block.

CONNECTIVE TISSUE DISORDERS

These disorders share the propensity for the body to produce antibodies against itself, resulting in inflammatory responses. Those most commonly occurring in fertile women include systemic lupus erythematosus (SLE), progressive systemic sclerosis, and rheumatoid arthritis (RA).[24] Remember, these are systemic disorders and affect many different organ systems that must be considered during preoperative evaluation.

Systemic Lupus Erythematosus

Since the majority of patients with SLE are young women, it is not uncommon for a parturient to present with this disease.[25] Typical findings of SLE include rash, arthritis, and pleuritis. However, renal failure, pulmonary hemorrhage, thrombosis, myocarditis, and cerebritis also occur. Flares and remissions are typical. Treatment is largely symptomatic, unless a life-threatening exacerbation requires administration of glucocorticoids. Although pregnancy does not appear to influence the course of SLE, the pregnant patient with SLE is more likely to experience preterm delivery, intrauterine growth retardation, and intrauterine demise. Preeclampsia also occurs more commonly in these patients and should be investigated.

Mild anemia and thrombocytopenia may occur with SLE. Occasionally, Coombs-positive hemolytic anemia occurs. Lupus anticoagulant, an autoantibody, occurs in some patients with SLE[25, 26] and prolongs the PTT. However, lupus anticoagulant associates with thrombosis, not hemorrhage. Laboratory confirmation of lupus anticoagulant is made by correction of the PTT with the addition of platelet-rich plasma (phospholipid dependency).

Patients with SLE may also have antibodies to the coagulation factors that, when present, predispose the parturient to hemorrhage. Seek evidence of a bleeding tendency with a good history and physical examination. Look for evidence of bleeding or bruising (bruises, petechiae, bleeding from venipuncture sites or vagina). This is how the author assesses the suitability of these patients for regional anesthesia.

A careful history also determines the extent of the disease, organ involvement, and current medication. Examine the patient—in particular, the cardiovascular system (heart rate, blood pressure, neck veins; listen for murmurs or extra heart sounds), the respiratory system (rales, rhonchi), neurologic system (peripheral neuropathy). Order and check the results of urinalysis, blood urea nitrogen, serum creatinine, electrolytes, blood glucose, hemoglobin, platelets, prothrombin time, PTT, and fibrinogen. Patients taking corticosteroids may require supplementation. One regime is hydrocortisone 100 mg intravenously every 12 hours for 24 hours followed by dose tapering. The necessity for supplementation and the dosage regime depend on circumstances (vaginal delivery or cesarean section) and the dose required for disease control. Remember, the parturient may receive aspirin or prophylactic heparin if lupus anticoagulant antibody is present.

Prior to providing analgesia or anesthesia, conduct a full discussion of the risks and benefits of appropriate techniques. Document the discussion on the patient's chart.

Labor Analgesia

As described previously, prophylactic *low-dose* aspirin or heparin therapy does not contraindicate regional anesthesia, provided there is no evidence of an overt bleeding tendency, and following appropriate testing (see "Hematologic Disorders," earlier in this chapter). Intrathecal administration of narcotics (preservative-free morphine 250 μg with fentanyl 25 μg) as well as epidural analgesia is also suitable for stage 1 labor.[5]

Parenteral narcotics such as demerol or fentanyl, either intramuscularly or intravenously (intermittent, infusion, PCA), offer an alternative for those patients refusing or who are not considered candidates for regional anesthesia. Nitrous oxide and oxygen in a 50% mixture provides effective short-term analgesia for some patients. TENS may be a useful adjunct.

Anesthesia for Cesarean Section

Parturients with severe renal disease may require central venous pressure monitoring to guide fluid administration during cesarean section. Direct arterial pressure monitoring is useful if the blood pressure is poorly controlled. Ideally, the preoperative blood pressure should be maintained during anesthesia. Monitor hourly urine output. Rigidly control intravenous fluids and maintain a balance between fluid input and urine output. If the patient has marked positive fluid balance or symptoms of fluid overload, consider intravenous furosemide 20 to 40 mg. If the patient has been receiving steroids immediately antepartum, provide steroid coverage.

Although regional anesthesia (epidural, spinal) is suitable if no coagulopathy exists, patients with SLE may have vasculitis, and prolonged hypotension may decrease spinal cord blood flow, leading to an anterior spinal artery syndrome and permanent neurologic damage. Assess the risks and benefits of regional anesthesia, and if selecting epidural anesthesia, administer local anesthetics incrementally and, hopefully, avoid hypotension. Treat hypotension with additional fluid or ephedrine 5 to 10 mg.

General anesthesia, sometimes indicated for fetal distress or a maternal complication, requires the standard technique of preoxygenation, a rapid-sequence induction with thiopental and succinylcholine and endotracheal intubation with a cuffed tube during cricoid pressure. If the parturient has myocarditis and poor cardiac function, utilize a modified narcotic induction with fentanyl 4 to 5 μg/kg and thiopental 1 to 2 mg/kg. Alert the neonatologist for possible newborn depression.

Progressive Systemic Sclerosis

Systemic sclerosis has a lower prevalence and a later age of onset than SLE and occurs less commonly during pregnancy.[27] Progressive systemic sclerosis (scleroderma) is characterized by inflammation, vascular sclerosis, and fibrosis of the skin and viscera, with major changes occurring in the skin, musculoskeletal system, peripheral nervous system, heart, lungs, kidneys, and gastrointestinal system.

Thickening of the dermis and subcutaneous tissue binds the skin to the tissues underneath, limiting mobility. Weakness of proximal muscle groups occurs secondary to myopathy. Compression of nerves by thickened connective tissue may produce peripheral or cranial neuropathy. Esophageal involvement leads to hypomotility and symptoms of gastric reflux. Diffuse pulmonary interstitial fibrosis impairs diffusing capacity and decreases pulmonary compliance. Sclerosis of small coronary arteries and the conduction system may cause dysrhythmias and congestive heart failure. Systemic or pulmonary hypertension may result from sclerosis of small vessels in the kidney and pulmonary arteries. Raynaud phenomenon occurs commonly.

Anesthetic Implications (Table 19–8)

Venous access may be difficult owing to skin thickening. A small nick in the skin with a separate needle a millimeter or two away from the vein, followed by insertion of the venous cannula, simplifies placement. Occasionally, a central venous catheter may be necessary for venous access owing to impossible peripheral venous cannulation. Early intravenous placement is essential.

Skin thickening and peripheral vasoconstriction may limit pulse oximetry and auscultation or palpation of the blood pressure. Use of an indwelling arterial catheter should be discouraged owing to vasoconstriction with compromised circulation to the hand. Ultrasonic blood pressure devices overcome this problem.

Labor Analgesia

Regional analgesia-anesthesia may be technically difficult because of skin thickening and limited joint flexion. Examine the patient in both the sitting and the lateral positions to

TABLE 19–8
Anesthetic Implications of Progressive Systemic Sclerosis

Involved System	Anesthetic Implication
Skin	Positioning owing to limited joint mobility Intubation difficulties Venous access problems Monitoring (pulse oximetry, automatic blood pressure) difficulties
Vascular	Systemic, pulmonary hypertension Dysrhythmias Congestive heart failure Monitoring (pulse oximetry, blood pressure) limitations
Gastrointestinal	Gastric reflux—increased risk of pulmonary aspiration
Neurologic	Peripheral neuropathy
Musculoskeletal	Myopathy (weakness)
Pulmonary	Pulmonary interstitial fibrosis Hypoxia

determine which is best for the procedure. Epidural anesthesia may improve lower limb perfusion but risks hypotension as a result of vasodilatation. Titrate small doses of local anesthetic, 3 to 5 ml, in low concentrations (0.125 to 0.25% bupivacaine) to establish analgesia. Treat hypotension with intravenous fluid and ephedrine. Since ephedrine may produce vasoconstriction, administer in 2- to 5-mg increments. Direct-acting vasopressors, such as phenylephrine, and ergot preparations should be used cautiously to avoid excessive hypertension and vasospasm.

Anesthesia for Cesarean Section

Regional anesthesia, despite the risk of hypotension, is preferable to general anesthesia because of the significant risks of difficult intubation, hypoxia, and gastroesophageal reflux in this patient population.

Skin tightening and thickening may impede mouth opening, making intubation difficult. Awake fiberoptic laryngoscopy and intubation may be necessary. Avoid nasal intubation, since telangiectasia and congestion of the nasopharynx increase the risk of nasal hemorrhage. Furthermore, potential gastroesophageal reflux increases the risk of pulmonary aspiration during general anesthesia, especially during difficult intubation. Administer ranitidine, a nonparticulate antacid, and possibly metoclopramide preoperatively. Pulmonary interstitial fibrosis increases the risk of hypoxia, and as discussed, monitoring with pulse oximetry may be an unreliable option. Monitoring the oxygen saturation on the ear lobe may be more reliable than on the extremities. To counteract these potential problems, increase the inspired oxygen concentration to maintain satisfactory oxygen saturation (above 95%). A volatile anesthetic agent such as isoflurane 0.75% reduces the incidence of awareness while the addition of a narcotic such as fentanyl produces analgesia. Use a peripheral nerve stimulator and monitor neuromuscular function during administration of muscle relaxants, especially when myopathy exists. It may be necessary to use maximal voltage amplitude to obtain a visible twitch. The train-of-four responds normally to muscle relaxants. Provide eye protection, since eyelid closure may be poor secondary to skin thickening.

These patients easily develop hypothermia. Utilize warm intravenous fluids and warm humidified gases during general anesthesia and maintain room temperature at 20° C. Position patients with care owing to their contractures and joint changes to avoid injury.

Rheumatoid Arthritis

Although RA is generally considered a disease of older adults, 80% of patients have an onset between the ages of 35 and 50 years.[28] Although the hallmark of RA is symmetric joint involvement, it is a systemic disease that includes cardiac and pulmonary involvement. Organ involvement is generally secondary to vasculitis.

Anesthetic Implications (Table 19–9)

The degree of joint involvement in RA correlates with anesthetic problems. Marked deformities of small and large joints may exist secondary to scarring and fibrosis. In rare instances, hip involvement may necessitate cesarean section owing to limited leg abduction. Anesthesia consultation prior to admission for delivery is desirable to allow assessment of the degree of joint involvement, especially airway involvement. Cervical spine x-rays (flexion, extension views) are

TABLE 19-9
Potential Anesthetic Problems in the Rheumatoid Parturient

Positioning	Limited movement of joints Difficulty in inserting epidural anesthesia
Intubation	Temporomandibular joint limitation Cricoarytenoid involvement Atlantoaxial instability
Medications	Corticosteroids Aspirin

particularly useful for assessing the risk of atlantoaxial instability, especially for those patients with a history of neck pain and transient upper limb neurologic symptoms. A lead apron shields the fetus during the procedure.

Deformity, rigidity, and pain may preclude optimal positioning of the patient for intubation or regional anesthesia. Padding of involved joints may be necessary.

Patients with RA frequently receive aspirin or corticosteroids. Corticosteroid therapy may require supplementation. Aspirin interferes with platelet function. However, the bleeding time is unreliable in assessing the risk of bleeding secondary to aspirin. Evidence of a bleeding disorder should be sought through a careful history and physical examination.

Labor Analgesia

The usual spectrum of analgesic options are available for labor. Remember, epidural analgesia provides excellent joint pain relief, as well as labor pain relief, so care must be taken with positioning to ensure that involved joints are not placed into abnormal, harmful positions. Document preexisting peripheral neuropathy prior to instituting the block and discuss possible complications with the patient.

Anesthesia for Cesarean Section

Regional anesthesia may be preferable to general anesthesia, especially when abnormalities of the cervical spine or temporomandibular joints exist. Involvement of the temporomandibular, cricoarytenoid, and cervical spine (atlantoaxial joint) may make intubation difficult, if not impossible.[29] Temporomandibular joint dysfunction limits mouth opening, and cricoarytenoid dysfunction narrows the glottic opening. Atlantoaxial instability and posterior subluxation make extension of the neck hazardous. Ask the patient to demonstrate acceptable positioning of head and neck prior to anesthetic induction of general anesthesia.

To assess the airway, ask the patient to open her mouth. An opening of greater than 4 cm between the upper and the lower teeth indicates good temporomandibular function. Ask the patient to speak. Hoarseness or stridor suggest cricoarytenoid dysfunction requiring a smaller endotracheal tube, which should be immediately available. Finally, ask the patient to flex and extend her neck. Paresthesias or pain may indicate atlantoaxial instability. When evidence of airway or cervical spine involvement exists along with a contraindication to regional anesthesia, perform awake intubation under topical anesthesia or fiberoptic laryngoscopy.

Move these patients carefully to avoid damaging inflamed joints. Remember, damage to the cervical spinal cord can occur with head and neck manipulation, and these considerations also apply to patients having regional anesthesia. However, the major problem encountered with regional anesthesia is identification of the epidural or spinal space owing to problems in positioning the patient for the block. The sitting position may prove easier for both the patient and the anesthesiologist. Careful positioning to avoid trauma to inflamed joints and cervical spinal cord is important during block placement.

MUSCULAR DISORDERS

Muscular Dystrophy (Myotonia)

Muscular dystrophy, an inherited muscle disorder, mainly affects males and only rarely presents during pregnancy. The myotonic disorders are characterized by an inability to relax the muscle (myotonia) and muscle weakness. Importantly, cardiac muscle may also be involved in these disorders, resulting in cardiac dysrhythmias and valvular disease. Progressive weakness of the diaphragm and muscles of respiration can occur and ultimately reduce expiratory reserve volume, vital capacity, minute volume, and maximal breathing capacity.

Complications associated with pregnancy include hydramnios, prolonged labor, retained placenta, and postpartum hemorrhage secondary to uterine hypotonia.[30] The neonate may also be affected by myotonia.

Labor Analgesia

These patients are sensitive to the central respiratory depressant effects of narcotics and sedatives. This is a nonspecific effect and possibly related to central nervous system (CNS) involvement by the disease. If narcotics are required, the author suggests using intravenous PCA with fentanyl rather than intramuscular meperidine. PCA (fentanyl 20 μg bolus with a 5- to 10-minute lockout time) allows administration of small narcotic doses while providing a relatively rapid onset of effect. When the patient becomes sleepy during PCA, she stops drug administration, allowing accurate titration. Monitor oxygen saturation and consider supplemental oxygen when these parturients receive narcotics during labor.

Epidural analgesia is the anesthetic method of choice. Unless indicated for other reasons, avoid epidural opioids, since systemic absorption may produce central respiratory depression in this population.

Anesthesia for Cesarean Section

Regional anesthesia avoids many of the problems of general anesthesia and is the preferred technique for operative delivery. However, muscle contractures can occur despite regional anesthesia (spinal, epidural) but are rare once the block is fully established. Contractures in the surgical field cause problems. Contracture may also occur during general anesthesia with nondepolarizing muscle relaxants, as surgical stimulation and electrocautery may trigger percussion myotonia. Treat contracture with local anesthetic infiltration of the affected muscle or intravenous quinidine (300 to 600 mg). Monitor the electrocardiogram carefully when using quinidine, as complete heart block may occur.

Potential sustained muscle contracture and difficult or impossible ventilation and intubation contraindicate succinylcholine. Furthermore, these patients demonstrate enhanced sensitivity to nondepolarizing muscle relaxants. Titrate these agents and use a peripheral nerve stimulator. As discussed, contracture may occur during general anesthesia even when nondepolarizing muscle relaxants are utilized. Surgical stimulation and electrocautery may trigger percussion myotonia.

Again, administer CNS depressants such as thiopental, midazolam, and narcotics with care (discussed earlier).

Myasthenia Gravis

Myasthenia gravis is an autoimmune disorder, involving the neuromuscular junction,[31] characterized by increased muscle weakness following repetitive skeletal muscle use. During pregnancy, partial recovery occurs with improvement in approximately one third of patients, whereas one third worsen and one third remain stable. Respiratory and bulbar involvement increases the risk of respiratory complications, including hypoventilation and pulmonary aspiration of gastric contents.

Medical treatment consists of cholinesterase inhibitor therapy, and these medications should be continued throughout labor and delivery. Administer these medications intramuscularly or intravenously and maintain adequate serum levels. Continue close monitoring of muscular function postpartum, as exacerbations of myasthenia may occur with changing drug requirements.

Complications of medication therapy include myasthenic crisis (weakness due to insufficient medication) and cholinergic crisis (weakness due to medication). Importantly, aminoglycoside antibiotics and magnesium sulfate can precipitate weakness in these parturients. Medical consultation is useful in determining drug requirements. Be prepared to ventilate.

Labor Analgesia

Regional anesthesia offers the benefits of good pain relief, minimal or no systemic medication, and anesthetic flexibility for a forceps-assisted or cesarean delivery. Chloroprocaine and other ester local anesthetics are metabolized by pseudocholinesterase, and their action may be prolonged by anticholinesterase medication. Although these agents are not contraindicated, they are probably best avoided.

Anesthesia for Cesarean Section

Both regional and general anesthesia can be used in the myasthenic patient. One must be alert to significant weakness with a high regional block and closely monitor the patient's oxygen saturation and ability to cough. When significant bulbar involvement exists, general anesthesia with endotracheal intubation may be safer than regional for the parturient because of the threat of aspiration.

Patients with myasthenia are sensitive to nondepolarizing muscle relaxants, and the response to succinylcholine varies.[32] If succinylcholine is required for rapid-sequence intubation, use 1.5 to 2.0 mg/kg, since the ED_{50} is increased.[32] Nevertheless, Phase II block may occur with this dose and must be treated appropriately. If muscle relaxation is required during surgery, use one half of the usual dose of atracurium or vecuronium and closely monitor the degree of relaxation with a peripheral nerve stimulator. However, muscle relaxants may be unnecessary and should be avoided when possible. If nondepolarizing relaxants are used, reverse neuromuscular blockade with incremental intravenous neostigmine 0.5 mg or pyridostigmine 1.0 mg, and monitor with the nerve stimulator.

Acquired Immunodeficiency Syndrome

Acquired immunodeficiency syndrome (AIDS) is a virus-induced illness that impairs the body's ability to defend itself against infection by viruses, fungi, parasites, and some bacteria. The virus, known as the "human immunodeficiency virus" (HIV), is transmitted through blood, semen, breast milk, and possibly other body fluids.

Although often considered a disease of homosexual men, AIDS is also transmitted heterosexually and is a leading cause of death in women of reproductive age.[33] Transplacental transmission of the virus to the fetus is thought to occur in the first trimester but may also be transmitted at delivery. Breast milk is another possible mode of newborn transmission.

Because of the increased incidence of HIV infection in the population, all hospitals should institute universal precautions to protect hospital personnel from possible infection through handling contaminated materials.[34]

General Considerations

Since it is impossible to identify all parturients infected with HIV, universal blood and body fluid precautions should be routine in the obstetric setting. Remember, although parturients with overt AIDS are frequently cachectic and febrile, parturients who are HIV positive can appear healthy. Protect yourself!

AIDS is a multisystem disease. Of particular importance to the anesthesiologist is the potential involvement of the neurologic, respiratory, and hematologic systems.[35] Neurologic symptoms may occur either with the initial infection or as the disease progresses. CNS symptoms include headache, behavioral changes, seizures, hallucinations, and sleep disorders. Diarrhea, increased sweating, and syncope may be symptoms of autonomic dysfunction. Limb weakness, sensory changes, pain, and herpes zoster indicate involvement of the peripheral nervous system. Clinical neuropathy and myopathy occur in 40% of infected adults and autopsy evidence indicates neurologic involvement in 80% of HIV-positive patients.

Protecting the parturient and the fetus/newborn from opportunistic infections is vital. Wear a gown, sterile gloves, and masks when handling the cachectic, critically ill patient to reduce the risk of introducing pathogens to the patient (reverse isolation).

Health care personnel are at risk from exposure to the blood and body fluids of the HIV-positive parturient.[34] Barrier protection (gown, gloves, goggles) should be used when dealing with infected material or when there is a risk of contamination from splashing during invasive procedures.[36] Do not recap needles or reattach syringes. Immediately dispose of material in a puncture-resistant container.

Protect other parturients from infected material from HIV-positive parturients by utilizing single-dose drug vials and disposable equipment. Do not use a drug-containing syringe for multiple patients, consistent with universal precautions. When necessary, reuse equipment only following appropriate sterilization.[36]

Obtain a routine hemoglobin, platelet count, and coagulation profile prior to initiating anesthesia, since these patients may be anemic, with decreased platelet count or a coagulopathy. Electrolytes and arterial blood gases may be indicated, especially when evidence of significant muscle wasting or pulmonary involvement exists (Table 19–10).

Choice of Anesthetic: Regional Versus Other

Owing to the high incidence of neurologic disease in patients who are HIV positive, anesthesiologists often reluctantly provide regional anesthesia. The reasons for this reluctance are fears of introducing a pathogen (i.e., HIV) into the CNS, fear of litigation (anesthesia could be blamed for neurologic symptoms), and the availability of alternate techniques.

However, a preliminary report[37] suggests that regional anesthesia is safe for HIV-positive parturients. Fifteen HIV-positive parturients who received regional anesthesia (14 epidurals, 1 spinal) were prospectively followed for 6 months to determine whether there were any adverse sequelae. No neurologic or infectious complications occurred in these patients. The author would have no hesitation in providing regional anesthesia to HIV-positive parturients.

Parenteral narcotics, inhalational agents, intravenous ketamine (increments of 5 mg), and TENS are alternatives (see Table 19–1) to regional anesthesia (epidural, intrathecal narcotics) for labor analgesia. General anesthesia is suitable for cesarean section.

Labor Analgesia

Be sensitive to the needs of a known HIV-positive parturient. She may be experiencing the pain of labor and may feel rejected and guilty. Support from family and friends may be lacking. Do not be judgmental! Discuss with the patient available alternatives and the advantages and disadvantages of each technique.

Obtain informed consent that addresses the issue of the neurologic complications associated with AIDS and what is known about regional anesthesia and AIDS. Document the discussion.

An experienced anesthesiologist should perform the block, reducing the risk of trauma from multiple punctures. Usual doses of local anesthetics are required.

Continuous epidural infusions minimize the need for repeated top-ups and decreases the potential risks to health care workers and the patient from repeated contact. Evidence indicates that epidural blood patch does not increase the risk of neurologic complications for these patients.[38]

Alternative techniques for labor analgesia include narcotics, TENS, and self-administered nitrous oxide and oxygen in a 50:50 mixture. Explanations and reassurance are an effective supplement to analgesia.

TABLE 19–10
Medical Problems of Anesthetic Importance in Parturients With AIDS

Problem	Importance
Thrombocytopenia	Contraindication to regional anesthesia
Respiratory disease	Hypoxia
Neurologic disease	? Contraindication to regional anesthesia
Psychosis	Informed consent
Opportunistic infections	Sterilization of equipment
Muscle wasting	Altered response to muscle relaxants

Abbreviation: AIDS = acquired immunodeficiency syndrome.

Anesthesia for Cesarean Section

As discussed earlier, providing there is no contraindication, evidence suggests that regional anesthesia is safe for the parturient with AIDS. Since epidural-intrathecal morphine associates with recrudescence of herpes simplex type I (cold sores)[39] and HIV-positive parturients are susceptible to opportunistic infections, it may be advisable to avoid epidural or intrathecal morphine.

General anesthesia is problematic for the HIV-positive parturient. Many of these patients have CNS disease and may be sensitive to the effects of CNS depressants. Utilize smaller doses. Pulmonary disease may increase the propensity for hypoxia, so administer an $F_{I_{O_2}}$ of at least 0.5. Significant muscle wasting or myopathy increases the patient's sensitivity to nondepolarizing muscle relaxants, and smaller doses may be required. Titrate and monitor the muscle relaxant. In patients with myopathy, succinylcholine might produce a massive potassium release, causing cardiac arrhythmias. Check electrolytes preoperatively. A peripheral nerve stimulator is useful to monitor neuromuscular block and to allow titration of the muscle relaxant. The author would use succinylcholine in the patient without a myopathy but would avoid it in the patient with myopathy (see Table 19–5).

Disposable circuits, soda lime, and circuit filters lessen the risk of anesthesia machine contamination. Wear gloves during intubation and change these immediately following intubation. Provide good anesthetic care to parturients who are HIV positive while protecting yourself and others from possible infection. These goals can best be achieved by sensitive handling of these patients, by maintaining an awareness of their needs and their medical problems, and by protecting ourselves during the provision of anesthetic care.

TEN PRACTICAL POINTS

1. A history and physical examination is the best screening test for coagulation abnormalities prior to regional anesthesia.

2. Regional anesthesia is contraindicated in parturients with a coagulopathy or receiving *therapeutic* heparin.

3. Check platelet counts in parturients with acquired immunodeficiency syndrome (AIDS), systemic lupus erythematosus (SLE), or a history of easy bruising or bleeding.

4. Epidural analgesia is *not* contraindicated in parturients with spinal cord injury, multiple sclerosis, or AIDS or who are receiving prophylactic (low-dose) heparin and aspirin.

5. Regional anesthesia is the best technique to avoid autonomic hyperreflexia in parturients with spinal cord injury.

6. Succinylcholine is contraindicated in parturients with a recent spinal cord injury (less than 12 months) and those with myotonic dystrophy.

7. Parturients with myasthenia gravis have a variable response to succinylcholine. Use *standard* doses for intubation and monitor the response with a nerve stimulator.

8. Parturients with myasthenia gravis and multiple sclerosis are sensitive to the nondepolarizing muscle relaxants.

9. Beware when positioning patients with rheumatoid arthritis, spinal cord injury, and progressive systemic sclerosis.

10. AIDS, myasthenia gravis, idiopathic thrombocytopenic purpura, myotonia dystrophica, and SLE may result in neonatal problems.

REFERENCES

1. Kafer ER: Respiratory and cardiovascular functions in scoliosis and the principles of anesthetic management. Anesthesiology 52:339, 1980.
2. Crosby ET, Halpern SH: Obstetric epidural anaesthesia in patients with Harrington instrumentation. Can J Anaesth 36:693, 1989.
3. Feldstein G, Ramanathan S: Obstetrical lumbar epidural anesthesia in patients with previous posterior spinal fusion for kyphoscoliosis. Anesth Analg 64:83, 1985.
4. Coalson DW, Glosten B: Alternatives to epidural analgesia. Semin Perinatol 15:375, 1991.
5. Leighton BL, DeSimone CA, Norris MC, et al: Intrathecal narcotics for labor revisited: The combination of fentanyl and morphine intrathecally provides rapid onset of profound, prolonged analgesia. Anesth Analg 69:122, 1989.
6. Daley MD, Rolbin S, Hew E, Morningstar B: Continuous epidural anaesthesia for obstetrics after major spinal surgery. Can J Anaesth 37:S112, 1990.
7. Norris MC, Leighton BL: Continuous spinal anesthesia after unintentional dural puncture in parturients. Reg Anesthesia 15:285, 1990.
8. Baker ER, Cardenas DD, Benedetti TJ: Risks associated with pregnancy in spinal cord–injured women. Obstet Gynecol 80:425, 1992.
9. Crosby E, St. Jean B, Reid D, et al: Obstetrical anaesthesia and analgesia in chronic spinal cord–injured women. Can J Anaesth 39:487, 1992.
10. Abouleish EI, Hanley ES, Palmer SM: Can epidural fentanyl control autonomic hyperreflexia in a quadriplegic parturient? Anesth Analg 68:523, 1989.
11. Baraka A: Epidural meperidine for control of autonomic hyperreflexia in a paraplegic parturient. Anesthesiology 62:688, 1985.
12. Warren TM, Datta S, Ostheimer GW: Lumbar epidural anesthesia in a patient with multiple sclerosis. Anesth Analg 61:1022, 1982.
13. Douglas MJ: Coagulation abnormalities and obstetric anaesthesia. Can J Anaesth 38:R17, 1991.
14. Douglas MJ: Potential complications of spinal and epidural anesthesia for obstetrics. Semin Perinatol 15:368, 1991.
15. Scott DB, Hibbard BM: Serious non-fatal complications associated with extradural block in obstetric practice. Br J Anaesth 64:537, 1990.
16. Rodgers RPC, Levin J: A critical reappraisal of the bleeding time. Semin Thromb Haemost 16:1, 1990.
17. Burrows RF, Kelton JG: Thrombocytopenia at delivery: A prospective survey of 6715 deliveries. Am J Obstet Gynecol 162:731, 1990.
18. Gatt S: Haematological disorders responsible for

maternal bleeding in late pregnancy. Anaesth Intensive Care 18:335, 1990.
19. Milaskiewicz RM, Holdcroft A, Letsky E: Epidural anaesthesia and Von Willebrand's disease. Anaesthesia 45:462, 1990.
20. Lubbe WF, Liggins GC: Role of lupus anticoagulant and autoimmunity in recurrent pregnancy loss. Semin Reprod Endocrinol 6:181, 1988.
21. Uzan S, Beaufils M, Breart G, et al: Prevention of fetal growth retardation with low-dose aspirin: Findings of the EPREDA trial. Lancet 337:1427, 1991.
22. Kleiman SJ, Wiesel S, Tessler MJ: Patient-controlled analgesia (PCA) using fentanyl in a parturient with a platelet function abnormality. Can J Anaesth 38:489, 1991.
23. Horlocker TT, Wedel DJ: Anticoagulants, antiplatelet therapy, and neuraxis blockade. Anesth Clin North Am 10:1, 1992.
24. Friedman SA, Bernstein MS, Kitzmiller JL: Pregnancy complicated by collagen vascular disease. Obstet Gynecol Clin North Am 18:213, 1991.
25. Davies SR: Systemic lupus erythematosus and the obstetrical patient—Implications for the anaesthetist. Can J Anaesth 38:790, 1991.
26. Malinow AM, Rickford WJK, Mokriski BLK, et al: Lupus anticoagulant. Implications for obstetric anaesthetists. Anaesthesia 42:1291, 1987.
27. Younker D, Harrison B: Scleroderma and pregnancy. Anaesthetic considerations. Br J Anaesth 57:1136, 1985.
28. Klipple GL, Cecere FA: Rheumatoid arthritis and pregnancy. Rheum Dis Clin North Am 15:213, 1989.
29. Crosby ET, Luis A: The adult cervical spine: Implications for airway management. Can J Anaesth 37:77, 1990.
30. Blumgart CH, Hughes DG, Redfern N: Obstetric anaesthesia in dystrophia myotonica. Anaesthesia 45:26, 1990.
31. Rolbin SH, Levinson G, Shnider SM, et al: Anesthetic considerations for myasthenia gravis and pregnancy. Anesth Analg 57:441, 1978.
32. Baraka A: Anaesthesia and myasthenia gravis. Can J Anaesth 39:476, 1992.
33. Chu S, Buehler J, Berkelman R: Impact of the human immunodeficiency virus epidemic on mortality in women of reproductive age, United States. JAMA 264:225, 1990.
34. Centers for Disease Control: Recommendations for preventing transmission of human immunodeficiency virus and hepatitis B virus to patients during exposure-prone invasive procedures. MMWR 40:357, 1991.
35. Douglas MJ: Management of the parturient with AIDS. *In* Janisse T (ed): Pain Management of AIDS Patients. Boston, Kluwer Academic, 1991, pp 61–71.
36. Kristensen MS, Sloth E, Jensen TK: Relationship between anesthetic procedure and contact of anesthesia personnel with patient body fluids. Anesthesiology 73:619, 1990.
37. Hughes SC, Dailey PA, Landers D, et al: The HIV+ parturient and regional anesthesia: Clinical and immunologic response. Anesthesiology 77:1036, 1992.
38. Tom DJ, Gulevich SJ, Shapiro HM, et al: Epidural blood patch in the HIV-positive patient. Anesthesiology 76:943, 1992.
39. Crone LAL, Conly JM, Storgard C, et al: Herpes labialis in parturients receiving epidural morphine following cesarean section. Anesthesiology 73:208, 1990.

TWENTY

Anesthesia for Non–Birth-Related Surgery During Pregnancy

Gertie F. Marx, M.D.   I. David Elstein, M.D.

More than 2% of pregnant women require anesthesia for emergent or urgent surgery during the course of gestation.[1] Most of the indications for such operations are nonobstetric, but cervical cerclage and intrauterine fetal surgery are related to the pregnancy itself.

Anesthesia administered to a pregnant woman is unique because it involves two recipients. The well-being of both mother and fetus as well as the preservation of the pregnancy is of concern. Maternal considerations center on pregnancy-induced physiologic alterations and their effect on anesthetic and adjuvant requirements. Fetal considerations revolve around the maintenance of normal uteroplacental perfusion, maintenance of normal maternal-fetal gas and substrate exchange, avoidance of potentially harmful drugs, and prevention of preterm labor.

The overall effects of maternal anesthetization on mother, fetus, and uterus can be classified as physiologic and pharmacologic. Physiologic alterations associated with gestation result from hormonal, metabolic, and mechanical causes. Those changes related to hormonal and metabolic developments begin shortly after conception; those resulting from the upward pressure of the enlarging uterus commence in mid pregnancy. Thus, the type and extent of these alterations vary with the duration of gestation.

PHYSIOLOGIC CONSIDERATIONS

Maternal Stress

Maternal fear, anxiety, and pain exert adverse effects on mother and fetus consequent to enhanced secretion of stress hormones. High plasma catecholamine levels not only raise the mother's arterial pressure but also increase peripheral and uterine vasoconstriction, with the resultant decrease in uterine blood flow threatening the fetus (Fig. 20–1).[2] It is therefore imperative to allay the patient's fear and anxiety and to relieve her pain. A comprehensive, reassuring preanesthetic visit is mandatory and may, in fact, be more effective than drugs in achieving this goal. The safety of modern anesthesia for mother and baby should be emphasized, but the possibility of fetal complications resulting from the surgical manipulation, blood loss, or the underlying disease (viremia, bacteremia) should not be withheld. There is, however, no contraindication to using drugs for premedication as long as potentially teratogenic substances are avoided during the first trimester (discussed later in this chapter). The authors recommend the use of 75 to 100 mg of secobarbital or pentobarbital orally or intramuscularly for sedation and meperidine 50 to 75 mg intramuscularly or intravenously for pain relief.

During general anesthesia, endotracheal intubation should be achieved expertly, and in hy-

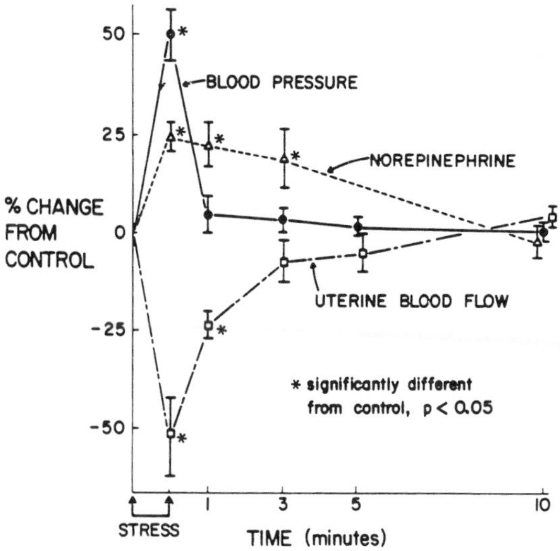

Figure 20–1. In awake pregnant ewes, a brief electrically induced stress (application to the skin of a uniform electrical stimulus of 30 V with frequency of 167 Hz) produced a 25% increase in maternal plasma norepinephrine level, a 50% increase in mean maternal arterial pressure, and a 52% decrease in uterine blood flow. Thus, maternal stress appears to reduce uterine perfusion secondary to release of endogenous norepinephrine. All values subsequent to control are given as mean percentage changes ± SE. (From Shnider SM, Wright RG, Levinson G, et al: Uterine blood flow and plasma norepinephrine changes during maternal stress. Anesthesiology 50:524–527, 1979.)

pertensive patients, the response to laryngoscopy should be dampened by pretreatment with an opioid (fentanyl 2.0–2.5 μg/kg or alfentanil 10 μg/kg) or labetalol (10 to 20 mg), injected intravenously shortly before induction of anesthesia. The patient's awareness should be prevented by ensuring an adequate depth of narcosis.

Maternal Position

From mid pregnancy on, the enlarged uterus compresses both the inferior vena cava and the lower aorta when the gravida lies supine. Obstruction of the vena cava reduces venous return to the heart. In the unanesthetized state, most women are capable of compensating for the resultant decrease in stroke volume by increasing peripheral vascular resistance and heart rate.[3] During anesthesia, however, these compensatory mechanisms are reduced or abolished, so that significant hypotension will rapidly ensue.

Obstruction of the lower aorta and its branches decreases renal and uteroplacental blood flow. During the third trimester, kidney function and urine output are significantly lower in the supine than the lateral position.[4] Reduced uteroplacental flow can severely affect the fetus. For example, fetal oxygenation diminishes following the mother's assumption of the supine position,[5] whereas fetal arrhythmias indicative of uteroplacental insufficiency have been completely abolished by turning the mother from a supine to a lateral position.[6]

As practiced during cesarean section, aortocaval compression and its sequelae are preventable by avoiding the supine position. When examinations or operations necessitate the supine posture, the uterus must be shifted away from the great abdominopelvic vessels without delay, usually to the left. This can be accomplished by elevating the right hip with a wedge or sandbag, by a 15- to 30-degree left-down tilt of the table, or by a combination of the two.

Vascular Tone

During gestation, vascular tone depends more on sympathetic control than it does in the nongravid state. Hypotension develops more readily and more markedly consequent to the sympathetic blockade accompanying spinal or extradural anesthesia. This increased dependence on sympathetic tone, combined with the effect of caval compression, makes the pregnant woman more susceptible to arterial hypotension at levels of regional blockade or depths of general anesthesia that would not affect maintenance of normal blood pressure in healthy, nongravid patients.

Hypotension resulting from sympathetic blockade can be minimized by increasing circulating blood volume with an intravenous preload of balanced electrolyte solution (8 to 10 ml/kg in early gestation to 12 to 15 ml/kg toward term).[7] Intravenous ephedrine 5 to 10 mg is a safe and dependable adjunct to hydration; its action is predominantly cardiac and, therefore, does not affect uterine blood flow.[8] However, without adequate hydration, ephedrine is not effective.[9] In contrast to ephedrine, peripherally acting vasopressors increase vascular resistance and consequently reduce uterine perfusion.[8] Yet, in pregnant women in whom positive cardiac inotropy and chronotropy are potentially hazardous, for example, in the presence of mitral valve lesions, phenylephrine in small doses (50 to 80 μg increments or microdrip infusion of 10 μg/minute) is more rational.[10]

Maternal hypotension invariably reduces uterine arterial blood flow and must be prevented to protect the fetus. Three measures are required: a sufficient maternal circulating blood volume, maternal normoglycemia (discussed later), and after the 20th week of gestation, adequate uterine displacement.

Metabolism

Pregnancy alters all metabolic functions, and the most pertinent change involves carbohydrate metabolism. Pregnant women live in a state of "accelerated starvation." First, the fuel demands of the fetus are met primarily by the consumption of glucose, and second, insulin secretion in response to glucose is augmented. As early as 15 weeks' gestation, maternal blood glucose levels following an overnight fast are considerably lower than those in women in the nongravid state. Optimal blood glucose levels in pregnant women range from 80 to 100 mg/dl (4.44 to 5.55 mmol/L). Hypoglycemia is defined as a blood glucose concentration below 60 mg/dl (3.33 mmol/L), whereas in nongravid individuals, the critical level is 50 to 40 mg/dl (2.2 mmol/L).[11]

The fetus depends on a constant supply of glucose to provide energy for its cellular metabolism. Maternal hypoglycemia will inevitably lead to fetal hypoglycemia. Fetal blood glucose concentrations are between 20 and 30 mg/dl (1.1 and 1.7 mmol/L) lower than those of the mother, and fetal hypoglycemia is defined as a blood glucose concentration of 40 mg/dl (2.2 mmol/L) or lower.[12]

Maternal hypoglycemia is unphysiologic for both mother and fetus. During anesthesia, the usual compensatory response to low blood glucose concentrations, particularly the release of epinephrine, is blocked. Thus, in healthy parturients undergoing elective cesarean section under regional analgesia, postblock hypotension has been difficult to reverse until after the patients' low blood glucose concentrations were normalized.[13] The fetal response to hypoglycemia is variable, but it primarily affects the heart rate (bradycardia, late decelerations).[14, 15]

Thus, hypoglycemia should be avoided for maternal and fetal reasons. Determinations of blood glucose are easily performed at the bedside. Test strips and glucometers rapidly provide information that can be used to gauge the amount of dextrose to be infused before the start of anesthesia. In general, the authors recommend the intravenous infusion of 200 to 300 ml of dextrose-containing electrolyte solution prior to anesthesia for all operations in nondiabetic pregnant women. If intraoperative blood glucose determinations are available, a concentration between 70 and 110 mg/dl (3.9 and 6.1 mmol/L) should be maintained. Since the fetus will not be delivered at this time, mild to moderate degrees of hyperglycemia are harmless.

Gastric Function

Pregnancy-induced alterations in gastric function are threefold. First, gastric tone and motility are reduced by the action of progesterone, resulting in a retardation of gastric emptying; delayed gastric emptying is evident as early as 8 to 11 weeks' gestation.[16] Second, stomach and intestines are gradually displaced cephalad by the enlarging uterus, and the axis of the stomach is shifted from the vertical to the horizontal. This increases intragastric pressure and changes the angle of the gastroesophageal junction, leading to incompetence of the junction's "pinchcock" mechanism. Third, gastric secretory activity of acid, chloride, and pepsin declines during the early part of pregnancy but increases to above-normal levels in the latter part of gestation. Aspirates of gastric juice collected for 45 minutes from fasting pregnant women yielded 70 ± 20 ml in the first trimester, 36 ± 12 ml in the second trimester, and 107 ± 28 ml in the third trimester, compared with 63 ± 8 ml in nongravid controls.[17] These physiologic alterations increase the danger of pulmonary inhalation of gastric contents during general anesthesia. In a comparison of obstetric and nonobstetric anesthesia malpractice claims, aspiration accounted for 4% of the obstetric cases but for only 1% of the nonobstetric suits.[18] Chemical aspiration (Mendelson's) pneumonitis is particularly prevalent during the third trimester consequent to the high gastric acidity.

To minimize the incidence and sequelae of

this complication, the authors recommend various measures:

1. Postponement of urgent but nonemergent surgery for 6 to 8 hours following the last intake of solid food.

2. Metoclopramide (Reglan) to increase the rate of gastric emptying. This is indicated mainly in women who ingested solid food within 4 to 6 hours before anesthesia. Dose: 10 mg intravenously slowly 20 to 30 minutes before anesthesia.

3. Ranitidine (Zantac) or cimetidine (Tagamet) to inhibit gastric acid secretion. This is indicated particularly in women prone to heartburn, a symptom of high gastric acidity and low esophageal sphincter tone. Dose: Ranitidine 50 to 100 mg intravenously 30 to 40 minutes before anesthesia or intramuscularly 90 minutes before anesthesia; cimetidine 200 mg intravenously 30 to 40 minutes before anesthesia or 300 mg intramuscularly 90 minutes before anesthesia.

4. A nonparticulate oral antacid such as cooled 0.3 M sodium citrate (Bicitra) to neutralize gastric acid present. This should be used for all patients regardless of whether general or regional anesthesia is chosen. Dose: 30 ml 20 to 30 minutes before anesthesia.

5. Rapid-sequence induction and endotracheal intubation with expert cricoid pressure. This is mandatory beginning in the early second trimester for operations in the supine position and from the early first trimester for surgery in the lithotomy position.

(There are no reports of human teratogenicity following the use of metroclopramide, ranitidine, or cimetidine, but none of these three drugs was subjected to a well-controlled study in pregnant women.[19])

Respiratory Gases

Oxygen levels fall more rapidly in gravid than in nongravid subjects. First, oxygen consumption rises progressively during pregnancy, to reach a 20% increase at term. Second, from the fifth month on, functional residual capacity gradually decreases, leading to reduced oxygen storage. These two factors result in an exaggerated fall in arterial oxygen tension during periods of hypoventilation and aventilation. In 12 healthy term-pregnant women, well oxygenated via endotracheal tube, arterial oxygen tension declined 139 ± 38 mmHg (18.5 + 5.1 kPa) during 60 seconds of apnea with exposure to room air, whereas in comparable nongravid patients, the decrease was only 58 ± 39 mmHg (7.7 ± 5.2 kPa) ($p < .05$).[20]

The oxygenation of the fetal blood mirrors that of the mother's blood. Oxygen tensions in both rise with maternal inhalation of oxygen concentrations greater than 21% and fall during inhalation of concentrations less than 21%.[21]

To prevent hypoxemia, which affects maternal and fetal brain function, the following measures are recommended:

1. During general anesthesia: Thorough preoxygenation, expert endotracheal intubation, utilize at least 50% oxygen.

2. During regional anesthesia: Supplemental oxygen, preferably humidified,[22] via nasal cannulas or transparent face mask.

Alveolar and arterial carbon dioxide levels are reduced to approximately 32 to 34 mmHg (4.3 to 4.5 kPa) during most of gestation consequent to a hormonally induced increase in the gravida's resting ventilation. Further hyperventilation, however, is potentially hazardous, regardless of whether active or passive, as hypocapnia and alkalemia result. Hypocapnia and alkalemia tend to produce hypoxemia.[23, 24] Hypocapnia constricts the cerebral and uteroplacental vasculature, thus reducing blood flow. Alkalemia, in turn, shifts the hemoglobin-oxygen dissociation curve to the left, thus impairing the release of oxygen to maternal tissues and fetal blood. In addition, active hyperventilation by a pregnant woman produces oxygen debt.[25] Until the carbon dioxide tension falls below 28 mmHg (3.7 kPa), the development of alkalosis is forestalled by a compensatory decrease in sodium bicarbonate.

Maternal hypoventilation is equally undesirable because the ensuing hypercapnia leads to a primary respiratory and secondary metabolic acidemia in mother and fetus. Furthermore, carbon dioxide is a potential uterine stimulant.[26]

Thus, the mother's respiratory minute volume should be kept at a normal level; Pa_{CO_2} should not fall below 28 mmHg (3.7 kPa) and should not rise above 36 mmHg (4.8 kPa).

PHARMACOLOGIC CONSIDERATIONS

Pharmacologic considerations apply to the mother, the uterus, and the fetus.

The Mother

Pregnancy alters the response to anesthetic and adjuvant drugs. Reduced drug requirements, manifest during both regional and general anesthesia, constitute the most relevant change. During the last trimester, regardless of maternal position and despite effective uterine displacement, local anesthetic requirements for spinal or lumbar extradural block decrease by one fourth to one third.[27] Thus, administering spinal block for cesarean section, the authors use 7 to 11 mg of hyperbaric tetracaine or 12 mg of hyperbaric bupivacaine, but for nongravid hysterectomy, 12 to 15 mg of tetracaine or 16 mg of bupivacaine are instilled. Decreased requirements begin in the first trimester. Following injection of 20 ml of 2% lidocaine with epinephrine 1:200,000, the upper level of analgesia was significantly higher in 23 women 8 to 12 weeks' pregnant than in 12 comparable nonpregnant women. The average extradural dose requirement per spinal segment was 21.3 ± 2.1 mg lidocaine in the pregnant group; the corresponding value for the controls was 27.1 ± 2.4 mg ($p < .001$) (Fig. 20–2).[28]

Similarly, bupivacaine toxicity was found to occur at lower doses in pregnant ewes than in nonpregnant ewes. The mean dose of bupivacaine resulting in cardiovascular collapse was significantly lower in the gravid sheep (5.1 ± 0.1 mg/kg) than the nongravid animals (8.9 ± 0.9 mg/kg) ($p < .05$). Furthermore, bupivacaine blood concentrations at the onset of respiratory and circulatory arrest were lower in the pregnant group, being 5.2 ± 0.7 μg/ml and 5.5 ± 0.8 μg/ml, respectively, versus 7.5 ± 0.9 μg/ml and 8.0 ± 0.9 μg/ml, respectively, in the nonpregnant group ($p < .05$).[29] A recent study did not confirm the difference in bupivacaine cardiotoxicity between pregnant and nonpregnant sheep.[57] Nevertheless, to increase the safety of epidural anesthesia, a 3-ml test dose containing epinephrine 1:200,000 is recommended; if injected into the intravascular compartment, transient tachycardia will ensue; if injected into the intrathecal space, a discernible sensory block will result. Subsequent doses should be fractionated; that is, following each injection of 5 ml of local anesthetic, signs and symptoms of intravascular injection (tinnitus, perioral pallor, metallic taste in mouth) and intrathecal injection (abnormally high sensory and motor levels) should be elicited.

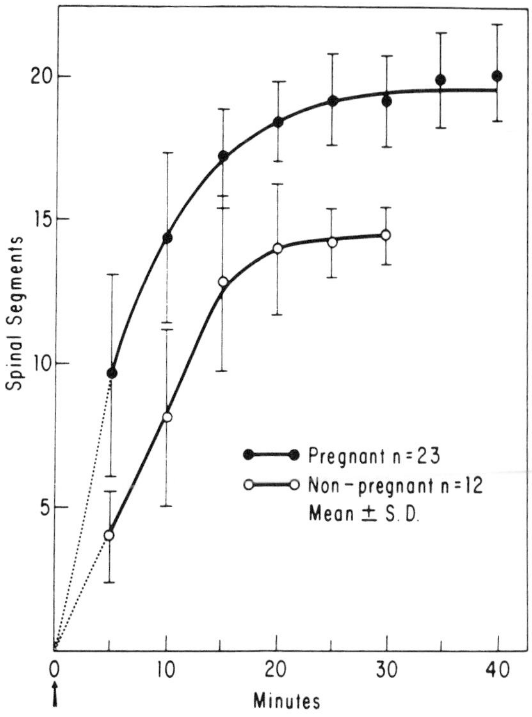

Figure 20–2. Rate of spread of epidural analgesia in nonpregnant women and comparable pregnant women in their first trimester (8–12 weeks). A line of best fit has been drawn. Injection time is denoted by the *arrow* at time zero. Thus, early pregnancy is already associated with an increased epidural spread of local anesthetic. (From Fagraeus L, Urban BJ, Bromage PR: Spread of epidural analgesia in early pregnancy. Anesthesiology 58:184–187, 1983.)

Inhalation induction and changes in the anesthetic depth occur with greater speed in pregnant women. Gestation enhances anesthetic input in two ways: Increased resting ventilation delivers more agent into the alveoli per unit time, and reduced functional residual capacity speeds replacement of lung air with inspired agent.

There are also alterations in the response to many intravenously administered agents, specifically prolongation of elimination half-lives consequent to the greater distribution volume resulting from the increase in plasma volume. Thus, the mean elimination half-life for thiopental was 26.1 hours in seven women following elective cesarean section as compared with 11.5 hours in five young gynecologic patients ($p < .025$);[30] this accounts for the prolonged sleepiness occasionally observed following barbiturate administration in pregnant women.

The Uterus

Two complications should be avoided: Increased uterine resting pressure (base tone) and stimulation of uterine contractility. Increased uterine base tone enhances uterine vascular resistance, which, in turn, decreases blood flow. (This, however, is not the only cause of reduced uterine perfusion.) Initiation of contractions may lead to premature labor.

Carbon dioxide markedly affects uterine function. Hypercarbia increases uterine tone and contractility,[26] whereas hypocarbia produces its effects through a reduction in uterine blood flow.[23] In an experimental setup, mechanical effects on cardiac output were predominantly responsible for the decreased uterine blood flow; but in the pregnant woman, the vasoconstriction associated with hypocarbia may additionally diminish uterine perfusion similar to the way it reduces blood flow in other vascular beds.

Halogenated inhalation agents tend to reduce uterine resting pressure. Halothane, enflurane, and isoflurane, studied on isolated human gravid and nongravid uterine muscle strips, were equally depressing in equipotent concentrations; the depressant effect was dose related and was markedly greater in the pregnant muscles.[31] In the intact postpartum human uterus, depression of spontaneous uterine activity began at anesthetic levels equivalent to 0.5 minimal alveolar concentration (MAC).[32] However, observations during second trimester terminations of pregnancy suggest that, during early gestation, even lower concentrations exert depressant effects so that administration of nitrous oxide and oxygen supplemented with intravenous drugs becomes the technique of choice for these procedures.

The response to ketamine by the human uterus varies with dose and period of gestation. In the first two trimesters, doses of 1.1 mg/kg or greater increased uterine resting pressure;[33] however, during the third trimester, doses of up to 1.8 mg/kg produced no adverse results.[34] Thus, in the doses used presently in pregnancy, which do not exceed 1 mg/kg, ketamine is devoid of adverse effects on uterine activity. The barbiturates, propofol, and the neuromuscular blocking agents do not affect uterine tone.

Uterine blood flow decreases consequent to maternal hypotension as well as through administration of vasopressors with predominantly α-adrenergic properties.[8] However, when administered in small doses (50 to 100 μg) to healthy parturients with healthy fetuses, phenylephrine had no biochemically or clinically observable adverse effects; although neither uterine conductance nor blood flow was investigated.[10] Phenylephrine is the drug considered preferable to ephedrine when—as already indicated—increases in heart rate or cardiac work are undesirable.

Epinephrine, accidentally injected into the maternal bloodstream or absorbed into the circulating bloodstream following addition to a local anesthetic solution, promptly induces uterine vasoconstriction, even in small amounts. Thus, the dosage of epinephrine added to a local anesthetic solution should be restricted; concentrations of 1:300,000 or 1:400,000 are preferable to the usual 1:200,000.

Although animal experiments have implicated inhalation agents with an increased incidence of fetal resorption and death, evaluations of human situations revealed an increased risk of spontaneous abortions mainly following intra-abdominal surgery, implicating the surgical manipulation or underlying disease as the cause.[35] In a retrospective review of fetal risk associated with incidental surgery during pregnancy, there was a higher incidence of spontaneous abortion in the first and second trimesters following obstetric and gynecologic procedures, but only after general anesthesia, not after spinal block.[36] This observation points to the importance of maximal relaxation of the abdominal musculature during intra-abdominal surgery to prevent any manual or retractor-induced stimulation of the uterus.

Uterine activity should be monitored by an external tocodynamometer as soon as the fundus is above the pelvic rim, provided the transducer does not encroach on the surgical field. This will give an early indication of the need for tocolytic drugs (β_2-adrenergic agonists, magnesium sulfate) to prevent premature delivery.

The Fetus

Human pregnancy is divided into three trimesters. For the fetus, the first trimester is the period of organogenesis, the second trimester that of growth, and the third that of maturation. The period of organogenesis, from the 13th to the 56th postconceptual day, is the critical time in which congenital malformations are caused by specific environmental factors called "teratogens." These include drugs and chemicals, infectious agents (viruses, treponema, parasites), and therapeutic radiation.[37]

All anesthetic and adjuvant drugs traverse the human placenta, albeit at different rates and in varying amounts. Inhalation agents have been detected in the fetal circulation within 2 minutes of maternal inhalation,[38] and intravenously injected drugs have been identified in fetal blood within 1 to 4 minutes of administration to the mother.[39, 40] Local anesthetics employed for major or minor regional block rapidly diffuse into the maternal circulation to be readily transmitted across the placenta.[41] Nevertheless, there is *no* evidence of human teratogenicity associated with *any* currently used anesthetic or adjunct drug. Data obtained from studies in small animals cannot be extrapolated to the human because of (1) species differences and (2) noncomparable anesthetic conditions. It is therefore not surprising that a woman, injured in a car accident at 6 weeks' gestation, was delivered at 35 weeks of a normal infant following administration of 17 general anesthetics (nitrous oxide or halothane).[42] It is also not astounding that the safety of anesthesia during pregnancy was confirmed in a review of 5405 cases compiled from three Swedish health care registries for the years 1973 to 1981.[43] The incidences of congenital malformations and stillbirths in the offspring of gravid women having an operation during the first trimester were not increased. An increased occurrence of low–birth weight infants was the result of both prematurity and intrauterine growth retardation. Although the incidence of neonates born alive but dying during the first week of life was increased, it appeared that the illness that necessitated surgery played a significant role in determining the results. Most importantly, no specific types of anesthesia or operations were associated with any adverse reproductive outcome.

The 1985 nitrous oxide "scare" was based on animal data that were not applicable to humans. Retrospective reviews revealed no evidence of fetal ill effects when the agent was employed for cervical cerclage;[44, 45] there was no difference in the incidence of inevitable abortion or of low–birth weight neonates between cases conducted under general anesthesia that included the administration of nitrous oxide (268 fetuses) and those managed under regional analgesia (115 fetuses).[45] Thus, there is no longer any doubt about the safety of nitrous oxide as an anesthetic during pregnancy.

Only one group of drugs occasionally employed by anesthesiologists is controversial; the safety of benzodiazepines ingested in early gestation remains questionable. A connection between these drugs and an increased risk of cleft lip or cleft palate is suspected.[46] Diazepam (Valium) intake during the first trimester has been associated with oral clefts,[47] although it is doubtful that one or two doses taken for sedation will cause the deficit. Nevertheless, it seems prudent to avoid diazepam and its relative midazolam (Versed) during the period of organogenesis. There may also be a small risk of congenital heart disease with the use of meprobamate (Equanil) and chlordiazepoxide (Librium).[48] The barbiturates and phenothiazines, in contrast, are considered generally safe.

After approximately the 16th week of gestation, continuous fetal heart rate monitoring should be undertaken whenever feasible. This may provide an early diagnosis of abnormal uteroplacental perfusion or of impaired maternal-fetal gas exchange—conditions that may or may not be treatable. Treatment consists of optimization of maternal physiologic variables (increase in oxygen-carrying capacity, improvement in oxygenation, normalization of carbon dioxide levels, glucose concentrations, body temperature) and of optimization of uteroplacental blood flow (shift of retractors and surgical instruments). It must, however, be recognized that there are benign drug-induced changes. A reversible decrease in variability is caused by many drugs, for example, narcotics, barbiturates, tranquilizers (Fig. 20–3). Furthermore, drugs that increase the maternal heart rate (e.g., atropine) will also raise the fetal heart rate, and drugs that lower the mother's heart rate (e.g., reserpine) will also decrease the fetus' heart rate. There are also drugs that reduce the fetus' heart rate more than the mother's (e.g., esmolol [Brevibloc]).[49] Thus, correct interpretation of the tracings is essential.

CHOICE OF ANESTHETIC METHOD

The same choice of anesthetic method is not possible for every kind of operation or every

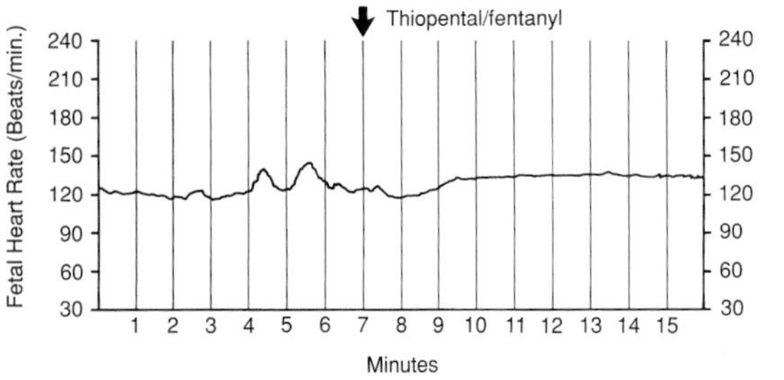

Figure 20–3. External fetal heart rate tracing during the induction of general anesthesia in a 20-year-old, 60-kg primigravida requiring emergency craniotomy for abscess formation. Induction was performed with thiopental 300 mg and fentanyl 250 μg. Fetal heart rate variability was lost within 1 minute of the injection of the induction agents.

type of patient. If, however, both regional and general anesthesia are feasible, the former is preferable to the latter, for both maternal and fetal reasons. Maternal advantages include maintenance of consciousness, minimal risk of aspiration, possibility of postoperative pain relief by epidural or spinal injection of local anesthetic or opioid, and rapid postanesthetic recovery permitting early ambulation. The fetal advantage is exposure to a lower amount of anesthetic drug.

A first trimester termination of pregnancy may be performed on an ambulatory basis under paracervical block and intravenous or intramuscular sedation. Of the local anesthetics, the ester-type drugs 2-chloroprocaine (Nesacaine) and prilocaine (Citanest) are safest for paracervical block, since the injections are made into a very vascular area. For the same reason, bupivacaine (Marcaine, Sensorcaine) is considered the least desirable drug; in fact, bupivacaine is contraindicated for "obstetric" paracervical block, as fetal deaths have occurred.

A second trimester termination of pregnancy requires more profound anesthesia; spinal, epidural, and general anesthesia are acceptable, with the choice depending on the patient's wishes. When general anesthesia is selected, endotracheal intubation is indicated, and as pointed out earlier, the halogenated agents should be avoided to prevent uterine "relaxation" with its risk of hemorrhage.

Cervical cerclage also may be performed utilizing spinal, epidural, or general anesthesia. A spinal block with tetracaine (Pontocaine), an ester (6 to 8 mg), is the only anesthetic technique without placental transfer of drug, a fact appreciated by many pregnant patients. Bupivacaine and lidocaine are safe alternatives. For patients desiring to be asleep, endotracheal intubation is mandatory; halogenated agents are not contraindicated, as there is no intrauterine manipulation.

For lower abdominal surgery, such as ovarian cystectomy or appendectomy, the authors prefer regional blockade because of its excellent muscular relaxation and contraction of the intestines. General endotracheal anesthesia is indicated for upper abdominal surgery including subcostal position of an inflamed appendix. Provision of maximal muscular relaxation is essential to facilitate surgical manipulations near the uterus.

Neurosurgical and intrathoracic procedures are performed as in nongravid patients with or without one of the special techniques outlined later.

For postanesthetic recovery, pregnant women should be cared for by trained postanesthesia care unit nurses, in either the obstetric unit or the regular operating room facility. Continued monitoring of maternal vital signs, uterine activity, and fetal well-being is essential.

SPECIAL TECHNIQUES

Both hypotensive and hypothermic techniques have been employed uneventfully during pregnancy. Controlled hypotensive anesthesia has been used predominantly for clipping of cerebral aneurysms to decrease the aneurysmal wall tension at the time of its clipping. Hypotension is commonly achieved by the combination of a halogenated agent with nitroglycerin, trimethaphan (Arfonad), sodium nitroprusside, or hydralazine (Apresoline). The depth of halothane or isoflurane anesthesia must be kept light (below 1 MAC) to prevent worrisome reductions in uteroplacental blood flow. In light planes of anesthesia, uteroplacental perfusion is maintained by the concomitant decrease in uterine vascular resistance. In deep planes, however, myocardial contractility is depressed, leading to reduced uterine blood flow and fetal impairment. Degree and duration of hypotension should be limited to the absolute minimum required, and the fetal heart rate should be monitored continuously for early recognition of impaired fetal tolerance.[50, 51] The authors prefer nitroglycerin or trimethaphan because of their short duration of action and lack of undesirable metabolic by-products.

Hypothermia was used as early as 1957 in a woman who was 8 weeks pregnant and who had a head injury; temperatures between 30° and 34° C were maintained for 7 days with recovery of the mother and delivery of a viable fetus at 28 weeks' gestation.[52] Since then, hypothermia has been employed for intracranial and cardiac operations.[53] Temperatures as low as 23° C have been tolerated by mother and fetus at gestational ages of 7 to 34 weeks, but temperatures of 28° to 30° C are considered safest. Such "moderate" cooling may, in fact, protect the fetus by reducing its oxygen requirement. Hypothermia is a potential cause of fetal bradycardia and ventricular dysrhythmias. During hypothermic cardiopulmonary bypass, fetal bradycardia may be due to fetal cooling and not to hypoxia or distress. Nevertheless, if fetal bradycardia occurs, pump flow and maternal mean arterial pressure may need to be increased.[54]

INTRAUTERINE FETAL SURGERY

Intrauterine fetal surgery has become a reality thanks to the diagnostic capabilities of modern ultrasonography. Procedures not requiring hysterotomy are mostly performed under local infiltration with or without sedation; if control of fetal movements is desired, direct injection of a neuromuscular relaxant into fetal muscle or umbilical vein is employed. Surgical correction of congenital anomalies is best undertaken under general anesthesia. Although regional block offers advantages to the mother, general anesthesia is preferred because fetal stress responses are blocked, fetal muscle tone is abolished, and uterine tone can be controlled. A light to moderate plane of halothane-oxygen or isoflurane-oxygen, supplemented by fentanyl and neuromuscular relaxants, is the anesthetic technique of choice. The effects of inhalational agents on the cardiovascular system of the human fetus have not as yet been ascertained. It is known that, despite the rapid placental transfer of these agents, their fetal levels remain lower than the maternal for a significant period after administration to the mother. Monitoring of the fetal heart rate and of fetal blood pH, glucose, and electrolytes is essential. Postoperative use of tocolytic drugs is mandatory to delay the onset of labor.[52]

A review of 17 cases, undertaken for one of four anomalies (bilateral hydronephrosis, diaphragmatic hernia, sacrococcygeal teratoma, cystic adenomatoid malformation), indicated that the risk to the mother of surgery and anesthesia was minimal and that future reproductive potential was not compromised. However, despite continued intravenous or oral tocolytic therapy, all deliveries occurred prematurely. Fetal outcome was disappointing; 6 of 8 fetuses with diaphragmatic hernia did not survive, and 2 neonates with pulmonary hypoplasia died at birth.[55, 56]

POSTPARTUM BILATERAL TUBAL LIGATION

The lack of specific complications associated with sterilization during cesarean section has led to the practice of performing bilateral tubal ligations immediately or soon after an uncomplicated vaginal delivery. Optimally, this is undertaken under continuous lumbar extradural analgesia started during labor and extended cephalad postpartum. If regional blockade was not administered before delivery, the rational choice lies between a single injection lumbar extradural block (approximate doses: bupivacaine 100 mg, lidocaine 400 mg, 2-chloroprocaine 600 mg) or a spinal block (hyperbaric bupivacaine 8 to 10 mg or lidocaine 50 to 80 mg). Mothers who desire to breast feed may prefer the spinal route because of the small dose of local anesthetic required. With use of a pencil-point needle, the incidence of postdural puncture headache has been significantly reduced.

General anesthesia is the least appropriate anesthetic method for early postpartum tubal ligation. Although the upward pressure on the stomach disappears with the birth of the fetus, all other pregnancy-induced gastrointestinal changes persist for at least 8 hours, possibly longer. Thus, the risk of pulmonary inhalation of gastric contents is not eliminated. The authors do not recommend utilizing general anesthesia for immediate postpartum tubal ligations. However, if circumstances dictate that this is the wisest course for medical considerations, the precautions for cesarean section anesthesia must be employed.

CONCLUSIONS

Elective surgery should not be undertaken during pregnancy, but there is no contraindication to the performance of indicated procedures. They should preferably be performed during the late second trimester; that is, following the period of organogenesis and before the period of increased risk of premature labor. General anesthesia, regional analgesia, and local infiltration methods may be safely employed provided the following recommendations are considered:

1. Mitigation of maternal stress.
2. Optimization of maternal physiologic variables including maintenance of normal glucose levels and carbon dioxide tensions and provision of increased oxygen tensions.
3. Optimization of uteroplacental blood flow.
4. Avoidance of potentially teratogenic sedatives.
5. Avoidance of anesthetic complications.
6. Provision of optimal surgical conditions.
7. Continuous monitoring of mother (according to American Society of Anesthesiologists' guidelines), uterine activity, and fetal well-being.
8. Intraoperative or postoperative tocolysis if indicated.

The anesthesiologist has control over most of these factors. Maintaining maternal cardiac output, providing an adequate oxygen content in the blood perfusing the placenta, and avoiding aortocaval compression and increases in uterine tone are the most important considerations for maternal and fetal well-being.

TEN PRACTICAL POINTS

1. First and foremost, never sacrifice maternal safety.
2. Regional anesthesia is preferable to general anesthesia—for maternal and fetal reasons—provided its use is feasible.
3. Beyond 20 weeks' gestation, displacement of the uterus from the great abdominopelvic vessels is essential for avoiding maternal and fetal hazards of aortocaval compression whenever a pregnant woman lies supine.
4. Utilize an intravenous crystalloid preload to increase circulating blood volume and minimize the incidence and severity of regional block–induced hypotension.
5. Maintain maternal blood glucose concentration above 70 mg/dl to prevent the maternal and fetal ill effects of hypoglycemia.
6. Antacids and expert cricoid pressure are essential to avoid pulmonary inhalation of gastric contents during the induction of general anesthesia.
7. Tracheal intubation must be performed expediently, as oxygen levels fall more rapidly in the gravid than the nongravid patient.
8. Currently employed anesthetic drugs are not teratogenic, but avoid benzodiazepines and other tranquilizers during the period of organogenesis.
9. Pregnancy reduces drug requirements for both regional and general anesthesia.
10. Minimize stimulation of uterine contractility during surgery by appropriate anesthetic selection, provision of optimal surgical conditions, and if indicated, tocolytic administration.

REFERENCES

1. Brodsky JB, Cohen EN, Brown BW: Surgery during pregnancy and fetal outcome. Am J Obstet Gynecol 138:1165–1167, 1980.
2. Shnider SM, Wright RG, Levinson G, et al: Uterine blood flow and plasma norepinephrine changes during maternal stress. Anesthesiology 50:524–527, 1979.
3. Lees MM, Scott DB, Kerr MG, Taylor SH: The circulatory effects of recumbent postural change in late pregnancy. Clin Sci 32:453–465, 1967.
4. Chesley LC, Sloan DM: The effect of posture on renal function in late pregnancy. Am J Obstet Gynecol 89:754–759, 1964.
5. Huch A, Huch R: Transcutaneous, noninvasive monitoring of Po_2. Hosp Pract 11:43–52, 1976.
6. Goodlin RC: Importance of the lateral position during labor. Obstet Gynecol 37:698–701, 1971.
7. Wollman SB, Marx GF: Acute hydration for prevention of hypotension of spinal anesthesia in parturients. Anesthesiology 29:374–380, 1968.
8. Ralston DH, Shnider SM, deLorimier AA: Effects of equipotent ephedrine, metaraminol, mephentermine, and methoxamine on uterine blood flow in the pregnant ewe. Anesthesiology 40:354–370, 1974.
9. Marx GF, Cosmi EV, Wollman SB: Biochemical status and clinical condition of mother and infant at cesarean section. Anesth Analg 48:986–993, 1969.
10. Ramanathan S, Grant GJ: Vasopressor therapy for hypotension due to epidural anesthesia for

cesarean section. Acta Anaesthesiol Scand 32:559–565, 1988.
11. Bergman M, Seaton TB, Auerhahn CC, et al: The incidence of gestational hypoglycemia in insulin-dependent and non–insulin-dependent diabetic women. NY J Med 86:174–177, 1986.
12. Gabbe SG, Quilligan EJ. Fetal carbohydrate metabolism: Its clinical importance. Am J Obstet Gynecol 127:92–103, 1977.
13. Marx GF, Domurat ME, Costin M: Potential hazards of hypoglycaemia in the parturient. Can J Anaesth 34:400–402, 1987.
14. Langer O, Cohen WR: Persistent fetal bradycardia during maternal hypoglycemia. Am J Obstet Gynecol 149:688–690, 1984.
15. Schiffmiller MW, Torbey M, Seidman SF: Fetal heart rate decelerations consequent to hypoglycemia. Anesthesiol Rev 16:47–49, 1989.
16. Simpson KH, Stakes AF, Miller M: Pregnancy delays paracetamol absorption and gastric emptying in patients undergoing surgery. Br J Anaesth 60:24–27, 1988.
17. Murray FA, Erskine JP, Fielding J: Gastric secretion in pregnancy. J Obstet Gynaecol 64:373–381, 1957.
18. Chadwick HS, Posner K, Caplan RA, et al: A comparison of obstetric and nonobstetric anesthesia malpractice claims. Anesthesiology 74:242–249, 1991.
19. Physicians' Desk Reference 1992, 46th ed. Montvale, NJ, Medical Economics Data, 1991, pp 1870, 2229, 1064.
20. Archer GW, Marx GM: Arterial oxygen tension during apnea in parturient women. Br J Anaesth 46:358–360, 1974.
21. Newman W, McKinnon L, Phillips L, et al: Oxygen transfer from mother to fetus during labor. Am J Obstet Gynecol 99:61–70, 1967.
22. Elstein ID, Marx GF: A humidification device for nasal oxygen. Anesthesiology 70:879, 1989.
23. Levinson G, Shnider SM, deLorimier AA, Steffenson JL: Effects of maternal hyperventilation on uterine blood flow and fetal oxygenation and acid-base status. Anesthesiology 40:340–347, 1974.
24. Miller FC, Petrie RH, Arce JJ, et al: Hyperventilation during labor. Am J Obstet Gynecol 120:489–495, 1974.
25. Gemzell CA, Robbe H, Stern B, Ström G: Observations on circulatory changes and muscular work during labor. Acta Obstet Gynaecol Scand 36:75–92, 1957.
26. Goldfarb WS: Contractions of the human uterus and a theory of labor. Q Rev Surg Obstet Gynecol 14:142–147, 1957.
27. Marx GF: Regional analgesia in obstetrics. Anaesthesist 21:84–91, 1972.
28. Fagraeus L, Urban BJ, Bromage PR: Spread of epidural analgesia in early pregnancy. Anesthesiology 58:184–187, 1983.
29. Morishima HO, Pedersen H, Finster M, et al: Bupivacaine toxicity in pregnant and nonpregnant ewes. Anesthesiology 63:134–139, 1985.
30. Morgan DJ, Blackman GL, Paull JD, Wolf LJ: Pharmacokinetics and plasma binding of thiopental. II. Studies at cesarean section. Anesthesiology 54:474–480, 1981.
31. Munson ES, Embro WS: Enflurane, isoflurane, and halothane and isolated human uterine muscle. Anesthesiology 46:11–14, 1977.
32. Marx GF, Kim YI, Lin CC, et al: Postpartum uterine pressures under halothane or enflurane anesthesia. Obstet Gynecol 51:695–698, 1978.
33. Galloon S: Ketamine for obstetric delivery. Anesthesiology 44:522–524, 1976.
34. Marx GF, Hwang HS, Chandra P: Postpartum uterine pressures with different doses of ketamine. Anesthesiology 50:163–166, 1979.
35. Shnider SM, Webster GM: Maternal and fetal hazards of surgery during pregnancy. Am J Obstet Gynecol 92:891–896, 1965.
36. Duncan PG, Pope WDB, Cohen MM, Greer N: Fetal risk of anesthesia and surgery during pregnancy. Anesthesiology 64:790–794, 1986.
37. Moore KL: The Developing Human: Clinically Oriented Embryology, 4th ed. Philadelphia, WB Saunders, 1988, pp 119, 145, 151.
38. Marx GF, Joshi CW, Orkin LR: Placental transmission of nitrous oxide. Anesthesiology 32:429–432, 1970.
39. Crawford JS, Rudofsky S: The placental transmission of pethidine. Br J Anaesth 37:929–933, 1956.
40. Finster M, Morishima HO, Mark LC, et al: Tissue thiopental concentrations in the fetus and neonate. Anesthesiology 36:155–158, 1972.
41. Shnider SM, Way EL: The kinetics of transfer of lidocaine (Xylocaine) across the human placenta. Anesthesiology 29:944–950, 1968.
42. Slater BL: Multiple anaesthetics during pregnancy. Br J Anaesth 42:1131–1134, 1970.
43. Mazze RI, Källén B: Reproductive outcome after anesthesia and operation during pregnancy: A Registry study of 5405 cases. Am J Obstet Gynecol 161:1178–1185, 1989.
44. Aldridge LM, Tunstall ME: Nitrous oxide and the fetus. A review and the results of a retrospective study of 175 cases of anaesthesia for insertion of Shirodkar suture. Br J Anaesth 58:1348–1356, 1986.
45. Crawford JS, Lewis M: Nitrous oxide in early human pregnancy. Anaesthesia 41:900–905, 1986.
46. Safra MJ, Oakley GP: Association between cleft lip with or without cleft palate and prenatal exposure to diazepam. Lancet 2:478–480, 1975.
47. Saxen I, Saxen L: Association between maternal

intake of diazepam and oral cleft. Lancet 2:498, 1975.

48. Milcovich L, Van den Berg BJ: Effects of prenatal meprobamate and chlordiazepoxide hydrochloride on human embryonic and fetal development. N Engl J Med 291:1268–1271, 1974.
49. Eisenach JC, Castro MI: Maternally administered esmolol produces fetal β-adrenergic blockade and hypoxemia in sheep. Anesthesiology 71:718–722, 1989.
50. Dhama MS, Goh M: Deliberate hypotension for clipping of cerebral aneurysm during pregnancy. Anesthiol Rev 12:20–22, 1985.
51. Donchin Y, Amirav B, Sahar A, Yarkoni S: Sodium nitroprusside for aneurysm surgery in pregnancy. Br J Anaesth 50:849–850, 1978.
52. Rowbotham GF, Bell K, Akenhead J, Cairns H: A serious head injury in a pregnant woman treated by hypothermia. Lancet 272:1016–1019, 1957.
53. Henre FW: Hypothermia for operations during pregnancy. Anesth Analg 44:424–428, 1965.
54. Strickland RA, Oliver WC, Chantigian RC, et al: Anesthesia, cardiopulmonary bypass, and the pregnant patient. Mayo Clin Proc 66:411–429, 1991.
55. Rosen MA: Anesthesia for procedures involving the fetus. Semin Perinatol 15:410–417, 1991.
56. Longaker MT, Globus MS, Filly RA, et al: Maternal outcome after open fetal surgery. A review of the first 17 human cases. JAMA 265:737–741, 1991.
57. Santos AC, Arthur GR, Wlody D, et al: Comparative systemic toxicity of ropivacaine and bupivacaine in nonpregnant and pregnant ewes. Anesthesiology 82:734–740, 1995.

T W E N T Y - O N E

Postoperative Analgesia in Obstetrics

James C. Eisenach, M.D.

Voluminous case reports, clinical studies, chapters, and reviews have been written concerning the treatment of pain after cesarean section. This reflects in large part the popularity of using the obstetric population as an acute pain model to test and compare pain treatments. As a result, a large variety of treatments, many new and experimental, are described and are commonly employed in women after cesarean section. The goal of this chapter is to guide the reader through the literature on post-cesarean pain, emphasizing practical approaches with demonstrated safety and pointing out pitfalls and dangers associated with these and other proposed methods. The first part of this chapter describes the problem being treated and defines goals of such treatment.

Pain after cesarean section is usually described as having two components: *incisional pain,* which is sharp, constant, and worsened by movement, deep breathing, coughing, and the like, and *uterine contraction pain,* which is less well localized, often described as gnawing or boring, and episodic. This distinction is important for two reasons. First, certain treatments that block only one type of pain (e.g., ilioinguinal nerve block for incisional pain) should not be expected to provide total pain relief and will require supplementation. Second, some treatments are more effective for one type of pain than the other (e.g., nonsteroidal anti-inflammatory drugs [NSAIDs] for uterine contraction pain), and changes in treatment can be guided by which pain is most bothersome to the patient.

Another aspect to consider about pain after cesarean section is its rapidly declining nature. A typical time course of pain intensity, measured by opioid usage, is demonstrated in Figure 21–1. Pain intensity rapidly declines after the first 24 hours, and many women receive only oral analgesics (NSAIDs alone or with a small amount of opioid) thereafter for pain relief. Clearly, one can provide better pain relief beyond the initial 24 hours by maintaining intravenous or epidural access, but it is far less obvious whether such invasive and costly measures provide real benefit during this period of waning pain intensity.

This brings us to the definition of goals of pain therapy after cesarean section. As regards duration of pain treatment, a number of easily

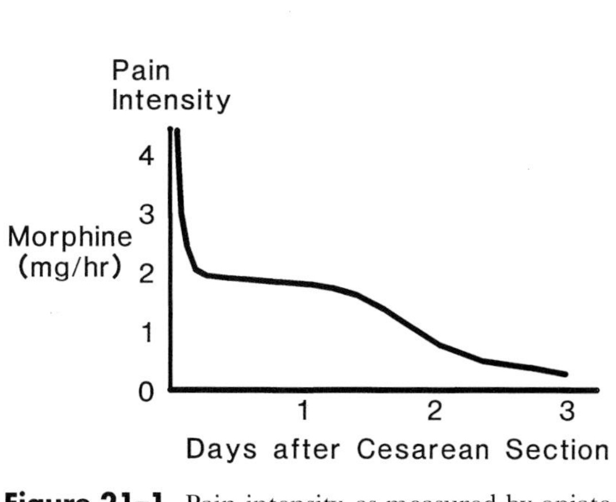

Figure 21–1. Pain intensity, as measured by opiate use (milligrams per hour [mg/hr] of morphine or equivalent systemically) in a typical patient after cesarean section.

available options exist to provide intense analgesia for 3 to 6 hours. For complete analgesia lasting 24 hours, fewer options are available, and these carry added economic costs and side effects. Still fewer options are available to provide complete pain relief throughout the 3- to 5-day hospital stay (Table 21–1). Intensity of analgesia from the various techniques is in the order: epidural-spinal opioid → intravenous (IV) patient-controlled analgesia (PCA) → intramuscular (IM) opioids = ilioinguinal block. Defining a goal for each patient simplifies the selection of a technique, although the method could range from continuous epidural morphine for 5 days—for a completely pain-free experience requiring no treatment—to a single dose of spinal fentanyl, providing 1 to 3 hours of pain relief.

Appropriate goals for pain treatment after cesarean section depend on the practice setting and the patient. Routine prolonged epidural catheterization for opioid administration may not be feasible or desirable in a low-risk population and a busy practice without dedicated postoperative pain management personnel. Other than practical constraints and patient preference, there is little to guide the choice of technique. For example, although complete pain relief diminishes the magnitude of the stress response and tissue catabolism in the postoperative state, such transient responses are well tolerated in a young healthy population, which constitutes the majority of women after cesarean section. Although some practitioners have suggested that women are discharged from the hospital earlier with spinal-epidural opioids than with other treatments, this difference is usually a matter of only a few hours, and the timing of discharge in this patient population is often mandated by social rather than medical factors. This is not to say that intensive analgesia therapy may not lessen morbidity or mortality in certain critically ill women after cesarean section, but it is unlikely to significantly alter these factors in healthy women. The goal in healthy women is to provide postoperative analgesia for 24 hours by simple means that are safe and effective and that provide a high degree of patient satisfaction.

Once a goal has been established, patient and "system" factors place constraints on the options available. Clearly, choice of intraoperative anesthetic technique determines which options are available. The remainder of this chapter is organized by description of analgesia options with each specific anesthetic technique. Important patient constraints include the desire for early ambulation and bathing, early social visits, and early removal of catheters. Minimizing sedation and newborn drug exposure is a concern for mothers who plan to breast feed during the postoperative period. System factors include the expense of apnea monitoring equipment, the invasive nature of this procedure and the difficulty in applying it to this ambulatory population, and the large number of patients cared for by each nurse, which makes intense monitoring for respiratory depression and sedation of a large proportion of patients difficult. This latter factor also limits the nurse's ability to respond effectively to as-necessary (PRN) IM opioid orders for postoperative analgesia. In the

TABLE 21–1
Goals and Options for Pain Management After Cesarean Section

Pain Relief	Duration	Options
Partial	1–3 days	Intravenous PCA alone or with agents below
Partial	1 day	Ilioinguinal nerve block Oral/intravenous NSAIDs
Complete	1–3 days	Epidural opiates by continuous infusion or repeated bolus
Complete	1 day	Epidural morphine (1 dose) or lipid-soluble opiates by continuous infusion Intrathecal morphine
Complete	2–6 hours	Epidural fentanyl Intrathecal fentanyl with epinephrine

Abbreviations: PCA = patient-controlled analgesia; NSAIDs = nonsteroidal anti-inflammatory drugs.

following discussion, the choice of technique includes considerations of these constraints.

THE PATIENT HAVING GENERAL ANESTHESIA

Peripheral Nerve Block

As in other areas of medicine, so also in obstetric analgesia, prevention is better than cure, and blockade of noxious sensory stimuli from reaching the central nervous system appears not only to provide excellent analgesia during the actual period of nerve block but also to prevent "central sensitization," which aggravates pain in the postoperative period.[1] Interestingly, peripheral nerve block is more effective than spinal-epidural block in this regard.

Two peripheral nerve blocks may be used for analgesia after cesarean section. Ilioinguinal nerve block, accomplished by depositing 5 to 8 ml of local anesthetic (usually 0.25% bupivacaine with epinephrine) bilaterally just above and below the fascia 2 cm from the anterior superior iliac spine on a line to the umbilicus (Fig. 21–2), will anesthetize the T12–L1 dermatomes. This is supplemented by bilateral subcutaneous infiltration (usually with 0.125% bupivacaine with epinephrine) from this injection site to the umbilicus to anesthetize the T11 dermatome.

Ilioinguinal nerve block decreases pain and diminishes postoperative opioid requirements after cesarean section.[2] Some suggest the pain relief obtained in these patients with this block is comparable to that achieved with intrathecal morphine.[3] However, in theory this block should not affect the visceral component of post–cesarean section pain, and the author's group's limited experience confirms this premise. Advantages of this therapy over others include no enhancement of opioid-induced side effects, no demonstrable neonatal effects, and only local bruising as a common side effect. Ideally, this block should be performed prior to skin incision. However, if it is performed before induction of regional or general anesthesia, this block may be painful, and if done after induction of general anesthesia, performance of this block would prolong the time from induction to delivery. Others would prefer to perform this block at the conclusion of surgery in order to avoid these problems and to avoid the distortion of lower abdominal anatomy present before delivery. Potential side effects include local bleeding, nerve trauma, and bowel perforation, the latter expected to be extremely uncommon in this population, since the enlarged uterus fills the pelvis. In addition, this block will not provide incisional pain relief for a vertical skin incision.

A second method of peripheral nerve block is infiltration of the wound with local anesthetic. In patients undergoing inguinal herniorrhaphy, this is as effective as ilioinguinal nerve block in decreasing postoperative pain[4] and would be expected to be so after cesarean section as well. There are few disadvantages to this technique except for distortion of local tissues, which may be bothersome to the surgeon regardless of whether infiltration is performed prior to skin incision or just before skin closure.

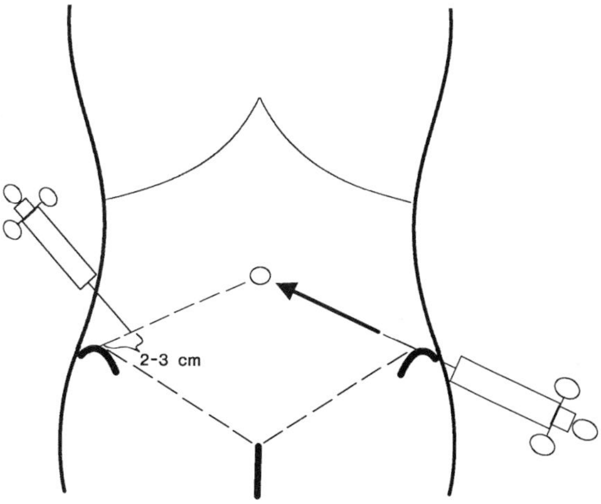

Figure 21–2. Technique for ilioinguinal nerve block. Bilateral injection of local anesthetic is performed in a fanning motion through the fascia at a point 2 to 3 cm along a line from anterosuperior iliac crest to umbilicus (shown on the patient's right), followed by bilateral subcutaneous infiltration of local anesthetic from this point to the umbilicus (shown on the patient's left).

Nurse-Administered Opioids

The multiple deficiencies and problems associated with PRN nurse-administered opioids for postoperative analgesia have been detailed in several recent reviews and are not repeated here. Advantages of this technique include low cost, long history of safety, and ease of use from the physician's standpoint. However, of all the methods discussed in this chapter, this is the least satisfactory to the patient, provides the poorest analgesia, and exposes the mother to at least as much opioid as any other technique.[5] Attempts have been made to enhance the efficacy of this therapy by adjusting the prescribed dose according to the amount of intravenous opioid required in the recovery room for pain control. This method is imprecise at best, and usually one is again left with a PRN order of a range of doses to be administered over a range of times, leading often to administration of the smallest dose prescribed and at the longest interval.

Intravenous Methadone

Methadone has the unique property among clinically available opioids of having a high lipid solubility, thereby achieving a rapid onset of effect following intravenous administration, and a long elimination half-life, leading to a long duration of effect, which approaches 12 hours. Some advocate titration of methadone in 5-mg increments in the recovery room for pain relief, such as with any analgesic, and observe prolonged (8 to 12 hours) pain relief without additional drug after this titration. Such long-lasting pain relief has not, however, been universally observed with this technique.[6] Published experience with this technique is limited, and appropriate therapy for breakthrough pain on the postpartum wards following methadone loading has not been clarified. Because of concern over the potential for opioid overdose with dosing on top of this methadone "basal infusion," the author's group has not utilized this technique, despite its potential advantage of simple titration in the recovery room and sustained analgesia.

Intravenous Patient-Controlled Analgesia

PCA provides better pain relief and is preferred by patients to nurse-administered PRN opioids after cesarean section.[5, 7] Opioid usage is similar with the two techniques; yet pain relief is better overall with PCA, and patients experience less pain at night with PCA than with nurse-administered PRN opioids (Fig. 21–3). The reasons for improved analgesia with PCA than with IM opioids despite similar overall doses is unclear, but they may relate to psychological factors or to a steadier level of pain relief produced by repeated small doses with PCA. Compared with a single epidural bolus of morphine 5 mg following cesarean section, women using PCA experience more pain but are equally satisfied,[5, 7] in part owing to the psychological benefits of being in control of their therapy, and perhaps owing to the high incidence of side effects with this method of epidural opioid therapy. Disadvantages of PCA include the bulkiness of these systems, the need for continued intravenous cannulation, the cost of the devices, and the chance of error owing to misprogramming. However, because of its advantages, the author's group uses IV PCA more often than any other technique for postoperative analgesia following cesarean section.

Factors important in the safety and efficacy of IV PCA therapy include the size of the bolus dose, the inclusion of basal infusion, and the choice of drug. Owen and colleagues showed

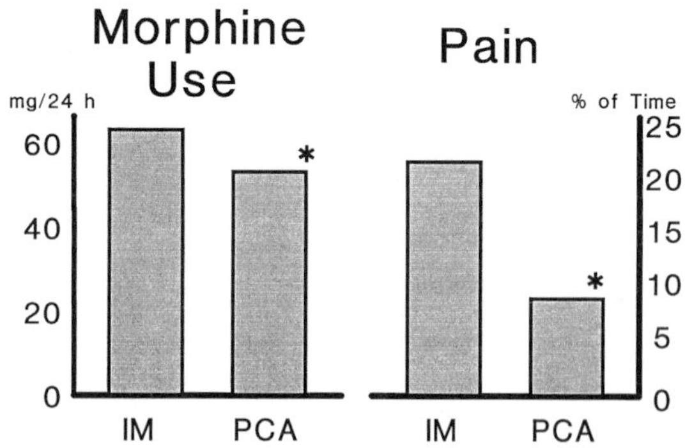

Figure 21–3. Comparison between intravenous patient-controlled analgesia (PCA) and as-needed nurse-administered intramuscular (IM) morphine following cesarean section. *Asterisk* indicates $p < .05$ in the PCA group versus the intramuscular group, demonstrating slightly decreased morphine use and better pain relief with PCA. (Modified from Eisenach JC, Grice SC, Dewan DM: Patient-controlled analgesia following cesarean section: A comparison with epidural and intramuscular narcotics. Anesthesiology 68:444–448, 1988.)

that, surprisingly, both the safety and the efficacy of PCA therapy in the postoperative period are affected by bolus dose.[8] Examining a narrow dose range (0.5, 1, 2 mg) with the ability to obtain the same total dose of morphine per hour, they observed similar opioid demand rates regardless of dose, a high degree of failure owing to inadequate analgesia in those receiving 0.5-mg boluses, and a high incidence of side effects, including significant respiratory depression in those patients receiving 2-mg boluses. Based on this literature, the author's group typically prescribes a bolus dose of 1 to 1.5 mg after cesarean section.

Should a basal infusion be added to PCA? Proponents of basal infusions cite advantages of more consistent analgesia and better sleep at night. Whereas the author's group does not dispute that an occasional patient may benefit from inclusion of a basal infusion with PCA, the group does not routinely use one for several reasons. First, studies comparing PCA alone with PCA plus basal infusion have demonstrated either no difference in quality of pain relief achieved or only minimal advantages to the infusion groups.[9, 10] Second, addition of a basal infusion may increase opioid usage to obtain the same degree of analgesia. Two studies demonstrate increases in opioid usage during the second postoperative day in patients receiving a basal infusion with PCA compared with PCA alone,[9, 10] supporting animal studies that suggest continuous opioid infusion hastens the development of acute opioid tolerance. Third, basal infusions may decrease the safety of the PCA technique.[11] This is true in part because continuous infusion removes patient feedback, inherent in the PCA technique, and is important because of the wide variability in patient opioid requirements. For this reason, the author's group does not routinely use basal infusions with PCA after cesarean section, and when such infusions are employed, the rate is limited to 0.5 mg/hour, which is less than would be used by 95% of the author's group's population.

A second way that basal infusions decrease PCA safety is by increasing the chance of human error in programming. This is in part due to the additional step required in programming the devices. Additionally, removal of patient feedback by basal infusion may increase the likelihood of morbidity should other errors occur. For example, the author's group is aware of a woman who recently received both epidural morphine and IV PCA. Despite orders that contradicted systemic opioids, PCA therapy was begun, including a basal infusion of morphine, 1 mg/hour. Six hours later, the patient was sedated and bradypneic, both of which cleared uneventfully with discontinuation of PCA. Without a basal infusion, it is unlikely the patient would have received any IV morphine, as she was reported to be pain free, and would have been less likely to experience these side effects.

Does it make a difference which opioid is chosen for PCA? Sinatra and associates recently compared morphine and oxymorphone by PCA after cesarean section and, aside from slightly more rapid onset of analgesia during the loading phase with oxymorphone, observed no significant differences between these drugs.[12] This same group then compared morphine with meperidine in a classic and thorough examination of issues important to the patient after cesarean section.[13] Again, no differences in efficacy were noted between these drugs. However, neonatal neurobehavioral scores were lower in breast-fed infants of mothers receiving meperidine than in those whose mothers received morphine, correlating with high accumulations of this drug's metabolite, normeperidine, in maternal plasma and breast milk. This effect is perhaps not surprising given the properties of normeperidine and its long half-life and demonstrates that maternally administered analgesics may interfere with newborn behavior. In addition, normeperidine is irritating to the central nervous system, explaining the seizures noted in patients receiving PCA meperidine postoperatively and providing yet another reason not to use this drug as first-line treatment with PCA. Based on these considerations, the author's group's typical IV PCA regimen in this patient population is outlined in Table 21–2.

Miscellaneous Techniques

A variety of other techniques, including transcutaneous electrical nerve stimulation, acupuncture, intranasally administered opioids, and NSAIDs, have been examined for postoperative analgesia in this setting. In general, these methods have been ineffective or only partially effective, often accompanied by significant side effects. NSAIDs, such as ketorolac, are likely to be effective in decreasing the dose and side

TABLE 21–2
PCA Guidelines

Drug	Morphine (second choice: oxymorphone; third choice: meperidine)
Dose	1 mg morphine (0.15 mg oxymorphone; 10 mg meperidine)
Lockout	10 minutes
Hourly limit	10 mg morphine (1.5 mg oxymorphone, 100 mg meperidine)
Basal infusion	0 (if desired for individual patient, 0.5 mg/hour morphine or equivalent)

Abbeviation: PCA = patient-controlled analgesia.

effects of opioids.[14] However, there is concern over large doses of potent NSAIDs in mothers who are breast feeding, because of neonatal transfer and potential cardiovascular complications in the neonate that have not been adequately studied to date. For this reason, the author's group does not use potent NSAIDs as a primary method of pain control in these patients.

THE PATIENT HAVING EPIDURAL ANESTHESIA

Previously Described Techniques

Epidural anesthesia does not preclude the use of any of the techniques discussed previously. Indeed, it is still rational to use peripheral nerve block to prevent "central sensitization" in such patients, and because of the problems with epidural opioids listed later, the author's group actually uses IV PCA morphine most commonly for postoperative analgesia in this group. Nonetheless, the presence of an epidural catheter adds a powerful option for pain treatment.

Epidural Morphine

Epidurally administered morphine 4 to 5 mg produces profound analgesia beginning 30 to 60 minutes after injection and lasting 12 to 24 hours after cesarean section. Because of its delayed onset, morphine should be administered well before the anticipated resolution of local anesthetic blockade and is typically administered immediately following delivery. Because of morphine's long duration and the desire of many women to have the epidural catheter removed, this drug is usually given as a single bolus, and the catheter is removed in recovery room. Of local anesthetics, only 2-chloroprocaine inhibits the analgesic action of opioids, including morphine.[15, 16] As a result, the author's group does not use epidural morphine if any 2-chloroprocaine has been administered in the preceding 6 hours. Although some physicians have observed an increased incidence of morphine-induced side effects when epinephrine has been added to the local anesthetic for intraoperative anesthesia,[17] the author's group has not.[16]

The most serious side effect from epidural morphine administration is respiratory depression, often occurring 6 to 12 hours after bolus injection, typically in the evening or night. Respiratory depression is thought to be due to cephalad spread of morphine with cerebrospinal fluid (CSF) circulation to brain stem sites. Although many institutions restrict epidural opioid therapy to intensively monitored settings for this reason, others have demonstrated safety on postoperative wards, provided adequate monitoring is instituted.[18] Most agree that hourly checks of respiratory rate and level of sedation are sensitive to detect any significant cases of respiratory depression, which occur with an incidence of approximately 1:1000 in the obstetric population.

Given that epidural morphine produces analgesia of variable duration and can produce delayed respiratory depression, how should one treat pain in the first 24 hours after epidural morphine injection? Although it is often stated that systemic opioid administration is a risk factor for epidural morphine–induced respiratory depression, review of the original surveys suggests an equal number of patients received systemic opioids and did *not* have respiratory depression. Because of this and large experience at other centers with the safety of administering opioid agonists *for pain* in this population after epidural morphine, the author's group allows 3 to 5 mg IV injections of morphine for pain in these patients. Alternatively, many patients experience only mild discomfort during this period, which could be treated by oral agents (e.g., acetaminophen). Although others would prefer to treat such pain with agonists-antagonists such as nalbuphine or butorphanol, limited efficacy and a high incidence of dysphoria and sedation with use of these agents make them less desirable.

Side effects, especially pruritus and nausea, are common with epidural morphine therapy. For an unknown reason, pruritus is especially common in the obstetric population, with most studies reporting an 80% incidence of pruritus and a 40% incidence of severe pruritus requiring treatment. Pruritus and scratching of the face may account for the cases of recrudescence of herpes labialis in the obstetric population,[19] which, although not dangerous, may interfere with the mother's contact with the newborn. Nausea can be treated symptomatically with intravenous promethazine (Phenergan), droperidol, or metoclopramide or with transdermal scopolamine,[20] the latter being particularly effective for cases of persistent nausea.

The cause of epidural morphine–induced pruritus is unknown, although it is thought to result from an action on opioid receptors, as it is reversed by naloxone. Pruritus may be prevented by continuous naloxone infusion (5 to 10 μg/kg/hour) or single naltrexone administration (3 to 6 mg orally), although in each case, the quality or duration of analgesia is decreased. Pruritus may also be treated with opioid antagonists, and the agonist-antagonist nalbuphine 5 to 10 mg IV has been reported to inhibit pruritus without affecting analgesia.[21] Coadministration of butorphanol with morphine was shown in one study to abolish morphine-induced pruritus.[22] However, other studies failed to replicate this observation,[23] and concerns over neurotoxicity from spinal butorphanol administration weaken the argument for its use. Interestingly, subhypnotic doses of propofol (10 mg IV) have been reported in double-blind studies to abolish morphine-induced pruritus,[24] perhaps by altering receptive fields of spinal cord neurons receiving sensory input. The author's group chooses to treat morphine-induced pruritus symptomatically with diphenhydramine 12.5 to 25 mg IV, and to resort only occasionally to naloxone therapy.

Epidural Fentanyl, Sufentanil, and Other Lipid-Soluble Agents

Epidural fentanyl 50 to 100 μg enhances intraoperative epidural anesthesia and provides 1 to 4 hours of pain relief following surgery. Unlike morphine, fentanyl is highly lipid soluble, correlating with a rapid onset of action (less than 20 minutes) but a much shorter duration than morphine.[25] Although this agent would appear ideal for providing pain relief in the first hours after surgery in the recovery room, this may just delay the IV opioid loading time to the postpartum ward, where pain relief is often achieved in a much slower fashion under less ideal monitoring. For this reason, the author's group uses epidural fentanyl as needed to enhance intraoperative analgesia but not routinely for postoperative analgesia.

Because of its limited duration, fentanyl must be administered by continuous infusion or intermittent bolus (typically patient-controlled epidural analgesia) for sustained pain relief. Unfortunately, when fentanyl is used in this manner, any advantages of its epidural administration are lost. Numerous studies demonstrate no difference between IV and epidural routes of administration for fentanyl, by either titrated infusion or PCA in the postoperative setting.[26, 27] Whether this is due to fentanyl's high lipid solubility and rapid systemic absorption or to its lack of synergy between spinal and supraspinal sites[28] is unclear, but there seems to be little rationale for routine use of epidural fentanyl alone beyond a dose in the operating room.

Fentanyl has been examined for epidural analgesia because of the concept that this lipid-soluble drug would not remain in the CSF long enough to circulate to the brain stem and depress respiration. Unfortunately, this appears not to be true. Lipid-soluble drugs appear rapidly in cervical CSF after lumbar (but not IV) administration,[29] and several cases of acute respiratory depression, 20 to 60 minutes after epidural fentanyl administration, have been reported.[30, 31] In addition, respiratory depression has been noted in a relatively high incidence of patients (4 : 1000) 2 to 10 hours after a titrated epidural fentanyl infusion was begun. These data suggest that should epidural fentanyl be chosen as the analgesic technique, respiratory monitoring should be equally vigilant as it is with epidural morphine.

Other lipid-soluble agents (sufentanil, butorphanol, nalbuphine) have been reported to produce analgesia after cesarean section. Not only do these agents suffer from the same disadvantages as fentanyl (Fig. 21–4) but they also

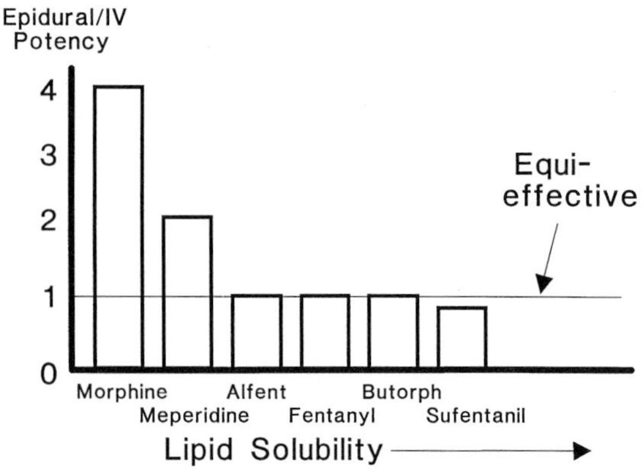

Figure 21–4. Ratio of potency epidurally versus intravenously of opiates with varying lipid solubility, from poorly lipid soluble (morphine) to highly lipid soluble (sufentanil), for postoperative pain. For clarity, the line drawn at a value of 1 indicates that the same dose would be required by either route. (*Abbreviations:* Alfent = alfentanil; butorph = butorphanol.)

either have not been tested for safety by this route or have been shown to be neurotoxic.[32] Therefore, they should not be used routinely until their safety is established. Similarly, relatively large doses of meperidine are required epidurally (300 to 600 mg/24 hour), raising the same issues as with IV PCA administration of this drug.

COMBINATION THERAPY

Opioids, local anesthetics, and α_2-adrenergic agonists act at different spinal sites to produce analgesia, and experiments in animals suggest that these classes of drugs interact synergistically. Cohen and coworkers have shown that addition of bupivacaine to fentanyl after cesarean section diminishes fentanyl dosage but results in evidence of unwanted local anesthetic blockade.[33] Addition of epinephrine to a reduced dose of bupivacaine also diminishes fentanyl dosage without demonstrable local anesthetic blockade.[34] Such combinations have several advantages over a pure opioid technique, but their use requires continued epidural catheterization and infusion, and their safety has not been assessed in large populations.

THE PATIENT HAVING SPINAL ANESTHESIA

Previously Described Techniques

All of the techniques described in those having general anesthesia are also applicable to patients following spinal anesthesia. In addition, many anesthesiologists are now using combined spinal-epidural techniques, in which the epidural space is identified with a curved-tip epidural needle, a spinal needle is inserted into the intrathecal space through the epidural needle, a spinal local anesthetic is injected, and an epidural catheter is inserted and secured. Several manufacturers are now producing epidural needles containing guide tubes or flanges for spinal needle insertion (Fig. 21–5). Of course, with the use of this technique, all of the options described in those having epidural anesthesia become available to these patients as well. However, although intrathecal "migration" of the epidural catheter appears unlikely with this technique, it is conceivable that a larger proportion of epidurally administered drug will reach the CSF owing to the dural puncture from the spinal needle than would occur with an intact dura. Since published experience with this technique for postoperative analgesia is relatively small, one should be alert for the possibility of

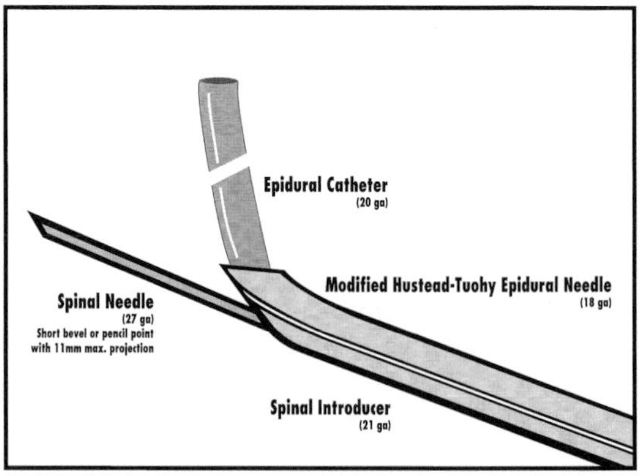

Figure 21–5. An example of a new, commercially available needle with dual cannulas for combined epidural/spinal technique. (Courtesy of Neurodelivery Technology, Inc., Lebanon, NH.)

exaggerated intensity of side effects from epidurally administered drugs.

Choice of Local Anesthetic

In most cases, the author prefers to use hyperbaric 0.75% bupivacaine for spinal anesthesia for cesarean section. Although the duration of anesthesia is longer with this agent than with lidocaine, in the author's group's experience, most patients are discharged from the recovery room within 90 minutes with either agent. Thus, even for relatively fast surgeons, this drug does not appear to prolong recovery room time. In addition, a major pain stimulus in the recovery room is frequent and vigorous uterine massage. Lingering sensory blockade with bupivacaine during this period diminishes the dose of IV opioid required for treatment.

Spinal Morphine

An extremely small dose of morphine, 0.2 mg, provides excellent and prolonged pain relief after cesarean section, similar to a 4- to 5-mg dose epidurally.[35] However, the side effects described with epidurally administered opioids are at least as intense, if not more so, following spinal administration, as might be expected from the observation than CSF morphine concentrations are two to four times higher after 0.25 mg morphine spinally than after 6 mg epidurally.[36] In addition, there is concern that spinal administration of morphine is more likely to result in delayed respiratory depression than is epidural administration, although this may have reflected the relatively large doses (0.5 to 1 mg) injected spinally in the initial reports. Spinal morphine–induced pruritus may be more resistant to treatment with naltrexone than epidural administration,[37] and nausea occurs more commonly and is more bothersome as well. For these reasons, the author's group rarely uses spinal morphine after cesarean section.

Other Spinal Opioids and Epinephrine

Fentanyl 10 to 20 μg or sufentanil 3 to 5 μg produces analgesia that outlasts the period of spinal bupivacaine anesthesia by about 1 hour and also diminishes intraoperative pain with exteriorization of the uterus during surgery.[38] Side effects from this small dose of fentanyl are unusual and short-lived, although respiratory depression occurring within 1 hour of fentanyl administration has been reported.[39] Interestingly, lipid-soluble opioids can reach cervical and brain stem sites rapidly after intraspinal injection (see discussion under "Epidural Fentanyl, Sufentanil, and Other Lipid-Soluble Agents," earlier in this chapter), which explains this phenomenon. These patients should therefore be continuously monitored for 60 minutes after the fentanyl injection, which almost always encompasses the intraoperative period, where such monitoring is part of routine practice anyway.

Although epinephrine does not dramatically prolong the duration of spinal bupivacaine anesthesia, it does extend the duration of spinal fentanyl analgesia by an additional 2 to 3 hours.[40] For this reason, if the goal is to provide 4 to 5 hours of complete analgesia, both fentanyl (10 to 20 μg) *and* epinephrine (200 μg) should be added to spinal bupivacaine. In some individuals, addition of epinephrine may prolong the duration of sensory and motor blockade by as much as 60 to 90 minutes, thereby delaying the time to discharge to the recovery room. Addition of epinephrine to spinal fentanyl does not, however, appear to alter the incidence of fentanyl-induced side effects, which are relatively infrequent in any case.

SUMMARY

In conclusion, a variety of options are available for postoperative analgesia in obstetrics. For women having general anesthesia for cesarean section, IV PCA with morphine without a basal infusion is the author's group's preferred technique; and if morphine dose is a concern, it can be reduced by intraoperative performance of ilioinguinal nerve blocks. For women having epidural anesthesia, the author's group prefers IV PCA with morphine because of its excellent patient satisfaction and few side effects, although many would choose single-bolus epidural morphine for 12 to 24 hours of more profound pain relief. Epidural morphine–induced side effects may be prevented by oral naltrexone or treated either symptomatically or with opiate antagonists. In contrast to single-dose morphine, continuous epidural infusion of lipid-soluble opioids appears to offer few advantages over IV PCA. For women having spinal anesthesia, the author's group prefers either IV PCA or the addition of spinal fentanyl and epinephrine to bupivacaine, the latter providing intense pain relief for 4 to 5 hours. Others use spinal morphine 0.2 mg for prolonged pain relief, but at the cost of a high incidence of side effects. Choice of analgesia technique depends ultimately on the patient, the anesthesiologist, and nursing constraints and preferences.

TEN PRACTICAL POINTS

1. Decide what your goal is—complete pain relief for the patient during the whole hospitalization or good pain relief in the recovery room.
2. After general anesthesia, consider an ilioinguinal block.
3. In general, for IV PCA, morphine and oxymorphone are preferred over meperidine. Do not routinely use a basal infusion.
4. The epidural morphine dose is 4 to 5 mg as a single bolus. Continuous infusion offers few advantages.
5. Avoid 2-chloroprocaine if you plan to give epidural opioids.
6. Have a standing order form for treatment of nausea, pruritus, and breakthrough pain.
7. Monitor the patient's respiratory rate and level of sedation for 24 hours after infusing epidural morphine.
8. Lipid-soluble opioids (e.g., fentanyl, sufentanil) are just as effective intravenously as epidurally for prolonged infusions, and these agents can depress respiration by either route.
9. The spinal morphine dose is 0.20 mg.
10. Spinal morphine has a high incidence of side effects in women after cesarean section.

REFERENCES

1. Wall PD: The prevention of postoperative pain. Pain 33:289–290, 1988.
2. Bunting P, McConachie I: Ilioinguinal nerve blockade for analgesia after caesarean section. Br J Anaesth 61:773–775, 1988.
3. Witkowski TA, Leighton BL, Norris MC: Ilioinguinal nerve blocks: An alternative or supplement to intrathecal morphine [Abstract]. Anesthesiology 73:A692, 1990.
4. Casey WF, Rice LJ, Hannallah RS, et al: A comparison between bupivacaine instillation versus ilioinguinal/iliohypogastric nerve block for postoperative analgesia following inguinal herniorrhaphy in children. Anesthesiology 72:637–639, 1990.
5. Eisenach JC, Grice SC, Dewan DM: Patient-controlled analgesia following cesarean section: A comparison with epidural and intramuscular narcotics. Anesthesiology 68:444–448, 1988.
6. Grochow L, Sheidler V, Grossman S, et al: Does intravenous methadone provide longer-lasting analgesia than intravenous morphine? A randomized, double-blind study. Pain 38:151–157, 1989.
7. Harrison DM, Sinatra R, Morgese L, Chung JH: Epidural narcotic and patient-controlled analgesia for post–cesarean section pain relief. Anesthesiology 68:454–457, 1988.
8. Owen H, Plummer JL, Armstrong I, et al: Variables of patient-controlled analgesia. 1. Bolus size. Anaesthesia 44:7–10, 1989.
9. Owen H, Kluger MT, Plummer JL: Variables of patient-controlled analgesia. 4. The relevance of bolus dose size to supplement a background infusion. Anaesthesia 45:619–622, 1990.
10. Hansen LA, Noyes MA, Lehman ME: Evaluation of patient-controlled analgesia (PCA) versus PCA plus continuous infusion in postoperative cancer patients. J Pain Symp Management 6:4–14, 1991.
11. Parker RK, Holtmann B, White PF: Patient-controlled analgesia. Does a concurrent opioid infusion improve pain management after surgery? JAMA 266:1947–1952, 1991.
12. Sinatra R, Chung KS, Silverman DG, et al: An evaluation of morphine and oxymorphone administered via patient-controlled analgesia (PCA) or PCA plus basal infusion in postcesarean-delivery patients. Anesthesiology 71:502–507, 1989.
13. Wittels B, Scott DT, Sinatra RS: Exogenous opioids in human breast milk and acute neonatal neurobehavior: A preliminary study. Anesthesiology 73:864–869, 1990.
14. Pavy T, Medley C, Murphy DF: Effect of indomethacin on pain relief after thoracotomy. Br J Anaesth 65:624–627, 1990.
15. Camann WR, Hartigan PM, Gilbertson LI, et al: Chloroprocaine antagonism of epidural opioid analgesia: A receptor-specific phenomenon. Anesthesiology 73:860–863, 1990.
16. Eisenach JC, Schlairet TJ, Dobson CE II, Hood DH: Effect of prior anesthetic solution on epidural morphine analgesia. Anesth Analg 73:119–123, 1991.
17. Douglas MJ, Kim JHK, Ross PLE, McMorland GH: The effect of epinephrine in local anaesthetic on epidural morphine–induced pruritus. Can Anaesth Soc J 33:737–740, 1986.
18. Ready LB, Loper KA, Nessly M, Wild L: Postoper-

ative epidural morphine is safe on surgical wards. Anesthesiology 75:452–456, 1991.
19. Crone L-AL, Conly JM, Clark KM, et al: Recurrent herpes simplex virus labialis and the use of epidural morphine in obstetric patients. Anesth Analg 67:318–323, 1988.
20. Loper KA, Ready LB, Dorman BH: Prophylactic transdermal scopolamine patches reduce nausea in postoperative patients receiving epidural morphine. Anesth Analg 68:144–146, 1989.
21. Davies GG, From R: A blinded study using nalbuphine for prevention of pruritus induced by epidural fentanyl. Anesthesiology 69:763–765, 1988.
22. Lawhorn CD, McNitt JD, Fibuch EE, et al: Epidural morphine with butorphanol for postoperative analgesia after cesarean delivery. Anesth Analg 72:53–57, 1991.
23. Gambling DR, Huber C, Howell P, Kozak S: Epidural butorphanol does not reduce side effects from epidural morphine post cesarean section [Abstract]. Proceedings of the 23rd Annual Meeting of the Society for Obstetric Anesthesia and Perinatology, Boston, 1991.
24. Gorgeat A, Wilder-Smith OHG, Saiah M, Rifat K: Subhypnotic doses of propofol relieve pruritus induced by epidural and intrathecal morphine. Anesthesiology 76:510–512, 1992.
25. Blanco J, Blanco E, Carceller JM, et al: Epidural analgesia for post-caesarean pain relief: A comparison between morphine and fentanyl. Eur J Anaesth 4:395–399, 1987.
26. Loper KA, Ready LB, Downey M, et al: Epidural and intravenous fentanyl infusions are clinically equivalent after knee surgery. Anesth Analg 70:72–75, 1990.
27. Ellis DJ, Millar WL, Reisner LS: A randomized double-blind comparison of epidural versus intravenous fentanyl infusion for analgesia after cesarean section. Anesthesiology 72:981–986, 1990.
28. Roerig SC, Hoffman RG, Takemori AE, et al: Isobolographic analysis of analgesic interactions between intrathecally and intracerebroventricularly administered fentanyl, morphine and D-Ala2-D-Leu5-enkephalin in morphine-tolerant and nontolerant mice. J Pharmacol Exp Ther 257:1091–1099, 1991.
29. Gourlay GK, Murphy TM, Plummer JL, et al: Pharmacokinetics of fentanyl in lumbar and cervical CSF following lumbar epidural and intravenous administration. Pain 38:253–259, 1989.
30. Wells DG, Davies G: Profound central nervous system depression from epidural fentanyl for extracorporeal shock wave lithotripsy. Anesthesiology 67:991–992, 1987.
31. Brockway MS, Noble DW, Sharwood-Smith GH, McClure JH: Profound respiratory depression after extradural fentanyl. Br J Anaesth 64:243–245, 1990.
32. Rawal N, Nuutinen L, Prithvi Raj P, et al: Behavioral and histopathologic effects following intrathecal administration of butorphanol, sufentanil, and nalbuphine in sheep. Anesthesiology 75:1025–1034, 1991.
33. Cohen S, Amar D, Pantuck EJ, et al: Continuous epidural-PCA post–cesarean section: Buprenorphine-bupivacaine 0.03% versus fentanyl-bupivacaine 0.03% [Abstract]. Anesthesiology 73:A975, 1990.
34. Cohen S, Amar D, Pantuck EJ, et al: Continuous epidural-PCA post–cesarean section: Buprenorphine-bupivacaine 0.015% with epinephrine versus fentanyl-bupivacaine 0.15% with and without epinephrine [Abstract]. Anesthesiology 73:A918, 1990.
35. Chadwick HS, Ready LB: Intrathecal and epidural morphine sulfate for postcesarean analgesia—A clinical comparison. Anesthesiology 68:925–929, 1988.
36. Jorgensen BC, Andersen HB, Engquist A: CSF and plasma morphine after epidural and intrathecal application. Anesthesiology 55:714–715, 1981.
37. Abboud TK, Lee K, Zhu J, et al: Prophylactic oral naltrexone with intrathecal morphine for cesarean section: Effects on adverse reactions and analgesia. Anesth Analg 71:367–370, 1990.
38. Hunt CO, Naulty JS, Bader AM, et al: Perioperative analgesia with subarachnoid fentanyl-bupivacaine for cesarean delivery. Anesthesiology 71:535–540, 1989.
39. Palmer CM: Early respiratory depression following intrathecal fentanyl-morphine combination. Anesthesiology 74:1153–1155, 1991.
40. Malinow AM, Mokriski BLK, Nomura MK, et al: Effect of epinephrine on intrathecal fentanyl analgesia in patients undergoing postpartum tubal ligation. Anesthesiology 73:381–385, 1990.

TWENTY-TWO

Resuscitation/Critical Care

Robert C. Chantigian, M.D.

Although infrequent, resuscitation of the newborn or the mother may be required. The general approach is similar for all patients, namely, the ABCs (airway, breathing, circulation and color, diagnosis and drugs). However, the newborn and the mother have special needs that dictate slightly different treatment regimens. This chapter presents a practical approach to newborn and maternal resuscitation.

Local hospital policies should clearly delineate who is responsible for resuscitation of the newborn or mother. In most hospital settings, the pediatrician assumes primary responsibility for the newborn. In hospitals in which a pediatrician is not always available, other physicians, such as the obstetrician, the family physician, or the anesthesiologist, must assume a primary role. Anesthesiologists can help stabilize the newborn until a pediatrician or a transport team from a pediatric center arrives. However, when the anesthesiologist is providing maternal care and the newborn requires resuscitation, the American Society of Anesthesiologists recommends that the benefit to the newborn must be compared with the risk of briefly leaving the mother, who is the primary responsibility.[1]

During maternal resuscitation, the obstetrician, family physician, internist, or anesthesiologist may need to assume the primary role.

NEWBORN RESUSCITATION

Before delivery, the maternal and fetal histories should be reviewed to identify potential problems that may require special treatment, special equipment, or additional trained personnel at delivery. In some cases, transferring the mother and fetus to an obstetric center with a pediatric intensive care unit is the most appropriate action. Recognition of significant problems can help establish realistic expectations for all concerned.

Maternal factors can indirectly affect oxygen delivery to the fetus by either decreasing oxygen content of maternal blood or decreasing uterine or placental perfusion. These factors include respiratory disease, anemia, hemorrhage, cardiovascular disease, pregnancy-induced hypertension (PIH), and diabetes mellitus. Maternal drug use may directly compromise the fetus.

Fetal problems that often require special intervention include hypoxia-asphyxia (e.g., severe late or variable deceleration patterns with low fetal scalp pH values, umbilical cord prolapse), meconium-stained amniotic fluid, prematurity, multiple gestation, and congenital birth defects (e.g., chromosomal abnormalities, anencephaly, diaphragmatic hernia, structural congenital heart disease, pleural effusions, neural tube defect, and hydrops). Many of these fetal problems can be identified antenatally through chorionic villus sampling, amniocentesis, percutaneous umbilical cord blood sampling, or ultrasound (see Chapter 3).

Certain fetal problems lead to poor outcome despite appropriate intervention. Anencephaly, some chromosomal abnormalities (e.g., trisomy 13 or trisomy 18), and some congenital anomalies (e.g., Potter syndrome) are associated with early neonatal death. Some structural congenital heart lesions are associated with circulation patterns that make adaptation to extrauterine life difficult, if not impossible. Newborns with diaphragmatic hernias have a survival rate of only about 50% with appropriate treatment. With severe thick meconium aspiration, some newborns die despite appropriate care. In very premature newborns (e.g., those less than 24 weeks' estimated gestational age [EGA] or those weighing less than 750 gm), survival is uniformly low.

This section on newborn resuscitation reviews the important aspects of fetal history and newborn anatomy and physiology related to resuscitation, newborn resuscitation techniques, and normal newborn care. Two conditions that frequently arise in obstetrics and often require resuscitation (meconium aspiration and respiratory distress syndrome [RDS]) are discussed.

Newborn

Estimated Gestational Age

"Term" newborns are usually defined as those being delivered between 37 and 42 weeks' EGA. Newborns born prior to 37 weeks are "preterm"; those born after 42 weeks are "postterm." Establishing the EGA is important for several reasons. First, knowledge of fetal EGA prior to delivery helps predict newborn survival as well as the potential need for intervention (Fig. 22–1).[2] Second, the differential diagnosis of potential newborn problems varies with gestational age. For example, respiratory symptoms resulting from RDS occur more commonly in preterm newborns than in term newborns; RDS rarely causes respiratory symptoms in postterm newborns. Third, by knowing the EGA, fetal weight can be estimated (Table 22–1).[2, 3] Knowledge of the estimated fetal weight

TABLE 22–1
Estimated Gestational Age and Approximate Newborn Mean Weights

Gestational Age (weeks)	Mean Weight (gm)
22	500
27	1000
30	1500
33	2000
35	2500
37	3000
40	3400
42	3500

Data from Williams RL, Creasy RK, Cunningham GC, et al: Fetal growth and perinatal viability in California. Obstet Gynecol 59:624–632, 1982; and Brenner WE, Edelman DA, Hendricks CH: A standard of fetal growth for the United States of America. Am J Obstet Gynecol 126:555–564, 1976.

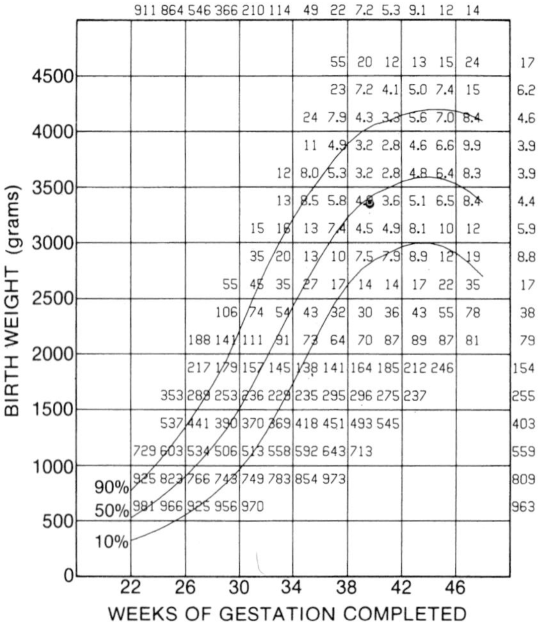

Figure 22–1. Birth weight percentiles and perinatal mortality rate (per 1000) for single births in California, 1970–1976. The birth weight–gestational age–specific mortality rates are computed on 2-week and 250-gm weight intervals; the values are placed within the square corresponding to the appropriate birth weight–gestational age grid. For example, the perinatal death rate for newborns weighing from 500 to 750 gm and of 22 to 24 weeks' estimated gestational age was 981 per 1000 deliveries. (The *black dot* indicates the mean birth weight–gestational age combination.) (Modified from Williams RL, Creasy RK, Cunningham GC, et al: Fetal growth and perinatal viability in California. Reprinted with permission from The American College of Obstetricians and Gynecologists [Obstetrics and Gynecology, 1982, Vol 59, pp 624–632].)

aids resuscitative efforts, particularly if resuscitation must proceed prior to establishing the actual newborn weight. Drug dosages, endotracheal tube diameter, and placement depend on infant size. For instance, a 27-week EGA newborn, whose estimated weight is 1000 gm, will need a 2.5-mm internal diameter (ID) endotracheal tube inserted 7 cm if intubation is necessary (Tables 22–1 and 22–2). However, extrapolation of the estimated fetal weight from the EGA assumes normal fetal growth. In some cases, the fetus is markedly smaller (e.g., because of intrauterine growth retardation) or larger (e.g., owing to maternal diabetes mellitus) than estimated from the EGA.

Anatomic Considerations

The head of the newborn is usually the largest anatomic diameter to pass through the birth canal. In vaginal breech deliveries, the dilating wedge, the breech, is smaller than the aftercoming head. Head entrapment may occur and lead to fetal hypoxia or asphyxia. Newborn intubation may be facilitated by placing a small towel under the shoulders, especially for newborns with a large caput and for premature newborns in whom head size is relatively larger than that in term newborns.

The newborn's tongue is relatively large, making intubations more difficult, especially in the newborn with hypoplastic mandible (e.g., Pierre Robin syndrome). Nasopharyngeal placement of an endotracheal tube bypasses the tongue and aids ventilation if oral intubation is not possible.

The cricoid cartilage is the narrowest part of the trachea. An endotracheal tube of 2.5-mm ID can be used safely to intubate a preterm newborn, 3.0-mm ID for a term newborn, and 3.5-mm ID for a postterm newborn. Although larger tubes may fit,[4] choosing a smaller tube initially may be advantageous, so that an airway can be quickly established. If resistance is met just past the vocal cords, the tube is too large. If a large air leak exists, a larger endotracheal tube can be placed once the newborn is given several breaths of oxygen. Smaller endotracheal tubes may save some time.

The distance from the vocal cords to the carina is approximately 3 cm in the smallest preterm newborn and about 6 cm in the term newborn.[4, 5] If intubation of the newborn is indicated, advancing the tip of the endotracheal tube about 2.5 cm past the vocal cords (i.e., to the first black mark from the tip of the endotracheal tube) positions the endotracheal tube tip in the mid trachea. The average distance of the tip from the newborn lips is about 7 cm for 1000-gm newborns, 8 cm for 2000-gm newborns, 9 cm for 3000-gm newborns, and 10 cm for newborns weighing more than 3000 gm (Table 22–2).

Respiratory Physiology

The fetus initiates diaphragmatic respiratory movements as early as 11 weeks' gestation.[6] Respiratory movements become more vigorous and more organized as the gestation advances.

The fetal lungs produce alveolar fluid at a rate of 3 ml/kg/hour. Fluid flows out through the trachea into the amniotic fluid, with complete turnover of lung fluid volume occurring every 10 hours.[7] Because of this flow, the surfactant (essential to prevent alveolar collapse) produced by the lung's alveolar epithelial type II cells can be measured in the amniotic fluid, and

TABLE 22–2
Newborn Weight, Endotracheal Tube Size, and Distance From Lips to Mid Trachea for Intubation

Mean Weight (gm)	Endotracheal Tube Size (mm internal diameter)	Endotracheal Tube Distance Lips to Mid Trachea (cm)
1000	2.5	7
2000	2.5–3.0	8
3000	3.0–3.5	9
>3000	3.5–4.0	10

lung maturity can be estimated.[8] Surfactant has several components, including lipids, proteins, and carbohydrates; its production starts at about 24 weeks' EGA. Lecithin concentration increases with gestational age, whereas the sphingomyelin concentration remains relatively constant in the amniotic fluid. When the concentration of lecithin in the amniotic fluid is equal to two to three times the concentration of sphingomyelin, the alveoli can better maintain their patency (i.e., the lungs are usually "mature"), and RDS is less likely to develop.

The stimulus to take the first breath involves several factors, including chest wall recoil at delivery, tactile stimulation, umbilical cord clamping, sympathetic stimulation, and arterial hypercarbia and hypoxemia.[9, 10]

Extrauterine breathing normally begins within 30 seconds of delivery (average 9 seconds).[11] The normal newborn breathes at a rate of about 30 to 40 breaths per minute, but for the first hour, respiratory rates may be as high as 90 breaths per minute. This rate decreases with time in normal newborns.[12]

Although some degree of hypoxia is a common finding in all newborns as a result of the normal birthing process, severe hypoxia, if present, will depress the newborn's respiratory center through the first week of life. Thereafter, hypoxia acts as a respiratory stimulant.[13]

The tidal volume of a normal newborn's first breath varies widely from 12 to 67 ml. After breathing is established, the tidal volume is about 15 to 20 ml or about 6 to 8 ml/kg.[14] If intubation and ventilation of the newborn become necessary, the required tidal volume is small! Proper tidal volumes are indicated by slight chest wall movement and adequate breath sounds and, if assisted ventilation is performed, with airway pressures of 15 to 20 cmH_2O.[4] Excessively high airway pressures can cause decreased cardiac output and barotrauma. Barotrauma can lead to air leaks and lung damage.

Oxygen consumption is about 6 to 7 ml oxygen/kg/minute (about double that of adults). Oxygen saturation gradually increases over the first 10 minutes of life. Porter and colleagues[15] examined oxygen saturation values in 100 normal newborns and found the oxygen saturations to be 78 ± 11% at 1 minute, 84 ± 8% at 5 minutes, and 89 ± 6% at 10 minutes.

Slight nasal flaring, rales, and mild retractions are common and usually clear spontaneously in less than 1 hour.[12] Persistence or worsening of these signs may indicate respiratory distress.

Cardiovascular Physiology

Newborns undergo major circulatory changes at birth. The intrauterine fetal circulation shifts first to a transitional circulation and eventually to the adult circulation (Fig. 22–2). The fetal circulation has high pulmonary vascular resistance (owing to the low arterial oxygen levels and the unexpanded lungs) and low systemic vascular resistance (owing to the placenta). The resultant pressure differential encourages blood flow through the two right-to-left shunts, the foramen ovale and the ductus arteriosus.

Breathing and clamping the umbilical cord initiate transitional circulation. With breathing, the lungs fill with air, arterial blood oxygen concentration increases, pulmonary vascular resistance decreases, and pulmonary blood flow increases. This increases blood flow to the left atrium, elevates the left atrial pressure, and leads to functional closure of the foramen ovale. When the umbilical cord is clamped, systemic vascular resistance increases, systemic blood pressure rises, and blood flow across the ductus arteriosus decreases. Functional closure of the ductus arteriosus in term newborns occurs physiologically in 10 to 15 hours, whereas anatomical closure takes 2 to 3 weeks. If hypoxia or acidosis develops before the ductus arteriosus anatomically closes, the ductus may reopen, reestablishing a right-to-left shunt. The adult circulation is established when these two shunts close.

The newborn heart rate is quite labile for the first 30 minutes, with rates ranging from 100 to 200 beats per minute (bpm). Thereafter, the heart rate stabilizes to about 120 to 140 bpm and varies with newborn activity.[12]

Blood pressure in the newborn is lower than that in the adult and varies with newborn size (Table 22–3).[16, 17]

Term newborn blood volume is approximately 80 to 100 ml/kg. If blood volume decreases by 10%, blood pressure falls by 20%. If blood volume decreases by 20%, blood pressure falls by 50%. The normal hemoglobin level is 15 to 20 gm/100 ml (hematocrit 45 to 60%).

Nervous System Physiology

The central nervous system is not fully developed at birth but develops rapidly over the next

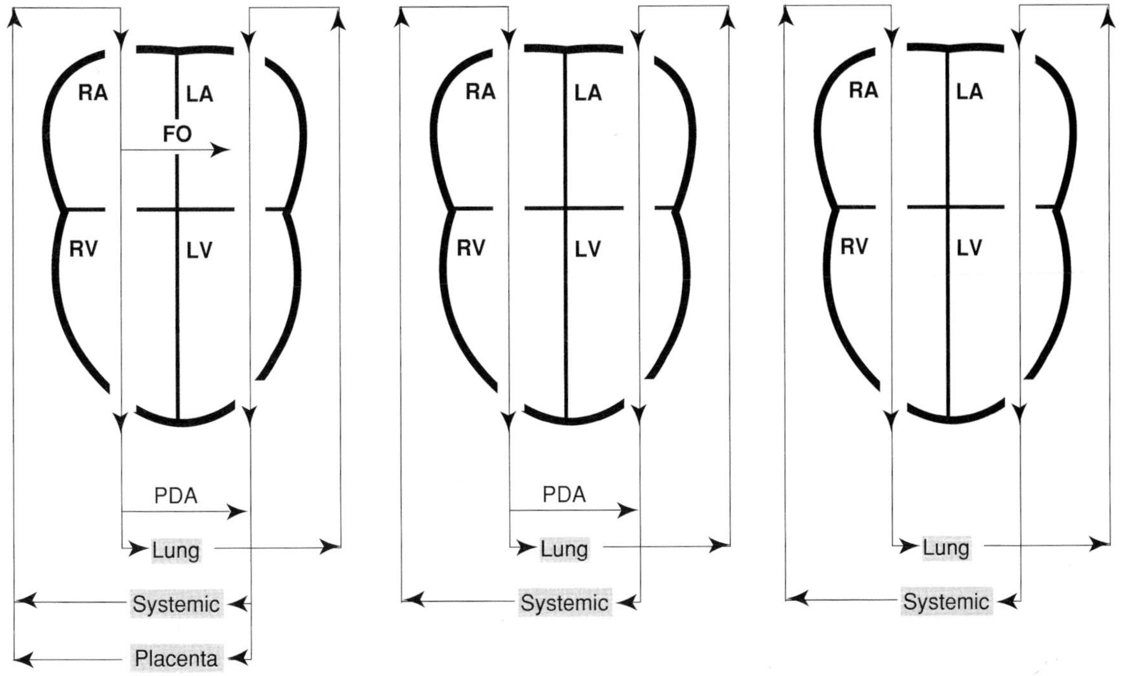

Figure 22–2. Fetal, transitional, and adult circulation patterns. (*Abbreviations:* RA = right atrium; LA = left atrium; FO = foramen ovale; RV = right ventricle; LV = left ventricle; PDA = patent ductus arteriosus.)

few years. This is evident by the primitive neurologic reflexes often seen at birth, such as the Moro and Babinski reflexes, and by the increase in neurons and maturation of central synapses during the first year of life.

TABLE 22–3
Systolic, Diastolic, and Mean Blood Pressures in Newborns for the First 12 Hours of Life

Birth Weight (gm)	Systolic (mmHg)	Diastolic (mmHg)	Mean (mmHg)
750	35–55	15–35	25–40
1500	40–60	20–40	30–50
2500	45–70	25–45	35–55
3500	55–75	30–50	40–60

Data from Kitterman JA, Phibbs RH, Tooley WH: Aortic blood pressure in normal newborn infants during the first 12 hours of life. Pediatrics 44:959–968, 1969; and Versmold HT, Kitterman JA, Phibbs RH, et al: Aortic blood pressure during the first 12 hours of life in infants with birth weights 610 to 4220 grams. Pediatrics 67:607–613, 1981.

Among the immature centers at birth are the respiratory and temperature-regulating centers. Some newborns develop apnea and bradycardia (A and B) spells, which are pauses in respiration greater than 20 seconds associated with heart rate slowing. These spells relate to the immature respiratory center and are more common in low–birth weight newborns (25% incidence in newborns weighing less than 2500 gm).[18]

Newborns begin losing body heat immediately after delivery. Wet newborns exposed to room air lose nearly five times more heat than dry, warmed newborns.[19] Most newborns should be dried rapidly immediately after delivery to help prevent heat loss and also to help stimulate breathing. However, when significant meconium is present, drying begins after tracheal suctioning. After drying, place the newborn in either a warm blanket (normal, vigorous newborns) or under a radiant heater if resuscitation or other care is needed (depressed or premature newborns).

The normal newborn is usually awake and responsive to sound, tactile stimulation, and other environmental stimuli for the first 15 to

60 minutes of life. This responsiveness is followed by a sleep cycle.[12]

The retinal vessels are not completely developed until about 44 weeks' EGA.[20] Retinopathy of prematurity, originally called "retrolental fibroplasia," may develop in newborns given oxygen therapy at birth. It is more likely to occur in premature newborns and is related to prolonged elevation of the newborn's increased oxygen tension (Pa_{O_2}) (e.g., greater than 100 mmHg). It is not related to the inspired oxygen concentration (FI_{O_2}) of the newborn.[21] In initial newborn resuscitation, the effects of hypoxia on the brain is of greater concern than retinopathy of prematurity. After the newborn is stabilized, the oxygen level is decreased as tolerated, especially in preterm newborns.

Metabolic Physiology

Blood glucose levels normally range between 40 and 60 mg/100 ml in newborns.[22] Hypoglycemia occurs in about 5% of newborns and is defined as a blood sugar level less than 30 mg/100 ml in term newborns and less than 20 mg/100 ml in preterm newborns. Because hypoglycemia is often asymptomatic and glycogen stores in the newborn are small, glucose levels should be determined during prolonged resuscitation.

The fetus lives at oxygen pressures of 20 to 30 mmHg and carbon dioxide pressures of 40 to 50 mmHg. Within a few minutes of delivery, the newborn establishes oxygen and carbon dioxide levels similar to those of adults (Table 22–4).[23, 24] These values can be useful in evaluating umbilical cord gases and newborn blood gases drawn after delivery.

The normal calcium level is 7 to 11 mg/100 ml.

The normal magnesium level is 1.5 to 2.8 mEq/L.

Predelivery Resuscitation

Evaluation of the fetus before delivery is based primarily on fetal heart monitoring, including the baseline fetal heart rate (FHR), FHR variability, and the detection of deceleration patterns. If an ominous FHR pattern develops, further evaluation, such as fetal scalp stimulation or fetal scalp capillary pH, is often performed to help determine whether prompt delivery is indicated (Table 22–5) (see Chapter 3).

When fetal distress is present, resuscitation should begin in utero. Predelivery resuscitation is directed at increasing fetal oxygen delivery by increasing the oxygen content of the maternal blood, improving placental perfusion, and resolving cord compression. To increase the oxygen content of maternal blood, administer 100% oxygen by face mask. In severely anemic mothers, mild fetal distress is often relieved by administering blood to the mother; blood administration followed by iron supplementation can be considered in cases of extreme prematurity (e.g., EGA less than 24 weeks) where prolonging the pregnancy may improve the chances of fetal survival.

Placental perfusion can be improved by relieving aortocaval compression, treating a low maternal cardiac output secondary to bradycardia (e.g., with atropine), reversing maternal hypotension with fluid or a vasopressor (e.g., with ephedrine), and changing maternal position

TABLE 22–4
Normal Umbilical Cord Gases and Newborn Arterial Blood Gases After Birth

	Cord at Delivery		Arterial After Delivery		
	Vein	*Artery*	*10 minutes*	*30 minutes*	*60 minutes*
PO_2 (mmHg)	30	20	60	68	70
PCO_2 (mmHg)	40	50	40	35	35
pH	7.35	7.25	7.25	7.33	7.36

Data from Modanlou H, Yeh S-Y, Hon EH: Fetal and neonatal acid-base balance in normal and high-risk pregnancies. Obstet Gynecol 43:347–353, 1974; and Yeomans ER, Hauth JC, Gilstrap LC III, Strickland DM: Umbilical cord pH, PCO_2, and bicarbonate following uncomplicated term vaginal deliveries. Am J Obstet Gynecol 151:798–800, 1985.

TABLE 22–5
Fetal Monitoring Parameters

Fetal Heart Rate (beats per minute)	
Bradycardia	<120
Normal	120–160
Tachycardia	>160
Fetal Heart Rate Variability (beats per minute)	
Decreased	<10
Normal	10–25
Marked	>25
Deceleration Patterns	
Early	Compression of the fetal head
Variable	Umbilical cord compression
Late	Uteroplacental insufficiency
Fetal Capillary pH	
Normal	7.25–7.40
Preacidotic	7.20–7.24
Acidotic	<7.20

and moving the fetus off the placenta or umbilical cord. Because the placenta is better perfused when the uterine muscle is relaxed (i.e., has less tone), decrease the frequency of uterine contractions by stopping an oxytocin infusion or by administering terbutaline.

If cord compression exists, fetal perfusion can often be improved by changing maternal position or by performing an amnioinfusion. In cases of umbilical cord prolapse for which cesarean delivery should be rapidly performed, manual elevation of the fetal head and administration of a β mimetic (e.g., terbutaline) may help relieve the umbilical cord compression and delay significant fetal compromise or fetal death. In addition to these interventions, preparations should be made to resuscitate the newborn by obtaining additional assistance and by checking resuscitation equipment prior to delivery (Table 22–6).

Routine Newborn Care and Resuscitation

Although causes of newborn distress may differ, the approach to resuscitating the newborn is the basic ABCs: airway, breathing, circulation and color, diagnosis and drugs. Figure 22–3 presents an overview of the current approach used by the American Heart Association/American Academy of Pediatrics to resuscitate newborns in the delivery or birthing room.[4] This section reviews and expands on this approach.

The Apgar score documents the newborn's adaptation to extrauterine life and response to indicated therapy during the immediate postpartum period. Five signs are evaluated at 1 and 5 minutes after delivery. Each sign is assigned a value of 0, 1, or 2 and totaled, to yield a score of 0 to 10 (Table 22–7).[25] If the 5-minute score is 6 or less, additional scores are obtained at 10, 15, and 20 minutes. Normal newborns score 7 to 10, moderately depressed newborns 4 to 6, and newborns who are severely depressed score 0 to 3. Resuscitation should *never* be delayed to assign the Apgar scores!

Of the five signs evaluated, heart rate and respiratory effort are much more significant than muscle tone and reflex irritability; color has the least significance.[26] As a result, some researchers use an Apgar minus color (A − C) score.[27]

The predictive value of the Apgar score for newborn acidosis and future neurologic outcome is poor.[28, 29] In fact, over 80% of surviving newborns with low 10-minute Apgar scores (0 to 3) were free from major handicaps at 7 years of age![29] Perhaps the enormous growth of nervous tissue that occurs after birth is the reason for these findings.

By itself, a low Apgar score indicates newborn depression. However, the reason for a low score may include inaccurate scoring, prematurity, drug effects, congenital abnormalities, esophageal intubation, nasopharyngeal suctioning, and asphyxia.

Airway

At delivery, the individual delivering the newborn suctions the infant's mouth and nose with a bulb syringe or a suction catheter. As the newborn is dried and placed on an infant warmer or the mother's abdomen, suctioning of the mouth and nose continues until all obvious secretions are removed. This maintains a clear upper airway.

However, oropharyngeal and nasopharyngeal suctioning can produce a vagal response (sinus bradycardia, nodal rhythm, heart block, cardiac arrest) and occasionally apnea. This occurs mainly in depressed newborns when suction catheters are passed nasally during the first few minutes of life. Therefore, many physicians

TABLE 22–6
Predelivery Resuscitation

Procedure

A. Increase oxygen content of the maternal blood
   1. Administer oxygen to the mother
   2. If the mother is severely anemic and time permits, administer blood
B. Increase maternal perfusion of the placenta
   1. Check for adequate uterine displacement (avoid aortocaval compression)
   2. Check maternal heart rate (if low, administer atropine)
   3. Check maternal blood pressure (if low, increase blood pressure with a non–dextrose-containing crystalloid or colloid solution or administer a vasopressor such as ephedrine)
   4. Change maternal position (especially with late decelerations)
   5. Decrease uterine contractions (allow more time for placental perfusion)
      a. If oxytocin is infusing, turn it off
      b. Consider the administration of terbutaline (β mimetic), which decreases uterine tone and frequency of contractions
C. Increase fetal perfusion
   1. Change maternal position (especially with variable decelerations)
   2. Amnioinfusion may help alleviate cord compression
   3. If a prolapsed cord exists, manual elevation of the fetal head out of the pelvis can relieve the cord compression; β mimetic (e.g., terbutaline) administration can help by decreasing uterine tone and contractions
D. Get ready for delivery and newborn resuscitation
   1. Call for additional trained medical personnel
   2. Be prepared for an emergency cesarean delivery if vaginal delivery is not possible within a reasonable period of time
   3. Check newborn resuscitation equipment—presence and function!

Equipment

Airway Equipment

Suction bulb
Bag and mask connected to an oxygen source
Laryngoscope with a #0 and #1 Miller blade
2.5-, 3.0-, 3.5-mm internal diameter endotracheal tubes with stylets (make sure the stylets are not extending past the tip of the endotracheal tubes)
Suction catheters

Breathing

Stethoscope

Circulation

Electrocardiograph
Blood pressure equipment
Pulse oximeter
Sterile umbilical vessel catheterization tray with 3.5- and 5-French catheters
24-gauge intravenous catheters

Drying and Drugs

Radiant heater and towels
Resuscitation drugs (see Table 22–9)

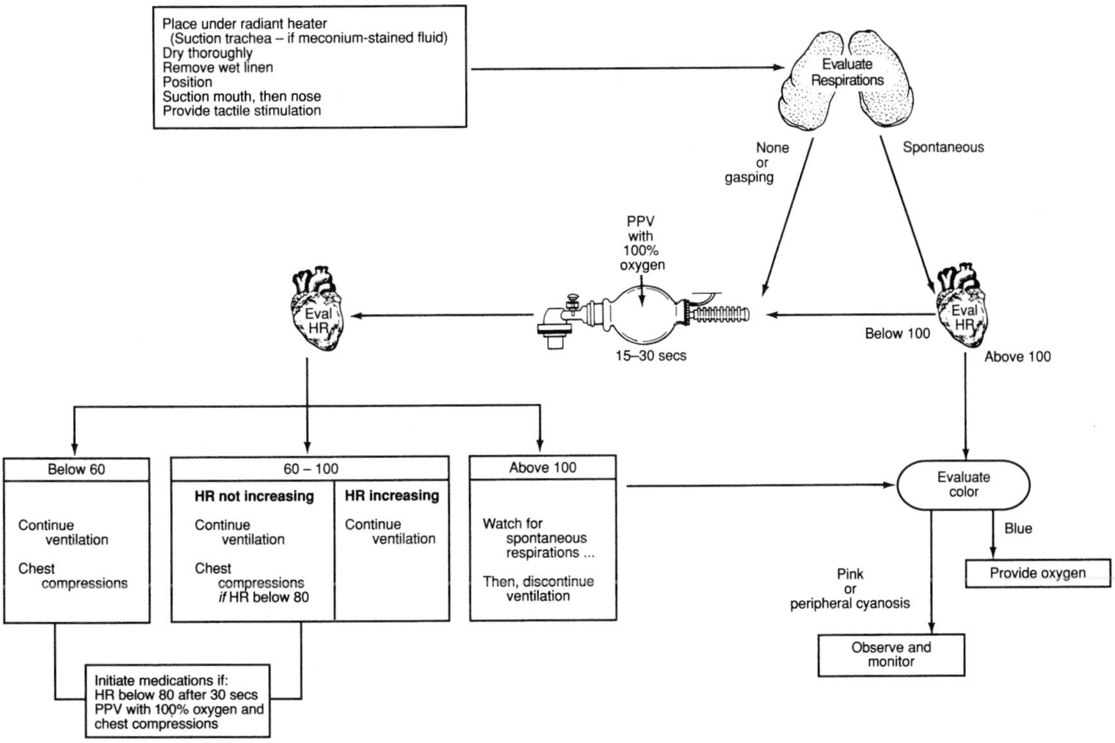

Figure 22–3. Overview of resuscitation in the delivery room. (*Abbreviations:* PPV = positive-pressure ventilation; HR = heart rate.) (From Bloom RS, Cropley C: Overview of the program. *In* Chameides L [ed]: Textbook of Neonatal Resuscitation, 2nd ed, p O-5. Dallas, American Heart Association, 1990. Reproduced with permission. Textbook of Neonatal Resuscitation, 1987, 1990. Copyright © American Heart Association.)

avoid the use of transnasal suction catheters within 5 minutes of delivery. The vagal response does not seem to occur with the use of bulb syringes. If bradycardia or apnea occurs, suctioning should be stopped and tactile stimulation performed to raise the heart rate and respiratory rate to normal. Rarely, bag-mask ventilation or chest compressions, or both, will be necessary to restore the heart rate to normal.[30]

Prior to or at the time of delivery, the newborn may inhale amniotic fluid or meconium-stained fluid, causing respiratory distress secondary to airway obstruction. In these newborns, intubate and suction the airway to clear the trachea and permit gas exchange in the

TABLE 22–7
The Apgar Score

Sign	0	1	2	Total
Heart rate	Absent	<100	>100	______
Respiratory effort	Absent	Slow, irregular	Good, crying	______
Reflex irritability*	No response	Grimace	Cough or sneeze	______
Muscle tone	Flaccid	Some flexion	Active motion	______
Color	Blue or pale	Pink body with blue extremities	Completely pink	______
			SUM†	______

*Reflex irritability is the response seen after the newborn's oropharynx and nares are suctioned with a suction catheter.
†Normal = 7–10; mild to moderate depression = 4–6; severe depression = 0–3.

lungs. When thick meconium staining occurs, routinely intubate and suction the trachea. However, when the meconium-stained fluid is thin or watery and the newborn is vigorous, intubation need not be routinely performed.

Rapid endotracheal intubation is often important to establish a route for administration of several emergency drugs and can usually be established faster than intravascular access. The mnemonic "ONES" describes the drugs that can be administered via the endotracheal tube for newborn resuscitation: oxygen, naloxone, epinephrine, and surfactant.

Thus, intubation of the newborn's trachea is performed for three main reasons: (1) to clear an obstructed airway, (2) to establish a patent airway for respiratory support, and (3) to provide a route for administration of several emergency drugs. Refer to Table 22–2 for endotracheal tube size selection and oral insertion distance. After endotracheal intubation is performed, one must confirm tube position by auscultating for bilateral breath sounds, observing chest expansion and improvement in the newborn's condition. If the newborn appears to deteriorate at any time during resuscitation, immediate reassessment of tube placement is *imperative.* Proper reassessment often requires direct laryngoscopic visualization of the endotracheal tube passing through the vocal cords. Bilateral breath sounds may be absent for several reasons, including main stem intubation, pneumothorax, hypoplastic lungs, or diaphragmatic hernia. A chest x-ray can help confirm endotracheal tube position as well as establish a diagnosis for newborns with respiratory compromise.

Newborns are obligate nasal breathers. Newborns with bilateral choanal atresia will be unable to ventilate adequately when the mouth is closed owing to the airway obstruction.[31] An oral airway may be needed to keep the upper airway patent.

Rarely, an infant is born with laryngeal stenosis or atresia. In this situation, a tracheostomy is required to establish an airway.[32]

Breathing

Breathing is evaluated as the newborn is dried. To stimulate breathing, gently slap the newborn's feet or rub the newborn's back. Drying helps stimulate breathing and prevent heat loss.

When respirations are established, watch the chest and abdomen for proper excursion. Since hypoxia induces bradycardia in the newborn, the adequacy of breathing can be evaluated by checking the heart rate. If the heart rate is above 100 bpm, ventilation is probably adequate. Heart rates below 100 bpm must be considered a sign of hypoxia and inadequate ventilation until proved otherwise, and assisted ventilation is indicated. Once breathing appears adequate, observe the newborn for signs of respiratory compromise, such as nasal flaring, grunting, retractions (sign of decreased lung compliance), and tachypnea (respiratory rates above 60). If mild, these signs usually resolve within the first hour. If these signs are persistent or progressive, significant respiratory compromise may be developing, and intervention may become necessary.

When spontaneous ventilation is inadequate, initiate bag-mask ventilation or endotracheal intubation and ventilation with 100% oxygen. To guide tidal volumes, watch for bilateral chest expansion and listen for breath sounds. If a pressure gauge is available on the resuscitation bag equipment, watch airway pressures and chest movements. Normal newborn airway pressures are 30 to 40 cmH_2O for the first breaths and they decrease rapidly to 15 to 20 cmH_2O. Newborns with decreased lung compliance (e.g., those with RDS) may require endotracheal intubation and pressures as great as 20 to 40 cmH_2O for adequate ventilation.[4] In many newborns, only a few breaths will be needed to stimulate breathing. If respiratory depression persists for more than 30 seconds, ventilate the newborn at a rate of 40 to 60 breaths per minute. This elevated respiratory rate (normal respiratory rate is 30 to 40 breaths per minute) helps to rapidly decrease the carbon dioxide levels that are elevated after inadequate ventilation. Administer 100% oxygen until the newborn is pink or a pulse oximeter or arterial blood gas reveals an oxygen saturation of 85 to 95%. If the oxygen saturation is greater than 95%, decrease the FI_{O_2} using an oxygen blender where available.

If narcotic depression is suspected as the cause of respiratory depression in a newborn with depressed respirations (e.g., one born to a mother who received a narcotic), naloxone may be needed. If very large doses of a narcotic have been administered to the mother (e.g., 25 μg/kg bolus of fentanyl), the newborn may develop chest wall rigidity; this is reversible with naloxone.[33]

Circulation and Color

Once the airway and breathing are established, evaluate the heart rate by palpating the base of the umbilical cord for the pulse or by auscultating the chest for heart sounds. Cord pulsations are present in most newborns during the first few minutes of life, but these may cease within 15 minutes.[12]

Bradycardia (heart rate less than 100 bpm) with the accompanying obligatory decrease in cardiac output is poorly tolerated. If the newborn is bradycardic, initiate positive-pressure ventilation (PPV) with 100% oxygen. If the heart rate is less than 60 bpm, pulmonary perfusion is inadequate, and chest compressions are necessary in addition to PPV with 100% oxygen. Endotracheal intubation is usually indicated.

Chest compressions are performed by pressing on the lower third of the sternum,[4, 34] to a depth of ½ to ¾ of an inch and at a rate of 120 compressions per minute.[4, 35] Compressions are performed using either the two-finger method (Fig. 22–4*A*)[4, 35] or the thumb method (see Fig. 22–4*B*)[4, 36] and produce aortic systolic pressures above 70 mmHg.[35, 36] When the heart rate rises above 60 bpm, chest compressions are stopped. If the heart rate does not continue to rise, resume chest compressions until the heart rate is above 80 bpm. If the heart rate then continues to rise, stop chest compressions. In all cases, continue PPV until the heart rate rises above 100 bpm. Survival for term newborns requiring cardiopulmonary resuscitation (CPR) (cardiac arrest) is just over 50%.[37] Survival rates are extremely poor when newborns weighing less than 1500 gm require CPR.[38]

The newborn's color and oxygen saturation are evaluated once the heart rate is greater than 100 bpm. Central cyanosis is often apparent immediately after delivery and usually clears spontaneously within a few minutes after breathing is established. If cyanosis is marked, oxygen is blown over the mouth and nose of the spontaneously breathing newborn. One must continuously observe the breathing pattern when oxygen is blown over the face, as some newborns will breath-hold when the cold gas hits their face.[39] Mild tactile stimulation and removal of the cold gas usually restores a normal breathing pattern. In the apneic newborn, 100% oxygen is administered by ventilation with a mask or endotracheal tube to correct cyanosis. In most cases, when respirations become adequate, cyanosis resolves and the need for supplemental oxygen ceases.

Increased Pa_{O_2} of the newborn assists closure of the cardiac shunts. In general, if oxygen therapy improves cyanosis, the cause of the cyanosis is more commonly respiratory. When oxygen

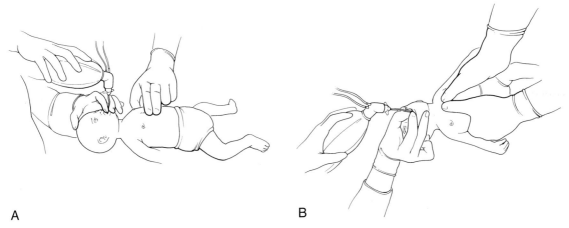

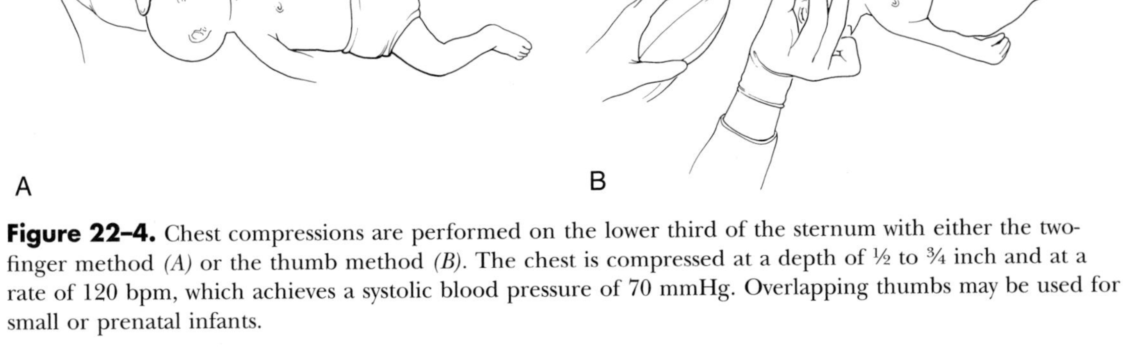

Figure 22–4. Chest compressions are performed on the lower third of the sternum with either the two-finger method *(A)* or the thumb method *(B)*. The chest is compressed at a depth of ½ to ¾ inch and at a rate of 120 bpm, which achieves a systolic blood pressure of 70 mmHg. Overlapping thumbs may be used for small or prenatal infants.

does not improve cyanosis, a large cardiac (right-to-left) shunt may exist. Here treatment is often difficult and may require drugs (e.g., tolazoline) or cardiac surgery to lower pulmonary artery pressures and enhance pulmonary blood flow. This requires neonatal intensive care.

A systolic blood pressure less than 50 mmHg in a term newborn after a normal heart rate is established requires treatment, usually with volume expansion for hypovolemia, with sodium bicarbonate for severe metabolic acidosis, or with inotropic drugs for decreased myocardial contractility.

An electrocardiographic monitor, blood pressure cuff, and pulse oximeter can be quickly placed on newborns who require active resuscitation. These should be available in a pediatric resuscitation room.

Diagnosis and Drugs

For most newborns, evaluation with the ABCs can be done within a few seconds and will reveal healthy, well-adjusting newborns. Vigorous term newborns can be suctioned and dried on the mother's abdomen immediately after delivery. Other routine newborn care, such as clamping the umbilical cord, weighing the newborn, and administering eye care, can be performed a few minutes later. If the mother prefers, the newborn can be placed in an infant warmer for routine care, then wrapped in warm linen and returned to her.

On occasion, a newborn will need assistance in establishing its airway, breathing, or circulation as outlined previously. These newborns should be stabilized and sent directly to the nursery for further observation.

In a small percentage of newborns, further assistance will be necessary. The cause of the problem and the need for drug treatment are often apparent. However, in some newborns, the problem is more subtle and a systematic evaluation is necessary (Table 22–8). Initial studies usually include prompt chest x-ray, arterial blood gases, hemoglobin/hematocrit, and glucose levels. Commonly administered drugs and their recommended dosages are summarized in Table 22–9. Preferably, the pediatrician or neonatologist will direct therapy.

Intravascular access can be established with a 24-gauge catheter inserted into a peripheral vein. Access can also be established by having trained personnel cannulate the umbilical vein or one of the two umbilical arteries. For umbilical cannulations, a 3.5-French catheter is used in a preterm newborn, and a 5.0-French catheter in a term or postterm newborn.

Whenever oxygen therapy is indicated after birth, 90 to 100% oxygen is used initially, and then this is decreased to the minimal oxygen concentration tolerated to keep the oxygen saturation at a level of about 85 to 95% or Pa_{O_2} levels of 50 to 80 mmHg.

If respiratory depression is secondary to narcotic administration, administer naloxone (0.1

TABLE 22–8
Differential Diagnosis of Newborn Problems

Airway Obstruction
Foreign material (e.g., mucus, meconium, blood)
Anatomic obstructions (e.g., choanal atresia, Pierre Robin syndrome, cystic hygroma, laryngeal stenosis or atresia)
Aspiration (e.g., meconium, amniotic fluid)

Respiratory Disease
Respiratory distress syndrome
Space-occupying lesions in the chest
- Air (e.g., pneumothorax, lung cysts)
- Bowel (e.g., diaphragmatic hernia)
- Fluid (e.g., pleural effusion)
- Tumors

Phrenic nerve paralysis
Pulmonary hypoplasia

Cardiovascular Disease
Congenital heart disease
Persistent fetal circulation
Hypovolemia
Anemia (e.g., erythroblastosis fetalis)

Neurologic Disease
Immature respiratory center (apnea and bradycardia spells)
Central nervous system insult (e.g., asphyxia, intracranial hemorrhage)

Infectious Disease
Sepsis
Group B β-hemolytic streptococcus

Metabolic Disorders
Hypoglycemia

Drugs
Narcotics
Magnesium sulfate
Anesthetics and other central nervous system depressants

TABLE 22-9
Resuscitation Drugs for the Newborn

Oxygen
Indication—hypoxia, bradycardia
Concentration—100% or with a blender 21–100%
Dose—start with 100%; decrease the concentration as tolerated to keep the oxygen saturation between 85 and 95%
Route*—inhalation via mask, hood, or ET

Naloxone
Indication—respiratory depression owing to narcotics
Concentration—0.4 mg/ml or 1.0 mg/ml
Dose—0.1 mg/kg
Route*—ET, IV, IM, or SQ
Do *not* administer naloxone if maternal-fetal drug addiction is suspected

Epinephrine
Indication—bradycardia, cardiac arrest
Concentration—1:10,000 (0.1 mg/ml)
Dose—0.1–0.3 ml/kg administered rapidly
Route*—ET or IV
Repeat as needed every 5 minutes

Volume Expansion
Indication—hypovolemia
Dose—10 ml/kg over 5–10 minutes
  Crystalloid (saline, lactated Ringer solution)
  Colloid (5% albumin)
  Blood (O-negative)
Route*—IV
Repeat as needed

Sodium Bicarbonate
Indication—suspected or documented metabolic acidosis
Concentration—0.5 mEq/ml or 4.2% solution
Dose—2 mEq/kg (or 4 ml/kg) given over at least 2 minutes
Route*—IV
Further doses based on blood gas results
Adequate ventilation must be established *before* bicarbonate is administered

Table continued on following page

mg/kg) rapidly via the endotracheal tube, intravenously, intramuscularly, or subcutaneously.[4] Because naloxone has a shorter half-life than most narcotics, this large dose is given to help prolong its action. Naloxone should *not* be administered if the newborn is thought to have a narcotic addiction (maternal narcotic abuse), as this may precipitate acute withdrawal. These addicted newborns with respiratory depression should receive ventilatory support and prompt neonatal consultation.

Epinephrine is indicated for bradycardia after chest compressions are started.[4, 40] If the heart rate is not improving after 30 seconds of CPR, epinephrine (0.1 to 0.3 ml/kg of a 1:10,000 solution) is administered rapidly down the endotracheal tube to increase heart rate and cardiac output. Epinephrine can be diluted with 1 to 2 ml of normal saline solution to aid delivery down the endotracheal tube. This dose may be repeated every 5 minutes in the absence of a good response. Once intravascular access is obtained, epinephrine can be administered parenterally. If the epinephrine response is poor, intravascular volume may be low or metabolic acidosis may exist.

Volume expansion is indicated for hypovolemia. Weak pulses coexisting with a good heart rate, hypotension, poor response to resuscitation after adequate ventilation, or pallor per-

TABLE 22-9
Resuscitation Drugs for the Newborn *Continued*

Dopamine
Indication—poor cardiac contractility
Concentration—The following concentration is most commonly used:

$$\frac{6 \times \text{weight (kg)} \times \text{desired dose } (\mu g/kg/minute)}{\text{desired fluid volume (ml/hour)}} = \text{mg dopamine/100 ml of D5W}$$

Dose—5 μg/kg/minute and increased up to 20 μg/kg/minute as needed
Route*—IV with an infusion pump
Check to make sure the patient is not volume depleted before using dopamine

Dextrose
Indication—hypoglycemia
Concentration—10% in water (D10W)
Dose—bolus dose of 200 mg/kg (2 ml/kg) over 1 minute followed by a maintenance dose of 8 mg/kg/minute
Route*—IV

Calcium
Indication—hypermagnesemia, hypocalcemia
Concentration—10 mg/ml of calcium chloride (dilute 100 mg/ml to 10 mg/ml)
Dose—10–20 mg/kg over 3–5 minutes
Route*—IV
Repeat as clinically indicated

Surfactant
Indication—respiratory distress syndrome
Dose: beractant (Survanta) 4 ml/kg, colfosceril (Exosurf) 5 ml/kg
Route*—ET over about 5 minutes

Abbreviation: D5W = 5% dextrose in water.
**Routes of administration:* ET = endotracheal tube; IM = intramuscular; IV = intravascular, includes umbilical vein, umbilical artery, and peripheral vein; SQ = subcutaneous.

sisting after oxygen therapy are often signs of hypovolemia.[4] The circulatory volume is expanded with an initial dose of 10 ml/kg of lactated Ringer solution, normal saline solution, 5% albumin, or type O-negative blood (cross-matched with the mother's blood if time permits to decrease the chance of a transfusion reaction). This dose corresponds to about 10% of the normal circulating blood volume. The dose is infused over 5 to 10 minutes. If time permits, the hemoglobin/hematocrit levels will help direct the administration of blood versus crystalloid, plasma, or albumin. This dose may need to be repeated.

To reverse suspected or documented severe metabolic acidosis (i.e., pH < 7.00 or base deficit greater than 15 mEq/L), sodium bicarbonate (0.5 mEq/ml or 4.2% solution) is administered via the intravascular access. The initial dose is 2 mEq/kg (or 4 ml/kg) given over at least 2 minutes.[4] Further bicarbonate dosages are based on blood gas results using the following formula:

$$\text{mEq bicarbonate} = \frac{0.3 \times \text{weight (kg)} \times \text{base deficit (mEq/L)}}{4}$$

This formula gives one fourth of the amount of bicarbonate needed to completely neutralize the acidosis, as complete neutralization is not necessary. After each dose of bicarbonate is administered, the response is evaluated. Concentrations of 0.5 mEq/ml are recommended over the standard adult concentration of 1.0 mEq/ml, since higher concentrations may be associated with intracranial bleeding. Remember, adequate ventilation must be established before bicarbonate is administered; otherwise, hypercarbia may result, since CO_2 is formed from the administered bicarbonate combining with the hydrogen ions from the acidosis.

Dopamine increases cardiac contractility, which may become compromised during prolonged resuscitative efforts.[4] Dopamine should be administered intravenously using an infusion pump once intravascular volume has been normalized. The initial dosage is 5 μg/kg/minute, which can be increased up to 20 μg/kg/minute. It can be prepared at various concentrations; commonly, dopamine is added to dextrose 5% in water (D5W) using the following formula:

$$\frac{6 \times \text{weight (kg)} \times \text{desired dose } (\mu g/kg/minute)}{\text{Desired fluid volume (ml/hour)}} = \mu g \text{ dopamine}/100 \text{ ml of D5W}$$

Dextrose is used to treat hypoglycemia. In asymptomatic newborns, D5W oral solution may be tried. If parenteral glucose is administered, a bolus dose of 200 mg/kg (2 ml/kg of dextrose 10% in water [D10W]) over 1 minute is followed by a maintenance dose of 8 mg/kg/minute.[41]

Calcium chloride is administered to newborns with hypocalcemia or to depressed newborns with elevated magnesium ion blood concentrations resulting from maternal magnesium sulfate administration. Calcium chloride prepared in a concentration of 100 mg/ml is diluted to 10 mg/ml with normal saline solution. Ten to 20 mg/kg of calcium chloride is administered intravenously over 3 to 5 minutes and is repeated as needed.

With suspected RDS, surfactant is administered down the endotracheal tube to improve lung function.[42] An endotracheal tube with a side injection port simplifies drug administration. The dose of surfactant is 4 to 5 ml/kg and is administered with several manual inflations of oxygen. The dose is given slowly (over about 5 minutes) or else a marked transient fall in oxygen saturation results. The author has found that increasing the $F_{I_{O_2}}$ for a few breaths prior to the administration of the surfactant attenuates the fall in oxygen saturation. Presumably this increases the oxygen reserve in the lung prior to administering the relatively large volume of drug.

Newborn Conditions Requiring Resuscitation

Meconium Aspiration

Meconium is composed of the sterile contents of the fetal gastrointestinal tract and includes swallowed amniotic fluid, desquamated cutaneous cells, and gastrointestinal secretions such as bile salts (which give meconium its green color). The passage of meconium may be a normal physiologic event related to the increasing maturity of the fetus or may be a sign of fetal distress. When the fetus is stressed (i.e., experiencing hypoxia), an increase in gastrointestinal motility with relaxation of the anal sphincter may occur, permitting meconium passage, which stains the normally clear amniotic fluid. Overall, the mortality rate for newborns with meconium-stained amniotic fluid is double the rate for unstained newborns (3.3% versus 1.7%).[43]

About 10 to 15% of all live newborns have meconium-stained amniotic fluid.[43-50] Of these, about two thirds have thin, watery, greenish amniotic fluid; the remainder have thick, pea soup–appearing amniotic fluid. Aspiration occurs when the stained amniotic fluid is aspirated into the trachea. This occurs in about 20 to 50% of newborns with meconium-stained amniotic fluid.[46, 48, 49] Aspiration can occur in utero[51] or when the newborn starts to breathe at the time of delivery.[50]

Clinical signs of respiratory distress secondary to aspirated meconium define the meconium aspiration syndrome (MAS), which occurs in about 0.5 to 30% of all stained live newborns.[44-47, 49, 51, 52] Signs are predominantly respiratory and relate initially to mechanical airway obstruction, with the gradual development of chemical pneumonitis over 48 hours.[53] The severity of respiratory compromise usually parallels the amount and thickness of meconium aspirated. When a small amount is aspirated, tachypnea and mild cyanosis are common, resulting from peripheral airway obstruction with atelectasis and ventilation-perfusion abnormalities. When a large amount of meconium is aspirated, the newborn is often severely depressed, with profound cyanosis and irregular, gasping respirations. Occasionally, complete airway obstruction leads to death.

Two other conditions that occur in some newborns with MAS are pulmonary air leaks (pneumothorax or pneumomediastinum) and persistent fetal circulation (pulmonary hypertension with a right-to-left shunt through a patent foramen ovale and ductus arteriosus).

Prevention of MAS begins before delivery. The obstetrician watches closely for intrapartum signs of fetal distress and implements therapeutic measures accordingly. Uncorrected fetal distress may lead to meconium passage and cause the fetus to gasp in utero, allowing the meconium-stained fluid to enter the trachea or lungs. However, most cases in which meconium is detected prenatally are not associated with fetal distress. Finally, fetal distress in the presence of meconium does not necessarily indicate poor outcome.[48, 54]

Table 22–10 summarizes the approach to meconium-stained newborns at the time of delivery.

After delivery of the head and before delivery of the shoulders, the obstetrician suctions the mouth and nose of all newborns with a DeLee suction catheter or with a bulb syringe.[4, 44–49, 54, 55] Immediately following delivery, the newborn's mouth is suctioned again and the trachea is intubated and suctioned, preferably before the newborn takes a breath (each breath may move tracheal meconium distally). Suction is applied to the endotracheal tube with a suction device attached to the endotracheal tube connector (Fig. 22–5). The negative pressure generated by the suction equipment should probably be around 100 to 120 mmHg.[4, 49] As suction is applied, the endotracheal tube is removed. If meconium is aspirated into the endotracheal tube from the newborn's trachea, intubation and suctioning may need to be repeated until the trachea is clear of meconium.

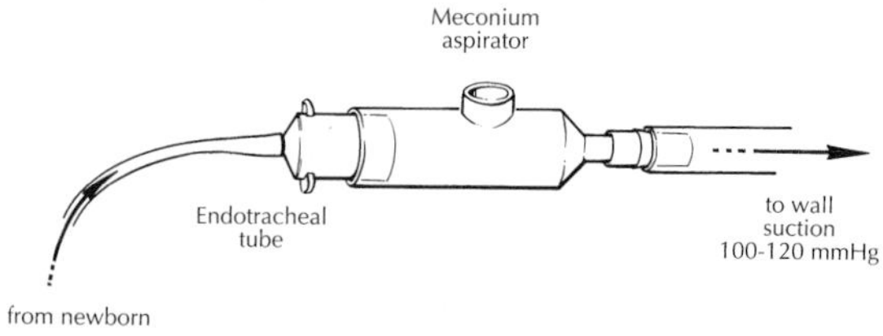

Figure 22–5. Suctioning the meconium-stained neonate. After the newborn's trachea is intubated with a 3.0- or 3.5-mm internal-diameter endotracheal tube, a meconium aspirator is attached to the tube. Wall suction, reduced to a negative pressure of about 100 mmHg, is applied to the aspirator, a finger is placed over the side hole of the aspirator, and the trachea is suctioned.

Although laryngoscopy and endotracheal intubation are important in the management of meconium-stained newborns, intubation may have adverse effects, including bradycardia, laryngeal trauma, and rarely, esophageal perforation.[56] The heart rate should be monitored during intubation, as bradycardia may be the result of fetal hypoxia or may develop as a result of vagal stimulation during laryngoscopy. If the newborn is severely depressed, 100% oxygen by PPV and occasionally chest compressions may rarely be needed before the trachea is completely clear of all meconium.

The need to intubate all newborns with meconium staining has been questioned.[47, 49, 55] Most clinicians now feel that after the mouth and

TABLE 22–10
Summary of Initial Approach to Meconium-Stained Newborns* at the Time of Delivery

Thin Meconium (two thirds of stained)	Thick Meconium (one third of stained)
Suction mouth and nose	Suction mouth and nose
Intubation usually not needed (intubate only if respiratory or cardiac distress is seen)	Intubate and suction the trachea of all newborns if possible (preferably before first breath)
	If meconium is aspirated, reintubate and suction until reasonably clear (if newborn is severely depressed, administer 100% oxygen by positive-pressure ventilation and consider cardiopulmonary resuscitation if the heart rate is less than 60 beats per minute)
Dry the newborn	Dry the newborn
Administer oxygen as clinically needed	Administer oxygen as clinically needed
Pass a nasogastric or orogastric tube and aspirate the gastric contents	Pass a nasogastric or orogastric tube and aspirate the gastric contents
Chest x-ray usually not needed	Obtain a chest x-ray if clinically indicated

*Meconium-stained newborns account for 10–15% of all deliveries.

nose are suctioned, the vigorous newborn (i.e., one who is breathing) with thin meconium does not benefit from tracheal intubation and suctioning. Endotracheal intubation and suctioning are recommended only for newborns with thick meconium staining or newborns with meconium who are severely depressed (Fig. 22–6).[50] Because the thickness of the meconium may be difficult to assess, the trachea should be intubated and suctioned if any question exists.

Once initial tracheal suctioning has been performed, the newborn is dried and oxygen administered if the newborn is cyanotic. Next, a DeLee suction catheter is passed to empty the stomach of any swallowed meconium. This helps prevent aspiration of meconium if emesis occurs subsequently.

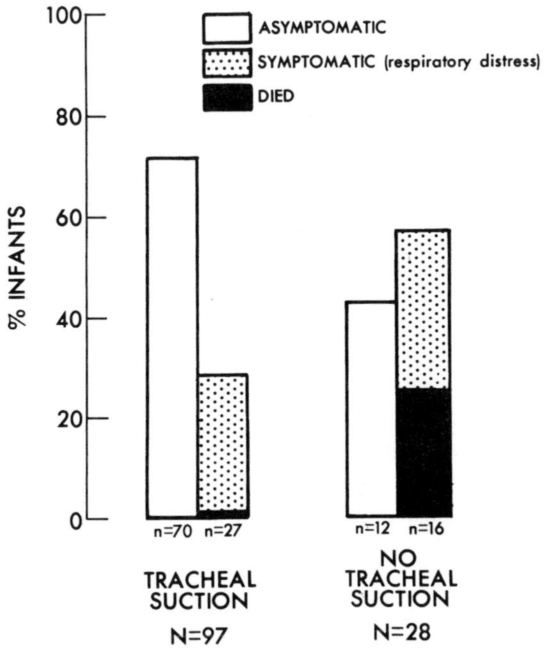

Figure 22–6. Comparison of percentage of incidence of respiratory distress and percentage of mortality in 97 infants who received tracheal suction in the delivery room and 28 infants who did not (numbers of infants appear below columns). Note that 1 infant (also with Down syndrome and an endocardial cushion defect) in the tracheal-suction group died and 7 infants in the no-tracheal-suction group died. All infants had moderate or severe meconium staining and were admitted to the neonatal intensive care unit for observation. (From Ting P, Brady JP: Tracheal suction in meconium aspiration. Am J Obstet Gynecol 122:767–771, 1975.)

If respiratory distress is present after a few minutes of therapy, a chest x-ray may be obtained. If the chest x-ray is normal, most newborns do well. Newborns with air leaks, patchy areas of consolidation, or atelectasis have a higher incidence of respiratory failure and death. Coarse infiltrates, if present, usually clear within 12 to 36 hours.[46, 52, 57]

After the newborn is stabilized, chest physical therapy may help loosen meconium-stained secretions that cannot be reached by tracheal suction. Tracheobronchial lavage with saline solution is not beneficial and may actually increase respiratory distress in some cases.[44] Similarly, glucocorticoid treatment for meconium aspiration is not of benefit[50, 58] and, in one study, decreased survival.[58]

Clinical signs suggesting pulmonary air leaks are respiratory distress, a shift in the cardiac impulse, and tracheal deviation. Small amounts of extra-alveolar air are usually asymptomatic and resolve spontaneously. Large pneumothoraces associated with cardiopulmonary distress may require needle aspiration and placement of a chest tube with suction.

Newborns with persistent fetal circulation are profoundly cyanotic and often do very poorly.[45, 52] Mechanical hyperventilation combined with a pulmonary vasodilator, such as tolazoline, may be required to establish adequate blood flow to the lungs. Mechanical hyperventilation produces a respiratory alkalosis, which is helpful, but it is associated with an increase in the incidence of pneumothoraces. Hypotension accompanying therapy is treated with volume expansion and, if necessary, dopamine. Remember, hypoxia, acidosis, or hypothermia can lead to an increase in pulmonary artery pressure and can increase the right-to-left shunt.

Newborns with mild meconium aspiration usually have a benign clinical course with resolution of any clinical signs within 24 to 72 hours.[52] With massive aspiration, repeated tracheal suctioning and ventilatory support may be needed. Unfortunately, despite appropriate airway management, some newborns die.[44, 45, 47–49, 52, 55]

Respiratory Distress Syndrome

Newborns born prematurely often develop a respiratory disease known as "respiratory distress syndrome" (RDS) secondary to insufficient pulmonary surfactant.[59]

The incidence of RDS varies inversely with the gestational age of the newborn and occurs more frequently in infants delivered by cesarean section than in those delivered vaginally. For vaginally delivered newborns, the incidence of RDS is 65% at 25 to 30 weeks' EGA, 35% at 31 to 32 weeks, 21% at 33 to 34 weeks, 5% at 35 to 36 weeks, and less than 1% after 37 weeks.[60] It also occurs more commonly in males and in newborns of diabetic mothers, and it is often more severe in the second born of twins (occasionally, the second twin develops RDS and the first twin does not).[60, 61]

Clinical signs relate to a decrease in lung compliance owing to progressive alveolar collapse and respiratory failure.[62, 63] The two signs most apparent are chest wall retractions and tachypnea (a respiratory rate above 60). The severity of chest wall retractions (suprasternal, intercostal, subcostal) depends on the respiratory effort generated by the newborn and the severity of the lung disease. Although many normal newborns have tachypnea at birth, it improves over several minutes. In RDS, the tachypnea increases and reflects progressive alveolar collapse. Other signs include nasal flaring, grunting, hypoxemia, hypercarbia, acidosis, and hypotension. The onset of clinical symptoms varies. Some newborns have difficulty initiating respirations (too weak to expand their noncompliant lungs), the rest develop respiratory symptoms over the next few hours.

Before exogenous surfactant therapy was available (in the 1980s), about 15% of newborns with RDS died.[64] Pathologic findings include firm collapsed lungs, collapsed alveoli, hyaline membranes seen on the alveolar walls, and low concentrations of pulmonary surfactant. Now surfactant can be administered into the trachea of newborns at risk for RDS immediately after birth (immediate prophylaxis)[65] or in newborns with established RDS (rescue therapy).[66] Results demonstrate a decrease in complications from respiratory support, such as pulmonary air leaks, and, more importantly, an overall decrease in infant mortality.[65, 66]

Treatment of a premature newborn with suspected RDS begins in the delivery room or, if available, in a pediatric resuscitation room. Treatment is usually performed by the pediatrician, but if the pediatrician is not immediately available, the initial care can be started by the anesthesiologist. As in all newborns, routine care (ABCs and drying) begins treatment. Respiratory care is the initial priority for these small newborns. The goal is to maintain the oxygen saturation at approximately 90%, the Pa_{O_2} between 50 to 80 mmHg, the Pa_{CO_2} below 55 mmHg, and the pH above 7.20. Methods to maintain these parameters vary. If the newborn has minimal signs of RDS, for example, respiratory rate below 60 with a heart rate above 100 bpm and mild retractions, the Pa_{CO_2} and pH are often normal, and a lowered Pa_{O_2} is the only blood gas abnormality. This can often be corrected with only supplemental oxygen administered by oxygen hood. If the newborn appears to be having respiratory difficulty as demonstrated by significant retractions, tachypnea, bradycardia, or cyanosis, intubation of the newborn and continuous PPV with 100% oxygen can be started. Positive airway pressure helps open collapsed alveoli. Usually only a mild elevation in airway pressures will be needed (e.g., 8 cmH_2O). Once more alveoli open, the concentration of oxygen needed to maintain an 85 to 95% saturation is much lower and the oxygen concentration should be rapidly decreased. Surfactant can be administered easily down the endotracheal tube by the anesthesiologist to help stabilize the newborn's lung function, if the transport team's or the pediatrician's arrival is delayed.

A baseline chest x-ray helps rule out other causes of respiratory compromise, such as diaphragmatic hernia, congenital lung cyst, lung hypoplasia, and pneumothorax. The chest x-ray seen in RDS shows a diffuse reticulogranular or "ground-glass" appearance and air bronchograms. These changes are related to the alveolar atelectasis (granular) and the ectatic air ducts (reticular).[60, 62, 63] This appearance is diagnostic for RDS within 1 hour in severe cases, within 4 hours in moderate cases, and within 8 hours for all cases of RDS.[60]

Group B β-hemolytic streptococcal infections are potentially lethal and may present with signs resembling those of RDS.[67] Because of the similarity, antibiotics are often started after cultures are obtained in newborns with respiratory difficulty. Therapy is directed by the pediatrician.

Any newborn with stabilized RDS who suddenly deteriorates requires a systematic evaluation to rule out and correct other complications, including pneumothorax, extubation, main stem intubation, or a plugged or kinked endotracheal tube.

Once stabilized, the preterm newborn often requires transfer to a neonatal intensive care facility for further management of the RDS as well as management of other problems of prematurity (e.g., apnea and bradycardia spells, feeding problems).

MATERNAL RESUSCITATION AND CRITICAL CARE

In the United States, maternal mortality progressively decreased from 376 maternal deaths per 100,000 live births in 1940 to 37 per 100,000 in 1960, and to 7.4 per 100,000 in 1986. The leading causes of maternal death from 1979 to 1986 were hemorrhage (30.2%), pulmonary embolism (23.4%), PIH (18.1%), infection (7.6%), cardiomyopathy (3.4%), anesthesia (3.3%), and other unspecified causes (14.0%) (Table 22–11).[68]

Many of the maternal conditions that lead to maternal mortality or morbidity require intensive care and have been described in other sections of this book, including anesthesia-related problems, embolism (amniotic fluid, venous, and air), bleeding, and PIH. This section reviews the basic approach to maternal resuscitation, the use of invasive monitors, and specific maternal conditions, including pulmonary aspiration of gastric contents, pulmonary edema, cardiac arrhythmias, cardiac arrest, and magnesium sulfate toxicity.

Although the basic approach to the mother is the same as in any patient, namely, the ABCs, the fetus must also be considered. If a potentially lethal maternal situation develops, delivery should be considered to reduce the physiologic demands on the mother or to save the life of a viable fetus.

TABLE 22–11
Causes of Maternal Deaths in the United States 1979–1986 (% per category)

Hemorrhage		30.2
Ruptured ectopic	11.2	
Placental abruption	4.8	
Uterine bleeding	3.1	
Uterine rupture/laceration	2.6	
Disseminated intravascular coagulation	2.1	
Placenta previa	1.7	
Retained placenta and products of conception	1.4	
Other	3.3	
Pulmonary Embolism		23.4
Thrombotic	12.1	
Amniotic fluid	10.0	
Air	1.0	
Other	0.3	
Pregnancy-Induced Hypertension		18.1
Preeclampsia	8.5	
Eclampsia	8.5	
Other	1.1	
Infection		7.6
Cardiomyopathy		3.4
Anesthesia		3.3
Aspiration	0.8	
Other	2.5	
Other Causes		14.0
TOTAL		100.0

Modified from Atrash HK, Koonin LM, Lawson HW, et al: Maternal mortality in the United States, 1979–1986. Reprinted with permission from The American College of Obstetricians and Gynecologists (Obstetrics and Gynecology, 1990, Vol 76, pp 1055–1060).

Maternal Resuscitation

Airway

Evaluate the airway. Secure the airway in unconscious patients with an endotracheal tube to prevent aspiration of maternal gastric contents or initiate mechanical ventilation. Although the upper airway is slightly edematous in most pregnant women, a 7.0- or a 7.5-mm ID endotracheal tube usually easily passes the vocal cords orally (with adequate sedation and muscle paralysis). On rare occasions, excessive upper airway edema (as seen in PIH) requires smaller endotracheal tubes in order to pass the edematous vocal cords.[69] As in all patients, confirm endotracheal tube position by auscultating the lung fields while watching for appropriate chest expansion and improvement in the mother's condition. Remember that esophageal intubation can produce bilateral breath sounds! Auscultate mainly to determine whether the endotracheal tube is past the carina or whether other pulmonary disease is also present (e.g., pneumothorax, bronchospasm). Any time proper endotracheal tube position is in question, proper position must be confirmed by direct laryngoscopic visualization of the tube passing through the vocal cords, by measuring an appropriate end-tidal CO_2 concentration, or by passing a fiberoptic bronchoscope through the endotracheal tube and observing the carina.

The nasal mucosa is edematous and more vascular in the pregnant woman. Extreme care must be exercised when placing a nasal airway or when a nasal endotracheal intubation is performed, as epistaxis commonly results.

Breathing

Maternal respiratory anatomy and physiology undergo profound changes during pregnancy.[70, 71] Tidal volume increases and functional residual capacity decreases by about 20%. Minute ventilation normally increases by about 15% by the third month of pregnancy and by 45% by the ninth month, primarily because of the stimulatory effects of elevated progesterone levels. At term, the tidal volume increases by 40% and the respiratory rate increases by 10%, producing a fall in maternal Pa_{CO_2} to approximately 27 to 32 mmHg and increasing the Pa_{O_2} slightly. A mild respiratory alkalosis results that is compensated by a fall in bicarbonate levels (about 3 to 5 mEq/L), keeping the maternal pH near normal (pH 7.40 to 7.45). Thus, a Pa_{CO_2} of 32 mmHg at term is normal!

Indications for intubation and mechanical ventilation include a respiratory rate greater than 35 breaths per minute, Pa_{CO_2} exceeding 50 mmHg, and Pa_{O_2} less than 60 mmHg (90% saturation) when supplemental 100% oxygen by face mask is used. Although PPV can potentially reduce oxygen delivery to the fetus in utero by reducing uterine blood flow, the beneficial effects of increasing maternal Pa_{O_2} and reducing maternal Pa_{CO_2} toward normal (Pa_{CO_2} 30 to 32 mmHg) in the critically ill mother outweigh any potential problems.

Significant maternal alkalosis, whether induced by respiratory or metabolic factors, may also compromise the fetus by decreasing fetal umbilical P_{O_2} and Pa_{O_2}. Maternal alkalosis shifts the maternal oxyhemoglobin dissociation curve to the left, which increases the maternal hemoglobin affinity for oxygen and makes less oxygen available for fetal transfer.[72]

Although newborns can develop retrolental fibroplasia as a result of elevated blood oxygen concentrations, administering 100% oxygen to the mother does not place the fetus at risk. Fetal umbilical Pa_{O_2} levels do not exceed 65 mmHg even when maternal Pa_{O_2} levels reach 500 mmHg.[73] Elevated maternal Pa_{O_2} levels do not cause retrolental fibroplasia.

In summary, begin ventilation with 100% oxygen. A tidal volume of 10 ml/kg pregnant body weight with a respiratory rate of 10 breaths per minute is an appropriate starting point for mechanical ventilation.[74] The goal is to achieve a Pa_{O_2} above 100 mmHg, a Pa_{CO_2} below 50 mmHg, and a pH around 7.40 to 7.45.

Circulation

After securing the airway and beginning ventilation, initially assess the maternal blood pressure and heart rate. In critically ill patients in whom cardiovascular function needs to be better defined, an arterial line and a central venous pressure line or pulmonary artery catheter connected to a cardiac output computer should be placed to evaluate the four physiologic variables that affect the cardiac output (preload, contractility, heart rate and rhythm, and afterload).[75, 76] Because pregnancy changes some of these values, a brief review of these physiologic changes follows.

Maternal cardiac output increases rapidly after conception and reaches a level of 30 to 50% above baseline values by 20 to 32 weeks' EGA, where it remains stable until term.[77–80] During labor, cardiac output increases further, peaking immediately after delivery (60 to 80% above prelabor levels).[81] Although cardiac output increases, mean maternal blood pressure may decrease during the second trimester, returning to near-normal in the third trimester.[77, 79] Early studies suggested a fall in cardiac output after 28 to 32 weeks' gestation, but these decreases were due to the effect of unrecognized aortocaval compression.

Maternal positioning (owing to the adverse effects of the enlarged uterus pressing on the vena cava and the aorta) can profoundly influence cardiac output and blood pressure in pregnant women past 20 weeks' EGA. When the pregnant woman changes from the supine to the lateral position, cardiac output increases by about 10% at 22 weeks, 15% at 30 weeks, and 30% at term.[80] Significant aortocaval compression can cause the supine hypotensive syndrome manifested by dizziness, nausea, maternal hypotension, tachycardia, shortness of breath, decreased uterine blood flow, and possible fetal distress.[82, 83] Because of the effects of aortocaval compression, all patients past 20 weeks' EGA who are receiving intensive care should avoid the supine position and be treated in the lateral or supine position with left uterine displacement.

Preload, estimated by the central venous pressure or by the pulmonary artery wedge pressure, remains unchanged during pregnancy.[78] Hemorrhage, dehydration, and aortocaval compression decrease preload, whereas fluid administration and venoconstriction increase preload. In patients with PIH, preload is usually low but is occasionally high.[76]

Contractility, as reflected by the ejection fraction or by left ventricular stroke work index, is unchanged during pregnancy.[77–79] Peripartum cardiomyopathy[84] reduces contractility. PIH may also decrease contractility.[76]

Heart rate typically increases 10 to 15 bpm throughout pregnancy.[77–80] Although increased stroke volume (owing to an increase in end-diastolic volume) accounts for the initial rise in cardiac output, increased heart rate maintains the higher cardiac output throughout pregnancy.

Afterload declines 20 to 30% during pregnancy as a result of peripheral vasodilatation and increased uterine blood flow.[78, 79] However, in some patients with PIH, afterload increases.[76]

During CPR, the uterus must be displaced to the left or the table should be tilted to the left 15 to 30 degrees.[85, 86] Sternal compressions are performed at a depth of 1.5 to 2 inches and a rate of 80 to 100 per minute. If CPR is needed after 24 weeks' EGA, rapid delivery of the fetus by cesarean section should be considered (see "Cardiac Arrest," later in this chapter). If rapid delivery is not possible, open-chest cardiac massage may be indicated to achieve a higher cardiac output than that possible with closed-chest massage.[87]

Invasive Monitoring

The indications for invasive monitoring are the same as those in the nonpregnant patient.

Arterial lines are useful for monitoring the blood pressure, particularly when potent cardiovascular medications with short duration of action are administered (e.g., sodium nitroprusside, nitroglycerin, dopamine). The arterial line can also be used in patients from whom several blood samples are to be drawn over time (e.g., blood gases in a patient with respiratory compromise, PIH patients for clotting studies or magnesium levels). The arterial line may help limit the number of punctures a patient must endure. Avoiding repeated venipunctures spares veins for future intravenous access.

Central venous lines provide intravenous access, allow monitoring of central venous pressure, and help guide fluid therapy in the patient with a normal heart.

Pulmonary artery catheters are placed in patients with significant cardiovascular compromise. The information they provide aids in the evaluation of cardiovascular function, which helps guide fluid management and selection of cardiovascular medications.

Maternal Problems Requiring Resuscitation

Pulmonary Aspiration of Gastric Contents

Although aspiration of gastric contents into the lungs is relatively uncommon (1.5:1000),[88] it continues as a major cause of morbidity and mortality in the obstetric population. The mortality rate for gastric aspiration approaches 10%.[89] If unconsciousness occurs, the pregnant patient experiences greater risk for aspiration of gastric contents compared with the nonpregnant patient because of the hormonal and mechanical changes of pregnancy.

Aspiration of gastric contents may produce two patterns of lung injury.[88] The first pattern results from aspirated food particles causing partial or complete obstruction of the airways. In complete obstruction, death occurs from suffocation. Partial obstruction of the airway leads to atelectasis and ventilation-perfusion abnormalities producing decreased Pa_{O_2} and increased Pa_{CO_2}. Symptoms include coughing, dyspnea, cyanosis, and tachycardia. The chest x-ray often reveals atelectasis, usually of the right lung field, with an associated mediastinal shift.

The second and more common pattern of lung damage results from aspirated acidic gastric fluid (pH less than 2.5) that causes bronchiolar spasm and peribronchiolar congestion and exudate. The aspirated fluid irritates the airways, producing asthma-like symptoms of dyspnea, wheezing, cyanosis, tachypnea, and tachycardia. Arterial blood gases reveal decreased Pa_{O_2} and increased Pa_{CO_2}. The chest x-ray may show irregular, soft mottling infiltrates, usually without a mediastinal shift. If the fluid is more neutral (water, saline solution, or neutralized vomitus), the lung damage is milder and recovery takes only a few hours. In more severe cases, an adult RDS picture may develop. Occasionally, cardiac failure and pulmonary edema will develop.

The risk of aspiration and lung damage increases with low gastric pHs (i.e., pH less than 2.5) or high gastric volumes (i.e., greater than 25 ml). Because it is difficult to know which patients have low gastric pHs or high gastric volumes, all pregnant women with recent food ingestion or signs of heartburn or who are past 20 weeks' EGA are considered at risk for aspiration.

To decrease the potential for damage caused by the aspiration of gastric contents, efforts are made to increase the gastric pH (e.g., with oral antacids or H_2-receptor antagonists) or to decrease the gastric volume (e.g., with metoclopramide) in all obstetric patients who will lose consciousness (e.g., those who will receive induction of general anesthesia). In patients who are already unconscious, an endotracheal tube should be inserted to help prevent gastric fluid from entering the lung, and some authorities recommend insertion of an oral or nasogastric tube to empty gastric contents.

Oral antacids rapidly increase gastric pH.[90, 91] Nonparticulate antacids are preferred over particulate antacids because aspiration of particulate antacids induces significant pulmonary damage.[92] Currently, two commercially available clear antacid preparations are available. Thirty milliliters of sodium citrate and citric acid (Bicitra)[93] or two tablets of sodium bicarbonate and potassium bicarbonate and citric acid (Alka-Seltzer effervescent)[94] dissolved in 30 ml of water are administered before a general anesthetic. Administer antacids within 1 hour of the induction of general anesthesia.[95]

The H_2-receptor antagonists cimetidine and ranitidine decrease gastric acid production and elevate gastric pH.[96] However, they take time to work—several hours after oral administration (300-mg cimetidine, 150-mg ranitidine) and 45 to 60 minutes after intravenous administration (300-mg cimetidine, 50-mg ranitidine). Because of the possibility of cardiovascular complications, the intravenous preparations are administered over 15 to 20 minutes.

Metoclopramide (10 mg intravenously) speeds gastric emptying[97] but requires at least 30 minutes before a significant reduction in gastric volume occurs. Because metoclopramide also increases lower esophageal sphincter tone without increasing gastric pressure, it can be administered immediately prior to the induction of general anesthesia to decrease the chance of regurgitation of gastric contents during induction.[98]

Treatment depends on the type of aspiration but consists primarily of supportive therapy. If the airway is completely obstructed, the Heimlich maneuver may clear the airway. When possible, secure the airway with an endotracheal tube, and suction with a suction catheter or with a bronchoscope to remove obstructing particles or to confirm the diagnosis of aspiration. Because aspirated fluid rapidly moves to the lung periphery, the damage may be extensive, and attempts to neutralize the aspirated fluid with saline solution lavage are ineffective.[99]

Administer oxygen by face mask and maintain an adequate Pa_{O_2} (e.g., above 60 mmHg). If maintenance of Pa_{O_2} requires high concentrations of oxygen, intubation, suctioning, and PPV may be indicated.

Will prophylactic positive end-expiratory pressure (PEEP) limit the lung damage after aspiration of gastric contents? In a human prospective clinical study in which PPV was started as soon as practical after aspiration, prophylactic PEEP (8 cmH_2O pressure for 24 hours compared with no PEEP) did not reduce the incidence of adult respiratory distress syndrome or death.[100] Currently, PEEP is used only as needed to help oxygenate and ventilate the patient.

Bronchospasm accompanying aspiration may be resistant to treatment with bronchodilators.[99] Because the bronchospasm may be due to a strong parasympathetic response, intravenous atropine has been suggested.[101]

Corticosteroids are not recommended. Although corticosteroids do not decrease mortality in patients who aspirate, they are associated with an increased incidence of gram-negative pneumonias.[102]

In some cases, cardiac failure develops, requiring invasive cardiopulmonary monitoring and inotropic agents (e.g., dopamine).

With the acid aspiration, an afebrile recovery often occurs, since the pulmonary insult is usually due to an irritative mechanism and not to an infectious disease.[88] If fever develops, infection should be suspected, and antibiotics may be required. Prophylactic antibiotics are generally not indicated.

Pulmonary Edema

Pulmonary edema occurs occasionally in obstetric patients. It frequently develops in patients with underlying cardiovascular disease who cannot compensate for the physiologic stresses of pregnancy or as a direct complication of pregnancy.

Various physiologic mechanisms produce pulmonary edema and include cardiac failure (excessively increased preload, decreased myocardial contractility, increased afterload, and arrhythmias, especially in patients with structural valvular lesions), a low colloid osmotic pressure, or increased pulmonary capillary permeability. Excessive fluid therapy,[103] cardiac failure, and some cases of PIH[75, 76] can elevate preload. Patients with myocardial infarction, peripartum cardiomyopathy,[84] amniotic fluid embolism[104] and some with PIH[5, 76] may have impaired contractility. Afterload increases in many patients with PIH.[75, 76] Colloid osmotic pressure can be markedly reduced in patients with nephropathy or PIH.[75, 76] Increased capillary permeability occurs in many patients with aspiration of gastric contents,[88, 99] PIH,[75, 76] tocolytic therapy for prevention of preterm labor,[103, 105] sepsis,[106] transfusion reactions,[107] and allergic drug reactions (Table 22–12).

TABLE 22–12
Conditions Associated With Pulmonary Edema

Cardiovascular Disease
Cardiac failure
Myocardial infarction
Arrhythmias, especially with structural valvular lesions
Pregnancy Related
Pregnancy-induced hypertension
Peripartum cardiomyopathy
Amniotic fluid embolism
Tocolysis for prevention of preterm labor
Other Conditions
Aspiration of gastric contents
Excessive fluid therapy
Sepsis
Some transfusion reactions
Allergic drug reactions
Nephropathy

Initiate supportive treatment while seeking the underlying cause. Elevate the patient's head and chest and administer oxygen. Because preload is elevated in most cases of pulmonary edema, drugs that decrease preload, such as furosemide, nitroglycerin, or morphine, should be administered while determining the cause. Patients with pulmonary edema may be quite anxious, making morphine appear attractive. However, morphine also depresses respirations; therefore, adequate ventilation must be ensured. Severe pulmonary edema may require intubation and PPV with 100% oxygen. Use pulse oximetry and arterial blood gas results to assess the severity of respiratory compromise. Arterial lines ensure arterial blood gas samples and make multiple analysis more acceptable to the patient. A pulmonary artery catheter can assist evaluation of cardiac function and guide therapy, especially in patients with amniotic fluid embolism, those with PIH, those receiving tocolytic therapy, and in those with underlying cardiovascular disease in whom treatment is often difficult.

Each patient's care must be individualized after the cause is determined. In addition to lowering preload, myocardial contractility may need to be increased with administration of dopamine, digoxin, and other inotropes. Elevated afterload can be decreased with nitroprusside and hydralazine. Albumin can help increase a low colloid osmotic pressure, but because it also expands the circulating blood volume and elevates preload, it must be given slowly and its effects carefully evaluated. In patients refractory to therapy, delivery may be necessary to decrease the physiologic demands on the mother's cardiovascular and respiratory systems and to improve chances for both maternal and fetal survival.

Cardiac Arrhythmias

Cardiac arrhythmias can develop during pregnancy as a result of a variety of conditions, with some underlying medical conditions exacerbated by the increased cardiovascular demands of pregnancy (Table 22–13). The approach to arrhythmia management in the pregnant patient is similar to the approach in the nonpregnant patient. Define the specific arrhythmia (with an electrocardiograph or Holter monitor), and then determine the cause and hemodynamic significance of the arrhythmia.

Most arrhythmias are not significant and do not require treatment. However, if the arrhythmia is hemodynamically significant, reduced cardiac output may produce dizziness, confusion, loss of consciousness, hypotension, cardiac ischemia, dyspnea, or pulmonary edema in the mother. Additionally, because the fetus depends on an adequate maternal cardiac output, inadequate placental perfusion may ultimately lead to intrauterine fetal distress and occasionally fetal demise. When these signs and symptoms are present, aggressive management of the arrhythmia is warranted. Treatment of the underlying cause (e.g., oxygen administration for hypoxia, thyroidectomy for hyperthyroidism) or nonspecific treatment, such as left uterine displacement, CPR, cardiovascular drugs, or electricity (e.g., pacing, cardioversion, defibrillation), and occasionally delivery may be indicated.

When using drugs, the benefits must be compared with the risks for the mother and the fetus, especially for acute life-threatening conditions. For example, when maternal cardiac output or maternal blood pressure is low (causing decreased placental perfusion and fetal distress) and refractory to routine treatments (such as left uterine tilt, fluid and ephedrine administration), the rise in cardiac output and blood pressure that develops after the administration of epinephrine may be more significant than the associated uterine artery vasoconstriction.

Digoxin, quinidine, procainamide, β blockers (e.g., propranolol, metoprolol, atenolol), labetalol, and lidocaine are relatively safe during pregnancy. Disopyramide, mexiletine, verapamil, and amiodarone require more study to determine their safety, and phenytoin should be used only in the acute setting, since chronic use in the first few months of pregnancy is associated with an increased risk of congenital malformations (e.g., fetal hydantoin syndrome).[108]

Adenosine has recently been released and will probably be found safe owing to its extremely short half-life ($t_{1/2}$ less than 10 seconds).[42] It has been used, without any serious side effects, to treat paroxysmal supraventricular tachycardia in a pregnant woman.[109] However, more studies are needed before it can be considered safe for use during pregnancy.

Arrhythmias refractory to drug therapy, such as atrial fibrillation,[110] atrial flutter with 1:1 conduction,[111] paroxysmal atrial tachycardia,[112] and ventricular fibrillation,[113] have been successfully treated during pregnancy with cardioversion or defibrillation. Currents up to 400 joules appear safe for the fetus.[112] When cardioversion is performed, sedation with a small dose of narcotic, barbiturate, or tranquilizer is commonly used.

TABLE 22–13
Causes of Cardiac Arrhythmias

Cardiovascular Disease
Congenital heart disease
Valvular heart disease
Cardiomyopathy
Myocardial infarction
Pulmonary or amniotic fluid embolism
Pulmonary Disease
Pneumonia
Pneumothorax
Asthma
Endocrine Disease
Thyrotoxicosis
Other Conditions
Severe anemia
Electrolyte disturbances
Drug effects
Caffeine
Nicotine
β mimetic
Hypoxia
Unknown

Cardiac Arrest

Cardiac arrests occur rarely during pregnancy (1 in 30,000 pregnancies).[86] Pulmonary embolism (amniotic fluid, blood clot, air), cardiac disease (myocardial infarction, valvular heart disease, cardiomyopathy, arrhythmias), hemorrhage, PIH, hypoxia, severe hypotension, drug toxicity (magnesium sulfate, local anesthetics), sepsis, and trauma are among the causes.

As with all patients suffering a cardiac arrest, initiate basic and advanced cardiac life support.[114] Intubation, ventilation with 100% oxygen, and chest compressions begin therapy. In order to ensure effective cardiac output, left uterine displacement is indicated if the fetus is over 20 weeks' gestation. The cause of the arrest should be determined and treatment instituted.

However, CPR in the pregnant patient may not be sufficient for maternal or fetal survival owing to the adverse physiologic effects of pregnancy, including increased oxygen and cardiac output demands and aortocaval compression. If the fetus is potentially viable (e.g., over 24 or 25 weeks' gestation), immediate cesarean delivery of the fetus should be considered if a favorable maternal response to treatment is not rapidly seen. After reviewing newborn and maternal outcome as a factor of time after CPR is started, Katz and coworkers[85] suggested that cesarean section should be initiated within 4 minutes and delivery should occur within 5 minutes to achieve a favorable outcome. Although the mother or the newborn[115–117] will occasionally survive and be neurologically normal after prolonged CPR (e.g., greater than 15 minutes), the sooner the delivery is accomplished, the more favorable the outcome for *both* the mother and the newborn.[85]

Rapid cesarean delivery may be the most important part of maternal resuscitation.[85, 86, 116, 118] Presumably, cesarean delivery enhances maternal survival by four mechanisms. First, removing the fetus relieves aortocaval compression and helps venous return. Second, with the contraction of the uterus, some blood may enter the circulation and may help increase venous return. Third, without the fetus, the low cardiac output associated with chest compressions may be more adequate for the mother. Fourth, chest compressions are more effective when the patient is in the supine position (after 20 weeks' EGA, CPR must be performed with lateral tilt owing to the adverse effects of aortocaval compression).

Magnesium Sulfate Toxicity

Magnesium sulfate is used as a tocolytic to treat pregnant women in preterm labor[119] and as an anticonvulsant both to treat and to prevent seizures in pregnant women with PIH.[120, 121] Although magnesium is an effective drug, toxicity may occasionally develop, requiring resuscitation of the patient.

In addition to its tocolytic and anticonvulsant properties, magnesium depresses deep tendon reflexes and muscle tone and can produce respiratory and cardiovascular depression.[122] Magnesium's effects vary depending on the blood level (Table 22–14). Magnesium does not produce central nervous system sedation at levels up to 15 mEq/L.[123] As long as deep tendon reflexes (e.g., patellar, biceps) are present, there is no immediate danger of magnesium toxicity. The patellar reflex decreases owing to sensory blockade in patients receiving epidural or spinal anesthetic; thus, in these patients, examine the biceps deep tendon reflex.

Magnesium sulfate (1 gm = 8.12 mEq) is commonly administered intravenously as a 4-gm bolus over 15 to 20 minutes, followed by a 2- to 4-gm/hour infusion. It may also be administered intramuscularly.

Toxicity develops with elevated blood levels of drug and may be the result of administering an intravenous dose too rapidly, miscalculating, overdosing, or normal dosing in a patient with renal failure (magnesium is excreted almost entirely in the urine).

Magnesium also potentiates the effects of depolarizing and nondepolarizing neuromuscular-blocking agents.[124, 125]

Calcium is the antidote for magnesium toxicity and will reverse the pharmacologic effects almost instantaneously. The common initial dosage is 1 gm of calcium chloride. It is repeated as needed.

SUMMARY

Fortunately, the need for resuscitation of the newborn or the mother is infrequent. When it

TABLE 22–14

Effect	Serum Level (mEq/L)*
Normal level	1.5–2.5
Therapeutic level	4–8
Loss of deep tendon reflexes (e.g., patellar or biceps reflex)	10
Respiratory depression	10–15
Cardiac arrest	15–25

*1 mEq/L = 1.2 mg/dl.

occurs, prompt treatment is the key. By knowing the basic physiologic differences of the newborn, by understanding the changes in physiology that occur in the pregnant patient, and by utilizing the basic ABC approach to resuscitation, appropriate care can be initiated. The underlying cause can then be established and definitive therapy started.

TEN PRACTICAL POINTS

1. Remember the basic ABCs.
2. Neonatal bradycardia (<100 bpm) is a sign of hypoxia until proved otherwise.
3. For newborn intubation, use an endotracheal tube with a 2.5-mm ID for the preterm newborn and 3.0-mm ID for term and post-term newborns.
4. The trachea can be used as a rapid route for drug administration. The mnemonic "ONES" indicates four drugs that can be administered via the endotracheal tube: oxygen, naloxone, epinephrine, and surfactant.
5. With meconium-stained amniotic fluid, intubate and suction only those newborns with thick meconium staining or those with respiratory distress.
6. Intubate any mother who cannot protect her airway to prevent aspiration of gastric contents, a common cause of maternal morbidity.
7. If any patient deteriorates after endotracheal intubation, immediately reassess tube position.
8. Epidural or spinal anesthesia can abolish the patellar reflex. Do not use this reflex to monitor for magnesium sulfate toxicity.
9. Avoid aortocaval compression in all mothers past 20 weeks' EGA, especially during CPR.
10. If cardiac arrest occurs and the fetus is potentially viable, a rapid cesarean section can produce a live newborn and also facilitate maternal resuscitation.

REFERENCES

1. American Society of Anesthesiologists: Guidelines for regional anesthesia in obstetrics. *In* American Society of Anesthesiologists 1996 Directory of Members, 61st ed. Park Ridge, IL, American Society of Anesthesiologists, 1996, pp 405–406.
2. Williams RL, Creasy RK, Cunningham GC, et al: Fetal growth and perinatal viability in California. Obstet Gynecol 59:624–632, 1982.
3. Brenner WE, Edelman DA, Hendricks CH: A standard of fetal growth for the United States of America. Am J Obstet Gynecol 126:555–564, 1976.
4. American Heart Association, American Academy of Pediatrics: Textbook of Neonatal Resuscitation. Elk Grove Village, IL, American Heart Association and American Academy of Pediatrics, 1990.
5. Loew A, Thibeault DW: A new and safe method to control the depth of endotracheal intubation in neonates. Pediatrics 54:506–508, 1974.
6. Manning FA: Fetal breathing movements as a reflection of fetal status. Postgrad Med 61:116–122, 1977.
7. Olver RE, Strang LB: Ion fluxes across the pulmonary epithelium and the secretion of lung liquid in the foetal lamb. J Physiol 241:327–357, 1974.
8. Van Golde LMG, Batenburg JJ, Robertson B: The pulmonary surfactant system: Biochemical aspects and functional significance. Physiol Rev 68:374–455, 1988.
9. James LS, Weisbrot IM, Prince CE, et al: The acid-base status of human infants in relation to birth asphyxia and the onset of respiration. J Pediatr 52:379–394, 1958.
10. Harned HS Jr, MacKinney LG, Berryhill WS Jr, Holmes CF: Effects of hypoxia and acidity on the initiation of breathing in the fetal lamb at term. Am J Dis Child 112:334–342, 1966.
11. Milner AD, Vyas H: Lung expansion at birth. J Pediatr 101:879–886, 1982.
12. Desmond MM, Franklin RR, Vallbona C, et al: The clinical behavior of the newly born. I. The term baby. J Pediatr 62:307–324, 1963.
13. Ceruti E: Chemoreceptor reflexes in the newborn infant: Effect of cooling on the response to hypoxia. Pediatrics 37:556–564, 1966.
14. Karlberg P, Cherry RB, Escardo FE, Koch G: Respiratory studies in newborn infants. II. Pulmonary ventilation and mechanics of breathing in the first minutes of life, including the onset of respiration. Acta Paediatr 51:121–136, 1962.
15. Porter KB, Goldenhamer R, Mankad A, et al: Evaluation of arterial oxygen saturation in pregnant patients and their newborns. Obstet Gynecol 71:354–357, 1988.
16. Kitterman JA, Phibbs RH, Tooley WH: Aortic blood pressure in normal newborn infants during the first 12 hours of life. Pediatrics 44:959–968, 1969.
17. Versmold HT, Kitterman JA, Phibbs RH, et al: Aortic blood pressure during the first 12 hours of life in infants with birth weights 610 to 4220 grams. Pediatrics 67:607–613, 1981.

18. Daily WJR, Klaus M, Meyer HBP: Apnea in premature infants: Monitoring, incidence, heart rate changes, and effect of environmental temperature. Pediatrics 43:510–518, 1969.
19. Dahm LS, James LS: Newborn temperature and calculated heat loss in the delivery room. Pediatrics 49:504–513, 1972.
20. Quinn GE, Betts EK, Diamond GR, Schaeffer DB: Neonatal age (human) at retinal maturation. Anesthesiology 55:A326, 1981.
21. Roberton NRC, Gupta JM, Dahlenburg GW, Tizard JPM: Oxygen therapy in the newborn. Lancet 1:1323–1329, 1968.
22. Cornblath M, Reisner SH: Blood glucose in the neonate and its clinical significance. N Engl J Med 273:378–380, 1965.
23. Modanlou H, Yeh S-Y, Hon EH: Fetal and neonatal acid-base balance in normal and high-risk pregnancies. Obstet Gynecol 43:347–353, 1974.
24. Yeomans ER, Hauth JC, Gilstrap LC III, Strickland DM: Umbilical cord pH, PCO_2, and bicarbonate following uncomplicated term vaginal deliveries. Am J Obstet Gynecol 151:798–800, 1985.
25. Apgar V: A proposal for a new method of evaluation of the newborn infant. Anesth Analg 32:260–267, 1953.
26. Apgar V, Holaday DA, James LS, et al: Evaluation of the newborn infant—Second report. JAMA 168:1985–1988, 1958.
27. Marx GF, Mahajan S, Miclat MN: Correlation of biochemical data with Apgar scores at birth and at 1 minute. Br J Anaesth 49:831–833, 1977.
28. Sykes GS, Johnson P, Ashworth F, et al: Do Apgar scores indicate asphyxia? Lancet 1:494–496, 1982.
29. Nelson KB, Ellenberg JH: Apgar scores as predictors of chronic neurologic disability. Pediatrics 68:36–44, 1981.
30. Cordero L Jr, Hon EH: Neonatal bradycardia following nasopharyngeal stimulation. J Pediatr 78:441–447, 1971.
31. Fearon B, Dickson J: Bilateral choanal atresia in the newborn: Plan of action. Laryngoscope 78:1487–1499, 1968.
32. Hoka S, Sato M, Yoshitake J, Kukita J: Management of a newborn infant with congenital laryngeal atresia. Anesth Analg 69:535–536, 1989.
33. Jarvis AP, Arancibia CU: A case of difficult neonatal ventilation. Anesth Analg 66:196, 1987.
34. Finholt DA, Kettrick RG, Wagner HR, Swedlow DB: The heart is under the lower third of the sternum. Am J Dis Child 140:646–649, 1986.
35. Moya F, James LS, Burnard ED, Hanks EC: Cardiac massage in the newborn infant through the intact chest. Am J Obstet Gynecol 84:798–803, 1962.
36. Todres ID, Rogers MC: Methods of external cardiac massage in the newborn infant. J Pediatr 86:781–782, 1975.
37. Steiner H, Neligan G: Perinatal cardiac arrest. Quality of the survivors. Arch Dis Child 50:696–702, 1975.
38. Lantos JD, Miles SH, Silverstein MD, Stocking CB: Survival after cardiopulmonary resuscitation in babies of very low birth weight. Is CPR futile therapy? N Engl J Med 318:91–95, 1988.
39. Brown WU Jr, Ostheimer GW, Bell GC, Datta SS: Newborn response to oxygen blown over the face. Anesthesiology 44:535–536, 1976.
40. Lindemann R: Resuscitation of the newborn. Endotracheal administration of epinephrine. Acta Paediatr Scand 73:210–212, 1984.
41. Lilien LD, Pildes RS, Srinivasan G, et al: Treatment of neonatal hypoglycemia with minibolus and intravenous glucose infusion. J Pediatr 97:295–298, 1980.
42. Physicians' Desk Reference, 46th ed. Montvale, NJ, Medical Economics Company, 1992.
43. Fujikura T, Klionsky B: The significance of meconium staining. Am J Obstet Gynecol 121:45–50, 1975.
44. Carson BS, Losey RW, Bowes WA Jr, Simmons MA: Combined obstetric and pediatric approach to prevent meconium aspiration syndrome. Am J Obstet Gynecol 126:712–715, 1976.
45. Davis RO, Philips JB III, Harris BA Jr, et al: Fatal meconium aspiration syndrome occurring despite airway management considered appropriate. Am J Obstet Gynecol 151:731–736, 1985.
46. Gregory GA, Gooding CA, Phibbs RH, Tooley WH: Meconium aspiration in infants—A prospective study. J Pediatr 85:848–852, 1974.
47. Wiswell TE, Tuggle JM, Turner BS: Meconium aspiration syndrome: Have we made a difference? Pediatrics 85:715–721, 1990.
48. Dooley SL, Pesavento DJ, Depp R, et al: Meconium below the vocal cords at delivery: Correlation with intrapartum events. Am J Obstet Gynecol 153:767–770, 1985.
49. Falciglia HS: Failure to prevent meconium aspiration syndrome. Obstet Gynecol 71:349–353, 1988.
50. Ting P, Brady JP: Tracheal suction in meconium aspiration. Am J Obstet Gynecol 122:767–771, 1975.
51. Brown BL, Gleicher N: Intrauterine meconium aspiration. Obstet Gynecol 57:26–29, 1981.
52. Bacsik RD: Meconium aspiration syndrome. Pediatr Clin North Am 24:463–478, 1977.
53. Tyler DC, Murphy J, Cheney FW: Mechanical and chemical damage to lung tissue caused by meconium aspiration. Pediatrics 62:454–459, 1978.
54. Yeomans ER, Gilstrap LC III, Leveno KJ, Burris

JS: Meconium in the amniotic fluid and fetal acid-base status. Obstet Gynecol 73:175–178, 1989.

55. Cunningham AS, Lawson EE, Martin RJ, Pildes RS: Tracheal suction and meconium: A proposed standard of care. J Pediatr 116:153–154, 1990.
56. Topsis J, Kinas HY, Kandall SR: Esophageal perforation—A complication of neonatal resuscitation. Anesth Analg 69:532–534, 1989.
57. Yeh TF, Harris V, Srinivasan G, et al: Roentgenographic findings in infants with meconium aspiration syndrome. JAMA 242:60–63, 1979.
58. Frantz ID III, Wang NS, Thach BT: Experimental meconium aspiration: Effects of glucocorticoid treatment. J Pediatr 86:438–441, 1975.
59. Avery ME, Mead J: Surface properties in relation to atelectasis and hyaline membrane disease. AMA J Dis Child 97:517–523, 1959.
60. Auld P, Hodson A, Usher R: Hyaline membrane disease: A discussion. J Pediatr 80:129–140, 1972.
61. Arnold C, McLean FH, Kramer MS, Usher RH: Respiratory distress syndrome in second-born versus first-born twins. A matched case-control analysis. N Engl J Med 317:1121–1125, 1987.
62. Kleinberg F: The management of respiratory distress syndrome. Chest 70:643–649, 1976.
63. Inselman LS: Respiratory distress syndrome. Pediatr Ann 7:243–251, 1978.
64. Morales WJ, Diebel ND, Lazar AJ, Zadrozny D: The effect of antenatal dexamethasone administration on the prevention of respiratory distress syndrome in preterm gestations with premature rupture of membranes. Am J Obstet Gynecol 154:591–595, 1986.
65. Corbet A, Bucciarelli R, Goldman S, et al: Decreased mortality rate among small premature infants treated at birth with a single dose of synthetic surfactant: A multicenter controlled trial. J Pediatr 118:277–284, 1991.
66. Long W, Corbet A, Cotton R, et al: A controlled trial of synthetic surfactant in infants weighing 1250 g or more with respiratory distress syndrome. N Engl J Med 325:1696–1703, 1991.
67. Ablow RC, Driscoll SG, Effmann EL, et al: A comparison of early-onset group B streptococcal neonatal infection and the respiratory distress syndrome of the newborn. N Engl J Med 294:65–70, 1976.
68. Atrash HK, Koonin LM, Lawson HW, et al: Maternal mortality in the United States, 1979–1986. Obstet Gynecol 76:1055–1060, 1990.
69. Jouppila R, Jouppila P, Hollmen A: Laryngeal oedema as an obstetric anaesthesia complication. Case reports. Acta Anaesth Scand 24:97–98, 1980.
70. Prowse CM, Gaensler EA: Respiratory and acid-base changes during pregnancy. Anesthesiology 26:381–392, 1965.
71. Weinberger SE, Weiss ST, Cohen WR, et al: Pregnancy and the lung. Am Rev Respir Dis 121:559–581, 1980.
72. Levinson G, Shnider SM, deLorimier AA, Steffenson JL: Effects of maternal hyperventilation on uterine blood flow and fetal oxygenation and acid-base status. Anesthesiology 40:340–347, 1974.
73. Baraka A: Correlation between maternal and foetal P_{O_2} and P_{CO_2} during caesarean section. Br J Anaesth 42:434–438, 1970.
74. Burger GA, Datta S, Chantigian RC, et al: Optimal ventilation in general anesthesia for cesarean delivery. Anesthesiology 59:A420, 1983.
75. Sibai BM, Mabie BC, Harvey CJ, Gonzalez AR: Pulmonary edema in severe preeclampsia-eclampsia: Analysis of thirty-seven consecutive cases. Am J Obstet Gynecol 156:1174–1179, 1987.
76. Clark SL, Cotton DB: Clinical indications for pulmonary artery catheterization in the patient with severe preeclampsia. Am J Obstet Gynecol 158:453–458, 1988.
77. Katz R, Karliner JS, Resnick R: Effects of a natural volume overload state (pregnancy) on left ventricular performance in normal human subjects. Circulation 58:434–441, 1978.
78. Clark SL, Cotton DB, Lee W, et al: Central hemodynamic assessment of normal term pregnancy. Am J Obstet Gynecol 161:1439–1442, 1989.
79. Capeless EL, Clapp JF: Cardiovascular changes in early phase of pregnancy. Am J Obstet Gynecol 161:1449–1453, 1989.
80. Ueland K, Novy MJ, Peterson EN, Metcalfe J: Maternal cardiovascular dynamics. IV. The influence of gestational age on the maternal cardiovascular response to posture and exercise. Am J Obstet Gynecol 104:956–864, 1969.
81. Ueland K, Hansen JM: Maternal cardiovascular dynamics. III. Labor and delivery under local and caudal analgesia. Am J Obstet Gynecol 103:8–18, 1969.
82. Bieniarz J, Maqueda E, Caldeyro-Barcia R: Compression of aorta by the uterus in late human pregnancy. I. Variations between femoral and brachial artery pressure with changes from hypertension to hypotension. Am J Obstet Gynecol 95:795–808, 1966.
83. Bieniarz J, Crottogini JJ, Curuchet E, et al: Aortocaval compression by the uterus in late human pregnancy. II. An arteriographic study. Am J Obstet Gynecol 100:203–217, 1968.
84. Cunningham FG, Pritchard JA, Hankins GDV, et al: Peripartum heart failure: Idiopathic car-

diomyopathy or compounding cardiovascular events? Obstet Gynecol 67:157–168, 1986.
85. Katz VL, Dotters DJ, Droegemueller W: Perimortem cesarean delivery. Obstet Gynecol 68:571–576, 1986.
86. Rees GAD, Willis BA: Resuscitation in late pregnancy. Anaesthesia 43:347–349, 1988.
87. Stephenson HE Jr: Pathophysiological considerations that warrent open-chest cardiac resuscitation. Crit Care Med 8:185–187, 1980.
88. Mendelson CL: The aspiration of stomach contents into the lungs during obstetric anesthesia. Am J Obstet Gynecol 52:191–205, 1946.
89. Gibbs CP, Rolbin SH, Norman P: Cause and prevention of maternal aspiration. Anesthesiology 61:111–112, 1984.
90. Roberts RB, Shirley MA: Reducing the risk of acid aspiration during cesarean section. Anesth Analg 53:859–868, 1974.
91. Gibbs CP, Spohr L, Schmidt D: The effectiveness of sodium citrate as an antacid. Anesthesiology 57:44–46, 1982.
92. Gibbs CP, Schwartz DJ, Wynne JW, et al: Antacid pulmonary aspiration in the dog. Anesthesiology 51:380–385, 1979.
93. Gibbs CP, Banner TC: Effectiveness of Bicitra as a preoperative antacid. Anesthesiology 61:97–99, 1984.
94. Chen CT, Toung TJK, Haupt HM, et al: Evaluation of the efficacy of Alka-Seltzer effervescent in gastric acid neutralization. Anesth Analg 63:325–329, 1984.
95. Dewan DM, Floyd HM, Thistlewood JM, et al: Sodium citrate pretreatment in elective cesarean section patients. Anesth Analg 64:34–37, 1985.
96. Joyce TH III: Prophylaxis for pulmonary acid aspiration. Am J Med 83(Suppl 6A):46–52, 1987.
97. Bylsma-Howell M, Riggs KW, McMorland GH, et al: Placental transport of metoclopramide: Assessment of maternal and neonatal effects. Can Anaesth Soc J 30:487–492, 1983.
98. Brock-Utne JG, Dow TGB, Welman S, et al: The effect of metoclopramide on the lower oesophageal sphincter in late pregnancy. Anaesth Intensive Care 6:26–29, 1978.
99. Hamelberg W, Bosomworth PP: Aspiration pneumonitis: Experimental studies and clinical observations. Anesth Analg 43:669–676, 1964.
100. Pepe PE, Hudson LD, Carrico CJ: Early application of positive end-expiratory pressure in patients at risk for the adult respiratory distress syndrome. N Engl J Med 311:281–286, 1984.
101. Colebatch HJH, Halmagyi DFJ: Reflex airway reaction to fluid aspiration. J Appl Physiol 17:787–794, 1962.
102. Wolfe JE, Bone RC, Ruth WE: Effects of corticosteroids in the treatment of patients with gastric aspiration. Am J Med 63:719–722, 1977.
103. Jacobs MM, Knight AB, Arias F: Maternal pulmonary edema resulting from betamimetic and glucocorticoid therapy. Obstet Gynecol 56:56–59, 1980.
104. Clark SL, Montz FJ, Phelan JP: Hemodynamic alterations associated with amniotic fluid embolism: A reappraisal. Am J Obstet Gynecol 151:617–621, 1985.
105. Benedetti TJ, Hargrove JC, Rosene KA: Maternal pulmonary edema during premature labor inhibition. Obstet Gynecol 59:33S–37S, 1982.
106. Anderson RR, Holliday RL, Driedger AA, et al: Documentation of pulmonary capillary permeability in the adult respiratory distress syndrome accompanying human sepsis. Am Rev Respir Dis 119:869–877, 1979.
107. Popovsky MA, Abel MD, Moore SB: Transfusion-related acute lung injury associated with passive transfer of antileukocyte antibodies. Am Rev Respir Dis 128:185–189, 1983.
108. Rotmensch HH, Rotmensch S, Elkayam U: Management of cardiac arrhythmias during pregnancy. Current concepts. Drugs 33:623–633, 1987.
109. Wolf EJ, Egan JFX, Rodis JF, Vintzileos AM: Intravenous adenosine for the treatment of maternal paroxysmal supraventricular tachycardia. J Maternal-Fetal Med 1:121–123, 1992.
110. Vogel JHK, Pryor R, Blount SG Jr: Direct-current defibrillation during pregnancy. JAMA 193:970–971, 1965.
111. Sussman HF, Duque D, Lesser ME: Atrial flutter with 1:1 A-V conduction. Report of a case in a pregnant woman successfully treated with DC countershock. Dis Chest 49:99–103, 1966.
112. Ogburn PL Jr, Schmidt G, Linman J, Cefalo RC: Paroxysmal tachycardia and cardioversion during pregnancy. J Reprod Med 27:359–362, 1982.
113. Curry JJ, Quintana FJ: Myocardial infarction with ventricular fibrillation during pregnancy treated by direct current defibrillation with fetal survival. Chest 58:82–84, 1970.
114. Emergency Cardiac Care Committee and Subcommittees of the American Heart Association: Guidelines for cardiopulmonary resuscitation and emergency cardiac care. JAMA 268:2172–2302, 1992.
115. Lopez-Zeno JA, Carlo WA, O'Grady JP, Fanaroff AA: Infant survival following delayed postmortem cesarean delivery. Obstet Gynecol 76:991–992, 1990.
116. DePace NL, Betesh JS, Kotler MN: "Postmortem" cesarean section with recovery of both mother and offspring. JAMA 248:971–973, 1982.

117. Selden BS, Burke TJ: Complete maternal and fetal recovery after prolonged cardiac arrest. Ann Emerg Med 17:346–349, 1988.
118. Marx GF: Cardiopulmonary resuscitation of late-pregnant women. Anesthesiology 56:156, 1982.
119. Hollander DI, Nagey DA, Pupkin MJ: Magnesium sulfate and ritodrine hydrochloride: A randomized comparison. Am J Obstet Gynecol 156:631–637, 1987.
120. Sibai BM, Lipshitz J, Anderson GD, Dilts PV Jr: Reassessment of intravenous $MgSO_4$ therapy in preeclampsia-eclampsia. Obstet Gynecol 57:199–202, 1981.
121. Pritchard JA, Cunningham FG, Pritchard SA: The Parkland Memorial Hospital protocol for the treatment of eclampsia: Evaluation of 245 cases. Am J Obstet Gynecol 148:951–963, 1984.
122. Mordes JP, Wacker WEC: Excess magnesium. Physiol Rev 29:273–300, 1978.
123. Somjen G, Hilmy M, Stephen CR: Failure to anesthetize human subjects by intravenous administration of magnesium sulfate. J Pharmacol Exp Ther 154:652–659, 1966.
124. Ghoneim MM, Long JP: The interaction between magnesium and other neuromuscular blocking agents. Anesthesiology 32:23–27, 1970.
125. Sinatra RS, Philip BK, Naulty JS, Ostheimer GW: Prolonged neuromuscular blockade with vecuronium in a patient treated with magnesium sulfate. Anesth Analg 64:1220–1222, 1985.

TWENTY-THREE

Medical-Legal Aspects of Obstetric Anesthesia

David M. Dewan, M.D.

For those who practice obstetric anesthesia, the hazards of malpractice litigation appear real. The Obstetric Anesthesia National Survey in 1986 revealed that over 70% of obstetricians and anesthesiologists believe the risk of malpractice claims increases for obstetric anesthesia providers.[1] This chapter explores, from a nonattorney's perspective, why the risk for obstetric anesthesia providers may be greater, what constitutes malpractice, what prompts suits, and some principles that may assist the anesthesia practitioner in preventing suits or may offer protection when suits arise.

In the author's opinion, obstetric patients and their families are likely litigators. Logic dictates that despite appropriate care, bad outcomes—either maternal or fetal, especially in light of the emergent nature of deliveries—inevitably occur. Indeed, as discussed in Chapter 2 dealing with risk and outcome, anesthesia is a persistent contributor to maternal mortality, accounting for up to 10% of maternal deaths. Disappointingly, as previously discussed in the same chapter, much of this mortality is considered preventable and subject to litigation. Unfortunately, poor neonatal outcomes are inevitable, and regardless of the degree of contribution by anesthesia to the adverse outcome, the obstetric anesthetist, as a coprovider of care, will likely be closely scrutinized as a potential litigant. The Obstetric Anesthesia Closed Claims Survey revealed that, although fewer claims involving newborn brain damage were anesthesia-related, the payment rate was not significantly different from that for other obstetric anesthesia claims.[2] Considering the financial impact of caring for an injured mother or baby, litigation may be the family's only choice for financial survival.

The inevitability of adverse outcomes is in stark contrast to the low antenatal risk perceived by the patients. Most obstetric patients are young and healthy, with high expectations. Furthermore, the aggressive move by hospitals to compete for obstetric care can contribute to unrealistic expectations. Indeed, *Hospital Risk Management* suggests that advertisements that speak to the quality of care at an institution blur the line between a patient's responsibility for his or her own care and the hospital's liability.[3] As a result of advertising, expectations may rise above what can be delivered. Simultaneously, advertising may lower the esteem of the hospital and physicians in the eyes of the jury in the event of litigation. Neither physicians nor hospitals should promise what they cannot deliver. Finally, poor maternal outcomes occurring in a healthy population are usually noticed and questioned, and poor neonatal outcomes, even when expected, are emotionally charged. Litigation should not be surprising, and thus it is imperative that anesthesia providers understand what constitutes malpractice.

MALPRACTICE

Malpractice allegations involve torts or wrongs. Torts are classified as either *intentional* or, more commonly, *negligent.*

TABLE 23–1
Intentional Torts

Assault	Deceit
Battery	Invasion of privacy
Breach of contract	Libel
False imprisonment	Slander
Fraud	

Intentional torts (Table 23–1) are specific acts. Adverse outcomes are not essential for proving guilt regarding intentional torts. For example, a properly performed hysterectomy, without consent, represents battery and perhaps assault, irrespective of whether the surgical procedure is carried out in a competent fashion. Traditionally, the presence of fear during assault delineates it from battery, which can occur in an unconscious patient.

In contrast to intentional torts, negligent torts involve deviating from the "standard of care." By definition, a negligent tort is "doing that which an ordinarily prudent person would not do under similar circumstances, or failure to do that which an ordinarily prudent person would do under similar circumstances."[4] In other words, the anesthesia care provider does not live up to her or his responsibility. Implicit in this concept is that at some point during physician-patient interaction, anesthesia care providers establish a contract between themselves and the patient with obligations for both parties. The contract is initiated either by interviewing the patient preoperatively and devising a proposed anesthetic plan or, alternatively, by initiating care under urgent circumstances when time does not permit the usual preoperative assessment. This contract obligates the anesthesia provider to (1) provide care, (2) respect confidences, (3) not unilaterally discontinue care, and (4) maintain standards. In turn, patients are required to follow medical advice. These are the contractual obligations that define duties without delineating outcome.

The first three obligations are straightforward, and the fourth major obligation, maintenance of standards, represents the crux of most litigation. In this instance, the plaintiff's attorney attempts to demonstrate deviations from the "standard of care." Successful suits must prove four specific items.

1. They must prove that a contract between the anesthesia care provider and the patient existed. Did the anesthesia care provider assume responsibility for the plaintiff's anesthetic?

2. They must demonstrate a breach of duty, a deviation from the standard of care. This area involves expert witnesses. Both the plaintiff and the defense attorneys investigate the anesthetic in detail and document the events. The defendant will, during this course of investigation, explain what happened and state why the chosen course of action was appropriate. Usually, a number of defense "expert witnesses" support the anesthetic plan and execution, attempting to convince the lay jury that the selected anesthetic conduct was appropriate and was representative of what was reasonably expected under the circumstances. Simultaneously, the plaintiffs engage a series of "expert witnesses" whose duty is to identify areas of weakness or perceived errors in the anesthetic conduct that they consider deviations from the standard of care. They attempt to demonstrate why the course of action was *not* reasonable under the circumstances. In summary, both sides attempt to define acceptable practice—the standard of care. The defendant attempts to show compliance; the plaintiffs attempt to demonstrate noncompliance. For example, an anesthesiologist, in the presence of severe fetal distress, may elect to proceed with a cesarean section utilizing mask general anesthesia following a failed intubation. If aspiration occurs, the plaintiff's attorney and expert witnesses might claim that waking the patient from anesthesia and proceeding with a regional anesthetic was the appropriate course of action. The defendant will claim that proceeding with mask anesthesia was necessary for preserving fetal life. *Ultimately, the jury decides.*

3. After proving a deviation exists, the next obligation of the plaintiff's attorney is to demonstrate or prove patient injury. Inappropriate action, without injury, is not malpractice. For example, performing a cesarean section, electively utilizing mask anesthesia, is not recompensable malpractice unless the patient suffers adverse sequelae secondary to anesthetic course.

4. The final obligation is to provide proximate cause. In other words, the plaintiffs must show that a deviation from the standard of care caused the patient's injury. Performing a cesarean section utilizing mask anesthesia would not

be the proximate cause of a postoperative footdrop.

Unless all four elements are proved, malpractice does not exist. Unfortunately, the concept of proximate cause may change. According to Bruce Fagel, M.D., J.D., a plaintiff attorney, the concept of proximate cause may be changed for "substantial factor."[5] In this instance, a course of action may not have to be the proximate cause, it may simply be a "substantial factor." According to Fagel, substantial factor "is more than a slight, trivial, negligible, or theoretical factor in producing a particular result."

DEFINING THE STANDARD OF CARE

"Standards of care" vary in different regions of the country and change with time. As dissemination of medical information and continuing education become more readily available and subspecialty training grows, the concept of appropriate care changes. In contradistinction to the early days when physicians practiced in relatively isolated areas and the accepted standard was a community standard and a physician's care compared with care provided by others in the same community, today's standard of care is gradually evolving into a national standard. In the author's state, physicians are compared, in terms of practice standards, with physicians practicing in *similar* communities of similar size and similar areas of the state. It makes a difference whether you practice in a rural 100-bed hospital or a 1000-bed urban hospital, although the plaintiff, nevertheless, attempts to prove otherwise. Your state may differ. The author suspects, ultimately, that courts will consider all board-certified anesthesiologists capable of delivering one standard of care. Finally, practice is also defined by time. Care in 1980 is not care in 1990. For the present, the important message remains that continuing education is vital for protecting oneself in litigation. Do not be out there by yourself!

Two additional areas require comment. First is the concept of *res ipsa loquitur.* In usual negligence cases, as discussed earlier, the burden rests with the plaintiff to prove negligence. However, the doctrine of res ipsa loquitur, "the thing speaks for itself," shifts the burden of proof to the defendant. The premise is that some injuries and outcomes are so outrageous and flagrant that they clearly could not happen without negligence. In this instance, the defendants must prove they were not negligent. Expert witnesses are not required to define a standard of care. The court and lay jury unilaterally determine guilt or innocence without expert opinions. Res ipsa loquitur is rarely invoked.

Failure to obtain consultation is another pitfall for anesthesia providers. The anesthesia provider, in the absence of an intentional tort, guarantees his or her *skills,* not outcome, when treating a patient. The anesthetist should be careful about guaranteeing results. For example, one should not say "I won't damage your teeth" or "You won't remember anything." These statements guarantee results and become a contractual obligation. In this setting, a difficult intubation will not be a defense for a chipped tooth. A broken tooth implies a broken contract—an intentional tort. However, in the absence of a contractual outcome, the anesthesia provider's obligation is to live up to a particular level of training. Nevertheless, a lack of training or knowledge does not allow the anesthesia care provider to abdicate responsibility. "I didn't know" is not always a defense. If a patient requires skill or knowledge beyond the capability or expertise of the anesthesia care provider, and there is sufficient time, appropriate consultation is mandatory. Failure to obtain appropriate consultation is a negligent omission.

CONSENT PROBLEMS

The concept of adequate consent is an evolving philosophy. Traditional consent forms probably represented a carte blanche for the surgeon and anesthesia team to use their discretion to perform an appropriate procedure and anesthetic. Today, these forms protect the caregiver from committing the intentional torts, assault and battery. Allegations of *negligence* regarding consent address the concept of informed consent, a practice in which the patients are given information and treatment alternatives and participate in selection of the treatment. Informed consent issues address *what information* was given. Unfortunately, as with the standard of care, what constitutes informed consent varies from court to court. However, current practice demands a more bipartisan decision-making process than in the past.

As with res ipsa loquitur, anesthesia suits involving informed consent are unusual. According to the American Society of Anesthesiologists (ASA) Closed Claims project, informed consent was an issue in only 37 of 3269 claims.[6] The review identified three patterns of inadequate consent. One pattern was the anesthesia care team's ignoring patient requests. In this instance, although the complications were not clearly linked to anesthetic care, the patients received sizable settlements. The second type of failed consent was the unexpected alteration in anesthetic plan dictated by emergent changing conditions. In obstetric anesthesia, the intrapartum anesthetic discussion of epidural anesthesia might wisely include the potential requirement of general anesthesia in the presence of fetal distress. The third group were allegations that potential complications were not discussed. Reliably performing and documenting a consent process, as discussed earlier, offers protection in this instance. Finally, the report noted that inadequate consent was associated with a greater frequency of plaintiff payments and a greater payment amount.

Unfortunately, even proper informed consent has many pitfalls, some of which are unique to the obstetric patient. In order to obtain appropriate consent, the patient has to have the ability (1) to comprehend information, (2) to deliberate a decision, and (3) to communicate a decision. However, even when properly informed, patients may misunderstand, not understand, or forget the information. For instance, within 1 day of signing consent forms for chemotherapy, radiation therapy, or surgery, only 60% of patients understood the purpose and nature of the proposed procedure, and only 55% could identify major risks or complications.[7] Labor complicates the consent process. For example, do intrapartum analgesics or the presence of pain, or both, preclude informed consent? At the author's institution, a randomized investigation compared the capacity of laboring patients to evaluate and retain information presented either verbally or verbally supplemented with *written* information.[8] In this series, both groups of patients were able to recall important information disseminated during consent 5 to 7 months later. Only 2 of 82 patients believed they were unable to give adequate consent. Knapp pointed out the court's liberal position on obtaining consent in laboring patients.[9] To his knowledge, there were no successful suits alleging improper informed consent involving anesthetic administration to obstetric patients. Nevertheless, reliably and uniformly participating in and documenting the consent process offer protection in the rare instance where a suit is filed. At the author's institution, although we do not have a separate anesthesia consent form for obstetric anesthesia use, there is a checklist on our preoperative evaluation forms that documents that the major risks of regional and general anesthesia were discussed.

How much information should be transmitted? When assessing appropriate consent, two of the more common measurement parameters include the prudent person test and material risks. *Material risk* considers the frequency and severity of potential injury when deciding appropriate disclosure. "Materiality is, in essence, the product of risk and its chance of occurring."[10] For example, minor complications that occur commonly, most likely do not necessarily deserve disclosure. In contrast, major injuries that occur, albeit rarely, require disclosure. For example, venous thrombosis at an intravenous site does not require disclosure. Potential dural puncture headache following spinal anesthesia is an appropriate area of discussion.

The prudent person test for consent addresses patient bias regarding complications. Already injured patients may, when asked on the witness stand whether additional information regarding their particular complication would have deterred them from accepting the anesthetic course, say yes. However, they already have the injury and bias exists. Rather than ask the patient, the court may apply the prudent person test. The prudent person test asks whether a hypothetical prudent person (not the patient) would potentially arrive at a different decision if given additional information.

Unique to obstetric patients is the consent issue that arises when there is court-ordered maternal intervention. For example, what is the anesthetic consent process when a laboring patient refuses a court-ordered cesarean section for a jeopardized fetus and refuses consent? Is she also refusing anesthesia? Despite a number of cases in the literature discussing this scenario, the liability of the anesthesia team has never been addressed. However, allowing transportation to the operating room and submitting to the induction of general or regional anesthesia implies consent. Nevertheless, potential liability exists. At present, the best that can be done is be aware of this rare problem and rely on the risk manager's advice.

In summary, defined adequate consent varies from court to court and no firm guidelines exist. Reliably performing and documenting that a discussion of anesthetic options and potential complications took place offers the best protection.

CLAIMS EXPERIENCE

The ASA Closed Claims Survey provides insight regarding litigation involving obstetric patients.[2] Obstetric claims involve a disproportionate percentage of all claims against anesthesia, supporting the perception that the obstetric anesthesiologist carries greater legal risk. Although 4.4% of all anesthetics are administered for cesarean section, cesarean section claims constitute 8% of all anesthetic claims. According to the survey, the most common complications evoking suits involving obstetric anesthesia care were maternal death (22%), newborn brain damage (20%), and headache (12%). Among nonobstetric claims, patient death (39%), nerve damage (16%), and brain damage (13%) constituted the leading initiators of litigation. However, if claims for newborn injury are eliminated from comparison, there are no significant differences in the percentage of claims regarding patient-maternal brain and nerve damage between obstetric and nonobstetric patients. Claims for maternal death nevertheless constitute a smaller portion of *obstetric* claims than patient deaths for *nonobstetric* patients. Importantly, obstetric claims for which payments were made produced a mean payment of $203,000 versus $85,000 for nonobstetric claims, and more payments exceeded $200,000. The explanation for the greater mean payment among obstetric patients was the greater frequency of high-paying brain injury suits because the combination maternal *and* newborn brain injury increased the number of payments for this high-payment category. Furthermore, the younger age of obstetric patients probably increased the dollar amount of payments. Forty-two percent of claims for maternal death involved general anesthesia, and not surprisingly, these cases were associated with more severe injuries and resulted in greater payment amounts than those involving regional anesthesia.

Obstetric claims involved a significantly greater number of minor injuries such as headache, backache, and pain during anesthesia than nonobstetric claims (eightfold), probably secondary to the prevalence of regional anesthesia among suits. Amazingly, 56% of headache claims resulted in payment. The authors speculated that the high payment rate for minor injuries among obstetric patients may be the result of unrealistic expectations and a general dissatisfaction with the care provided for postpartum emotional disturbances. The lessons are clear for the practitioner: Pay attention to minor complaints and aggressively treat pain during regional anesthesia.

The survey also supported the risk associated with delivering a brain-damaged infant. Whereas 76% of all obstetric claims were considered anesthesia-related, only 50% of newborn brain injury claims were considered anesthesia-related. Nevertheless, the payment rate for newborn brain injury did not differ significantly from the payment rate for other obstetric claims, despite the lessened anesthetic contribution. Obviously, providing appropriate care does not guarantee freedom from litigation. Surprising factors associated with litigation were (1) nonavailability of anesthesia for obstetrics, (2) not informing the obstetrician by telephone of a coincident disease during pregnancy, (3) inadequate preloading, and (4) delay in availability of anesthesia services.

Suits involving aspiration and convulsions were more prevalent among obstetric cases. Difficult tracheal intubation, esophageal intubation, and pulmonary aspiration constituted 13% of all obstetric claims, consistent with the belief that tracheal intubation and aspiration are leading causes of maternal anesthetic mortality. The incidence of aspiration claims were fourfold over those in the nonobstetric group. Two cases of pulmonary aspiration occurred during regional anesthesia and, amazingly, seven involved mask anesthesia, although the year of these suits was not listed. Not surprisingly, suits involving convulsions associate predominantly with epidural anesthesia. Disturbingly, 83% of the obstetric claims involving convulsions associated with regional anesthesia produced neurologic injury or death to the mother or the newborn, or both. Three claims involved management complications of high/total spinal anesthesia and 5 of 11 equipment problems involved epidural catheters and other ventilatory equipment.

Overall, the standard of care was judged comparable among obstetric and nonobstetric claims (46% of obstetrics and 39% of nonobstetrics met the standard of care). However, remember, this does mean that in perhaps over half the cases in which claims were made, the obstetric anesthesia care provider did *not* meet the standard of care. However, the imperfections of our legal system are exemplified by the fact that 30% of payments were made when the standard of care was met, and when the standard of care was *not* met, *only* 56% of patients received compensation. Anesthesia care was judged to be less than appropriate in half the cases in which general anesthesia was the primary anesthetic technique and in one third in which regional anesthesia was the primary technique in both obstetric and nonobstetric suits. Regarding anesthesia and payment for nerve damage, payments are essentially the same regardless of whether the standard of care is met. Meeting the standard of care does not reduce the payment rate for nerve damage. Finally, the authors concluded that obstetric anesthesia claims reveal a medical-legal risk profile distinctly differently from nonobstetric claims. There are reasons for worry.

Further insight into the current legal climate and the anesthesiologist's potential role is exemplified in a number of additional papers. Brennan and coworkers[11] reported in the *New England Journal of Medicine* that adverse events occurred in 3.7% of all hospitalizations. Of adverse events, 27.6% were due to negligence and 2.6% of adverse events caused permanent disabling injury and 13.6% led to death. Not surprisingly, more severe injuries were more likely to have been caused by negligence. However, when malpractice claims are matched to inpatient medical records, and consistent with the obstetric experience, the civil justice system unreliably compensates injured patients and rarely identifies and holds health care providers accountable for substandard medical care. Ward identified that 27% of *obstetric* claims were indefensible because of breaches in the standard of care or absence of documentation, or both.[12] Physicians must accept some blame. Nevertheless, Sloan and associates noted that physicians with adverse claims experienced from incidents between 1975 and 1980 had worse claims experience from incidents between 1981 and 1983, suggesting there are some recurrent bad offenders.[13] Finally, Tinker and colleagues' examination of the role of monitoring devices in prevention of anesthetic mishaps identified the severity of injuries scores that were the same for preventable mishaps occurring during regional or general anesthesia, suggesting that monitoring devices might be equally efficacious for preventing serious negative outcomes during regional or general anesthesia.[14]

RECOMMENDATIONS

Failure to consult or refer, failure to appropriately use equipment and laboratory tests, failure to respond expeditiously to "clinical distress," failure to document, too much reliance on inexperienced nurses or residents, and inappropriate maternal expectations are among the factors cited by Depp as common deficiencies in obstetrics.[15] Gibbs and coworkers identified questionable resident supervision as a potential problem on labor and delivery.[1] Considering the obstetric claim profile, physicians should improve obstetric coverage, but whether this is possible in this health care climate of cost cutting and hospital competition is unclear.

The Harvard Risk Management Survey identified problems existing in anesthesia care that are particularly applicable to obstetrics.[16] The survey identified minimal intraoperative and postoperative monitoring, remote anesthetizing locations, poor equipment standards (including checkout, maintenance, and repair), poor records, and inadequate preoperative and postoperative visits as risk factors for anesthesia care. If the legal problems among obstetric anesthesia care are addressed, attention should be directed to providing equal care and monitoring standards in the obstetric suite and the main operating room, attempting, as much as possible, to ensure that the obstetric patient receives appropriate and timely care.

TEN PRACTICAL POINTS

1. Know that obstetric anesthesia is a high-risk area with a distinct claim profile.
2. Have policies and procedures in place for

dealing with the administration of anesthesia on labor and delivery.

3. Maintain standards for labor and delivery that are equivalent to the primary surgical suite and postanesthesia care unit.

4. Clearly define the roles for personnel involved in neonatal resuscitation.

5. Have personnel readily available to deal with obstetric and anesthetic complications on labor and delivery.

6. Do a preoperative assessment, discuss anesthetic options and risks, and *document* the interview!

7. Include labor and delivery in continuing education programs.

8. Do a postanesthetic follow-up and be attentive to "minor" complaints and complications.

9. Have a quality assurance program in place.

10. Do not promise or imply perfect outcomes such as pain-free labor.

REFERENCES

1. Gibbs C, Krischer J, Peckham B, et al: Obstetric anesthesia: A national survey. Anesthesiology 65:298–306, 1986.
2. Chadwick H, Posner K, Caplan R, et al: A comparison of obstetric and non-obstetric anesthesia malpractice claims. Anesthesiology 74:243–229, 1991.
3. Make sure advertising brings in patients, not lawyers. Hospital Risk Management 14(7):85–88, 1992.
4. Dornette WHL: Legal aspects of anesthesia. Clin Anesth 8:400, 1971.
5. Fagel B: Peripartum malpractice. Presented at the Society for Obstetric Anesthesia and Perinatology Symposium, "The compromised fetus: Medical and legal issues," May 1993, Palm Springs, CA.
6. Caplan RA, Posner KL: Informed consent in anesthesia liability: Evidence from the Closed Claims Project. American Society of Anesthesiologists News Letter 59(6):9–12, 1995.
7. Cassileth B, Zupkis R, Sutton-Smith K, March V: Informed consent—Why are its goals imperfectly realized? N Engl J Med 302:896–900, 1980.
8. Grice SC, Eisenach JC, Dewan DM, Robinson ML: Evaluation of informed consent for anesthesia for labor and delivery. Anesthesiology 69:A664, 1988.
9. Knapp R: Legal view of informed consent for anesthesia during labor. Anesthesiology 72:211, 1990.
10. Winkjer vs. Herr 22 N.W. 2nd 579,588 N.D. 1979.
11. Brennan TA, Leapell, Laird NM, et al: Incidence of adverse events and negligence in hospitalized patients: Results of the Harvard Medical Procedure Study I. N Engl J Med 324:370–376, 1991.
12. Ward CJ: Analysis of 500 obstetric and gynecologic malpractice claims: Causes and prevention. Am J Obstet Gynecol 165:298–306, 1991.
13. Sloan FA, Mergenhagen PM, Burfield WB, et al: Medical malpractice exposure of physicians—Predictable or haphazard? JAMA 262:3291–3297, 1989.
14. Tinker JH, Dull DL, Caplan RA, et al: Role of monitoring devices in prevention of anesthetic mishaps: A closed claims analysis. Anesthesiology 71:541–546, 1989.
15. Depp R: Experts reveal sources of perinatal liability, solutions. Hospital Risk Management 7:109–132, 1985.
16. Harvard launches risk management initiative. Hospital Risk Management 7(8):97–108, 1985.

Index

Note: Page numbers in *italics* refer to illustrations; page numbers followed by t indicate tables.

B

C

D

E

M

P

S